Register Now for O... to Your Boo...

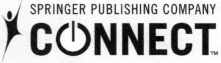

SPRINGER PUBLISHING COMPANY
CONNECT™

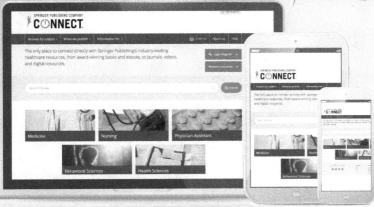

Your print purchase of *A New Era in Global Health,* **includes online access to the contents of your book**—increasing accessibility, portability, and searchability!

Access today at:

**http://connect.springerpub.com/content/book/978-0-8261-9012-3
or scan the QR code at the right with your smartphone
and enter the access code below.**

B492E7GK

*Scan here for
quick access.*

LS

SPRINGER PUBLISHING COMPANY
View all our products at springerpub.com

A New Era in Global Health

William Rosa, MS, RN, LMT, AHN-BC, AGPCNP-BC, CCRN-CMC, is a nurse, author, and educator. He graduated with his bachelor of science degree in nursing, magna cum laude, from New York University (NYU) Rory Meyers College of Nursing in 2009. While working as a critical care bedside clinician for 4 years at NYU Langone Medical Center (NYULMC), climbing to the top rung of the clinical ladder, he became committed to excellence in patient care delivery, advocacy for positive change within the profession, and the elevation of consciousness for nurses and nursing. After graduating as valedictorian of his master of nursing program at the Hunter–Bellevue School of Nursing at Hunter College, New York, New York, in 2014, he moved into the role of nurse educator for critical care services at NYULMC.

He is a graduate of the Caritas Coach Education Program (CCEP) offered by the Watson Caring Science Institute (WCSI), the Integrative Nurse Coach Certificate Program (INCCP) offered by the International Nurse Coach Association, and the Clinical Scene Investigator (CSI) Academy of the American Association of Critical-Care Nurses (AACN). To date, these experiences have inspired over 150 publications in peer-reviewed and non-peer-reviewed journals, book chapters, newspapers, magazines, and international social media platforms such as SpringBoard and The Huffington Post. Mr. Rosa's first book, *Nurses as Leaders: Evolutionary Visions of Leadership,* was released by Springer in 2016.

Mr. Rosa has been recognized with the Association for Nursing Professional Development's national 2015 Excellence in Professional Development Change Agent/Team Member Award and the 2015 national AACN Circle of Excellence Award, and he was the winner of the 2012 National League for Nursing (NLN) Student Excellence Paper Competition. Most recently he has been named a national 2017 Rising Star in Nursing by *Modern Healthcare* and one of America's Most Amazing Nurses by *The Doctors* television show and *Prevention* magazine. Mr. Rosa will be awarded the international Daniel J. Pesut Spirit of Renewal Award by Sigma Theta Tau Interntational in 2017. He is a Fellow of the New York Academy of Medicine.

He has become passionate about cultivating a healthy environment in which nurse leaders can thrive through his participation in the Nurse in Washington Internship and his organizational positions as U.S. board of advisors' member for the Nightingale Initiative for Global Health (NIGH), New York City chapter leader and national Nominating Committee member the American Holistic Nurses Association (AHNA), and secretary for the New York City chapter of the Association for Nursing Professional Development.

Mr. Rosa is soon to be a Robert Wood Johnson Future of Nursing Scholar in the University of Pennsylvania's PhD in nursing program. He most recently worked as a Palliative Care Medicine Fellow at Memorial Sloan Kettering Cancer Center in New York, and in Kigali, Rwanda, as visiting faculty at the University of Rwanda and as an intensive care unit clinical educator at the Rwanda Military Hospital, Human Resources for Health Program in partnership with the NYU Rory Meyers College of Nursing.

A New Era in Global Health

Nursing and the United Nations 2030 Agenda for Sustainable Development

William Rosa, MS, RN, LMT, AHN-BC, AGPCNP-BC, CCRN-CMC

Editor

SPRINGER / PUBLISHING COMPANY

NEW YORK

Springer Publishing Company, LLC
11 West 42nd Street
New York, NY 10036
www.springerpub.com

Acquisitions Editor: Margaret Zuccarini
Senior Production Editor: Kris Parrish
Compositor: Exeter Premedia Services Private Ltd.

ISBN: 978-0-8261-9011-6
e-book ISBN: 978-0-8261-9012-3

17 18 19 20 / 5 4 3 2 1

The author and the publisher of this Work have made every effort to use sources believed to be reliable to provide information that is accurate and compatible with the standards generally accepted at the time of publication. The author and publisher shall not be liable for any special, consequential, or exemplary damages resulting, in whole or in part, from the readers' use of, or reliance on, the information contained in this book. The publisher has no responsibility for the persistence or accuracy of URLs for external or third-party Internet websites referred to in this publication and does not guarantee that any content on such websites is, or will remain, accurate or appropriate.

Library of Congress Cataloging-in-Publication Data

Names: Rosa, William, 1982- editor.
Title: A new era in global health: nursing and the United Nations 2030
   Agenda for Sustainable Development / editor, William Rosa.
Description: New York: Springer Publishing Company, LLC, [2017] | Includes
   bibliographical references.
Identifiers: LCCN 2017004467 | ISBN 9780826190116 | ISBN 9780826190123 (e-book)
Subjects: | MESH: United Nations. | Nursing | Global Health | Conservation of
   Natural Resources
Classification: LCC RT86.5 | NLM WY 101 | DDC 362.17/3—dc23
LC record available at https://lccn.loc.gov/2017004467

Contact us to receive discount rates on bulk purchases.
We can also customize our books to meet your needs.
For more information please contact: sales@springerpub.com

Printed in the United States of America by McNaughton & Gunn.

For Michael

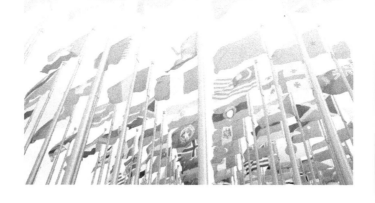

Contents

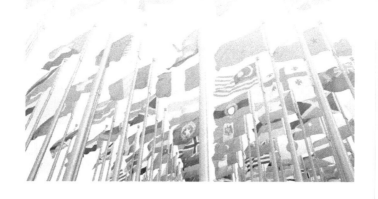

Contributors

Sarah Abboud, PhD, RN, Assistant Professor, Department of Women, Children, and Family Health Science, College of Nursing, University of Illinois at Chicago, Chicago, Illinois

Julie K. Anathan, RN, MPH, Associate Chief Nursing Officer, Seed Global Health, Boston, Massachusetts

Olivia Bahemuka, DNP, MSN, RN-BC, Visiting Clinical Instructor, College of Nursing, Human Resources for Health Program at the College of Medicine and Health Sciences, University of Illinois at Chicago, Chicago, Illinois, Kigali, Rwanda

Deva-Marie Beck, PhD, RN, International Co-Director, Nightingale Initiative for Global Health (NIGH), Neepawa, Manitoba, Canada

Busisiwe Rosemary Bhengu, PhD, RN, Honorary Associate Professor, University of KwaZulu-Natal (UKZN), Durban, South Africa

Suellen Breakey, PhD, RN, Assistant Professor, MGH Institute of Health Professions, Boston, Massachusetts

Kelly Burke, MPH, BSN, RN, Former Clinical Nurse Educator, University of Maryland, Baltimore, Maryland

Cathy Catrambone, PhD, RN, FAAN, President, Sigma Theta Tau—The Honor Society of Nursing, Chicago, Illinois

Maureen E. Connell, MPH, BSc (Hons), RN, Nurse Educator, Rwamagana, Rwanda

Christine M. Darling, MPA, Senior Operations Administrator, Sigma Theta Tau—The Honor Society of Nursing, Indianapolis, Indiana

Barbara Montgomery Dossey, PhD, RN, AHN-BC, FAAN, HWNC-BC, Co-Director, International Nurse Coach Association (INCA), Core Faculty, Integrative Nurse Coach Certificate Program (INCCP), North Miami, Florida

Carole Ann Drick, PhD, RN, AHN-BC, Director of Conscious Awareness, Co-Director of Golden Room Advocates, Austintown, Ohio

Linda A. Evans, PhD, RN, Program Director at the Center for Nursing Excellence, Brigham and Women's Hospital, Boston, Massachusetts

Helen Ewing, DHSc, MN, RN, Senior Manager for Nursing and Midwifery, Clinical Training Specialist—Clinton Health Access Initiative, Health Workforce Program, Monrovia, Liberia

Joyce J. Fitzpatrick, PhD, MBA, RN, FAAN, FNAP, Elizabeth Brooks Ford Professor of Nursing, Frances Payne Bolton School of Nursing, Case Western Reserve University, Cleveland, Ohio

Martha Hill, PhD, RN, Dean Emerita and Professor, Johns Hopkins University School of Nursing, Baltimore, Maryland

Elizabeth Holguin, MPH, MSN, FNP-BC, **RN,** PhD Candidate in Nursing and Health Policy, University of New Mexico College of Nursing, Albuquerque, New Mexico

Sara Horton-Deutsch, PhD, RN, PMHCNS, FAAN, ANEF, Caritas Coach, Heart-Math Trainer, Professor, University of Colorado, Denver, Denver, Colorado

Frances Hughes, RN, BA, MA, DNurs, Col (ret), JP, ONZM, Chief Executive Officer, International Council of Nurses, Queensland, Australia

Lynn Keegan, PhD, RN, AHN-BC, FAAN, Director, Holistic Nursing Consultants (HNC), Port Angeles, Washington

Hester C. Klopper, PhD, RN, MBA, FAAN, ASSAf, Deputy Vice Chancellor, Strategic Initiatives and Internationalization, Stellenbosch University, Cape Town, South Africa

Ann E. Kurth, PhD, CNM, MPH, FAAN, Dean, Linda Koch Lorimer Professor (inaugural chair), Yale University School of Nursing, New Haven, Connecticut

Jeanne M. Leffers, PhD, RN, FAAN, Professor Emeritus, University of Massachusetts, Dartmouth, Dartmouth, Massachusetts

Susan Luck, MA, RN, HNB-BC, CCN, HWNC-BC, Integrative Nurse Coach, International Nurse Coach Association, Bay Harbor Islands, Florida

Phalakshi Manjrekar, MScN, RN, Distinguished Nursing Director and Board Member, P. D. Hinduja National Hospital & Medical Research Centre, Mumbai, India

Tamara H. McKinnon, DNP, APHN, RN, Professor, The Valley Foundation School of Nursing, San Jose State University, San Jose, California

Afaf Ibrahim Meleis, PhD, FAAN, LL, Professor of Nursing and Sociology, University of Pennsylvania, Philadelphia, Pennsylvania

Patricia Moreland, PhD, CPNP, RN, Visiting Faculty, Master of Science in Nursing Program, Pediatric Track, School of Nursing and Midwifery, Human Resources for Health Program at the College of Medicine and Health Sciences, University of Illinois at Chicago, College of Nursing, University of Rwanda, Kigali, Rwanda

Karen H. Morin, PhD, RN, ANEF, FAAN, Professor Emeritus, the University of Wisconsin—Milwaukee; Visiting Professor, University of West Georgia, Tanner System School of Nursing, Carrollton, Georgia

Jasintha T. Mtengezo, MPH, BSN, RN, Certified Midwife, PhD Candidate, University of Massachusetts, Boston, Massachusetts

Sarah Oerther, MSN, MEd, RN, CSPI, Jonas Nurse Leader Scholar, PhD Candidate, Saint Louis University, School of Nursing, St. Louis, Missouri

Melissa T. Ojemeni, MA, RN, PCCN, PhD Candidate, Rory Meyers College of Nursing at New York University, New York, New York

Laura Ridge, ANP-BC, RN, PhD Candidate, Rory Meyers College of Nursing at New York University, New York, New York

William Rosa, MS, RN, LMT, AHN-BC, AGPCNP-BC, CCRN-CMC, Palliative Care Nurse Practitioner Fellow, Memorial Sloan Kettering Cancer Center, New York, New York

Judith Shamian, PhD, RN, LLD (Hons), DSci (Hons), FAAN, President of the International Council of Nurses (ICN), Geneva, Switzerland

Holly K. Shaw, PhD, RN, Director, UNDPI/NGO Executive Committee, Vice Chair, NGO Committee on Mental Health, Representative to UN DPI, Nightingale Initiative for Global Health, Sea Cliff, New York

Allison P. Squires, PhD, RN, FAAN, Associate Professor and Director of International Education, Rory Meyers College of Nursing at New York University, New York, New York

Michele J. Upvall, PhD, RN, CRNP, Professor of Nursing, Coordinator, MSN Nurse Educator Programs, University of Central Florida, Orlando, Florida

Cynthia Vlasich, MBA, RN, BSN, Director—Global Initiatives, Sigma Theta Tau—The Honor Society of Nursing, Indianapolis, Indiana

Jean Watson, PhD, RN, AHN-BC, FAAN, Distinguished Professor and Dean Emerita, College of Nursing Anschutz Medical Center, University of Colorado Denver, Denver, Colorado

Deborah Wilson, BSN, RN, CRNI, MSN/MPH Candidate, Johns Hopkins University, Baltimore, Maryland

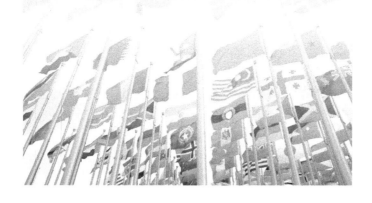

Foreword

As a physician, I recognize I am an unusual choice to write the foreword for a book on global nursing. However, as a colleague in health care delivery, I have spent my career learning about the power of nursing, celebrating how our work—my own work—is profoundly enhanced by strong partnerships with nursing colleagues. Since medical school, I have been humbled by the experience, knowledge, willing vulnerability, and compassion of the nurses with whom I have worked. I have consistently relied on their wisdom and experience on difficult nights in the intensive care unit. Now, as cofounder and CEO of Seed Global Health, a nonprofit that invests in nursing and medical training in sub-Saharan Africa, I have continued to be empowered by my nursing colleagues, learning from them about the needs of nursing globally, global nursing education, and investing in nursing leadership to promote the health and well-being of all.

Nelson Mandela famously said, "Education is the most powerful weapon with which to change the world." This concept is central to the work we do at Seed. Our hope is to use education to help improve quality of health care delivery in some of the most challenging settings globally. Seed partners with the U.S. Peace Corps to send nurses, midwives, and physicians abroad for 1 year as visiting faculty in sub-Saharan Africa. These U.S. health professionals embed as faculty: teaching, providing clinical mentorship, collaborating on practice improvement, and role-modeling quality care. Our approach is to partner with local health professionals and their institutions, helping to support their education and delivery priorities. Seed brings expertise in nursing, midwifery, and medicine, and the Peace Corps draws on 50-plus years of experience sending U.S. citizens abroad in service in an integrated and culturally sensitive way. Further, we collaborate with academic partners, like the Massachusetts General Hospital, to provide academic resources and recognition for the volunteers' work.

Nurses and midwives have been central to Seed's vision since its inception. We have been committed to investing in the nursing profession and its leadership because nurses are the core of most health systems. Little known (and even less recognized) health professionals other than physicians provide the vast majority of health care globally. Most often, it is nurses.

Martha Geodert, a 2015–2016 Seed–Peace Corps Global Health Service Partnership volunteer, is an example of a global nurse on the front lines of providing care. She lived and worked for a year in central Tanzania. She was only a visitor, working alongside her local colleagues who face tough challenges every day. Martha's story illustrates the difficult but deeply critical role she and her local counterparts play in providing comfort and care.

At our Close of Service Conference in June 2016, Martha showed a picture of a woman and shared the following:

> This was a woman that I'd cared for during labor and delivery. She'd come in with a single footling breach. I cried . . . for [two of my Tanzania-based Global Health Service Partnership OB/GYN colleagues] to be at my side—for any OB/GYN that would rapidly [intervene]. [This woman] was on our unit for 4 hours. I was trying to get this single footling breach delivered by caesarian section. The baby's heart rate finally fell from 130 down to 70. I ran over to get one of the OB/GYNs and the baby's femur was fractured during the process. [The infant] was transferred to the pediatric ward where we saw him the next day. The leg had not been set. The second day, the leg had not been set. Finally, the students and I set the leg. His pain was immediately decreased. And they saw for the first time, I think, that our role as nurse practitioners [and] nurse midwives is doing whatever needs to be done in consultation with our physician colleagues. And when there's a gap, we fill it. And you all know that we have filled this gap in a way that we would never perhaps do in the United States, but it is a very important way of responding. This mother took my face in her hands and her face in my hands, you know that there's a connection. When you come back day after day, she knows that she's been cared for and she knows that the students that were with her are also with her [now].

Martha shares not only the power of collaboration across the profession but also the skill, sixth sense, and deep commitment to the patient and his or her well-being, which nursing embraces. She demonstrates firsthand the powerful advocacy nurses ensure for their patients and the deep bond that is formed. Despite the presence of many nurses like Martha, or her counterparts, nurses are often underutilized, unempowered, or simply excluded from important discussions about patient care, or even policy. To provide an example, I attended one meeting at the Ministry of Health in an African nation to discuss launching our program for nursing and midwifery in their country. The director of nursing for the Ministry of Health arrived late because no one had told her about the time. She then sat in a back row of chairs—not at the table—and was never asked for her input. We need strong global nurse leaders who will address these interprofessional inequities and inspire a collaborative and inclusive model of care delivery worldwide.

The American Nurses Association (ANA, 2016) defines *nursing* as "the protection, promotion, and optimization of health and abilities, prevention of illness and injury, facilitation of healing, alleviation of suffering through the diagnosis and treatment of *human response*, and advocacy in the care of individuals, families, groups, communities, and populations." Nurses are at the intimate frontlines of patient care, whether at the bedside or advocating at the population level. They must be at the table for any meaningful discussion about health care delivery, health system strengthening, or changing health outcomes for the better.

In *A New Era in Global Health*, William Rosa and his fellow contributors help outline this poignant and essential role of nursing. They articulate the incredible strength and diversity of the nursing profession to serve as a change agent for individual, population, global, and planetary health. In the vein of Mandela's quote, *A New Era in Global Health* empowers us by archiving the profound ways that nursing can influence every aspect of our health, well-being, and wholeness.

This book is important. There remains today a paucity of literature on global nursing. Yet, nurses have been toiling on the front lines throughout all the dynamic shifts to health care and its systems in settings both resource rich and poor. In countries like the United States, for example, new practice systems have been implemented for quality improvement. In resource-limited settings like Tanzania, where Martha worked, new partnerships are blossoming to bolster nursing capacity, education, and numbers produced. Much more attention is required to explore these developments, their impact on health, and, ultimately, the field of nursing overall.

Mr. Rosa and his colleagues help close this gap. And they do so using a smart, salient approach by critically linking nursing to the United Nations 2030 Agenda, grounding the discussion in the Sustainable Development Goals (SDGs) and a greater transnational discourse. The SDG campaign has 17 all-encompassing goals, including reducing poverty, ensuring food security, improving health, and combating climate change, and 169 targets that create tangible benchmarks for which to both plan and strive. *A New Era in Global Health* brings nursing into the center of this effort, exploring the SDGs and also the profession's unique and vital contribution toward their realization.

When all is said and done, *A New Era in Global Health* reminds us that nurses are at the frontlines of the *human response* to all of these issues. We must continue to support the work of global nursing and promote nurses' involvement in practice, education, and policy arenas. This work guides us in understanding the potential impact of nursing across contexts and cultures—beyond paternalistic disciplinary scopes and limiting interprofessional hierarchies—in creating the safe and equitable world called for by the United Nations 2030 Agenda for Sustainable Development.

Vanessa B. Kerry, MD, MSc
Chief Executive Officer
Seed Global Health
Boston, Massachusetts

REFERENCE

American Nurses Association. (2016). What is nursing? Retrieved from http://www
.nursingworld.org/EspeciallyForYou/What-is-Nursing

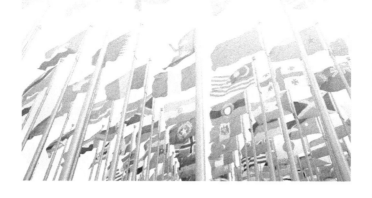

Preface

We stand at a critical moment in Earth's history. . . . To move forward we must recognize that. . . . we are one human family and one Earth community. . . . [I]t is imperative that we, the peoples of Earth, declare our responsibility to one another, to the greater community of life, and to future generations. (The Earth Charter Initiative, 2000)

It is a time for heightened and more universal considerations in the fields of global health and global nursing. It is, as the title of this book suggests, *A New Era in Global Health*, in which we, as human beings, are coming to truly understand—possibly more than ever before—our deep interconnectedness to nature and all people on the planet. We are currently witnessing firsthand the widespread consequences of our individual and collective choices on the planet, and beginning to see how the foundational premise of nursing—to preserve and protect human dignity in the promotion of good health and well-being—must now be expanded in order to create and sustain a more equitable and inclusive world. In this continually emerging age of technology, with the aid of media reporting, each one of us can now come face to face with the socioeconomic and political disparities that divide us and the violence and threats to safety that keep those without health, food, education, rights, or stability disproportionately disadvantaged. This new era is not about stand-alone theories or didactics, and it cannot be relegated to classroom and clinical settings. It is about taking informed and deliberate action—in real time and with a commitment to professional integrity—to improve the holistic welfare of all, and to expand and maximize the scope of practice for global nurses to include values-guided leadership, consistent and reliable advocacy, and outcomes-driven change agency in the transnational arena. The literature is overwhelmed by discourses on being a leader, advocate, and change agent; with haste and equipped with the necessary information, we must confidently put the discourses into action. The time is now and *A New Era in Global Health* is just one offering to help us get there.

On September 25, 2015, the United Nations General Assembly (UNGA) adopted the 2030 Agenda for Sustainable Development, a resolution that will continue to change how the world addresses poverty, ensures environmental stability, and procures a peaceful, just, civil society for all human beings on the planet. The purpose of this book is threefold: (a) to identify the opportunities global nurses must leverage in order to achieve this agenda, (b) to explore the implications and personal–professional responsibilities we all share to each of the agenda's 17 Sustainable Development Goals (SDGs), and (c) to create a vision for the future of global nursing that ensures health equity and improves the quality of life for all human beings on the planet.

Ultimately, the chapters throughout this text remind us that "global nursing" is not defined by working internationally or participating in mission trips, but requires a shift in consciousness and an evolving awareness regarding how our work contributes to outcomes not only in health sectors, but also in policy, education, economic relations, and environmental activism. Global nursing moves us toward a paradigm of shared humanity, a heightened understanding of healing and its meaning in an internationalized context, and the untapped potential of the profession to contribute wholly, intelligently, and courageously to each of the SDGs wherever, and in whatever context, we may find ourselves.

A New Era in Global Health arose from my experiences of living in East Africa and my personal–professional development while working in severely resource-constrained clinical and academic settings. Just after midnight on August 1, 2015—roughly 2 months before the UNGA adopted the Sustainable Development Agenda—I landed in Kigali, Rwanda. It would be a year that would change my understanding of the world and what it means to be of service. Over the next 12 months I would come face to face with my own frustrations about the dehumanizing impacts of poverty and confront the seemingly unending cycle of economic inequity that prevents men, women, and children from experiencing the quality of life they deserve. But I would also find myself celebrating the small moments of change and hope that spring forth from the resilience made possible through partnership. I would slowly come to surrender stingy and culturally impotent opinions regarding "the right way" to do things and "how it should be" in favor of contextually sensitive explorations and greater humility in my approach to human care.

I have come to realize firsthand the essential responsibilities global nurses have in forwarding the United Nations (UN) 2030 Agenda for Sustainable Development (2015; also referred to as the "Post-2015 Agenda" or the "2030 Agenda" for short). This transnational plan consists of 17 SDGs, also known as the "global goals," with 169 targets and seeks to:

- End poverty in all its forms everywhere by addressing widespread inequality and promoting socioeconomic opportunities for development
- Protect the planet and all species, preserve the Earth's natural resources, and combat climate change
- Create the possibilities of prosperous and fulfilling lives for all human beings worldwide while promoting a more harmonious existence with nature
- Foster peaceful, just, and inclusive societies that are free from fear and the threat of violence

- And build partnerships among all people and nations that will address the needs of the most vulnerable populations on the planet and represent our global solidarity

This agenda comes in the wake and achievements of the UN's Millennium Development Goals (MDGs) that were adopted and implemented from 2000 to 2015 (see Chapter 2 for complete listings of the SDGs and MDGs, Chapter 3 for a brief history of the UN, and the Appendix for the complete resolution, *Transforming Our World: The 2030 Agenda for Sustainable Development*). The preamble states:

> This Agenda is a plan of action for people, planet and prosperity. It also seeks to strengthen universal peace in larger freedom. We recognize that eradicating poverty in all its forms and dimensions, including extreme poverty, is the greatest global challenge and an indispensable requirement for sustainable development.
>
> All countries and all stakeholders, acting in collaborative partnership, will implement this plan. We are resolved to free the human race from the tyranny of poverty and want and to heal and secure our planet. We are determined to take the bold and transformative steps which are urgently needed to shift the world on to a sustainable and resilient path. As we embark on this collective journey, we pledge that no one will be left behind.
>
> The 17 Sustainable Development Goals and 169 targets which we are announcing today demonstrate the scale and ambition of this new universal Agenda. They seek to build on the Millennium Development Goals and complete what they did not achieve. They seek to realize the human rights of all and to achieve gender equality and the empowerment of all women and girls. They are integrated and indivisible and balance the three dimensions of sustainable development: the economic, social and environmental.
>
> The goals and targets will stimulate action over the next 15 years in areas of critical importance for humanity and the planet. (UN, 2015, p. 5)

These words lay the foundation for *A New Era in Global Health*.

Out of the Human Resources for Health Program experience in Rwanda and my personal immersion into the work of the 2030 Agenda came a collection for Springer Publishing Company's blog, SpringBoard, titled *The Public Health Nursing Series*. The series explored nursing's unique contributions to each of the UN's 17 SDGs. As the series progressed and the idea for this book was birthed, I realized that developing these ideas into book form would involve taking public health nursing prerogatives and applying them to a transnational context, inviting heightened considerations for the health and well-being of the global village. It would also require translating the ideals and values of public health nursing that I had employed in the series and expanding them in relation to my vision for equitable and ethical global nursing practice.

This book is designed to raise the awareness of fellow nursing colleagues about the opportunities that exist for them in aiding governments and health infrastructures to obtain the targets established by the SDGs. Additionally, it provides ample opportunities for the profession to integrate global considerations into nursing curricula, research efforts, and practice initiatives right now. In my experience, nurses are not fully aware of the opportunities available to them regarding the Post-2015 Agenda and are focused primarily on SDG 3, "Good Health and Well-Being." However, there are potential roles related to each of the 17 Global Goals that invite us to maximize the scope of global nursing and provide ample invitation to bring a nursing sensibility to interprofessional alliances. There exists a vast array of partnership options and innovative possibilities for nursing to define and pursue the future SDG health indicators (Benton & Ferguson, 2016).

This book is divided into three units. Unit I provides a background of emerging considerations in global nursing and global health for personal–planetary transformation, a brief history and future directions of the relationship between nursing and the UN, guidelines for global leadership and discussion of the importance of global citizenship, and ethics in the global health context. Unit I also identifies opportunities to create more inclusive models in education, research, and practice; explores ways to increase the role of international nursing organizations in realizing the 2030 Agenda; and provides exemplars of caring personal–professional relationships that are creating the peaceful and just societies mentioned earlier.

Unit II provides a primer on the 17 SDGs. Each of these chapters has been adapted from the original *Public Health Nursing Series* and expanded upon to include global considerations. Readers will find information about the SDG targets, options for how nursing can play direct and indirect roles in furthering the priorities of each goal, and the current initiatives under way that deserve global nursing's input and partnership if they are to be truly effective.

Lastly, Unit III articulates a vision for the future of global nursing and global health, one that moves from the firsthand global wisdom of nurses who guide us to further the SDGs in countries around the world; requires us to be reflective as individuals, as well as with partners, groups, organizations, and communities, as we commit to sustainable development; creates a collaboration consciousness to engender unity and peace; and illustrates a Post-2030 Agenda, beyond the SDGs, for planetary health.

A New Era in Global Health is designed for any nurse who wants to be "in the world" and develop concrete action plans to contribute effectively to the safe and inclusive global society envisioned by the UN's 2030 Agenda for Sustainable Development. It is more than a collection of chapters and case studies; it is a call to act on our leadership, advocacy, and change agency skills for the betterment of humanity and the planet. The breadth and depth of the Sustainable Development Agenda has an impact on the nursing care being delivered at bedsides in every nation around the world. It invites nursing to take its rightful place at the global and interprofessional tables that will determine the quality of future planetary health and well-being for all through policy development and cross-cultural partnerships. Nursing's willingness to actively champion the SDGs and their associated targets will determine much more than patient outcomes; it will curtail the deleterious consequences of poverty, hunger, and inequality; influence economic infrastructures worldwide; impact climate and environmental sustainability; and be integral to the possibility of creating a peaceful and just world.

Ultimately, this book is a call to action for all of us—the entire global village—to confront and untangle the myriad factors that prevent health equity and identify the opportunities for nurses to lead and integrate impactful, long-term change for all populations everywhere. It speaks to our professional legacy, the courage to transform outdated systems and worldviews, and an ethical commitment to evolve how we deliver compassionate and effective care across settings and contexts. It reflects an empowered, fully expressed, and globally conscious profession, and our current and potential contributions to sustainable development. *A New Era in Global Health* is about the impact of global nursing and the future of planetary well-being, which we will both individually and collectively determine and be accountable for through our action, as well as our inaction. It is about nations, governments, and health care systems worldwide. It is about you and it is about me.

This is, indeed, *A New Era in Global Health*.

William Rosa

REFERENCES

Benton, D., & Ferguson, S. L. (2016). Windows to the future: Can the United Nations' Sustainable Goals provide opportunities for nursing? *Nursing Economics, 34*(2), 101–103.

The Earth Charter Initiative. (2000). The earth charter. Retrieved from http://earthcharter.org/invent/images/uploads/echarter_english.pdf

United Nations. (2015). Transforming our world: The 2030 Agenda for Sustainable Development. Retrieved from https://docs.google.com/gview?url=http://sustainabledevelopment.un.org/content/documents/21252030%20Agenda%20for%20Sustainable%20Development%20web.pdf&embedded=true

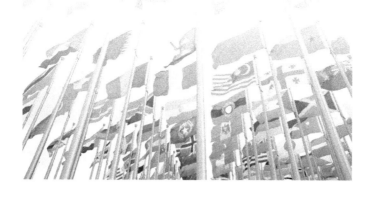

Acknowledgments

I wish to offer my first and humble thanks to the contributing authors who have helped to bring this book into existence. I share this accomplishment with each of you. Your wisdom and expertise are calls to action for all of us to become more globally conscious professionals.

My endless thanks to my collaborating team at Springer Publishing Company, Margaret Zuccarini, Kris Parrish, and Amanda Devine, for supporting me throughout my creative process and for ensuring the integrity of my vision every step of the way. And to Lucy Frisch, thank you for allowing me to write the *Public Health Nursing Series*: the SpringBoard blogs that birthed the idea for this book.

For all my interprofessional colleagues affiliated with the Human Resources for Health Program in Rwanda, I am so very thankful for your presence and contributions to my personal and professional life. Each one of you is ensuring the health and well-being of those we serve one day at a time. Thank you for expanding how I see and understand global health and for your contributions toward cocreating a safe and inclusive world. My deepest gratitude goes to Anne Jones and Patricia Moreland for being role models of compassionate global nursing and for being my dearest confidants and friends. You are both deeply loved and cared for.

For my closest friends and beautiful family, thank you for your support as I brought this work to life. You each give me countless reasons to be grateful and celebrate every day of my life.

Mom and Dad, I love you very much. Thank you for all that you do and all that you are. You always inspire me to remember that "No act of kindness, no matter how small, is ever wasted."

Michael, you are whole, perfect, and complete and I love you just as you are. This is for you.

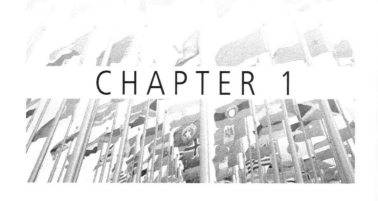

CHAPTER 1

Re-Membering Humanity: A First Step Toward One Health

William Rosa

Your job is not to be perfect. Your job is only to be human. . . . Our leaders and ourselves want everything, but we don't talk about the costs. . . . [W]hat is the cost of not daring? What is the cost of not trying? . . . We face huge issues as a world. . . . We can take the easier road, the more cynical road . . . based on . . . dreams of a past that never really was, a fear of each other, distancing, and blame. Or we can take the much more difficult path of transformation, transcendence, compassion, and love, but also accountability and justice. . . . Our lives are so short, and our time on this planet is so precious, and all we have is each other. So may each of you live lives of immersion. They won't necessarily be easy lives, but in the end, it is all that will sustain us. (Jacqueline Novogratz, founder and CEO, Acumen, 2010)

The altruistic values central to nursing as a global profession ask us to re-member humanity. To *re-member* another means to see, hear, and acknowledge them as a human being worthy of respect and care. Re-membering calls nurses to invite that person to be engaged in the policy, practice, education, and research interventions that directly impact their health and healing, and determine their overall welfare. It asks us to count all peoples—regardless of their race, ethnicity, faith, sexual orientation, disability, gender, education, or socioeconomic status—as equal and worthy members of the global village. Re-membering requires confronting the "truths" we think we know about the world, and inviting people to share their life's narrative in a way that expands and enlightens our understanding of their context and worldview.

Included throughout this text are exemplars of global nursing, global health, ethical stances on leadership and advocacy in the transnational context, and invitations to elevate and expand your definitions of the nursing profession, human rights, justice, and planetary health. This journey begins when we listen to each other, honor and celebrate one another's stories, and make the choice to partner in a way that benefits our collective welfare and global best interest. *A New Era in Global Health* addresses the health and dignity of human beings as a group, but extends far beyond us as a species toward a model of "One Health," which includes the well-being of animals, nature and its ecosystems, and the planet as an interdependent matrix. Planetary health may be the goal, but we start here by pausing to re-member one another and the dynamism of the human race.

While writing this introduction, I was shocked to see the headline of an article in *The New York Times*, which bleakly stated, "Over 100 Children Among 338 Killed in Aleppo Attacks This Week" (Saad & Cumming-Bruce, 2016). At that moment, more than 840 people were trapped in eastern Aleppo, Syria, and expected to die of wounds due to lack of medical resources and needed treatment, including 261 children. While food, water, and fuel resources dwindled, the health system was rapidly disintegrating, with only six minimally functional hospitals and fewer than 30 physicians available to care for the ill and injured (World Health Organization [WHO], 2016). Health workers and hospitals were being attacked and their supplies looted by rebel forces with alarming frequency, while those trapped in eastern Aleppo eagerly awaited aid and humanitarian assistance. The WHO (2016) was calling directly on all parties involved in the conflict to allow the immediate evacuation of the sick and wounded, permit access for the provision of medicine, medical supplies, fuel, and health workers to support medical staff in Aleppo, immediately halt attacks on health workers and facilities, respect the neutrality of health workers and health facilities, and cease removal of critical supplies from medical supplies deliveries. The BBC noted that the war in Syria had been raging for roughly 4.5 years, resulting in the death of over 250,000 Syrians and over 11 million people being forced from their homes due to violence and fear of bombings and bloodshed (Rodgers, Gritten, Offer, & Asare, 2016).

This is not a Syrian problem—it is humanity's. It is not about "them" or "those people," but about us and the kind of world we, as a human collective, continue to foster and create, whether by our direct participation in violent acts or our decision to remain passive in the face of them. Right now, a world exists where atrocities such as these can and do persist. The reasons are many: poverty, hunger, lack of education, inequality, and political injustice, to name a few. But the solutions are also formidable. They include addressing the root socioeconomic disparities that allow families to be poor and children to go hungry; restoring human dignity wherever it is lost or threatened; promoting equal laws and policies for all men, women, and children in all nations; building systems that deliver quality and inclusive education; and demonstrating that peace is possible through the development of compassionate, informed, deliberate, and unyielding global partnerships.

It begins and ends with each of us being bold, courageous, and daring enough to take full and radical accountability for the world in which we live. The realization of a safe and inclusive global village is not some visionary, futuristic pipe dream. It is a possibility that each of us can create each and every day; it is a choice we get to make right now.

And, you—what will you choose?

"WE ARE ALL THE SAME, YOU AND I"

During a recent visit to Cape Town, South Africa, I met a man named Thando. Thando is "Colored," a socially acceptable term in South Africa used to describe people of mixed race. He is from the Xhosa tribe, and his name in the Xhosa language means "love." Thando walked my family and me through the footsteps of his earliest memories and young adulthood in apartheid-era South Africa. He led us through District 6, an area from which non-White individuals and their families were forcibly removed as a result of the Group Areas Act of 1950 (Michigan State University, n.d.). In the 1950s and 1960s, the government enforced residential segregation in District 6 and countless other locations throughout the country, moving more than 860,000 Blacks, families of Indian descent, and coloreds—who were no longer considered suitable to live there—into geographically distant townships up to 19 miles away from their places of employment in the city center. Thando pointed out the Roeland Street Prison, the infamous, rat-infested "Black Hole" that was known for its deplorable conditions during the 20th century (The Heritage Portal, 2016). Thando's mother had been imprisoned there for apartheid resistance and was thereafter "correctively raped" by the police sergeant. Nine months later, a colored child was born who would, in his later years, become a global ambassador for shared humanity and love (as his name suggests).

Thando grew up in the Bonteheuwel township and became a freedom fighter against the apartheid government—quite literally standing off and engaging in violent acts against his father and other authorities who carried out the dehumanizing policies of the time. He was later exiled to Namibia and was able to return to South Africa only after the apartheid government commenced its disintegration. Thando now lives in New Rest, Gugulethu township, and is a warm and gentle man of integrity in his 60s who has witnessed the advancement of his nation toward a more unified way of living.

Though South Africa has come a long way, the road toward ultimate national inclusion and true equality will be a long and challenging journey for years to come. The National Planning Commission (NPC, 2011), in its *Diagnostic Overview* report, acknowledged the substantial inequities in educational outcomes, continued marginalization of the poor based on historical forced removal, and uneven public service performance across people of differing races and socioeconomic status. Ultimately, "South Africa remains a divided society" (NPC, 2011, p. 26). The broad implications of apartheid and residential segregation continue to create countrywide disparities in health care coverage, access, and delivery; education; and economic opportunity; and even in the attainment of the most basic human rights, such as food security, safety, and access to clean water and sanitation (Mahajan, 2014). The NPC's *National Development Plan* was implemented in 2013 as a multisector effort to promote national solidarity and invite a more unified vision for a country that has inherited a complex legacy of oppression, but is actively striving to reclaim the narrative toward a more socially just and inclusive future (NPC, 2013).

The possibility of hope is realized through individuals such as Thando. Many times throughout our visit, he would say to us some version of the following:

> Thank you for coming to South Africa. By seeing us, by listening to our stories and bearing witness to our history, you re-member us, all

of us who have been dis-membered and forgotten for so long. It is in you being here that we become human again. It is in you including us in the history of the country that we become a part of humanity. By being here with us, you can take us and our experiences back to where you come from and become ambassadors for us never to be forgotten again. And though I've never traveled to other countries, I am blessed because I get to see and know the world through you. We are all the same, you and I.

Thando is a living testament to the power of love and a commitment to peace. Unfortunately, his story of oppression, violence, poverty, and political injustice is not uncommon; in fact, it is a globally pervasive reality for countless men, women, and children. According to the United Nations High Commissioner for Refugees (UNHCR, 2001–2016a, 2001–2016b), there are currently 65.3 million forcibly displaced people worldwide, of which there are 21.3 million refugees, 10 million stateless people who have been denied a nationality and basic human rights, and roughly 1 million people each year seeking asylum and safety in foreign countries to avoid persecution. These statistics remind us there are millions of our fellow human beings whose daily lives are dictated largely by fear, uncertainty, inequality, and countless threats to their personal and collective well-being.

The United Nations (UN) 2030 Agenda for Sustainable Development is a transnational pact by UN Member States to re-member the Thandos of the world, a decision to directly invite all human beings into the global conversations that affect them and determine their overall health and dignity, in partnership and brotherhood, quite possibly for the first time in human history. The Agenda acknowledges their histories of being dis-membered and invites their narratives into a cohesive plan for improved welfare as a human right. It is a tremendous step in the right direction toward healing the global consequences of poverty and violence and the widespread apathy that has allowed cultural malignancies, such as apartheid and other forms of institutionalized discrimination, to blot human history with the shame of silence and inaction.

LIVING A LIFE OF IMMERSION: WHY IT MATTERS

Acumen is a charitable organization that seeks to invest in local entrepreneurs worldwide, promoting autonomy and human dignity through empowering knowledge and skills transfer, as an innovative solution to tackle poverty (Acumen, 2016). Founder and CEO Jacqueline Novogratz (2010) promotes living a life of immersion: a choice to be "in the world" with a compass of personal integrity, moral courage and leadership, and a commitment to social justice. A life of immersion does not require living in low- and middle-income countries (LMICs) or working internationally to realize a future of peace and prosperity for all. But it does call for an awareness of global interdependence and an understanding that what we do and don't do, what we say and don't say, and how we contribute and don't contribute to the broader social agendas of our time impact people in all parts of the world whom we may never see, meet, or even know exist. Living a life of immersion asks us to allow ourselves to be touched and changed by others' stories, be vessels and conduits for their own self-growth, share our experiences in constructive and positive ways for the betterment of all involved, and don a respectful and compassionate boldness in our service to a greater good. It is a courageous choice to re-member one another and to have the audacity to believe that "in a gentle way, [each of us] can shake the world" (Gandhi, n.d.). In many ways, this book supports Novogratz's (2010) advocacy for living a life of immersion.

A Reflection on Rwanda: An Immersion Exemplar

No, you don't have to work abroad to live a life of immersion. But for me, having the opportunity to live and work for a year in Kigali, Rwanda, was the awakening for which I had long been waiting. Rwanda, the story of its history and the resilience of its people, is a country that has forever changed my perspectives on what it means to be "in the world" as a global citizen. As a person, I could not have been prepared when I first arrived for the inspiring relationships that would deeply touch my heart or the experiences that would enlighten me to new ways of being, living, and working. As a professional—as a global nurse—it has been both a gratifying and grounding process of learning to collaborate across cultures, and developing practical and clinical dexterity in significantly resource-constrained environments. Rwanda has been a call to evolve my perspectives regarding nursing's role in procuring human betterment, and to become more intentional about our individual and collective personal–professional contributions to global health and well-being.

I arrived in Rwanda as a member of the Human Resources for Health (HRH) Program. This 7-year multi-investor global health initiative was started in 2012 and seeks to increase the number of skilled health care workers, heighten the quality of health worker training and education, improve the infrastructure of health facilities, and elevate the standards of how health care is managed and facilitated in Rwanda (Rwandan Ministry of Health [MOH], n.d.). The HRH Program is a consortium of U.S. medical centers and academic institutions of nursing, public health, and dentistry that partner with interprofessional Rwandan affiliates in practice, education, and research settings. Through these partnerships, the HRH Program strives to achieve its overall goals: to improve the delivery of quality health care services, foster in-country autonomy and sustainability, and decrease long-term dependence on foreign aid and intervention (Binagwaho et al., 2013). The HRH Program introduced a new model of foreign aid that promoted Rwanda's full government ownership through strong international coordination, low overhead, and direct alignment with the government's broader goals and needs (Sliney & Uwimana, 2014). A recent 4-year midterm review has demonstrated that the targets of the HRH Program are on track to be realized by its conclusion in 2019, and that, to date, outcomes demonstrate improved quality of education and mentorship opportunities, increased research capacity, increased access to health services for the Rwandan population, and improved quality of care, particularly for those suffering from HIV and chronic diseases (Rwandan MOH, 2016).

There can be a frequently lingering mindset of arrogance on the part of health care workers in service to global initiatives in LMICs, one that says, "We are here to make you better, to teach you how to do it right." During my orientation for

HRH, the dean of the School of Medicine, College of Medicine and Health Sciences at the University of Rwanda, said something to this effect:

> You are not here to teach me how to fish. I already know how to fish. You just fish differently. Let us not waste time with who fishes better but learn from each other what we can so that we might both grow in the best ways possible. Let's get into the boat together and find a mutually beneficial way of fishing that will sustain us.

There it was: I was not there to teach anyone how to fish. I was there to be a collaborator, lifelong student, and teacher where appropriate. I was called to be a leader in achieving a shared vision with similarly invested leaders and an advocate in coordination with like-minded advocates.

In my work as an intensive care unit clinical educator at the Rwanda Military Hospital, and later as faculty in the country's inaugural master of science in nursing program at the University of Rwanda, Kigali, I have been fortunate to contribute a small part to the honorable goals of the HRH Program. There have been countless lessons learned from my participation in global health delivery and a recalibration of what it means to be a global nurse. Some of my most influential shifts in perception include:

- An understanding that we live and work in a complex and globalized society. The HRH Program has granted me the privilege of collaborating not only with Rwandan colleagues but also with nurse leaders from India, South Africa, Kenya, Nigeria, Botswana, Uganda, the Democratic Republic of Congo, the United States, Canada, and across Europe. We must expand our concept of "nursing" to incorporate global implications and maximize health outcomes across countries and cultures. In fact, our responsibilities as nurses in this continually emerging and multidimensional transnational society supersede more narrowly focused and traditional definitions, and are growing to include those of teacher, leader, role model, and mentor (Murray, Wenger, Downes, & Terrazas, 2011).

- The maturing realization that, as human beings, despite the broad variances in race, ethnicity, and culture, "we are so much stronger together than apart and . . . so much more alike than different" (Mukamana, Niyomugabo, & Rosa, 2016, p. 4). We are, indeed, deeply interconnected, and our choices of action and inaction reverberate with myriad consequences throughout the world. How we live our lives—the translation of our individual ethos into daily practice— positively or negatively impacts the quality of life for people we may never meet or know worldwide. Adopting a holistic ethic of shared humanity and promoting a universal experience of dignity for all are foundational precepts of the art and science that constitute nursing (Dossey & Keegan, 2016; Watson, 2008, 2012). In accepting the widespread impact of our presence on the world, we come to understand our power as health care advocates and change agents, and the profession's obligation to improve health and well-being for all clients, communities, and nations.

- A reinterpretation of both "health" and "health care," not only as human rights, but also as contextually variant experiences for every human being on the planet. "Health" goes beyond physical, emotional, mental, and spiritual well-being, and carries with it a unique and personally derived meaning for every individual, informed by values, norms, and traditions but also dependent upon sociopolitical and economic welfare, as well as environmental influences (Kreitzer & Koithan, 2014). This definition of health as both integrative and inclusive supports a whole-person/whole-people approach to addressing the challenges of the global village. "Health care" is determined by a host of broad-spectrum factors at the local, national, and international levels. It is not simply about the delivery of high-caliber services or the implementation of evidence-based, validated protocols; it must be provided in a way that is meaningful and relevant for the recipient. In short, it must be given in a manner in which it can be received. This involves a steadfast allegiance to human-centered, as opposed to provider- or system-centered, care, and individualized treatment plans for clients and communities, despite time and resource constraints.

Without a doubt, the experience of living and working in Rwanda has informed me as to my role in advancing global health from a nursing perspective. Out of this work and the many lessons learned, I have become passionate about how nurses can better understand and pursue their commitment to healing, health, and well-being on a transnational scale. It requires a change in consciousness regarding how we see and understand nursing and a broadening of our scopes of practice to be inclusive of cross-cultural contexts and more universal, interconnected considerations.

ONE PLANET—ONE HEALTH

The One Health movement "recognizes that the health of humans, animals and ecosystems are interconnected. It involves applying a coordinated, collaborative, multidisciplinary and cross-sectoral approach to address potential or existing risks that originate at the animal-human-ecosystems interface" (One Health Global Network, 2012–2015). The UN 2030 Sustainable Development Agenda, through the 17 Sustainable Development Goals (SDGs) and 169 associated targets, calls for a worldwide adoption of One Health approaches in order to meet their mission to eradicate poverty and build a peaceful, safe, and inclusive global village (see Appendix in this text for the complete 2030 Agenda). Engaging the materials provided throughout this book through a lens of One Health will aid you in understanding the broader implications of the 2030 Agenda, as well as the more global possibilities for nurses and nursing to contribute to each of the 17 SDGs.

Key Paradigm Shifts (found in Box 1.1) were identified by Lueddeke (2016) in relation to the SDGs as helpful guideposts in moving these "good intentions" toward "concrete and measurable enabling actions at global and national levels" (p. 336). These Paradigm Shifts call us to embrace the international overarching mission of the 2030 Agenda while respecting and honoring individual nations' development plans, socioeconomic and political histories, and circumstances. They require us to find the meeting ground between thinking and acting locally and thinking and acting globally. Lueddeke's (2016) Paradigm Shifts include not only

Box 1.1	Key Paradigm Shifts: Fundamental Global Transformations in Mindset

- Recognizing global imbalances, in particular the reality that most people—about 5 billion out of c. 7.3 billion in 2015—live in LMICs and that there is an urgent need for geopolitical momentum to end extreme poverty and strive toward global economic and social justice, within and across all nations, underpinned by the SDGs, targets, and indicators, perhaps following an incremental 5-year target and timescale to 2030.

- Placing much more emphasis on humanitarian agendas at the highest global decision-making levels and collectively adopting and implementing the principles and practices espoused in the UN Earth Charter and the SDGs: prioritizing ecological integrity, democracy, nonviolence, and peace (The Earth Charter Initiative, 2012–2016).

- Turning from government and corporate demands for short-term gain, too often encompassing ruthless exploitation of resources (human and physical) in poor nations, to managing economic growth by adopting humane principles that underpin the UN Earth Charter and recognizing that government and corporate activity must operate for a higher purpose to sustain the planet and its species.

- Reorienting thinking from health as a strictly "human" concern to One Health that links all living species—human, animals (wildlife and domestic), plant, and the environment.

- Weaving the One Health concept throughout early childhood, under-/postgraduate education, and lifelong learning, including leadership development, fostering interdisciplinary collaborations and communications in all aspects and addressing many difficult problems facing the world.

- Shifting from a patient disease-driven (or "sickness") culture, dominated by costly centralized hospital care, to a holistic "health and well-being" culture, focusing on individual responsibility for health supported by families, communities, and information technology support that places a greater emphasis on prevention (physical, emotional) over curative measures, including global and national budgetary re-balancing.

- Replacing the unidimensional view of public health, based largely on 20th century assumptions and linear or reductionist practices, with a much more positive and broader socioecological, multidimensional orientation that has the potential of impacting significantly on social, economic, and political decision-making.

LMICs, low- and middle-income countries; SDGs, Sustainable Development Goals; UN, United Nations.
Source: Adapted from Leudekke (2016).

attention to One Health but also to *The Earth Charter* (The Earth Charter Initiative, 2000), a document with an extensive history that can be more thoroughly explored at earthcharter.org/discover/history-of-the-earth-charter. The charter itself is a globally conscious ethical framework, serving as a call to action and an invitation to build a more sustainable world through a commitment to ecological integrity, the eradication of poverty and related threats to human rights, and the recognition of planetary interdependence (The Earth Charter Initiative, 2012–2016).

Bringing a Nursing Sensibility to Global Paradigm Shifts

In essence, this book is largely about providing the needed resources and education to assist global nursing in successfully and strategically making these paradigm shifts. As previously noted, interprofessional and broadly inclusive collaborative initiatives are required to address the many dimensions and complexities of the 2030 Agenda. A major goal of *A New Era in Global Health* is to identify opportunities for global nurses to be a part of the solution: to be at the decision-making tables in equal partnership with multidisciplinary experts to most efficiently identify and implement sustainable interventions. We must not sacrifice our nursing sensibilities or intraprofessional identity in order to participate, but rather actively employ these assets to lead and cocreate the necessary changes. Nursing brings a humanistic and scientifically rooted, evidence-based contribution to the forefront of the discussions regarding the 2030 Agenda. We must not await invitation to participate in such initiatives, but actively and deliberately share our expertise—the art and science of nursing—in whatever forums we create for ourselves and in collaboration with invested partners, including but not limited to publication, advocacy, policy advancement, educational restructuring, the creation of new knowledge through research capacity building, and a global commitment to ethical, respectful, and unified professionalism. Table 1.1 provides

Table 1.1 Global Considerations Related to the Provisions of the American Nurses Association's (ANA's) *Code of Ethics for Nurses* (2015)

Provisions of the *Code of Ethics* (as identified by the ANA [2015]) As global nurses, we recognize the following provisions as an ethical starting point for our work:	Global Considerations Related to the Provisions of the ANA's *Code of Ethics* (2015) As global nurses, we:
Provision 1. *The nurse practices with compassion and respect for the inherent dignity, worth, and unique attributes of every person.*	• Re-member all people everywhere by listening to their stories and including them in the conversations and decisions that matter to them. • Honor the contextual and unique characteristics of those we serve. • Acknowledge the inherent worth of all species and ecosystems with respect for the interdependence of a globalized world.
Provision 2. *The nurse's primary commitment is to the patient, whether an individual, family, group, community, or population.*	• Redefine "patient" to include the planet, its natural resources, and all animal species. • Refine and recommit to our work as vanguards of planetary health on an ongoing basis. • Adjust personal practices and implement systems improvements that do not serve our "patient's" greater good.

(continued)

Table 1.1 Global Considerations Related to the Provisions of the American Nurses Association's (ANA's) *Code of Ethics for Nurses* (2015) (*continued*)

Provisions of the *Code of Ethics* (as identified by the ANA [2015]) As global nurses, we recognize the following provisions as an ethical starting point for our work:	Global Considerations Related to the Provisions of the ANA's *Code of Ethics* (2015) As global nurses, we:
Provision 3. *The nurse promotes, advocates for, and protects the rights, health, and safety of the patient.*	• Strive to defend the rights of animals and ecosystems unable to advocate. • Drive policy changes that procure global safety and preservation of nature's resources. • Protect the best interest of the "patient" through scholarly contributions, environmental activism, and interprofessional best practice and ongoing education.
Provision 4. *The nurse has authority, accountability, and responsibility for nursing practice; makes decisions; and takes action consistent with the obligation to promote health and to provide optimal care.*	• Bring a nursing sensibility to global decision-making tables. • Identify actions and methods that are not consistent with the promotion of health and optimal well-being for the "patient." • Foster interprofessional alliances that create an accountable and responsible global health sector.
Provision 5. *The nurse owes the same duties to self as to others, including the responsibility to promote health and safety, preserve wholeness of character and integrity, maintain competence, and continue personal and professional growth.*	• Engage in regular self-care practices, understanding that the quality of care for self is the basis for how we deliver care for others and the planet. • Take deliberate steps to restore integrity where it is lost at personal and global levels. • Choose to live a life of immersion that promotes universal inclusion of the human/planetary narrative and takes accountability for reclaiming it.
Provision 6. *The nurse, through individual and collective effort, establishes, maintains, and improves the ethical environment of the work setting and conditions of employment that are conducive to safe, quality health care.*	• Infuse all work settings with an ethical commitment to the preservation of dignity for all (including self and planet). • Improve mechanisms to promote safety and ensure that all health care is of the highest quality possible given the context and resources available. • Hold authorities responsible for implementing policies that are unethical through a commitment to social and environmental justice.
Provision 7. *The nurse, in all roles and settings, advances the profession through research and scholarly inquiry, professional standards development, and the generation of both nursing and health policy.*	• Maintain professional standards that expand the global scope of practice for nurses and create an environment for planetary health to flourish. • Identify planetary health determinants and collaborate with key stakeholders to improve the likelihood of good health for all. • Translate health ethics into health policy by educating policy makers and the general public about planetary considerations for well-being.

(*continued*)

Table 1.1 Global Considerations Related to the Provisions of the American Nurses Association's (ANA's) *Code of Ethics for Nurses* (2015) (*continued*)

Provisions of the *Code of Ethics* (as identified by the ANA [2015]) As global nurses, we recognize the following provisions as an ethical starting point for our work:	Global Considerations Related to the Provisions of the ANA's *Code of Ethics* (2015) As global nurses, we:
Provision 8. *The nurse collaborates with other health professionals and the public to protect human rights, promote health diplomacy, and reduce health disparities.*	• Address inequities and disparities in health, education, economic opportunity, and politics. • Clarify nursing's unique contributions to public and global health agendas through the dissemination of scholarly advancements and culturally inclusive health promotion. • Invite experts outside of the nursing profession to contribute to initiatives for a One Health approach to solutions that are attainable for all.
Provision 9. *The profession of nursing, collectively through its professional organizations, must articulate nursing values, maintain integrity of the profession, and integrate principles of social justice into nursing and health policy.*	• Teach and practice social justice as a central component of global nursing, global health, and global well-being for all beings on the planet. • Support professional organizations that promote the positive and visionary image of global nurses as leaders in the journey toward global health equity. • Participate with ethically aligned interprofessional organizations in order to maximize our collective impact and mobilize global unity.

Source: ANA (2015).

global considerations identified by this author for each of the nine provisions identified by the American Nurses Association's (2015) *Code of Ethics for Nurses*. These considerations aid us, as global nurses, to remain true to our professional mandates and responsibilities while ushering in the Key Paradigm Shifts articulated by Lueddeke (2016), which are necessary for the world to know and experience the achievement of the 17 SDGs.

AS WE BEGIN, RE-MEMBER . . .

A New Era in Global Health is an opportunity to create emergent and evolutionary possibilities for nursing, health care, and planetary health, using the UN 2030 Agenda as a guiding framework. By re-membering humanity—re-membering the Thandos and Aleppos of the world—we return to ourselves and clarify our individual and collective purpose in this unifying work. We must be able to take the risk: to immerse ourselves in the implications of planetary interdependence while being a part of the paradigm shift necessary to realize improved planetary health. We must be bold enough to maintain our intraprofessional identity while making evidence-based contributions to the collaborative efforts underway related to the UN Sustainable Development Agenda. We must dispel the myths that limit us and support each other in the development of globally relevant literacies in leadership and advocacy. Ultimately, global nursing must be committed to a vision of planetary health, beyond the SDGs and the year 2030.

And that is what we will learn, together, throughout *A New Era in Global Health*.

REFLECTION AND DISCUSSION

- In what ways is nursing responsible for re-membering humanity?
- What parts of myself and my narrative need to be re-membered?
- What are my fears, concerns, joys, and anticipations related to living a life of immersion?
- Where am I on the journey of shifting my mindset toward a more globally conscious and relevant paradigm?
- In addition to the global considerations listed above based on the ANA's *Code of Ethics for Nurses*, what other aspects of nursing practice need to be expanded upon to meet the transnational targets of the SDGs?

REFERENCES

Acumen. (2016). Who we are. Retrieved from http://acumen.org/about

American Nurses Association. (2015). *Code of ethics with interpretive statements.* Silver Spring, MD: Nursesbooks.org.

Binagwaho, A., Kyamanywa, P., Farmer, P. E., Nuthulaganti, T., Umubyeyi, B., Nyemazi, J. P., . . . Goosby, E. (2013). Human resources for health program in Rwanda: A new partnership. *New England Journal of Medicine, 369*(21), 2054–2059.

Dossey, B. M., & Keegan, L. (Eds.). (2016). *Holistic nursing: A handbook for practice* (7th ed.). Burlington, MA: Jones & Bartlett.

The Earth Charter Initiative. (2000). The earth charter. Retrieved from http://earthcharter.org/invent/images/uploads/echarter_english.pdf

The Earth Charter Initiative. (2012–2016). What is the earth charter? Retrieved from http://earthcharter.org/discover/what-is-the-earth-charter

Gandhi, M. (n.d.). BrainyQuote. Retrieved from http://www.brainyquote.com/quotes/quotes/m/mahatmagan150724.html

The Heritage Portal. (2016). Looking back at the Roeland Street Prison. Retrieved from http://theheritageportal.co.za/article/looking-back-roeland-street-prison

Kreitzer, M. J., & Koithan, M. (Eds.). (2014). *Integrative nursing.* New York, NY: Oxford University Press.

Lueddeke, G. R. (2016). *Global population health and well-being in the 21st century: Toward new paradigms, policy, and practice.* New York, NY: Springer Publishing.

Mahajan, S. (2014). *Economics of South African townships: Special focus on Diepsloot.* A World Bank study. Washington, DC: World Bank Group.

Michigan State University. (n.d.). Forced removals. Retrieved from http://overcomingapartheid.msu.edu/multimedia.php?id=65-259-6

Mukamana, D., Niyomugabo, A., & Rosa, W. (2016, June). Global partnership advances medical-surgical nursing in Rwanda. *Med-Surg Nursing Connection.* Retrieved from https://amsn.org/sites/default/files/documents/articles-events/amsn/msnc0616.pdf

Murray, J. P., Wenger, A. F. Z., Downes, E. A., & Terrazas, S. B. (2011). *Educating health professionals in low-resource countries: A global approach.* New York, NY: Springer Publishing.

National Planning Commission. (2011). Diagnostic overview. Retrieved from http://www.education.gov.za/Portals/0/Documents/Publications/National%20Planning%20Commission%20Diagnostics%20Overview%20of%20the%20country.pdf?ver=2015-03-19-134928-000

National Planning Commission. (2013). National development plan 2030. Our future—make it work. Executive summary. Retrieved from http://www.gov.za/sites/www.gov.za/files/Executive%20Summary-NDP%202030%20-%20Our%20future%20-%20make%20it%20work.pdf

Novogratz, J. (2010). Inspiring a life of immersion. Retrieved from https://www.ted.com/talks/jacqueline_novogratz_inspiring_a_life_of_immersion/transcript?language=en

One Health Global Network. (2012–2015). What is one health? Retrieved from http://www.onehealthglobal.net/what-is-one-health

Rodgers, L., Gritten, D., Offer, J., & Asare, P. (2016, March 11). Syria: The story of the conflict. Retrieved from http://www.bbc.com/news/world-middle-east-26116868

Rwandan Ministry of Health. (n.d.). Human resources for health program. Retrieved from http://www.hrhconsortium.moh.gov.rw

Rwandan Ministry of Health. (2016). Rwanda human resources for health program midterm review report (2012–2016). Internal Program Review Report.

Saad, H., & Cumming-Bruce, N. (2016, September 30). Over 100 children among 338 killed in Aleppo attacks this week, W.H.O. says. Retrieved from http://www.nytimes.com/2016/10/01/world/middleeast/aleppo-syria-civilians.html?_r=0

Sliney, A., & Uwimana, C. (2014). Rwanda Human Resources for Health Program. In M. J. Upvall & J. M. Leffers (Eds.), *Global health nursing: Building and sustaining partnerships* (pp. 208–218). New York, NY: Springer Publishing.

United Nations High Commissioner for Refugees. (2001–2016a). Figures at a glance. Retrieved from http://www.unhcr.org/en-us/figures-at-a-glance.html

United Nations High Commissioner for Refugees. (2001–2016b). Asylum seekers. Retrieved from http://www.unhcr.org/en-us/asylum-seekers.html

Watson, J. (2008). *Nursing: The philosophy and science of caring* (Rev. ed.). Boulder: University Press of Colorado.

Watson, J. (2012). *Human caring science: A theory of nursing* (2nd ed.). Sudbury, MA: Jones & Bartlett.

World Health Organization. (2016). WHO calls for immediate safe evacuation of the sick and wounded from conflict areas. Retrieved from http://www.who.int/mediacentre/news/releases/2016/health-workers-attacks/en

Global Nursing in an Interconnected World

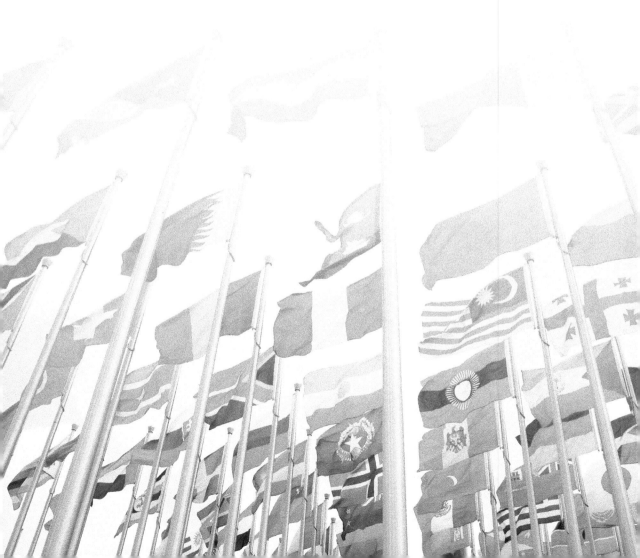

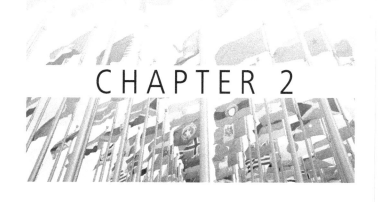

CHAPTER 2

Global Health and Global Nursing: Emerging Definitions and Directions

William Rosa

The nursing profession, that so-called "sleeping giant," is actually wide awake and ready to race ahead in clearly defined strategic directions. You are waiting for the starting gun. Even more so, you are waiting for someone to let up the reins that hold you back, the constraints that keep you from performing with the full set of competencies for which you were educated, trained, and licensed. . . . Given the enormous complexity of health challenges faced as the world transitions to the post-2015 era, no one . . . dares to ignore the full contribution that the nursing profession can make . . . the starting gun has sounded. (Chan, 2015)

THE SUSTAINABLE DEVELOPMENT GOALS: A NEW ERA

The heart of the United Nations (UN) 2030 Sustainable Development Agenda are the 17 Sustainable Development Goals (SDGs), along with their 169 targets, which went into effect on January 1, 2016. These targets articulate the depth of each goal, provide an outline for how the efforts of all people and governments around the world should be focused, and identify the indicators that should be consistently evaluated to demonstrate progress and alignment with the agenda. While the complete 2030 Agenda can be found in the Appendix of this text, Box 2.1 lists the 17 SDGs: the Global Goals that have given rise to a new era in global health, and to emerging considerations for global nursing and interprofessional health partners worldwide.

The SDGs are discussed in great detail throughout this book. They build on the achievements of the UN's Millennium Development Goals (MDGs), which addressed similar needs from 2000 to 2015 (see Chapters 3 and 4 for more information and history regarding the MDGs). Box 2.2 lists the eight MDGs.

The SDGs provide an integral and whole-person/whole-people plan to address all systems that threaten the welfare of human beings and their rights to health

| Box 2.1 | **Sustainable Development Goals** |

Goal 1. End poverty in all its forms everywhere.

Goal 2. End hunger, achieve food security and improved nutrition, and promote sustainable agriculture.

Goal 3. Ensure healthy lives and promote well-being for all at all ages.

Goal 4. Ensure inclusive and equitable quality education and promote lifelong learning opportunities for all.

Goal 5. Achieve gender equality and empower all women and girls.

Goal 6. Ensure availability and sustainable management of water and sanitation for all.

Goal 7. Ensure access to affordable, reliable, sustainable, and modern energy for all.

Goal 8. Promote sustained, inclusive, and sustainable economic growth, full and productive employment, and decent work for all.

Goal 9. Build resilient infrastructure, promote inclusive and sustainable industrialization, and foster innovation.

Goal 10. Reduce inequality within and among countries.

Goal 11. Make cities and human settlements inclusive, safe, resilient, and sustainable.

Goal 12. Ensure sustainable consumption and production patterns.

Goal 13. Take urgent action to combat climate change and its impacts.*

Goal 14. Conserve and sustainably use the oceans, seas, and marine resources for sustainable development.

Goal 15. Protect, restore, and promote sustainable use of terrestrial ecosystems, sustainably manage forests, combat desertification, and halt and reverse land degradation and halt biodiversity loss.

Goal 16. Promote peaceful and inclusive societies for sustainable development, provide access to justice for all and build effective, accountable, and inclusive institutions at all levels.

Goal 17. Strengthen the means of implementation and revitalize the Global Partnership for Sustainable Development.

*Acknowledging that the United Nations Framework Convention on Climate Change is the primary international, intergovernmental forum for negotiating the global response to climate change.

Source: Reprinted with permission from the United Nations (2015).

Box 2.2	**United Nations Millennium Development Goals**

Goal 1. Eradicate extreme hunger and poverty

Goal 2. Achieve universal primary education

Goal 3. Promote gender equality and empower women

Goal 4. Reduce child mortality

Goal 5. Improve maternal health

Goal 6. Combat HIV/AIDS, malaria, and other diseases

Goal 7. Ensure environmental sustainability

Goal 8. Develop a global partnership for development

Source: UN Millennium Project (2006).

and well-being (see Chapter 7 for more on the rationale for integral worldview in achieving the SDGs). They create new mechanisms for partnerships that will strengthen global solidarity and guide all countries to see their individual possibilities for prosperity in the context of a globalized and unified world. A global village of safety and inclusivity will not simply appear "someday"; it will be the result of cross-cultural collaboration such as the world has never known, requiring a new paradigm in which to bring nursing to the forefront of issues that extend beyond the traditional practice scope of the bedside or the classroom. It calls us to be *global* in our thinking and *planetary* in our doing.

The SDGs and the transnational efforts being rallied to ensure their achievement remind humanity that we are, indeed, interconnected and reliant on each other not only for today, but also for tomorrow. In other words, we need each other if we, and our children and the many generations to come, are to survive. This knowledge carries with it the great responsibility to maximize nursing's contributions beyond outdated and paternalistic systems to ensure the global betterment of humanity.

Establishing a Context for Global Nursing

The American Nurses Association (ANA, 2016) defines "nursing" as

> the protection, promotion, and optimization of health and abilities, prevention of illness and injury, facilitation of healing, alleviation of suffering through the diagnosis and treatment of human response, and advocacy in the care of individuals, families, groups, communities, and populations.

This explanation regarding the work of nurses and nursing identifies us as essential components in realizing the far-reaching and broad goals of global health initiatives. Global nursing requires us to take locally relevant concepts in our work and apply them in contextually relevant ways for partnering countries, the environment, and the planet as a whole.

Nursing, a profession that was referred to as a "must" by Nightingale (Dossey, 2010), is founded on three basic tenets: healing, leadership, and global action (Dossey, Selanders, Beck, & Attewell, 2005). Each of these concepts should be explored both personally and professionally in order to bring about the transformation envisioned by the SDGs. How do you integrate a healing perspective and intentionality into your work? What are the leadership skills and literacies you possess and can utilize right now? What are your opportunities for taking global action to raise awareness in your current position, with what you have right now, today?

The following is a list of recommendations (Beck, 2010; Beck, Dossey, & Rushton, 2014) that you can use not only to begin advancing your thinking toward a global paradigm, but also to start practicing nursing in a more globally inclusive and transculturally considerate manner:

- Prioritize health and the activation of positive health determinants in all human affairs and personal–professional efforts.
- Support the work of nurses and nurse caring so the collective may continue to achieve health goals worldwide.
- Invite interprofessional and cross-cultural collaboration to create contextually appropriate health care across communities.
- Think globally and promote health literacy at local levels for all people at all ages.
- Intelligently and responsibly utilize media to advance the global nursing and global health agenda.
- Promote the experience of health as holistic, integrative, and inclusive of all disciplines.
- Find your own calling; explore your own "must."

Beyond the steps we can take to represent a more global approach to nursing practice, we must establish a context for how we deliver nursing and promote its values to those we serve in order to sustain effectiveness in the global health arena long term. The profession should be selective regarding the definitions employed to describe practice, education, and research efforts, and deliberate about which strategies will be relied upon to guide future development and sustainability initiatives.

From Public Health to Global Health

The appropriate allocation of terms such as *public health*, *international health*, and *global health* has been an ongoing and vibrant discussion in the literature for some time (Farmer, Kim, Kleinman, & Basilico, 2013; Fried et al., 2010; Koplan et al., 2009). It may be helpful to consider these categories in terms of their geographical reach and focus. For example, *global health* is centered on health-related issues that extend beyond national borders; *international health* addresses health-related issues in a country other than one's own, and is particularly focused on low- and middle-income countries (LMICs); and *public health* tends to the population health issues of a specific country or community (Koplan et al., 2009). Koplan and colleagues (2009) further describe global health as a derivative of public and international health, which are outgrowths of hygiene and tropical medicine.

Global Health and *Global Nursing:* Emerging Definitions

In 2013, the Honor Society of Nursing, Sigma Theta Tau International (STTI) formed the Global Advisory Panel on the Future of Nursing (GAPFON) in order to create a future vision for nurses and midwives to effectively lead, contribute to, and advance global health (Klopper & Hill, 2015). Most recently, GAPFON conducted a literature review identifying the themes related to *global health* and *global nursing* in order to propose final definitions for both (Wilson et al., 2016).

Box 2.3 lists and describes the 13 themes identified by Wilson and colleagues (2016) related to the definition of *global health*. Based on the themes noted and the professional experiences of GAPFON members, the authors propose that global health:

> . . . refers to an area for practice, study, and research that places a priority on improving health, achieving equity in health for all people (Koplan et al., 2009), and ensuring health-promoting and sustainable sociocultural, political, and economic systems (Janes & Corbett, 2009). Global health implies planetary health, which equals human, animal, environmental, and ecosystem health (Kahn, Kaplan, Monath, Woodall, & Conti, 2014) and it emphasizes transnational health issues, determinants and solutions; involves many disciplines within and beyond the health sciences and promotes interdependence and interdisciplinary collaboration; and is a synthesis of population-based prevention with individual holistic care. (Koplan et al., 2009; Wilson et al., 2016, p. 1536)

In their literature review related to the definition of "global nursing," the GAPFON task force identified 11 themes listed and summarized in Box 2.4. Ultimately, Wilson and colleagues' (2016) proposed definition of "global nursing" is as follows:

> Global nursing is the use of evidence-based nursing process to promote sustainable planetary health and equity for all people (Grootjans & Newman, 2013). Global nursing considers social determinants of health, includes individual and population-level care, research, education, leadership, advocacy and policy initiatives (Upvall, Leffers, & Mitchell, 2014). Global nurses engage in ethical practice and demonstrate respect for human dignity, human rights and cultural diversity (Baumann, 2013). Global nurses engage in a spirit of deliberation and reflection in interdependent partnership with communities and other health care providers. (Upvall et al., 2014; Wilson et al., 2016, p. 1537)

In the end, global health and global nursing are all about communities—both local and global—striving to create a unified front for the sake of humanity. Wolf (2015) proposes that "global health action begins and ends in a community context . . . the collective expression of the health of individuals and groups . . ." (p. 86). The definitions proposed by the GAPFON task force assist nurses worldwide in locating their place and identifying their potential roles in global health and, more importantly, in regard to the UN 2030 Sustainable Development Agenda. Beyond these definitions are competencies that each global nurse can employ to effectively implement global health strategies and build innovative partnerships for the future of the global village.

Box 2.3   Themes Related to the Definition of "Global Health"

- *One health or planetary health:* a holistic approach to health that moves beyond the sole focus on human health to include priorities related to diverse species and the environment toward overall planetary well-being. It requires multidisciplinary efforts in research, practice, and education and cross-cultural collaboration in improving the quality of life for all.

- *Transnational:* the transcendence of national geopolitical borders in creating links between social determinants of health and corresponding solutions worldwide.

- *Collaboration:* refers to multidisciplinary partnerships both within and beyond health care in order to heighten awareness of the priorities beyond human health.

- *Equity:* the promotion of social justice and eradication of global health disparities for the benefit of all.

- *Health promotion, protection, and disease prevention:* a key component of global health that includes the delivery of adequate and quality medical care, but also takes into consideration sociocultural factors, demographics, global burden of diseases, technology, etc.

- *Population health and public health:* an expansive and globally relevant view of public health that recognizes a host of strategies for health improvement and advancement.

- *Determinants of health:* exploration of the social, political, and economic determinants of health problems.

- *International health:* a movement beyond just a focus on low- and middle-income countries to include discussions regarding interdependence and transnational solutions.

- *Global health improvement/health for all:* concern for the entire global village in promoting health and eradicating health inequities.

- *Interdependence:* a focus on the interconnectedness between nations and sectors: consideration of all stakeholders and their common vulnerabilities in addressing global health challenges.

- *Complex and comprehensive:* address the dynamic and varied components of global health, including but not limited to an adequate health workforce, appropriate financial infrastructures, policy frameworks, and social scales.

- *Individual-level health care:* addresses the need for both individual and population-based interventions and initiatives.

- *Glocal:* the interdependence of global and local health: strengthening individual populations to converge on a global scale, ultimately improving global health for all.

Source: Identified by Wilson et al. (2016).

| Box 2.4 | Themes Related to the Definition of "Global Nursing" |

- *Interdependence:* the ability for nurses to contextualize care and gain a comprehensive understanding of diverse and complex societies.

- *Collaboration:* refers to nursing's role in collaborating across disciplines and specialties, both within and beyond health care, to address more far-reaching global concerns to the populations being served.

- *Glocal:* challenges nurses to think and act locally and globally and to become avid contributors to the global agendas of the United Nations

- *Advocacy:* the goal of ensuring quality health for all, at both local and global levels through attention to education and the demonstration of respect for all clients and their needs.

- *Caring:* identifies caring as foundational to the nursing profession and in alignment with the legacy of Florence Nightingale.

- *Cultural competence:* a core competency in professional nursing in ensuring that care delivered is individualized, culturally sensitive, and inclusive of social determinants of health.

- *Respect for diversity:* an honoring of diversity and shared humanity through meaningful inclusion.

- *Partnerships:* presents nurses as equal partners in global health initiatives with colleagues across disciplines.

- *Equity:* brings a focus to the ethical responsibilities of nursing to create equitable and socially just environments for all people.

- *Holistic:* an inclusion of myriad perspectives in developing client-sensitive care, including but not limited to cultural, social, psychological, economic, and spiritual concerns that honor the whole person.

- *Sustainable:* refers to not only sustainability of the planet and ecosystems but also to the future directions of the nursing profession itself.

Source: Identified by Wilson et al. (2016).

Global Health Competencies: The Backbone of Implementation

But how to enact these concepts? How to put these broad-spectrum, evidence-based definitions into practice? Several global health competencies have been identified for nursing and their interdisciplinary partners (Warren, Breman, Budhathoki, Farley, & Wilson, 2016; Wilson et al., 2014). A list of global health competencies with their definitions, compiled by Clark, Raffray, Hendricks, and Gagnon (2016), appears in Table 2.1. These competencies are resultant of a systematic review that analyzed 15 articles related to global health and subsequently grouped the competencies into 12 diversely encompassing categories. By beginning to inform and educate self and others about the responsibilities regarding these competencies,

Table 2.1 Global Health (GH) Competencies With Descriptions

Global burden of disease	Understand the major causes of morbidity/mortality, epidemiology, relevant GH statistics, and major disease conditions/health problems.
Travel and migration	Recognize the effects of travel and migration on health status.
Determinants of health	Identify the social, economic, political, environmental factors that affect health status, including historical context and north–south dynamics.
Environmental factors	Include access to clean water, sanitation, population factors, environmental resources; as well as cost of global environmental change, urban overcrowding, and pollution as factors that affect health.
Cultural competency	Operate with sensitivity and respect in a diverse world and respect the history, context, values, and culture of communities.
Communication	Have comprehensive knowledge of languages, writing skills and the ability to communicate effectively across cultures and possession of consultation/advisory skills.
Health systems/delivery	Pay attention to low resource settings, and the effects of globalization and health policy on the delivery of health care and the evolution of health care systems.
Professionalism/ethics	Work ethically and responsibly in any environment. Recognize own biases, limitations, and abilities. Emphasize honesty, accountability, and cost consciousness.
Social justice/human rights	Base knowledge in the belief in a human right to health care. Acknowledge disparities in availability, accessibility, affordability, and quality of health care globally. Acknowledge the effect of legal systems on the just distribution of resources.
Partnership/collaboration	Foster empowerment and the creation of sustainable programs/partnerships. Encourage multidirectional sharing and exchange of experiences, with objectives aligned among partners, and an emphasis on teamwork and solidarity.
Management skills	Emphasize policy planning as well as program design, implementation, evaluation, management, problem solving, and critical thinking skills.
Key players	Know the key players in global health governance; the effects of nongovernmental organizations on health and health care; and the effects of multiagency policy making.

Source: Reprinted from Clark et al. (2016) with permission.

global nursing practice can begin to mold itself to meet the health requisites of the SDGs' targets and anticipate the related health care needs of global populations at large.

The competencies addressed in Table 2.1 will be recurrent themes throughout this text and all initiatives that seek to further the Post-2015 Agenda (see Chapter 32 for more information on integrating global health competencies into a global health practice).

Throughout this book, you are encouraged to recontextualize your practice and worldviews to the global scenario. As you move through the following sections and identify how you can become a vital component of global nursing, and more specifically to the realization of the SDGs, I invite you to consider:

- In what ways does my current role relate to global health? If it does not, in what ways can I expand the definition of my role to incorporate a sense of community and global health considerations?

- How does global nursing determine and influence the quality of global health delivery? How does global health delivery determine and influence the quality of global nursing?

- By the nature of my profession, how do I see myself as an integral contributor to the SDG journey?

- Right now, with the knowledge and resources within reach, how can I more strategically promote the tenets of global health and global nursing as defined by GAPFON?

- Where and why am I resistant to transforming my nursing practice into one of global significance? What support do I need to make the paradigm shift?

A UNIFIED FRONT FOR NURSING: EMERGING DIRECTIONS

Since 2000, the World Health Organization (WHO) has been creating and continually revising its global plan to strengthen and empower nursing and midwifery in meeting the health needs of people and nations worldwide. The WHO's (2016a) recent document, *Global Strategic Directions for Strengthening Nursing and Midwifery 2016–2020*, builds on the 2002 and 2011 strategic directions reports (WHO, 2002, 2011), as well as countless other worldwide initiatives by the WHO to improve human resources for health (WHO, 2016b), transform health professionals' education and training (WHO, 2013a), ensure and monitor universal health coverage (UHC; WHO, 2013b, 2015a), and provide quality care delivery to improve the health and well-being of populations (WHO, 2013c, 2014, 2015b, 2015c).

The 2016 to 2020 *Global Strategic Directions* urge the profession of nursing to implement systems and frameworks that will help all countries achieve UHC and the SDGs by 2030 (WHO, 2016a). This document helps nurses to operationalize the definitions and themes of global health and global nursing identified by the GAPFON task force. Following, by permission of the WHO, you can find the Background, Overview, and Thematic Areas identified by the WHO's (2016a) report. For further implementation strategies, as well as monitoring and evaluation criteria, you can access the full document online (www.who.int/hrh/nursing_midwifery/global-strategic-midwifery2016-2020.pdf?ua=1).

EXCERPTS FROM THE WHO'S (2016) *GLOBAL STRATEGIC DIRECTIONS* REPORT

Since the first *Strategic Directions for Strengthening Nursing and Midwifery Services 2002–2008*, there has been continued progress, as evidenced in the WHO nursing and midwifery progress reports, 2008–2012 and 2013–2015 (WHO, 2013d, 2015e), the WHO 2015 Executive Board report on health workforce and services (WHO, 2015f), and the Global Strategy on Human Resources for Health: Workforce 2030 (WHO, 2016b). However, more still needs to be done. The issues highlighted in this chapter are closely linked to those of the Global Strategy on Human Resources for

Health: Workforce 2030—being the overall framework for health workforce development—and they constitute the basis for the development of the thematic areas of the *Global Strategic Directions for Strengthening Nursing and Midwifery 2016–2020*.

The Availability, Accessibility, and Quality of the Nursing and Midwifery Workforce

There is a continued global shortage of human resources for health. The implementation of various global strategies, such as the Global Strategy for Women's, Children's and Adolescents' Health 2016–2030 and the Mental Health Action Plan 2013–2020, will also depend to a large extent on the health workforce capacities of the nursing and midwifery workforce. The social determinants of health, including laws, policies, human rights, gender equity, and governance mechanisms, can influence health risks and access to services. It is of utmost importance that the most marginalized and vulnerable populations have equitable access to quality care. The mere availability in numbers of the nursing and midwifery workforce is not sufficient. They must be equitably distributed, accessible by the population, and possess the required competencies and motivation to deliver quality care that is appropriate and acceptable to the sociocultural contexts and expectations of the served population.

The Vital Role of the Nursing and Midwifery Workforce in Building the Resilience of Communities to Respond to Diverse Health Conditions

Universal health coverage can help to ensure the availability of a sufficient, well-educated and motivated nursing and midwifery workforce to provide the required health services. The universal health coverage approach aims to promote strong, efficient, well-run health systems through the promotion of people-centered care, while applying a broad range of interventions related to health promotion, disease prevention, rehabilitation, and palliative care (WHO, 2012). This implies provision of a continuum of health interventions throughout the life course. Therefore, the agenda of universal health coverage places the nursing and midwifery workforce at the core of the health response. It is therefore critical to invest in all areas of nursing and midwifery workforce development.

Notable Achievements Have Been Made

Although progress has been made, political will and other resources are still needed to sustain and expand efforts. Two WHO progress reports on nursing and midwifery (2008–2012 and 2013–2015) highlight some major achievements in nursing and midwifery development. A summary is presented in Table 2.2.

In spite of these achievements there are major constraints, and more needs to be done at global, regional, and country levels in order to address policy levers that shape education, the health labor market, and the delivery of appropriate services.

The Nursing and Midwifery Workforce: Enablers for Health Service Delivery Priorities

There is demonstrable evidence substantiating the contribution of the nursing and midwifery workforce to health improvements, such as increased patient satisfaction, decrease in patient morbidity and mortality, stabilization of financial systems through decreased hospital readmissions, length of stay, and other hospital-related conditions, including hospital-acquired infections (Cho et al., 2014; Howard & Papa, 2012; Kendall-Gallagher, Aiken, Sloane, & Cimiotti 2011; Pintar, 2013), which consequently contributes to patient well-being and safety. The utilization of the nursing and midwifery workforce is cost-effective. Nurses and midwives usually act as first responders to complex humanitarian crises and disasters; protectors and advocates for the community; and communicators and coordinators within teams. They provide services in a broad range of settings and needs, including in underserved populations. Nurses' interventions and informed decision making in treatment of HIV, tuberculosis, and other chronic conditions have stimulated

Table 2.2 Achievements in Nursing and Midwifery Development

Area	Achievements
Primary health care and people-centered care	Primary health care models of care led by nurses and midwives such as (community/family) women-centered care and the midwifery model of care (Devane et al., 2010; Walsh & Devane, 2012) Meeting the needs of people with disabilities, chronic conditions and noncommunicable diseases, including the needs of those in need of palliative care Core competencies in primary health care being assessed Capacity building in areas of emergency and disaster responses, infection control, mental health, and substance abuse More involvement in community health services Nurse-led multidisciplinary and multiprofessional team growth
Workforce policy and practice	National strategic plans for nursing and midwifery Greater commitment to regulation, legislation, and accreditation Regulation, education, and practice standards More commitment to establishing reliable nursing and midwifery databases
Education	Adoption of competency-based training at preservice, continuous education, and faculty levels Progress toward advanced nursing and midwifery practice
Career development	Gradual improvement in developing upgraded bridging program Leadership, skill development, and presence in leadership positions
Workforce management	Agreements reached on needs to increase recruitment, retention, motivation, and participation supported by global initiatives on retention Implementing better technology and communication platforms for nursing and midwifery Workforce capacity building and dissemination of good and best practices
Partnerships	Move toward strengthening collaboration with donor partners and nongovernmental organizations to address challenges Much more synergy among WHO collaborating centers for nursing and midwifery development and other stakeholders, such as the International Council of Nurses and the International Council of Midwives Enhanced faculty development and fellowships being awarded through North–North and North–South partnership collaboration

WHO, World Health Organization.
Source: Adapted from WHO (2013d).

improved patient adherence to treatment and reduced waiting times and the number of missed appointments at health care clinics (Lloyd et al., 2013; Patel, Yotebieng, Behets, Driessche, Nana, & Van Rie, 2013; Purssell, 2014). Studies also show that midwifery, including family planning and interventions for maternal and newborn health, could avert a total of 83% of all maternal deaths, stillbirths, and neonatal deaths (Ten Hoope-Bender et al., 2014).

In addition, recent studies show that midwives can provide 87% of the needed essential care for women and newborns, when educated and regulated to international standards (Homer et al., 2014). It is also documented that educated, regulated, and supported midwives are the most cost-effective suppliers of midwifery services. However, limitations in the scope of practice for midwives, and gaps in inclusion of maternal health indicators in national data systems, have impeded efforts to scale up programs nationally (Smith, Currie, Cannon, Armbruster, & Perri, 2014). Substantial reductions in child deaths are possible, but only if intensified efforts to achieve intervention coverage are implemented successfully (Universal Health Coverage Post-2015: Putting People First, 2014).

Persistent Nursing and Midwifery Challenges Require Innovative and Transformative Strategies and Actions

There is continued need for quality nursing and midwifery education and competent practitioners. Responding to unhealthy lifestyle choices, risk factor reduction, and provision of a broad range of interventions in various practice conditions are critical in order to address natural and anthropogenic disasters and emerging and reemerging infections and diseases, including noncommunicable diseases. Governments and relevant stakeholders should ensure that the nursing and midwifery workforce is appropriately prepared and enabled to practice to their full scope. Nursing and midwifery education and practice are taking place in an era of progressive technological advancement, and its promotion is an important element for the future. Technology advances can support transformational outcomes of safe, integrated, high-quality, knowledge-driven, evidence-based care and educational approaches. Future approaches should embrace interprofessional education and collaborative practice, as was noted in resolution WHA64.7 (WHO, 2011) on strengthening nursing and midwifery, for which the integration of increased availability and growing capabilities of information and communication technologies was an imperative. In responding to nursing and midwifery workforce challenges, robust leadership, governance, and accountability are essential. Strategic planning based on collecting and monitoring data and indicators on country profiles can contribute to effective education, recruitment, deployment, retention (WHO, 2010), and management of the nursing and midwifery workforce. It is on this premise that the WHO *Global strategic directions for strengthening nursing and midwifery 2016–2020* are built.

OVERVIEW OF THE GLOBAL STRATEGIC DIRECTIONS FOR STRENGTHENING NURSING AND MIDWIFERY 2016–2020

The *Global Strategic Directions for Strengthening Nursing and Midwifery 2016–2020* provide a framework for WHO and various key stakeholders to develop, implement, and evaluate nursing and midwifery accomplishments to ensure available, accessible, acceptable, quality, and safe nursing and midwifery interventions at global, regional, and country levels. The global strategic directions enable all involved to demonstrate commitment, be accountable, and report progress on essential elements. Optimizing leadership, strengthening accountability and governance, and mobilizing political will for the nursing and midwifery workforce is key for their effective contribution to the SDGs and universal health coverage. The global strategic directions embrace strategic partnerships with key stakeholders at all levels as essential for their implementation.

The *Global Strategic Directions for Strengthening Nursing and Midwifery 2016–2020* present a vision, guiding principles, and four broad themes to guide growth of capabilities and maximize the contributions of the nursing and midwifery workforce to improve global health. The vision and the principles presented in this document reassert the Global Strategy on Human Resources for Health: Workforce 2030. Furthermore, the four themes reinforce the WHO Global Strategy on Human Resources for Health: Workforce 2030. Themes 1 and 2 are aligned to objectives 1 and 2 of the Global Strategy, while theme 3 is aligned to objective 3 of the Global Strategy, and theme 4 is aligned to objective 1. Figure 2.1 shows the conceptual framework for the *WHO Global strategic directions for strengthening nursing and midwifery 2016–2020*.

Vision

Vision: Accessible, available, acceptable, quality, and cost-effective nursing and midwifery care for all, based on population needs, in support of universal health coverage and the SDGs.

Figure 2.1 WHO *Global strategic directions for strengthening nursing and midwifery 2016–2020:* conceptual framework.

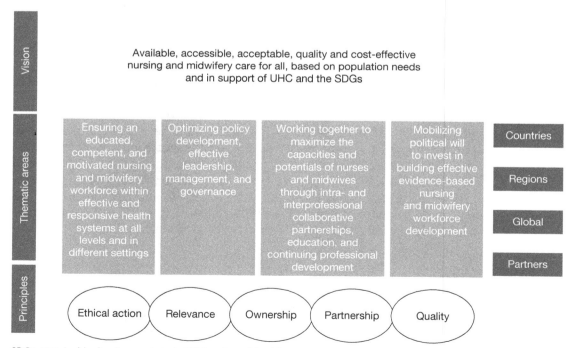

SDGs, sustainable development goals; UHC, universal health coverage; WHO, World Health Organization.

This vision is in line with the Global Strategy on Human Resources for Health: Workforce 2030, which seeks to accelerate progress toward universal health coverage and the UN SDGs by ensuring the universal accessibility, availability, acceptability, quality, and cost-effectiveness of nursing and midwifery care for all, based on population needs.

Thematic Areas

1. Ensuring an educated, competent, and motivated nursing and midwifery workforce within effective and responsive health systems at all levels and in different settings
2. Optimizing policy development, effective leadership, management, and governance
3. Working together to maximize the capacities and potentials of nurses and midwives through intra- and interprofessional collaborative partnerships, education, and continuing professional development
4. Mobilizing political will to invest in building effective evidence-based nursing and midwifery workforce development

Guiding Principles for Implementation

The guiding principles of the WHO *Global Strategic Directions for Strengthening Nursing and Midwifery 2016–2020* are in alignment with the previous versions and with the principles of the Global Strategy on Human Resources for Health: Workforce 2030. They are essential to guide individual and collaborative application of the 5-year WHO strategic directions for nursing and midwifery in different contexts. They are as follows:

- **Ethical action.** Planning, providing, and advocating safe, accountable high-quality health care services based on equity, integrity, fairness, and respectful practice, in the context of gender and human rights
- **Relevance.** Developing nursing and midwifery education programs, research, services, and systems guided by health needs, evidence, and strategic priorities
- **Ownership.** Adopting a flexible approach that ensures effective leadership, management, and capacity-building with active ownership, accountability mechanisms, engagement, and involvement of all beneficiaries in all aspects of the collaboration
- **Partnership.** Working respectfully together on common objectives, acting collaboratively with relevant stakeholders, and supporting each other's efforts
- **Quality.** Adopting mechanisms and standards based on evidence for best practice that promote relevant education and research, competent practice, effective professional regulation, and dynamic leadership

Target Audience

This document has been developed primarily to provide a framework for nursing and midwifery interventions within a WHO operational context. The main target audience includes WHO headquarters, regional and country offices, WHO collaborating centers for nursing and midwifery development, and key partners. However, it is envisaged that this framework can be used by any entity working on nursing and midwifery. In addition to existing global strategies and mandates, the development of this document has considered current regional strategic directions to ensure relevancy and consistency in approach. These WHO *Global Strategic Directions for Strengthening Nursing and Midwifery 2016–2020* are not exhaustive. Partners can implement activities on nursing and midwifery based on their mandates. The specific interventions indicated here are in support of the implementation of the WHO global strategic directions. It is envisaged that partnership collaboration will be cross-cutting.

THEMATIC AREAS OF THE GLOBAL STRATEGIC DIRECTIONS FOR STRENGTHENING NURSING AND MIDWIFERY 2016–2020

Theme 1. Ensuring an Educated, Competent, and Motivated Nursing and Midwifery Workforce Within Effective and Responsive Health Systems at All Levels and in Different Settings

In order to ensure that health services are accessible, acceptable, available, and of good quality, investing in the nursing and midwifery workforce is critical. The planning should involve not just increasing the quantity of providers but investment in improving their quality and relevance. This also entails ensuring enabling work environments, including through provision of adequate equipment and resources; decent working conditions; and fair compensation to help enhance recruitment and retention, as supported in the International Labour Organization (ILO) Nursing Personnel Convention, 1977 (No. 149), and the Nursing Personnel Recommendation, 1977 (No. 157); see ILO Nursing Personnel Convention (1977); ILO Nursing Personnel Recommendation (1977). Quality care also requires up-to-date, evidence-based education, regulation, and practice standards for nurses and midwives. Education includes continuing professional development to help maintain competence and advance practice.

Objective

To educate, recruit, deploy, and retain the right number of nursing and midwifery workforce with appropriate competencies, equipped with the necessary resources and governed by professional regulation.

Strategy

Align investments and coordinate plans for development of nursing and midwifery in workforce management; in pre- and in-service education; in regulation; and in guaranteeing positive practice environments.

Strategic Interventions
COUNTRIES

In alignment with national health priorities and workforce plans:

- Develop national costed plans for nursing and midwifery development with a minimum cycle of 4 to 5 years and an in-built monitoring and evaluation system.

- Integrate minimum data sets into national human resources for health observatories as a source of evidence-based decisions for the nursing and midwifery workforce.

- Develop and adopt, and support and monitor, quality management systems for nursing and midwifery services.

- Establish or strengthen and maintain national accreditation standards for nursing and midwifery education.

- Conduct a task analysis of the various cadres providing nursing and midwifery services to clarify their roles and scopes of practice.

- Review and implement competency-based curricula for educators, student nurses and student midwives, and preclinical teachers, taking into account quantity, quality, and relevance of the nursing and midwifery workforce to meet local and national changing health needs.

- Develop and implement a plan on improving working conditions to ensure positive practice environments.

REGIONS

- Consolidate evidence or update data on educational institutions, regulatory bodies, and regulatory information on licensing, registration, and scopes of practice to establish a baseline for the nursing and midwifery workforce.

- Support the establishment of a minimum data set for the nursing and midwifery workforce for regional human resources for health observatories, where applicable.

- Provide technical support to countries to develop key service indicators to assess nursing and midwifery care.

- Develop or disseminate competency-based prototype curricula for nursing and midwifery programs.

- Provide support to countries for the development and adoption of guidelines on establishing registration, licensure, education, and nursing and midwifery service delivery.

- Invest in the nursing and midwifery workforce, including through building capacity and ensuring appropriate skills and strategies for developing positive practice environments.

GLOBAL

- Develop a scope of practice framework for nursing and midwifery with the relevant skills mix to help achieve universal health coverage and the SDGs.

- Work with relevant WHO departments, teams, and partners to ensure that data are generated based on minimum data sets and are compiled and disseminated on actual supply, geographical distribution (numbers, skills mix, and competencies), and the population's demand for health services.

- Establish a template for assisting countries in developing and implementing national nursing and midwifery workforce plans through nursing and midwifery structures, for example, directorates and units.

- Develop composite indicators for measuring the overall development of nursing and midwifery in each country.
- Work with relevant WHO departments, teams, and partners to advocate the development of coordinated plans for investment in nursing and midwifery in line with the overall Global Strategy on Human Resources for Health: Workforce 2030.
- Disseminate the WHO nursing and midwifery educator competencies and promote their application at regional and country levels for preparing nursing and midwifery educators or to guide the development of new programs.

PARTNERS

Work in collaboration with educational and practice institutions, including regulatory bodies and nursing and midwifery associations, to:

- Implement, monitor, and evaluate the quality of education and training programs and practice in support of the WHO global strategic directions.
- Advocate and support the implementation of an enabling work environment.
- Coordinate investments to strengthen nursing and midwifery.
- Engage and support nursing and midwifery professional associations in planning and implementation of nursing and midwifery development.

Theme 2. Optimizing Policy Development, Effective Leadership, Management, and Governance

Health systems are dynamic and are undergoing rapid changes globally. In the midst of these changes, nursing and midwifery leaders act as positive change agents in creating effective and responsive health systems as they engage in policy formulation across the different sectors, including education, workforce management, data collection and management, and research. Consequently, leaders will be required to plan and manage health services and education and regulatory systems, and to establish sound governance structures.

Objective

To engage and have active participation of nursing and midwifery leaders at every level of policy formulation, program-planning development and implementation, including evidence generation for the purpose of informed decision making.

Strategy

Prepare nursing and midwifery leaders to meet the challenges of dynamic health systems by ensuring their competence in all aspects of nursing and midwifery development, including policy development, management, and evidence generation, in order to improve the quality of education and nursing and midwifery service delivery.

Strategic Interventions
COUNTRIES

In alignment with national health priorities and workforce plans:

- Advocate and set up mechanisms to raise the level of involvement of nurses and midwives in policy and decision making across the major sectors of service planning and management, education, and management of human resources.
- Engage professional associations of nurses and midwives in policy discussions and development.
- Obtain resources, and where necessary use regional support from WHO and competent national bodies, to update or establish programs for leadership preparation in all sectors of nursing and midwifery responsibility.
- Advocate effective systems of professional regulation, and strengthen and support the legislative authority to implement them.
- Establish and maintain robust systems for assessing the appropriate implementation of nationally agreed nursing and midwifery practice standards in health care delivery systems.
- Work to implement data collection and information systems to enable reliable reporting on the nursing and midwifery workforce status as relevant to local contexts, and to inform the national health workforce accounts.

REGIONS

- Promote and provide technical assistance to countries to support the establishment of a national nursing and midwifery department, headed by a nurse or midwife prepared in leadership and policy development roles.
- Review the relevance, adequacy, and effectiveness of professional regulatory systems and offer technical assistance to reform or introduce regulation where it does not exist.
- Invest in training to enhance policy formulation and set up a mentoring system to prepare and support nurses and midwives who are currently holding policy development responsibilities, or are seeking to enter this field across various areas of nursing and midwifery.
- Provide support and guidance to adapt, develop, and implement competency-based, action-oriented leadership preparation programs that deal with service planning and delivery, policy formulation, strategic planning, human resources management, materials and financial management, and communication and advocacy.

GLOBAL

- Sustain the WHO Global Forum for Government Chief Nursing and Midwifery Officers to enhance the leadership capacity of the nursing and midwifery workforce in countries.
- Engage governments through the WHO Global Forum on Government Chief Nursing and Midwifery Officers to share the evidence in support of nursing and midwifery workforce development.

- Review and analyze models of current governments' chief nursing and midwifery roles and promote context-sensitive approaches to introduce or strengthen these roles.
- Develop a competency framework for leadership roles in the various aspects of nursing and midwifery.
- Identify the best practices for good governance and develop a tool to enable countries to evaluate the status of their nursing and midwifery governance systems.

PARTNERS

- Seek participation from partners in monitoring and evaluating the implementation of the national nursing and midwifery development strategic plan.
- In collaboration with partners, promote and disseminate successes and lessons learned to all stakeholders, including politicians and key civil society groups, to strengthen perceptions of and raise commitment to supporting nursing and midwifery leadership development.

Theme 3. Working Together to Maximize the Capacities and Potentials of Nurses and Midwives Through Intra- and Interprofessional Collaborative Partnerships, Education, and Continuing Professional Development

The nursing and midwifery professions continue to evolve as their roles and responsibilities are influenced by local, national, regional, and global challenges. These challenges require nurses and midwives to enhance professional collaboration within and outside the health sector. Educational institutions along with regulatory and professional associations must also foster intra- and interprofessional learning in both their preservice and continuing professional development programs.

Objective

To optimize the nursing and midwifery impact on health systems at all levels through intra- and interprofessional collaboration and partnerships.

Strategy

Delineate, monitor, and evaluate roles, functions, and responsibilities of the nursing and midwifery workforce to advance collaborative education and practice.

Strategic Interventions
COUNTRIES

In alignment with national health priorities and workforce plans:
- Formulate, strengthen, and reinvigorate interdisciplinary and multisectoral technical working groups on interprofessional education and collaborative practice based on evidence.

- Strengthen collaborative practices at policy level to maximize effective nursing and midwifery input on health care.
- Develop or strengthen national nursing and midwifery strategies on interprofessional education and collaborative practice.
- Create interprofessional networks facilitated through web-based communities of practice to improve the quality of education, safety of practice, and capacities of the nursing and midwifery workforce.

REGIONS

- Develop tools and provide technical support to improve partnerships and work environments among health services, departments of health, professional associations, research and educational institutions, and communities.
- Develop a nursing and midwifery implementation research agenda responding to the needs of the region in collaboration with WHO collaborating centers, government nursing and midwifery leaders, nursing and midwifery associations, regulators, and nursing and midwifery educational institutions.

GLOBAL

- Identify key partners, including service users, through the development of a database of experts to support and build the capacity of the nursing and midwifery educational system and workforce to contribute to universal health coverage and the SDGs.
- Develop and disseminate an implementation toolkit for the WHO Framework for Action on Interprofessional Education and Collaborative Practice and other educational tools.
- Develop models for joint planning, implementation, monitoring, and evaluation of sustainable nursing and midwifery educational programs and services, including continuing professional development.
- Disseminate models of effective and sustainable partnerships at global, regional, and country levels.

PARTNERS

- Implement multiyear plans for strengthening the capacity of nursing and midwifery education and services developed for each region, coordinated by WHO with partner organizations taking the lead on specific objectives and activities identified in the plan.
- Create leadership opportunities and positions for interprofessional education and collaboration for nurses and midwives and mechanisms for involvement in leadership roles.

Theme 4. Mobilizing Political Will to Invest in Building Effective Evidence-Based Nursing and Midwifery Workforce Development

Building effective development of nursing and midwifery services and generating political commitment will require the involvement of governments, civil society, and other allied professions to ensure relevant education and research and evidence-based safe practice. Regulating health care professional practice and setting standards for education and practice can help to improve nursing and midwifery educational practice. As responsible and accountable stakeholders in the delivery of care, nurses and midwives must engage with the forces that drive health care and become more committed in policy making.

Objective

To establish structures that enable nurses and midwives to be empowered in order to achieve effective engagement and contribute to health policy development in order to increase nursing and midwifery workforce quantity and quality of service delivery.

Strategy

Build political support at the highest level of health systems and within civil society to ensure that the policies created to achieve universal health coverage and the SDGs encapsulate people-centered nursing and midwifery services.

Strategic Interventions

COUNTRIES

In alignment with national health priorities and workforce plans:

- Formulate and implement nursing and midwifery policies that ensure integrated people-centered services that are in line with universal health coverage and the SDGs.
- Establish a multisectoral group to support the development of nursing and midwifery policies.
- Develop and support nursing and midwifery interventions that lead to improved access to health care services through the creation of links among the public, nongovernmental, and private sectors to minimize barriers obstructing access to health services for vulnerable populations in urban, rural, and remote areas.
- Update nursing and midwifery curricula and ensure that nursing and midwifery students acquire effective leadership skills, including assertiveness, negotiation and advocacy, and ability to develop and influence health policy.
- Develop and implement national advocacy plans targeting policy makers and organizations.

REGIONS

- Engage ministries of health through regional committees to make commitments that support nursing and midwifery in their respective countries.
- Follow up on the commitments made by ministries of health in countries through periodic reviewing and reporting.

GLOBAL

- Disseminate existing global mandates and frameworks as reference materials for regional and country interventions for both health and nonhealth sectors.

- Develop frameworks for regional and country reporting on achievements in line with the global strategic directions.
- Support governments in strengthening the capacity of chief nursing and midwifery officers.
- Work with partners to develop advocacy and communication strategies and tools, for example, media packs.
- Collaborate with relevant partners to compile existing evidence in workforce development, with emphasis on evidence specific to nurses and midwives.

PARTNERS

- In support of the global strategic directions and with a view toward strengthening nursing and midwifery education and services, mobilize financial, human, and material resources and increase awareness and advocacy on priority issues.
- Collaborate with WHO to assist governments in the implementation of global mandates and the resolutions of WHO regional committees.

Source: Reprinted with permission from the WHO (2016a).

A SHIFT IN CONSCIOUSNESS AS STARTING POINT

Global nursing is not something that is happening "out there"; it is a "right here" conversation that demands "right now" conversations and "real time" solutions. This dialogue is the sounding gun referred to by Chan (2015) at the start of this chapter. The prior discussions on the SDGs and global health competencies, as well as the emerging definitions of global health and global nursing and the *Global Strategic Directions* for nursing and midwifery, provide countless reflection opportunities for every nurse to expand how they perceive their role as change agents and leaders in the transnational context. It is not only for nurses working in LMICs, but for every nurse making contributions to practice, research, and educational arenas to consider the cross-cultural, broad-spectrum implications of their daily work. It is a reminder for those seasoned global health professionals to be resolute in their determination to maximize the contributions of nurses in promoting positive advances for the profession and delivery of health care, and in advocating for human dignity. And it is also a spotlight on how nurses are redefining themselves and becoming global advocates for human betterment, beyond the bedside and the boardroom, on a transnational platform, through their ongoing collaboration with international affiliates committed to achieving the SDGs.

Colleague and member of the UN NGO/DPI Executive Committee (2014–2016), Holly K. Shaw, PhD, RN, shares,

> For me, the most important issue is that global nursing is not about mission trips or international travel. Global nursing involves every nurse everywhere: at home and abroad, in our own indigenous villages in

Uganda, Cambodia, New York, and Indiana. It is a (new) lens through which we view ourselves, our communities, our patients, our colleagues, and our students. (H. K. Shaw, personal communication, September 1, 2016; see Chapter 4 for more on Shaw's perspectives on global nurse citizenship)

This work requires clarity of vision and purpose and a humble acceptance that, at the end of the day, we are truly in this together. Beyond the surface differences that sometimes appear prominent, we share one world and one chance to get it right.

In 2007, Dr. Monica Sharma published an article for *Kosmos Journal* entitled, "Personal to Planetary Transformation," which is reprinted in full here. In it, she details the shift in consciousness required at both personal and planetary levels so that global initiatives seeking to build peaceful, just, safe, and inclusive societies, such as the 2030 Sustainable Development Agenda, can be achieved with integrity and compassion for all human beings everywhere. Sharma's (2007) platform interweaves seamlessly with the SDGs and their associated targets in a way that promotes human dignity and honors our global interdependence. The SDGs outline *who* needs to be accountable and *what* needs to be accomplished to improve quality of life for all; Sharma shows us *how* we can get there through a shift in consciousness and *why* it matters. Sourcing from Sharma's (2007) wisdom, one understands that it is not only possible to create a world that works for everyone but, in fact, it becomes an ethical obligation as global nurses to strive toward such a vision.

PERSONAL TO PLANETARY TRANSFORMATION

Our World

We are living in a time of whole system transition on a personal and planetary scale that affects every aspect of life as we know it. Patterns of possibility are emerging that have never before been available to all the earth's people and to the whole planet. Two million organizations are working toward ecological sustainability and social justice, according to Paul Hawken. Millions of individuals are self-organizing to make a better world in spite of the negative factors that threaten to destroy us. Technological innovations and collective wisdom have created unprecedented opportunities for change. The revolution in communication technologies and the Internet have made it possible to connect all people in the world for the first time in human history. The new science of consciousness is revolutionizing our attitudes and worldviews, and the interdependence of all life is now an established scientific fact.

Yet, in 2007 three billion people barely manage to eke out an existence. Poverty, malnutrition, lack of employment, and inadequate shelter, combined with an ever-widening gap between the rich and the poor, have resulted in human suffering and violence on a massive scale.

Almost a billion people live on less than a dollar a day. Each day is a life-and-death struggle for those faced with chronic hunger, illness, and environmental hazards in a world that has enough food to feed everyone, the money to tackle disease, and the power to make decisions to create a hazard-free environment. Over 40 countries are scarred by violent conflict. Three million people die of AIDS every year, and 40 million live with the virus. Some 115 million children of primary school age are denied schooling. At least 180 million children are engaged in the worst forms of child labor; there are some 300,000 child soldiers; 1.2 million children are trafficked every year—that is more than 3,000 a day; and 2 million children, mostly girls, are exploited in the sex industry.

We have the technology and the resources: so what is missing? Too few see how limited our current responses are for the enormity and complexity of global problems that ultimately affect human well-being. In explaining the causes of our global crises, we generally focus on economic, social, and political forces. Governments, corporations, the UN, civil society, and other institutions focus on financial and monetary parameters, technological (e.g., medical, educational, informational), political, administrative, military, diplomatic, legal, and economic resources, measures, and approaches. These approaches are necessary, but partial. Not until we see the global problematique as symptoms of a more fundamental, deeper rooted crisis can we begin to mount a more integral and profound response that is likely to move us forward in a more sustainable way. That crisis is in our individual and shared mind-sets, where psychological and cultural factors and forces reign. That crisis challenges all of us, in the Northern countries and in the Southern countries alike!

New Paradigm Design Sourced in Wisdom

> The world we have made as a result of the level of thinking we have done thus far creates problems that we cannot solve at the same level at which we have created them. . . . We shall require a substantially new manner of thinking if humankind is to survive. (Albert Einstein)

Evidence indicates that sourcing action from wisdom works. Wisdom is sourcing action from the deepest place within ourselves and generating appropriate action for meeting challenges. For example, extraordinary results were generated by the Leadership for Results Programme on HIV/AIDS of the United Nations Development Programme (UNDP). It reached 130 million people; over five thousand breakthroughs in 40 countries were reported. The corporate world offers examples of innovations sourced from transformational leadership that have successfully addressed the triple bottom line—profit, people, and planet. There are a few examples in civil society organizations, such as the Ashoka Foundation, where personal transformation manifests in significant transformation, and where interior deeper rooted forces are addressed along with systems and technological approaches. However, most of our responses are aimed at solving specific problems rather than whole systems.

We are not yet able to identify, distinguish, design, and generate responses that integrate the different domains related to the entangled hierarchies of any given situation. Three major impediments stand in the way. First, most of us do not even recognize the new generative patterns of response and therefore do not act upon them or support them. Second, our spirituality has been a personal matter that is often equated with religious practice. Most of us do not know how to provide the opportunity for "secular, sacred, strategic action." Third, the large-scale successes of leaders at the top have been based on narrowly focused interventions such as smallpox eradication or wealth creation. This was appropriate. But they have little experience in innovations that foster the expression of individual and collective wisdom in action. Considering the urgency of today's crises, interdependence and global complexity, we have no option but to learn to do things differently.

Figure 2.2 illustrates personal transformation manifesting in planetary transformation, where individual leadership uses appropriate technology and addresses systems transformation. This approach overcomes fragmentation and leads to synthesis. It includes the recognition that (a) the source of all strategies and action is wisdom—personal awareness and transformation; (b) global complex systems generate tangible consequences for people and our planet that must be addressed; (c) the use of technologies must be placed in the context of large-scale systems; and (d) the transformational approach must be sourced from wisdom for sustainable change. A few thoughtful people from governments, business, and civil society are now designing programs that incorporate these principles. They are asking piercing questions:

> Why are so many people poor and hungry when we have the technology and resources to prevent this? There are so many "good" people with "good" intentions, yet we don't seem to make a dent in the world's problems. Why?

These questions became so urgent for me that I began to reach out to others for effective responses. For 15 years, I held hundreds of conversations on every continent with people who formulate policy, design programs, and generate breakthroughs. I designed and implemented two successful large-scale programs: (a) UNDP's ongoing Leadership for Results Programme with several organizations in 40 countries; and (b) United Nations Children's Fund's (UNICEF) earlier maternal mortality reduction program in six countries in South Asia. What have I learned? We have been trying to solve complex societal problems at a surface level while neglecting the deeper dimensions of the problematique; and it is possible to design and implement programs differently.

Then I began to design a program based on the emergence of a new paradigm: the UN's current Leadership and Capacity Development Initiative for 60 countries. The basic assumption of the design is founded on the new sciences of psychology, neuroscience, and cosmology as well as successful applications in organizational development. New evidence in the science of consciousness is revealing our potential for deeper and higher states of consciousness that reveal our essential Oneness in an interdependent universe. Our "Oneness" can be the springboard for all action for humanity and the planet. Given the scientific, technological, and social tools at hand, in concert with the dramatic revolution in consciousness research and its applications, we have an opportunity never before available in human history to manifest a new paradigm for our planet and humanity.

Personal to planetary transformation is a unique design because it sources all action from the creative and sacred space of wisdom. It addresses immediate, systems, and root causes of a problem or condition. For example, in designing our responses to address HIV/AIDS, we made technical solutions available—condoms for safe sex, treatment for those with AIDS, safe blood for transfusion services, and clean instruments. We addressed systemic issues by including people living with HIV/AIDS in every planning session. But most importantly, we began our work by looking within toward our attitudes, our worldviews, and the spirit that informs our decisions even in the face of opposition. We asked: How can we provide services and care without stigma and discrimination? Or allocate resources for those in need who do not have a voice? How can we make love in a deeply respectful way, ensuring the safety of our partner? We understood that HIV/AIDS is more than a virus. It is about power relations in the bedroom and boardroom!

It is an art to simplify without being simplistic especially in the midst of complexity. We design our responses to diverse conditions to help people innovate, generate breakthroughs, and sustain the specific change that is needed. I have distinguished seven ways in which we act and organize ourselves for the best results, illustrated in Figures 2.2 and 2.3.

Figure 2.2 illustrates the first approach, and reflects the emerging paradigm we need for sustainable change. It uses approaches for personal transformation manifesting in planetary transformation (outer, middle, and inner circles as one seamless whole). The new paradigm must design and generate responses that integrate the different domains that are related to the entangled hierarchies of any given situation and that source from our individual and collective wisdom, addressing immediate, systems, and root causes.

Figure 2.3 reflects the six other ways we embark on strategic action:

1. Identify immediate causes and offer specific solutions with available technologies (inner circle). Examples are bed nets to deal with malaria, immunization to eradicate polio, roads to connect villages, reduced

---

Figure 2.2   **Personal to planetary transformation.**

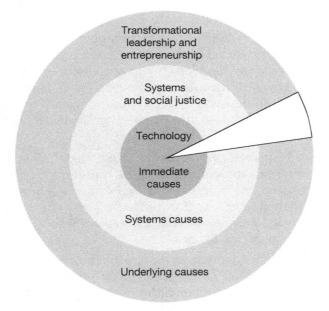

Source: Copyright 2007 by Monica Sharma.

| Figure 2.3 | **Ways of sourcing actions and results.** |

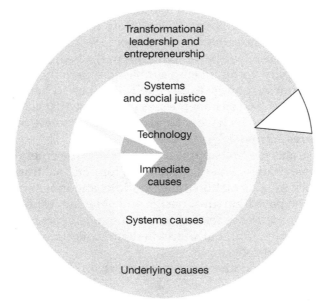

Source: Copyright 2007 by Monica Sharma.

sources of carbon emission to deal with global warming, and clinics to treat illness. However, when strategies are limited primarily to technological solutions for a specific problem, only the specific problem is resolved.

2. Identify the factors and structures that empower or disempower, and define ways to address systemic causes (middle circle). We formulate ethical norms, promote democracy, and encourage activists to fight for social justice. We establish rules and systems for financing, intellectual property rights, trade, health care, education, and so on. Much of what we have done in these areas heretofore has benefited a few while depriving many.

3. Embark on a journey of self-discovery (outer circle). Over the past two decades, numerous consciousness-based training programmers have been initiated, and books on personal self-awareness have proliferated. They have paved the way for different perspectives and actions. However, self-discovery alone will not transform the planet unless we also respond to larger challenges.

4. Promote social justice with concrete actions (inner and middle circles). In these cases, the "DNA" or the policy of the organization sources itself from principles related to human rights or healthy ecosystems. The Earth Charter and Amnesty International are examples.

5. Open our hearts and engage in charity or philanthropy (inner and outer circles). People often give support and resources generously, but

do not engage with systems issues. Their actions benefit some people, but do not address systemic causes—for example, providing a clinic without looking at the medical or health system or the pharmaceutical industry.

6. Open our hearts and engage in systems change (outer circle for self-discovery, middle and inner circles for action). Leaders are often deeply spiritual, offer themselves generously, and engage with systems issues. Their actions benefit people, and address systemic causes—for example, Mahatma Gandhi and the freedom movement in India. However, the strategy for change does not provide a platform for everyone to source action from deep within, so over time the actions fall short of the potential for significant sustainable change.

While working in the field, I observed that policy makers and program managers have discovered that integrating transformative practices actually strengthens the "technological" response. Hitherto, professionals engaged in development argued that time-bound results can be achieved only if the interventions are focused and specific. On the contrary, if technology and systems actions are skillfully synthesized with transformational approaches, not merely applied sequentially or separately, we can address the different factors needed for development simultaneously and hence much more effectively.

Emerging new leaders will understand both the visible and hidden sources of action and inaction, and the attitudes that determine them. They will understand factors and forces that create and legitimize structures, and the systems and cultural norms that inhibit or enhance progress. They will enhance their own personal awareness, realizing that this is the most critical element of social transformation. They will keep informed of the complex emerging global systems, and have courage to take action that creates a better world for everyone.

Global Architecture for Personal to Planetary Transformation

Today, the most urgent and sustainable response to the world's problems is to expand solutions for problems that are driven solely by technology, to responses that are generated from personally aware leadership. Evidence shows this is possible in business and in development, and a few large-scale initiatives are now under way.

The Leadership and Capacity Development Initiative of the UN is one of these expanded approaches that I am directing. This initiative builds on successes, and works with a worldwide constellation of like-minded organizations and individuals. The purpose is to foster sustainable transformation at every level of society. A pregnant space for emergence enables actions that are sourced from deep within. Key components and systems are in concert and are aligned to the larger purpose. All strategies and actions embody wisdom, courage, and compassion. This strategic resonance has the potential to generate a planetary paradigm shift. It has attracted hundreds of leading-edge individuals and organizations, and corporations and governments. We have identified the key players and organizations; and in this constellation we are working as universal partners for large-scale planetary change. The 11 components of our business plan follow.

1. Implement Transformational Leadership Programs for Change

The transformational leadership development programs are currently being implemented in 20 countries and are expanding rapidly. Transformation is the powerful unleashing of human potential to commit, care, and effect change for a better life. Using the best science, the programs are designed to apply at scale some 40 distinctions, frameworks, and conversations, woven into a unique methodology. Technologies for achieving the MDGs (and now the SDGs) and establishing businesses are integrated with technologies for leadership development and systems transformation. Effective, results-oriented stakeholder partnerships among government, civil society, and private sector support country-specific issues related to youth, women, and marginalized groups. The theme of the program is selected locally according to need. For example, last year Cambodia worked in the education sector, providing a platform for how my being, my essence, my stand, is the source of my action. Coaching and education programs are under way in 15 countries. Capacity is being developed in-country to "coach" transformational approaches with people who have generated breakthroughs and who have a stake in the future of their own country and society.

2. Support the New Archetypal Leaders

New archetypal leaders are emerging. Largely unnoticed, they are more like midwives giving birth to other people's ideas than "stars" of the show. They invest in their own spiritual (not necessarily religious) growth; they proactively inform themselves about the state of the world; they see patterns in addition to events; they have the courage to take on difficult issues; they act from a source of wisdom, compassion, and empathy, rather than charity and "doing good." They do not reflect the traditional sage, hero, or savior archetypes. They are informed sages, wise in the ways of the world; they are courageous nonviolent heroes with a cause; they are compassionate saviors, grateful to be able to serve . . . We are actively connecting with and supporting such sage–hero–saviors.

3. Source Deeper "Corporate Social Responsibility Plus"

Five corporations are in conversation with us, and more are engaging. They feel the urgency for renewal and increased effectiveness. They provide platforms for developing leadership competencies for their staff and managers; encouraging innovations and breakthrough initiatives through employees or members; developing capacity by using transformational approaches. Through individual insights and generative conversations, people set new pathways to address systems issues beyond the company, encouraging mechanisms that impact our planet positively and challenging those that impact negatively. Community service is not a matter of better "PR" for companies, but the source of employee engagement; partnership is not a matter of "technical support" for local civil society organizations, but the opportunity for one's own growth and contribution. Our intention is to deepen corporate engagement for social transformation with more corporate leaders.

4. Empower Grassroots

We are designing programs with six groups who have global presence and who aspire to touch the lives of three to five hundred million people—and eventually a billion. Our mutually reinforcing objectives using transformational leadership programs include strengthening grassroots voices and governance, addressing issues and concerns related to ecosystems, innovative strategies for education, and creating entrepreneurial opportunities.

5. Generate Financing

The purpose of this initiative is to create an understanding of, demand for, and subsequent funding by development partners, donors, and financiers, of transformational leadership as an integral and critical component of development and business. We encourage UN organizations, international financial institutions, multilateral and bilateral aid organizations, large international nongovernmental organizations (INGOs), and big foundations to embark on transformational leadership development in their own organizations. Specifically, donors, development agencies, and financiers could earmark funds for projects that include leadership development, and establish units within their organizations to learn, design, and implement transformational development and business. Currently, we are working with three multilateral organizations, a large umbrella INGO, and potentially two bilateral organizations. Concurrently, we seek additional partners. As we find leadership that recognizes and promotes the importance of this approach, the outcome will be massive and sustainable, a paradigm shift from "charity" to universal partnership. Shifting from promoting technologies as the major solution to current problems, we will build leadership competencies that draw upon the power and wisdom of people and politicians. There will be a new appreciation for humanity in current corporate philanthropy and donor support. In addition, financing will be available for new leadership to manifest social and planetary transformation.

6. Support Champions of Change

Influential people and institutions from civil society and business, development partners, and governments that distinguish the strategic nuances of programs where personal transformation manifests in planetary and social transformation, are actively championing this emerging paradigm. They articulate and promote the new paradigm and distinguish it from traditional ways of doing business. We are connecting individuals and institutions worldwide. Together we are actively supporting the numerous innovative risk-takers who change the status quo in order to create a new and positive future.

7. Connect Through Information Technology

With our partners in the constellation, we will link together the innovators of change who participate in this global effort to form a worldwide interconnected and collaborative group to share expertise in transformation. They will implement programs designed to generate measurable results using transformational approaches. We are seeking partnerships with groups who design and implement innovations, using cutting-edge information technology and transformative approaches.

8. Foster Change With Media Leadership

We are forming coalitions with media as well as working with individuals so that they can become influential leaders. Media activities in eight countries we are currently working with aim at scaling up social transformation by creating new icons and metaphors of leadership; voicing unvoiced questions about the root causes of underdevelopment; acknowledging women and men as leaders; shifting the cultural response paradigm from despair to courage, commitment, and positive lives. They are writing new stories of wisdom–courage–compassion in action from around the world.

9. Create Transformation Through Art

It is in art that our stories, songs, music, dance, and paintings reside and our renewal is expressed and created. Using transformational approaches, we have created a space for the emergence of artists to lead "possibilities and peace." We have identified artists in several countries who are poised to create a worldwide movement, using transformational art with a shared global vision of world development. Critical to these initiatives is overcoming the present culture of war and violence, and replacing it with the dynamics and directives of the culture of peace based on a sustainable and empowering development paradigm.

10. Identify Global Patterns and Share the Information

Often decisions are made on the basis of incorrect or incomplete information. This has become an increasingly critical problem in the era of "globalization." People need information on global and local patterns and systems, distinguishing between those that empower and those that disempower. Having access to correct and complete information, in a simple way, allows people to make choices. We are seeking partnerships with organizations that are making information on global patterns readily available in a coherent, understandable, and actionable way.

11. Measure for Momentum and a Paradigm Shift

Personal transformation manifesting in social and planetary transformation requires appropriate indicators and an evolving system of measurement. The current set of indicators used for most development efforts tells an incomplete story. It often omits stories of innovation, courage, transformation, and profound change. We are now partnering with eminent persons to see how national indices of progress can include the wisdom and contribution of people as an asset. We are looking at the vast body of knowledge to distill indicators of empowerment and planetary well-being sourced from wisdom, and then to promote our findings worldwide.

A World That Works for Everyone

The next 50 years will show whether the world as a whole can come together as one, resolving the many seemingly intractable problems we now face. Or will we continue to muddle through, from crisis to crisis, never solving the problems of humankind in a definitive and sustained way? Yesterday, we were engaged in resolving a crisis: HIV/AIDS. Today, we are focusing on global warming. Tomorrow, we may focus on nuclear waste. What remains constant in this changing world is the power of human wisdom.

There are challenges to overcome if personal transformation is to become an inherent part of whole systems change. If you say yes to any of the following questions, please step forward.

- Are you a champion of the emerging paradigm? Are you more like a midwife than a "star?" Can you distinguish the strategic nuances of programs where personal transformation manifests in planetary transformation? Do you promote new leadership?
- Do you have influence and resources to support the unknown risk-takers who are sourcing from a creative and sacred place? Are you supporting courageous activists who promote empowering systems and challenge disempowering ones?
- Risk-takers are innovating and changing the status quo in order to create new possibilities for a positive future. They need you. Will you respond?
- Are you a pioneer who dares to speak up and challenge the reliance on the "technology-only" paradigm? Are you willing to source all action from creative and sacred wisdom, despite the ridicule by experts?
- Are you a new architect who knows how to design large-scale programs that source from wisdom? Can you address simultaneously the practical problems embedded in complex world issues?
- Are you a corporate leader who generates innovation sourced from the creative and sacred space of the people you lead and the processes you change? Do you speak out in the world of business and commerce for changing systems and products that do not help humanity and the planet? Do you promote the practices that work for everyone?
- Are you a "consciousness scholar or teacher" who can stretch beyond our brand identity and serve selflessly from a space of wisdom?
- Are you willing to examine yourself deeply to understand how you are contributing to the global problematique? Do your actions and decisions subtly perpetuate gender, class, and ethnic inequalities resulting in the intolerable situation of 30% of us who cannot "make it?"

Never before in history have both opportunity and need been so great. Never before has "grow or die" been more apparent. And never before have the means existed to effect planetary transformation. Indeed, this is the time to pioneer results-oriented designs that can then be applied across the urgent and significant issues of our time. This is the time for mind-sets that foster the culture of peace. This is the time for a world that works for everyone.

Source: Reprinted from Sharma (2007).

FINAL THOUGHTS: PERSONAL–PROFESSIONAL OBJECTIVES FOR TRANSFORMATIVE OUTCOMES

As nurses, we need to establish a context of globally informed and globally relevant ideals if we are to be effective in contributing toward the achievement of the SDGs. This includes being selective in the language and definitions we employ, the paradigms we adopt, and challenges us to become increasingly conscious of our choices and their widespread implications in the areas of education, practice, research, advocacy, leadership, collaboration, and relationship building. Understanding that personal choices impact planetary outcomes can aid global nurses in fostering more satisfying, socially respectful, and culturally inclusive personal–professional endeavors. In doing so, nurses maximize their disciplinary-specific contributions to global health while remaining true to the caring ethic and scientific inquiry central to the profession. Table 2.3 offers objectives related to personal and professional development for personal and planetary transformation identified by this author. Each of these objectives is based on the business plan components of the UN Leadership and Capacity Development Initiative, as noted by Sharma (2007). These objectives urge us to use both individual and collective forces to keep our work as global nurses ethically grounded and focused on transforming both self and systems.

Table 2.3 Personal and Professional Objectives for Nurses and Nursing Related to the Business Plan Components of the United Nations Leadership and Capacity Development Initiative

Components (Sharma, 2007)	Personal Objectives: Individual	Professional Objectives: Collective
1. Implement transformational leadership programs for change	• Define *transformation* for self in relation to personal and professional life • Create action plans for individual leadership initiatives in current context • Understand individual role in promoting unity among government, civil society, and private sector stakeholders	• Drive organizational priorities toward principles based on safety and inclusivity • Promote colleagues' full self-expression for widespread professional advancement and overall well-being • Delineate outcome measures for transformational programs committed to leadership and capacity building
2. Support the new archetypal leaders	• Investigate personal intentions for being of service • Reflect on the meaning of *spiritual growth* and its role in self-development • Seek opportunities to see the larger patterns of humanity and include global considerations in personal decision making	• Support leaders who are ethically rooted, compassionate, and invested in contributing toward a unified planet • Create interprofessional alliances that inspire and nurture new sources of collective wisdom • Reframe professional mission and vision statements in terms of courageous and humanistic values
3. Source deeper "Corporate Social Responsibility Plus"	• Expand individual role in organizational well-being • Use personal influence for the betterment of colleagues and civil society • Engage with like-minded people across the spectrum regardless of position	• Invite partnerships with similarly invested organizations • Expand the corporate mind-set to include vulnerability and transparency through education and outreach • Broaden goals of service to include partnerships with communities and populations

(continued)

Table 2.3 Personal and Professional Objectives for Nurses and Nursing Related to the Business Plan Components of the United Nations Leadership and Capacity Development Initiative (*continued*)

Components (Sharma, 2007)	Personal Objectives: Individual	Professional Objectives: Collective
4. Empower grassroots	• Identify strengths and weaknesses related to communication strategies and self-marketing • Create opportunities to demonstrate leadership in multisector initiatives for improved environmental and organizational well-being	• Promote a culture of "grassroots" innovation by respecting all ideas and inviting creative solutions • Generate system-wide goals inclusive of other sectors and global initiatives
5. Generate financing	• Investigate personal financing to ensure responsible and globally considerate investments • Support financial donors and agencies interested in building partnerships across socioeconomic divides	• Draw on the wisdom of shared humanity as a mechanism for attaining responsible, ethical philanthropy and donor support • Invest in initiatives geared toward social and planetary transformation
6. Support champions of change	• Reflect on personal comfort with risk-taking • Redefine the status quo through self-expression and commitment to transformative practices • Advocate from a stance of inclusiveness	• Invite new and innovative leadership strategies • Create opportunities to hear all colleagues' voices and views • Restructure governing bodies to become safe forums and explore new paradigms of social development and progress
7. Connect through information technology	• Utilize social media responsibly and with consideration for the global village • Use technology to create new partnerships with innovators and visionaries around the world	• Create technology programs that return the profession of nursing toward its humanistic heritage • Seek partnerships to convey nursing's unique contributions to global health and well-being through technologically responsible mechanisms
8. Foster change with media leadership	• Engage with media outlets to promote a global dialogue of courage and positivity • Tell personal stories of accomplishments toward a transformative paradigm of health and well-being	• Invite media partners to be involved in nursing initiatives • Promote widespread dissemination of nursing advocacy, policy, practice, research, and education

(continued)

Table 2.3 Personal and Professional Objectives for Nurses and Nursing Related to the Business Plan Components of the United Nations Leadership and Capacity Development Initiative (*continued*)

Components (Sharma, 2007)	Personal Objectives: Individual	Professional Objectives: Collective
9. Create transformation through art	• Make time to self-express in a way that positively contributes to self and community • Share individual perspectives through creative expression • Align with like-minded artists, leaders, and professionals through community empowering art	• Promote the inclusion of art and creative expression as a professional priority • Create art initiatives that seek to translate professional ethics and values into varied modes of expression • Foster sensitive and empathic infrastructures that respect individual ideas and artistic expressions
10. Identify global patterns and share the information	• Identify individual opportunities to expand "global thinking" and "global doing" • Share information that highlights the interdependent nature of a globalized world	• Incorporate global developments in institutional and organizational work • Identify opportunities to connect professional goals to global solidarity
11. Measure for momentum and a paradigm shift	• Consider individual knowledge and wisdom as assets in planetary transformation • Evolve harmful practices that hinder self-growth and development toward a more peaceful paradigm for positive change • Empower self and others through compassionate ways of being	• Recalibrate outcome measures to include humanistic and qualitative data • Ensure professional practices reflect empowerment of the whole • Celebrate all accomplishments toward a unitary paradigm while continuing to envision profound change sourced in wisdom

In closing, I challenge you to read the following words closely, while considering what the world will need for personal to planetary transformation and how global nursing can partner to create and implement solutions through a commitment to the *Global Strategic Directions* (WHO, 2016a) and SDG attainment. The following are the UN Secretary-General, Ban Ki-moon's, remarks at the Summit for the Adoption of the Post-2015 Agenda:

Esteemed co-Chairs of this post-2015 Summit,
Mr. President of the General Assembly,
Distinguished Heads of State and Government,
Excellencies,
Distinguished guests,
Ladies and Gentlemen,
We have reached a defining moment in human history.
The people of the world have asked us to shine a light on a future of promise and opportunity.

Member States have responded with the 2030 Agenda for Sustainable Development.
The new agenda is a promise by leaders to all people everywhere.
It is a universal, integrated and transformative vision for a better world.
It is an agenda for people, to end poverty in all its forms.
An agenda for the planet, our common home.
An agenda for shared prosperity, peace and partnership.
It conveys the urgency of climate action.
It is rooted in gender equality and respect for the rights of all.
Above all, it pledges to leave no one behind.

Excellencies,
Ladies and Gentlemen,
The true test of commitment to Agenda 2030 will be implementation.
We need action from everyone, everywhere.
Seventeen Sustainable Development Goals are our guide.
They are a to-do list for people and planet, and a blueprint for success.
To achieve these new global goals, we will need your high-level political commitment.
We will need a renewed global partnership.
The Millennium Development Goals showed what is possible when we work together.
The Addis Ababa Action Agenda has given us a solid financing framework.
Let us build on these foundations.
To do better, we must do differently.
The 2030 Agenda compels us to look beyond national boundaries and short-term interests and act in solidarity for the long-term.
We can no longer afford to think and work in silos.
Institutions will have to become fit for a grand new purpose.
The United Nations system is strongly committed to supporting Member States in this great new endeavour.

Excellencies,
Ladies and Gentlemen,
We need to start the new era on the right foot.
I call on all governments to adopt a robust universal climate agreement in Paris in December.
I am encouraged that several countries are already working to incorporate the 2030 Agenda into their national development strategies.
But no-one can succeed working alone.
We must engage all actors, as we did in shaping the Agenda.
We must include parliaments and local governments, and work with cities and rural areas.
We must rally businesses and entrepreneurs.

We must involve civil society in defining and implementing policies—
and give it the space to hold us to account.
We must listen to scientists and academia.
We will need to embrace a data revolution.
Most important, we must set to work—now.

Excellencies,
Ladies and Gentlemen,
Seventy years ago, the United Nations rose from the ashes of war.
Governments agreed on a visionary Charter dedicated to "We the Peoples."
The Agenda you are adopting today advances the goals of the Charter.
It embodies the aspirations of people everywhere for lives of peace,
security and dignity on a healthy planet.
Let us today pledge to light the path to this transformative vision.
Thank you. (UN, 2016. Reprinted with permission.)

REFLECTION AND DISCUSSION

- What are the connections between the GAPFON task force definitions of "global health" and "global nursing" and my current work?

- How are the thematic areas identified by the WHO's (2016a) *Global Strategic Directions* applicable to my local community of nurses and nursing?

- What beliefs and values need exploration in order to shift toward a more planetary consciousness in my personal and professional life?

- What are my own objectives for personal growth and development in regard to social progress?

- In what ways am I an integral component of the transformative vision articulated by the Sustainable Development Agenda?

REFERENCES

American Nurses Association. (2016). What is nursing? Retrieved from http://www .nursingworld.org/EspeciallyForYou/What-is-Nursing

Baumann, S. L. (2013). Global health nursing: Toward a human science-based approach. *Nursing Science Quarterly, 26*, 365.

Beck, D.-M. (2010). Expanding our Nightingale horizon: Seven recommendations for 21st-century nursing practice. *Journal of Holistic Nursing, 28*(4), 317–326.

Beck, D.-M., Dossey, B. M., & Rushton, C. H. (2014). Global activism, advocacy, and transformation: Florence Nightingale's legacy for the twenty-first century. In M. J. Kreitzer & M. Koithan (Eds.), *Integrative nursing* (pp. 526–537). New York, NY: Oxford University Press.

Chan, M. (2015, June 20). *Global citizen, global nursing: Reshaping nursing for the future needs of citizens.* Keynote address presented at the International Council of Nurses Conference, Seoul, Republic of Korea. Retrieved from http://www.who.int/dg/speeches/2015/international-conference-nurses/en

Cho, E., Sloane, D. M., Kim, E.-Y., Kim, S., Choi, M., Yoo, I. Y., . . . Aiken, L. H. (2014). Effects of nurse staffing, work environments, and education on patient mortality: An observational study. *International Journal of Nursing Studies, 52*(2), 535–542.

Clark, M., Raffray, M., Hendricks, K., & Gagnon, A. J. (2016). Global and public health core competencies for nursing education: A systematic review of essential competencies. *Nurse Education Today, 40,* 173–180.

Devane, D., Brennan, M., Begley, C., Clarke, M., Walsh, D., Sandall, J., . . . Normand, C. (2010). *Socioeconomic value of the midwife: A systematic review, meta-analysis, meta-synthesis and economic analysis of midwife-led models of care.* London, UK: Royal College of Midwives.

Dossey, B. M. (2010). *Florence Nightingale: Mystic, visionary, healer* (Commemorative ed.). Philadelphia, PA: F. A. Davis.

Dossey, B. M., Selanders, L., Beck, D.-M., & Attewell, A. (2005). *Florence Nightingale today: Healing, leadership, global action.* Silver Spring, MD: American Nurses Association.

Farmer, P., Kim, J. Y., Kleinman, A., & Basilico, M. (2013). Introduction: A biosocial approach to global health. In P. Farmer, J. Y. Kim, A. Kleinman, & M. Basilico (Eds.), *Reimagining global health: An introduction* (pp. 1–14). Berkeley and Los Angeles: University of California Press.

Fried, L. P., Bentley, M. E., Buekens, P., Burke, D. S., Frenk, J. J., Klag, M. J., & Spencer, H. C. (2010). Global health is public health. *The Lancet, 375,* 535–537.

Grootjans, J., & Newman, S. (2013). The relevance of globalization to nursing: A concept analysis. *International Nursing Review, 60,* 78–85.

Homer, C. S., Friberg, I. K., Dias, M. A., Hoope-Bender, P., Sandall, J., Speciale, A. M., & Bartlett, L. A. (2014). The projected effect of scaling up midwifery. *The Lancet, 384*(9948), 1146–1157.

Howard, K. H., & Papa, N. (2012). Future-of-nursing report: The impact on emergency nursing. *Journal of Emergency Nursing, 38*(6), 549–552.

International Labour Organization Nursing Personnel Convention, 1977 (No. 149). (1977). Retrieved from http://www.ilo.org/dyn/normlex/en/f?p=1000:12100:0::NO::P12100_ILO_CODE:C149

International Labour Organization Nursing Personnel Recommendation, 1977 (No. 157). (1977). Retrieved from http://www.ilo.org/dyn/normlex/en/f?p=NORMLEXPUB:12100:0::NO::P12100_ILO_CODE:R157

Janes, C. R., & Corbett, K. K. (2009). Anthropology and global health. *Annual Reviews of Anthropology, 38,* 167–183.

Kahn, L. H., Kaplan, B., Monath, T., Woodall, L. J., & Conti, L. (2014). A manifesto for planetary health—Correspondence. *The Lancet, 383,* 1459–1460.

Kendall-Gallagher, D., Aiken, L. H., Sloane, D. M., & Cimiotti, J. P. (2011). Nurse specialty certification, inpatient mortality, and failure to rescue. *Journal of Nursing Scholarship, 43*(2), 188–194.

Klopper, H. C., & Hill, M. (2015). Global Advisory Panel on the Future of Nursing (GAPFON) and Global Health. *Journal of Nursing Scholarship, 47,* 3–4.

Koplan, J. P., Bond, T. C., Merson, M. H., Reddy, K. S., Rodriguez, M. H., Sewankambo, N. K., & Wasserheit, J. N. (2009). Towards a common definition of global health. *The Lancet, 373,* 1993–1995.

Lloyd, A. R., Clegg, J., Lange, J., Stevenson, A., Post, J. J., Lloyd, D., . . . Monkley, D. (2013). Safety and effectiveness of a nurse-led outreach program for assessment and treatment of chronic hepatitis C in the custodial setting. *Clinical Infectious Disease, 56*(8), 1078–1084.

Patel, M. R., Yotebieng, M., Behets, F., Driessche, V. K., Nana, M., & Van Rie, A. (2013). Outcomes of integrated treatment for tuberculosis and HIV in children at the primary health care level. *International Journal of Tuberculosis and Lung Disease, 17*(9), 1206–1211.

Pintar, P. A. (2013). An entrepreneurial innovative role: Integration of the clinical nurse specialist and infection prevention professional. *Clinical Nurse Specialist, 27*(3), 123–127.

Purssell, E. (2014). Shingles vaccination: Background and advice for community nurses. *British Journal of Community Nursing, 19*(9), 442–446.

Sharma, M. (2007). Personal to planetary transformation. *Kosmos Journal, Fall/Winter,* 31–37.

Smith, J. M., Currie, S., Cannon, T., Armbruster, D., & Perri, J. (2014). Are national policies and programs for prevention and management of postpartum hemorrhage and preeclampsia adequate? A key informant survey in 37 countries. *Global Health: Science and Practice, 2*(3), 275–284.

Ten Hoope-Bender, P., de Bernis, L., Campbell, J., Downe, S., Fauveau, V., Fogstad, H., . . . Van Lerberghe, W. (2014). Improvement of maternal and newborn health through midwifery. *The Lancet, 384*(9949), 1226–1235.

United Nations. (2015). Transforming our world: The 2030 agenda for sustainable development. Retrieved from https://sustainabledevelopment.un.org/post2015/transformingourworld

United Nations. (2016). The Secretary-General remarks at Summit for the adoption of the post-2015 development agenda. Retrieved from http://www.eg.undp.org/content/egypt/en/home/presscenter/speeches/the-secretary-general----remarks-at-summit-for-the-adoption-of-t.html

United Nations Millennium Project. (2006). What they are. Retrieved from http://www.unmillenniumproject.org/goals

Universal health coverage post-2015: Putting people first. (2014). *The Lancet, 384*(9960), 2083.

Upvall, M. J., Leffers, J. M., & Mitchell, E. M. (2014). Introduction and perspectives of global health. In M. J. Upvall & J. M. Leffers (Eds.), *Global health nursing: Building and sustaining partnerships* (pp. 1–17). New York, NY: Springer Publishing.

Walsh, D., & Devane, D. (2012). A metasynthesis of midwife-led care. *Qualitative Health Research, 22*(7), 897–910.

Warren, N., Breman, R., Budhathoki, C., Farley, J., & Wilson, L. L. (2016). Perspectives of nursing faculty in Africa on global health nursing competencies. *Nursing Outlook, 64*, 179–185.

Wilson, L., Callender, B., Hall, T. L., Jogerst, K., Torres, H., & Velji, A. (2014). Identifying global health competencies to prepare 21st century global health professionals: Report from the Global Health Competency Subcommittee of the Consortium of Universities for Global Health. *Journal of Law, Medicine & Ethics, 42*, 26–31.

Wilson, L., Mendes, I. A. C., Klopper, H., Catrambone, C., Al-Maaitah, R., Norton, M. E., & Hill, M. (2016). "Global health" and "global nursing": Proposed definitions from The Global Advisory Panel on the Future of Nursing. *Journal of Advanced Nursing, 72*(7), 1529–1540.

Wolf, K. A. (2015). The intersection of global health and community/public health nursing. In S. Breakey, I. B. Corless, N. L. Meedzan, & P. K. Nicholas (Eds.), *Global health nursing in the 21st century* (pp. 85–101). New York, NY: Springer Publishing.

World Health Organization. (2002). Strategic directions for strengthening nursing and midwifery services. Retrieved from http://apps.who.int/iris/bitstream/10665/42558/1/924156217X.pdf

World Health Organization. (2010). *Increasing access to health workers in remote and rural areas through improved retention: Global policy recommendations.* Geneva, Swizterland: Author. Retrieved from http://apps.who.int/iris/bitstream/10665/44369/1/9789241564014_eng.pdf

World Health Organization. (2011). Nursing & midwifery services strategic directions 2011–2015. Retrieved from http://www.wpro.who.int/hrh/documents/nursing_and_midwifery_services_strategic_directions.pdf

World Health Organization. (2012). Positioning health in the post-2015 development agenda [Discussion paper]. Retrieved from http://www.who.int/topics/millennium_development_goals/post2015/WHOdiscussionpaper_October2012.pdf

World Health Organization. (2013a). *Transforming and scaling up health professionals' education and training. World Health Organization Guidelines 2013.* Geneva, Swizterland: Author. Retrieved from http://apps.who.int/iris/bitstream/10665/93635/1/9789241506502_eng.pdf

World Health Organization. (2013b). *World Health Report 2013: Research for universal health coverage.* Geneva, Swizterland: Author. Retrieved from http://apps.who.int/iris/bitstream/10665/85761/2/9789240690837_eng.pdf

World Health Organization. (2013c). *Mental health action plan 2013–2020.* Geneva, Swizterland: Author. Retrieved from http://apps.who.int/iris/bitstream/10665/89966/1/9789241506021_eng.pdf

World Health Organization. (2013d). *WHO nursing and midwifery progress report 2008–2012.* Geneva, Switzerland: Author. Retrieved from http://www.who.int/hrh/nursing_midwifery/NursingMidwiferyProgressReport.pdf?ua=1

World Health Organization. (2014). *Every newborn: An action plan to end preventable deaths.* Geneva, Swizterland: Author. Retrieved from http://apps.who.int/iris/bitstream/10665/127938/1/9789241507448_eng.pdf?ua

World Health Organization. (2015a). *Tracking universal health coverage: First global monitoring report.* Geneva, Switzerland: Author. Retrieved from http://apps.who.int/iris/bitstream/10665/174536/1/9789241564977_eng.pdf

World Health Organization. (2015b). The global strategy for women's, children's and adolescents' health (2016–2030). Retrieved from http://www.who.int/pmnch/media/events/2015/gs_2016_30.pdf

World Health Organization. (2015c). *Strategies toward ending preventable maternal mortality (EPMM).* Geneva, Switzerland: Author. Retrieved from http://www.everywomaneverychild.org/images/EPMM_final_report_2015.pdf

World Health Organization. (2015d). *World report on ageing and health.* Geneva, Switzerland: Author. Retrieved from http://apps.who.int/iris/bitstream/10665/186463/1/9789240694811_eng.pdf

World Health Organization. (2015e). *WHO progress report on nursing and midwifery 2013–2015.* Retrieved from http://www.who.int/hrh/nursing_midwifery/nursing-midwifery_report_13-15.pdf?ua=1

World Health Organization. (2015f). *Health workforce and services. Draft global strategy on human resources for health: Workforce 2030. Report by the Secretariat.* Retrieved from http://apps.who.int/gb/ebwha/pdf_files/EB138/B138_36-en.pdf?ua=1

World Health Organization. (2016a). *Global strategic directions for strengthening nursing and midwifery 2016–2020.* Geneva, Switzerland: Author. Retrieved from http://www.who.int/hrh/nursing_midwifery/glob-strategic-midwifery2016-2020_EN.pdf

World Health Organization. (2016b). Global strategy on human resources for health: Workforce 2030. Draft for the 69th World Health Assembly. Retrieved from http://www.who.int/hrh/resources/16059_Global_strategyWorkforce2030.pdf

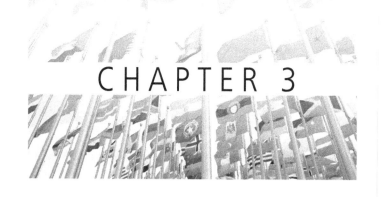

CHAPTER 3

A Brief History of the United Nations and Nursing: A Healthy World Is Our Common Future

Deva-Marie Beck

If the nurses and midwives of the world cannot become the lead advocates for global goals related to health—especially the health of women, girls, and vulnerable infants—who can? And who will? (Seth, 2009)

THE UNITED NATIONS AND ITS WIDE-RANGING MANDATES

Founded in the wake of World War II, the United Nations (UN) is an international organization currently composed of 193 Member States. The UN's most visible components are two of its six main organs. The widely recognized UN General Assembly is often featured in the news when heads of government and other Member State delegates and dignitaries consider current issues and sponsor, debate, and pass related UN resolutions.

Less known is the UN Security Council, consisting of five permanent members—China, France, the Russian Federation, the United Kingdom, and the United States—along with 10 rotating member nations, elected by the General Assembly to serve for 2 years (UN, 2016a).

The UN was established in 1945—with a charter famous for its opening words "We the peoples of the United Nations determined to save succeeding generations from the scourge of war" (UN, 2016b). Today, the UN scope is much wider than specific peacekeeping missions. The globally comprehensive UN System, headed by the very visible and oft-quoted UN secretary-general—and often referred to as the "UN family"—comprises several UN agencies and organizations, thematic programs, and funds working on scores of complex issues that address the overall welfare of all peoples, species, and the Earth itself (UN, 2016a).

Perhaps the best example of this wider mandate is the UN Economic and Social Council (ECOSOC), also established by the 1945 UN charter as another of the UN's main organs. It is the central platform for fostering discussion, debate, and forward plans on economic and social issues. Through this foundational role, UN ECOSOC convenes high-level meetings and related substantive sessions and initiates major UN summits and conferences. Through these platforms UN ECOSOC builds consensus among UN Member States and, in consultation with nongovernmental stakeholders, on ways forward, thus coordinating efforts to achieve globally agreed-upon goals. In this way and over time, UN ECOSOC has become the innovative heart of the UN system's aspirations for advancing sustainable development in three clear arenas—economic, social, and environmental (UN ECOSOC, 2016).

Within the UN family of organizations, many other agencies, programs, and funds take responsibility for thematic components within the UN ECOSOC mandates. For instance, the UN International Children's Fund, better known by its original acronym UNICEF, was founded in 1947 to meet the critical needs of children in postwar Europe and China. It has since been working to improve children's lives, with many programs reaching out to the differing needs of children in 192 countries (UNICEF, 2016).

Another inspiring example is the UN High Commissioner for Refugees, better known as UNHCR. Founded in 1950 to protect the rights and well-being of peoples who no longer had a place to live in the aftermath of World War II, the UNHCR—currently famous for supporting large camps of refugees fleeing strife in the Middle East and Africa—remains challenged with this same issue (UNHCR, 2016). The UNHCR logo is a prominent image on each tent of vast settlements seen in video footage of refugee camps in Greece, Lebanon, Jordan, and Turkey.

A fresh UN structural initiative is the Entity for Gender Equality and the Empowerment of Women—or UN Women for short—established in 2010. This was an historic step in accelerating UN goals that have long been focused on the overall needs and well-being of women and girls, achieving a major part of the UN reform agenda to gather resources and mandates for greater impact (UN Women, 2016a).

NIGHTINGALE, THE NURSE: FORERUNNER OF THESE MANDATES

Until very recently, nurses have rarely been seen or involved within this widest scope of the UN family. However, Florence Nightingale, the founder of modern secular nursing worldwide, also directly assisted British government representatives to participate in ratifying the First Geneva Convention. This leading-edge global document led to the establishment of the League of Nations in 1919 and, after a second worldwide war, the UN itself in 1945 (UN, 2016c).

Nightingale, working quite actively behind the scenes with the British government of her time, prepared briefing documents to facilitate Britain's involvement in the related 1864–1865 meetings of leading European nations in Geneva, Switzerland (Dossey, 2010; McDonald, 2015). Following her own profound experiences serving battlefield wounded and dying soldiers during the Crimean War (1854–1856), Nightingale became an expert devoted to discovering and establishing peacekeeping efforts. She also knew, from her own work as a nurse, that war is a major contributor to disease and that the absence of war is only a fraction of what is needed to achieve and sustain a peaceful, healthy world (Beck, 2010).

Nightingale envisioned what a world of good health would look like, and she worked tirelessly to both articulate and realize this vision. She anticipated the wider interconnected concerns we readily see, in substance today, as sustainable development milestones articulated through UN ECOSOC. Nightingale called for and worked to achieve better conditions and rights for women, children, the poor, and the hungry, and for better educational programs for people marginalized by culture and geography. She identified environmental health determinants, such as clean air and water, better homes, nutrition and sanitation, and social health determinants, such as poverty, education, human rights, family relationships, and employment—all interdependent locally to globally (Dossey, Selanders, Beck, & Attewell, 2005).

INTRODUCING GLOBAL CIVIL SOCIETY AND NGOS

Nightingale's own "good citizenship" commitment—aimed independently toward achieving all these causes—anticipated another key component that has evolved, over time, through the work of the UN family. This component is a more active collaboration, by the UN, with nongovernmental organizations (NGOs) working in common cause on these issues today. This "global civil society" is "a vast assemblage of groups operating across borders and beyond the reach of governments" (Keane, 2016).

An *NGO* is defined as any nonprofit, voluntary citizens' group that is organized on local, national, or global levels. Established as an idea as early as 1863—and also directly inspired by Nightingale's work—the International Federation of Red Cross and Red Crescent Societies today serves as one of the world's oldest citizen-based organizations and a prime example of how these should work (Dossey, 2010; IFRC, 2016). NGOs, focused on completing relevant tasks and driven by people sharing a common ideal, perform a wide range of services to achieve humanitarian goals. They bring concerns of ordinary citizens to governments by advocating for and monitoring policies. An essential role of many NGOs is the wider provision of information to increase citizen understanding and concern for key issues, thereby strengthening political will and encouraging political participation in the causes of their concerns (NGO Global Network, 2016).

Many NGOs, such as Amnesty International (AI) and Greenpeace International (GI), are organized around specific issues such as human rights and the environment (AI, 2016; GI, 2016), often providing needed analysis and expertise, serving as early-warning mechanisms, and helping to monitor and implement international agreements.

Another active global example, focused on the issue of world health through the lens of nursing, was founded earlier, in 1899, as the International Council of Nurses (ICN)—"the first and widest reaching international organization of health professionals"—based in Geneva, Switzerland (ICN, 2016). With the 1948 founding of the World Health Organization (WHO), a major UN specialized agency also based in Geneva, the ICN has focused its considerable UN NGO collaboration primarily with the WHO, whose primary role is to direct and coordinate international health (WHO, 2016a).

How NGOs Work With the UN

NGOs directly collaborate with the UN at two divisions of official participation. In each case, NGOs are encouraged to assign their own designated representatives and youth representatives (ages 18 to 30 years) who thus have access to many

Secretariat briefings and meetings on-site at UN headquarters and with other facets of the UN family.

The primary level of NGO participation directly interacts throughout the entire UN. This designation is called "UN ECOSOC consultative status," providing NGOs and their representatives with opportunities to collaborate specifically with UN ECOSOC and its administrative arm—the UN Department of Economic and Social Affairs (UN DESA, 2016a). To be considered eligible to apply for this accreditation, an NGO must demonstrate that its program of work has direct relevance to the aims and purposes of the UN. It must have been in existence for at least 2 years, with an established headquarters and a democratically adopted constitution. NGO leaders must also prove authority to speak for their members, through a representative structure and appropriate mechanisms of accountability and transparent decision-making processes. The basic resources of such an organization must be derived mainly from contributions of the national affiliates or from individual members. Today, more than 4,000 NGOs worldwide have achieved this ability to officially consult with and recommend solutions to UN ECOSOC and, through ECOSOC, to the overall UN system (UN DESA, 2016b).

During the founding decade of the UN, 41 already established NGOs were granted consultative status by UN ECOSOC (UN DESA, 2016b). As noted earlier, the ICN—founded in 1899 and working as an NGO for 46 years by then—also holds a specialized "Agency Roster" consultative status interacting specifically in consultation with WHO (UN, 2016e).

The more basic entry mode—to officially work with the UN to increase worldwide concern for its mandates and aims—is termed "UN DPI-NGO status" for its direct affiliation with the UN Department of Public Information (DPI). UN DPI was established in 1946 to promote global awareness and understanding of the work of the UN and now furthers this goal through multimedia tools such as radio, television, print, the Internet, and videoconferencing (UN, 2016d). Through conferences, weekly briefings, regular workshops, orientation programs, and a Resource Centre in both New York and Geneva, UN DPI reaches out to representatives of approximately 1,400 affiliated organizations with DPI-NGO status. This process aims to facilitate exchange of information, to develop partnerships around issues relating to global civil society, and to enhance NGO interaction with and understanding of the UN's work. This UN DPI-NGO affiliation can be applied for when an NGO fully demonstrates its ability to disseminate such information, at grassroots levels, on UN priority issues, such as sustainable development, creating a safer, more secure, and healthy world, empowering women and young people, and addressing poverty (UN DPI-NGO, 2016).

Why and How UN NGO Participation Developed

Steadily, the role and participation of NGOs have developed into a significant contribution to the UN from global civil society. One of the longest established channels for this cooperation has been through CoNGO—the Conference of NGOs in Consultative Relationship with the United Nations. Since its founding in 1948, CoNGO has aimed to be of primary support and a platform for the global community of informed, empowered, and committed NGOs. Based near the UN headquarters in New York City, Geneva, and Vienna, CoNGO facilitates, through various means, the development and accessibility of a dynamic and informed worldwide

NGO community. This facilitates NGOs to influence policies and actions at all levels of the UN. CoNGO also seeks to engage NGOs to continue their advocacy for the principles and goals these NGOs and the UN share (CoNGO, 2016). As of this writing, CoNGO's elected president, Cyril Ritchie, who has also been a lifelong civil society activist, has also—as noted later in this chapter—encouraged and facilitated the increased participation of nurses with the UN since the early 2000s.

Across the 1960s and 1970s, the UN family increasingly collaborated with UN NGOs to raise public awareness by establishing two "Development Decades." Much in keeping with the wide-ranging mandates of UN ECOSOC at that time, these Decades were designated as global tools to foster widespread understanding of the UN's advocacy concerning economic, social, and environmental issues beyond, yet including, its narrower "peacekeeping" role (Nations Encyclopedia, 2016a, 2016b). At the end of the 1960s, an outcomes review determined that a second Development Decade would be required, and that a more focused effort to mobilize global public opinion through increased UN NGO participation was also necessary. Thus, in 1969, the 24th session of the UN General Assembly unanimously passed the UN Resolution on the Mobilization of Public Opinion (UN, 2016f). This groundbreaking motion articulated a specific mandate establishing a UN Centre for Economic and Social Information (CESI) in New York and Geneva to collaborate with all UN agencies and components of the UN family to facilitate mass media and NGO involvement in support of global development (UN CESI, 1973).

UN NGO participation was also considerably strengthened during the UN Conference on the Human Environment (UN CHE) convened in Stockholm in 1972. This was the first major event to focus the world's attention on global ecological impacts upon the environment, aiming to forge a basic common outlook on how to address the challenge of preserving and enhancing the human environment (UN, 2016g).

While preparing for this "human environment" idea—one that was leading edge at the time—the Conference Secretary-General, Maurice Strong, was concerned that a growing number of youth and students from around the world were activating their plans to inundate the Conference with massive protests aimed specifically to disrupt the proceedings. Seeking to address this concern, Mr. Strong consulted UN/ CESI Geneva's initiator of "student coalitions for development," Wayne Kines, to facilitate broader participation of NGOs worldwide in the Stockholm event (W.L. Kines, personal communication, June 10, 2016). Mr. Kines own background included journalism, broadcasting, and the strategic nationwide information campaign created to support international development during the Canadian Centennial Celebration of 1967 (Nightingale Initiative for Global Health [NIGH], 2016a).

From field experience with student activism arising during the 1960s and early 1970s, Mr. Kines proposed more direct involvement and substantive contribution within the UN CHE. Hundreds of NGOs were thus invited to daily early morning briefings and encouraged to proactively join an NGO Declaration addressing critical issues on the Conference agenda and to bring their voices to be heard directly and officially at the "plenipotentiary" gathering of all UN Member State delegates. The precedent was thus established for all the NGOs, including for world youth and student NGOs, to actively debate, decide, and present directly to the Conference floor. The UN CHE event concluded with unanimous approval, from UN member state delegates, of all agenda recommendations and resolutions. The

Conference also proposed the 1972 founding of the UN Environment Programme (UNEP) by the UN General Assembly (W.L. Kines, personal communication, June 10, 2016). The dramatic increase in worldwide public concern for environmental issues is attributed to the unprecedented media attendance at UN CHE, to world-wide coverage of its resolutions, and to the birth of more meaningful participation of international NGOs at this Conference (Mwangi, 2005; Ruhlman, 2014).

As is discussed later in this chapter, Mr. Kines, who became founding Director of Communications working from UNEP headquarters in Nairobi, created media cam-paigns of environmental human health promotion and continued to facilitate increas-ingly direct participation of UN NGOs, including through many global channels within UN organizations. His early life volunteerism in health promotion and edu-cation strengthened his focus on grassroots citizen action for a healthy global envi-ronment, further evident in the Brundtland Report *Our Common Future* (UN, 1988). He also actively participated in primary health care initiatives in Central America and in empowering nurses and midwives to communicate more effectively—includ-ing through UN NGO channels—concerning the rural and urban determinants of health (W.L. Kines, personal communication, June 10, 2016; NIGH, 2016a).

The 1990s Decade of UN Summits: Focus on Key Issues

Although UN CESI was later dismantled by a shift in political priorities of UN Secretary-General Kurt Waldheim, NGO collaboration with the UN family of agencies and organizations has continued to grow and has been further strength-ened by NGO participants themselves (Ruhlman, 2014). Throughout the 1990s, a coordinated series of UN summits created increasing global awareness, participa-tion, and concern for key economic, social, and environmental issues (Emmerij, Jolly, & Weiss, 2001). Most newsworthy of these was the Earth Summit convened in Rio de Janieiro in 1992, as a 20-year follow-up to the 1972 Stockholm UN CHE. The Women's Summit in Beijing in 1995—and other summits focused on Children (New York, 1990); Human Rights (Vienna, 1993); Population (Cairo, 1995); and on Social Development (Copenhagen, 1995; UN, 2016g)—also stand as evidence of this vital trend.

As with the milestone Stockholm Conference, these thematic global summits were officially attended by many UN Member heads of state and government offi-cials addressing these specific topics. However, the follow-up of national govern-ments, committed to agreed-upon aims, has not always been effective. But the already thriving global civil society of affiliated UN NGOs was more actively preparing thousands of delegates to participate in these events. NGOs did fol-low through with renewed advocacy, even with public demonstrations, to increase greater awareness and action for the social, economic, and environmental causes they served (Ubuntu Forum Secretariat, 2009).

NIGHTINGALE AS GLOBAL ADVOCATE AND LEADER

First-Ever UN Summit "Tribute to Florence Nightingale"

Near the last of these global events was the UN Conference on Human Settlements, referred to as "Habitat II," convened in Istanbul in 1996 (United Nations Human Settlements Programme [UNHSP], 2016). It was at this conference that I came to actively participate, as a nurse and an officially attending UN NGO, and to begin research on the work of Florence Nightingale as a significant nursing activist and advocate for economic, environmental, and social causes at global levels. Starting in the early 1990s, while still practicing in critical care settings in Washington, D.C., I had become increasingly interested in learning more about and participating in global civil society activities (Beck, 2013). After attending several related 1995 NGO conferences at the Group of 7 (G-7) economic summit in Halifax, Canada, and at the World Bank, I coestablished a pilot program called "Wellness Dynamics" to introduce the global connections between health and related issues of economics, environment, education, society, and culture. Based on this work, I was encouraged to present this program at the UN headquarters in New York City for the final preparatory committee before the Istanbul Habitat II conference. While in New York, I was then invited to cohost several related meetings to be convened during that conference's international NGO forum and granted special conference-related UN NGO status to do so.

At the UN headquarters, Wayne Kines happened to be attending a study session on UN reform. As previously noted, Mr. Kines had already developed many innovative approaches to enlist world media in the mobilization of public opinion around UN causes and also to proactively engage UN NGOs. Upon meeting, he mentioned to me, as a nurse, that Florence Nightingale had begun her famous Crimean War nursing career in Istanbul (when it was Constantinople) and that the Scutari barracks hospital where she worked remained standing (Dossey, 2010). He suggested that a special NGO UN International Tribute to Florence Nightingale might be convened at this site during the upcoming Habitat II conference. Two weeks later, this suggestion was confirmed to be an official event; the proceedings would also involve leading Turkish nurses and nursing educators from the Turkish Red Crescent Society and the Florence Nightingale School of Nursing at Istanbul University (Beck, 2013, 2016).

My direct involvement in this project prompted me to look more closely at the significance of Nightingale's life. I asked myself, beyond Nightingale's service as a nurse for war-wounded and dying soldiers and her subsequent contribution to modern nursing education, did her life have any relevance to the concerned global civil society of the late 20th century? Would Nightingale's insights have relevance to a UN summit focused on "quality of life" wherever people live in "human habitats"? What would she have urged us, as aspiring world citizens, to do to make a difference regarding the many global challenges confronting the emerging 21st century? (Beck, 1996).

Following Nightingale's early nursing work in Turkey, she did indeed continue to focus, for four more decades, on the critical multifactorial global health issues of her time. She actually shifted political will by interacting with government leaders across the British Empire and beyond. She focused on the environments of both rural and urban peoples to improve health through active advocacy for better living conditions for women, children, and the poor. She collaborated with the media, while also broadly networking through written correspondence, with numerous friends, contacts, and colleagues around the world. In essence, Nightingale became fully functioning as a one-woman NGO, demonstrating the kind of activism and advocacy UN NGOs seek to achieve today (Beck, 2005).

At the UN's International Tribute to Nightingale at Scutari, convened months later at the UN Human Settlements summit in Istanbul (NIGH, 2016b), I spoke to the audience, envisioning emerging "global nursing" work and a new level of nursing collaborations that would soon evolve. "Nightingale saw 19th century problems and created 20th century solutions. We see 20th century problems and we can create 21st century solutions. That's why we are here today" (Beck, 1996).

Remembering Nightingale's Powerful Public Voice

By 1999, I had joined two other Nightingale scholars, Dr. Barbara Dossey and Dr. Louise Selanders, and met with them for the first time in London, at the centennial celebration of ICN's founding. We shared a realization, as well, that the centennial of Nightingale's death would be forthcoming in the year 2010. We agreed to act together and to encourage others to stage local celebrations worldwide, recognizing Nightingale's relevance to the new century at the 2000 millennium (NIGH, 2016c).

Seeking a fresh outlook on the Nightingale story, we focused on her specific work to establish worldwide networks and communications strategies—comprising her 14,000 letters and 200-plus official reports and books, which still exist today in text collections around the world. Her *Notes on Nursing: What It Is and What It Is Not* (Nightingale, 1860) was first written for public readership and became an immediate bestseller upon first printing. Only later was a revision of this text recognized as the first modern nursing textbook (Dossey, 2010).

Nightingale, while writing her own articles to submit to newspapers and magazines, was also consciously cultivating connections with media professionals of her time, ensuring that they understood, communicated, and shared her messages. She developed and refined her own media skills to impact public awareness, actively promoting health as a worldwide priority (Beck, 2010). Much in keeping with and anticipating the previously noted 1969 UN Resolution on the Mobilization of Public Opinion and the public global advocacy work of UN NGOs of our time, Nightingale used the media tools of her day to stimulate action for needed changes at national and international levels.

Dr. Dossey specifically addressed the significance of Nightingale's media skills the first time a service commemorating Nightingale was convened at the National Cathedral in Washington, D.C., in 2001, asking the audience to consider, "What would Nightingale have done with a fax machine, email, and the Internet?" (B. Dossey, personal communication, August 12, 2001).

NIGH and the *Nightingale Declaration for a Healthy World*

By the year 2003, Dr. Dossey, Dr. Selanders, and I addressed this question in an innovative manner, presenting our Nightingale research in Toronto at the 37th Biennial Convention of the Honor Society of Nursing, Sigma Theta Tau International (STTI). We, along with Dr. Larry Dossey, were hosted for dinner at the Royal Canadian Military Institute (RCMI), where nurses, who had followed Nightingale's Crimean War example by serving in both World Wars, were specifically remembered. Our RCMI host was Wayne Kines, and the conversation focused on how best to prepare for a Nightingale Centennial in 2010 (NIGH, 2016d).

Based on his own global media and NGO experience, Mr. Kines suggested that we begin by crafting a *Nightingale Declaration for a Healthy World*, with an opening text purposefully written to mirror the first words of the UN's founding charter, "We the peoples . . ." (see Figure 3.1). By recalling Nightingale's own exemplary work to communicate her concerns worldwide, the *Nightingale Declaration for a*

| Figure 3.1 | Nightingale Declaration for a Healthy World. |

"We the nurses and concerned citizens of the global community, hereby dedicate ourselves to achieve a healthy world.

We declare our willingness to unite in a program of action, to share information and solutions, and to improve health conditions for all humanity—locally, nationally and globally.

We further resolve to adopt personal practices and to implement public policies in our communities and nations

—making this goal achievable and inevitable, beginning today in our own lives, in the life of our nations, and in the world at large."

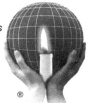

Please sign this *Declaration* @ www.nighvision.net/nightingale-declaration.html

Healthy World was thus written to emphasize shared nursing goals and purposes to address global needs. Its text encourages all nurses and all concerned citizens to commit to their own emerging individual and collective global advocacy—to call for the achievement of a healthy world, together and each in his or her own way (Dossey, Beck, & Rushton, 2011; NIGH, 2016e).

This shared commitment soon became the focal text for launching a Nightingale Declaration Campaign to gather collaborative support for celebrating the 2010 Nightingale centennial as the International Year of the Nurse. Thus it became an online declaration of more than 22,000 nurses, midwives, and concerned citizens from 106 nations. These included 1,000 leaders who signed on behalf of nursing groups totaling more than 3 million people (NIGH, 2016e).

Encouraged by all of this global activity, the authors of the *Nightingale Declaration* founded the Nightingale Initiative for Global Health, often called "NIGH"—an NGO formally registered in Washington, D.C. as NIGH USA, also incorporated in Canada as NIGH World (Beck, Dossey, & Rushton, 2013). Both founding documents reflect NIGH's unique twin mandate—to increase public awareness and concern for global health issues and to inform, engage, and empower nurses' and concerned citizens' participation in this grassroots-to-global NGO advocacy.

ESTABLISHING UN MILLENNIUM DEVELOPMENT GOALS

Meanwhile, global leaders were expressing renewed commitment to UN mandates, building on decades of work to attain interrelated social, economic, and environmental targets essential for a better world. The bellwether UN Millennium Summit, convened in New York City, adopted eight milestone Millennium Development Goals (MDGs) endorsed by the UN General Assembly in the year 2000 (see Chapter 2 for a complete list of the MDGs).

Of these eight MDGs, three were directly related to health and nursing—MDG 4: "Reduce Child Mortality," MDG 5: "Improve Maternal Health," and MDG 6: "Combat HIV/AIDS, TB, Malaria and Other Diseases." The remaining Goals, related to poverty and hunger, education, gender equality and empowerment, environmental sustainability, and global partnerships, are key factors as "health determinants." One or more specific targets for each MDG were set to be achieved across a specific timeframe, by the year 2015 (UN, 2011).

Overseen by the UN Development Programme (UNDP)—established in 1966 and headquartered in Manhattan—achievement of the MDGs was to become an unprecedented strength of focus from the UNDP offices directed principally from New York (UNDP, 2016). Thus, ratifying these MDGs, and focusing their outcomes from New York, would also establish a geographical challenge for many UN NGOs, specifically those working outside the United States, on achievement and advocacy for many of these goals.

Most of the eight MDGs were initiatives specifically associated with UN agencies based in other parts of the world. For example, MDG 3, "Achieve Universal Primary Education," was the focus of the UN Educational, Scientific and Cultural Organization (UNESCO), sited in Paris in 1945 (UNESCO, 2016). MDG 7, "Ensure Environmental Sustainability," was the focus of UNEP, founded in Nairobi, Kenya, in 1972 (Ruhlman, 2014).

Also, many UN NGOs, working on advocacy for these causes such as education and the environment, have long-established operational offices near UN agencies and programs related to these topics, located at distances from New York—that made it inconvenient for them to collaborate, in person, with UNDP and the UN headquarters.

This geographical challenge was particularly true for UN NGOs working on advocacy for the three MDGs focused on health. For instance, the ICN, for more than 50 years, had contributed their considerable health and nursing achievements and advocacy from their base in Geneva, Switzerland, near the WHO. In the year 2000, globally focused nursing leaders were those based in Geneva—rather than in New York—and less able to collaborate with the UN in achieving and advocating for the MDGs.

NIGH AND THE UNITED NATIONS

Establishing NIGH's Emerging UN Collaborations

In recognizing this geographical factor, NIGH has sought ways to have nursing leaders communicating, directly from the grassroots, to share their concerns and experience with all components in uniting to achieve the MDGs.

As NIGH was being established in the mid-2000s, its work focused on preparing for the 2010 Nightingale centennial. In early consultations with like-minded nursing organizations, we explored the idea of honoring Nightingale with a UN resolution naming 2010 as the International Year of the Nurse. Thus, NIGH's entire founding team began to build consensus for celebrating the 2010 International

Year of the Nurse and to strengthen this intention, through formal and informal meetings and presentations convened around the world, to propose such a UN resolution.

In Mumbai, one notable event occurred in celebrating the 100th anniversary of India's national nursing organization, the Trained Nurses Association of India (TNAI), whose headquarters in New Delhi are sited on a street named Florence Nightingale Lane (TNAI, 2016). While in Mumbai, I was invited to represent NIGH and speak to an audience of thousands. It was at this celebration that I also met, for the first time, with Phalakshi Manjrekar, who had already taken the lead to circulate the *Nightingale Declaration for a Healthy World* to nurses across India (NIGH, 2016f). Since then, Ms. Manjrekar has been actively serving on NIGH's development team and on NIGH World Board of Directors' Executive Committee guiding NIGH's growth. She is also a leading voice calling for the increased support and appreciation of India's nurses and their needs, and in the context of global nursing advocacy and public awareness (Manjrekar, 2016; NIGH, 2016g).

In the United States, NIGH cohosted a second Nightingale Tribute Service at the National Cathedral in Washington, D.C., in 2004. Exemplary nurse recipients of International Red Cross Florence Nightingale Medals were honored and two global nursing leaders were featured as keynote speakers: Dr. Rita Carthy, then Secretary-General of the Global Network of WHO Collaborating Centres for Nursing and Midwifery, and Dr. Daniel Pesut, then President of STTI (NIGH, 2016d).

During this period, I was invited to serve as rapporteur for the 2006 WHO Global Forum for Government Chief Nursing and Midwifery Officers in Geneva (WHO, 2006), where I also met and networked with the nursing leaders serving as WHO regional nursing officers for the six WHO regional headquarters in Brazzaville (in Africa), Cairo, Copenhagen, Manila, New Delhi, and Washington, D.C. I was privileged also to meet with nursing educators, serving as leaders at university schools of nursing, who have worked to build the growing Global Network of WHO Collaborating Centres for Nursing and Midwifery.

During that visit to WHO, Mr. Kines and I also met with WHO librarian Tomas Allen. Along with WHO archivist Marie Villemin, they arranged to give us access to the WHO's extensive historic photo archives featuring nurses and midwives around the world. I have since been able to creatively utilize these images in several of NIGH's multimedia presentations. First, in 2007, I shared a brief photo essay at a WHO regional meeting of nurses and midwives in Lusaka, Zambia. This led to then WHO Chief Nursing Officer Dr. Jean Yan inviting me to collaborate with a selected global nursing Task Force and to coproduce a video, featuring these historical images, to celebrate WHO's 60th Anniversary in 2008. *Nurses & Midwives: Now More Than Ever for a Healthy World!* was thus premiered at a WHO Regional meeting in China and then showcased at related conferences in Africa, Europe, North, and South America. In keeping with NIGH's mandate to increase global public awareness and engage nurses in this advocacy, this video remains available, online, in English, plus seven other language versions translated by nursing and health leaders based in Brazil, China, Jordan, Russian Federation, Switzerland, Turkey, and the United States (NIGH, 2016h).

NIGH at the United Nations

Based on NIGH's early approaches to increase public awareness of UN global man-dates and missions, we were awarded UN DPI-NGO status in 2009. We have since been fully utilizing this designation in leading-edge ways, as is explained further in the following text. By then, in 2009 and 2010, CoNGO's Cyril Ritchie had joined NIGH World board of directors and invited Mr. Kines and me to serve, as NIGH representatives, presenting at two UN Civil Society Development Forums. These and other NIGH initiatives, for the UN ECOSOC high-level Annual Ministerial Reviews, were convened in those years. In 2009, we presented in Geneva on panels specific to global health, and in 2010, we presented in New York City for panels focused on women's issues and gender equity. During that same time, Dr. Barbara Dossey joined us as three of NIGH's first official UN DPI-NGO representatives, giving voice to the capacity and commitment of nurses and midwives worldwide. We were invited to meet with then President of the UN General Assembly, Miguel d'Escoto Brockmann, who shared our concerns and urged us to continue. We also served as official observers at the UN ECOSOC high-level Annual Ministerial Review convened in the summer of 2010, again, in New York City. At that meeting, we networked with officials for the corporate role of nurses and midwives to be named, in ECOSOC documents, as essential to achieving the health-related MDGs (NIGH, 2016i).

Convening Meetings at and Near UN Headquarters

During those early years, with an aim to learn how to work more closely with the UN, and to discover if a UN resolution for the 2010 International Year of the Nurse was a feasible request, NIGH also convened meetings of its leadership team and related advisors both on-site and near UN headquarters in New York City. These meetings were hosted by then UN staffer Dr. Monica Sharma (NIGH, 2016e). One attendee of these meetings was Dr. Karen Morin, then serving on the board of STTI and soon to be president (2009–2011; NIGH, 2016f; see Chapter 5 for Dr. Morin's perspectives regarding global nurse leadership). Learning that NGOs could estab-lish closer official collaborative ties with the UN—as described earlier—Dr. Morin built upon what she learned at these early meetings to subsequently establish STTI's UN DPI-NGO status during her presidency and to pave the way for STTI's nursing presence at the UN, subsequently developing STTI's achievement of UN ECOSOC consultative status in 2012. These efforts have brought stronger and more meaningful UN collaborative potential to STTI's global membership of more than 135,000 nurse leaders (STTI, 2016; Wilson et al., 2016).

Determined to request a UN resolution for the 2010 International Year of the Nurse at the highest possible levels, NIGH's team focused this "task" with several leading UN ambassadors in Geneva and New York, as well as with leaders at UN ECOSOC and UN DESA. But advised that this resolution strategy was no longer popular at the UN General Assembly (it had become overused during numerous UN General Assembly sessions prior to this request), NIGH's team was prompted, instead, to establish an innovative strategy that would dramatically change the course of nursing's participation in achieving and advocating for UN mandates.

During our meeting with a lead UN DESA administrator, Nikhil Seth, he commended NIGH's UN NGO-DPI role and mandate to increase global public concern for UN issues. To build on what we were already achieving, Mr. Seth recommended that we—Mr. Kines, Dr. Dossey, and I—"turn the tables." Instead of asking the UN to honor nurses with a UN General Assembly resolution, Mr. Seth invited NIGH to take the global lead in assisting the UN to increase public awareness about the significance of achieving the UN MDGs. This included the goal most likely to fail in its specified targets—MDG 5: "Improve Maternal Health." Mr. Seth reasoned that nurses and midwives are the key experts who continually struggle to achieve infant and maternal health in marginalized and rural regions of the world. He encouraged NIGH's team to consider focusing on advocacy for UN MDGs because, as he noted, "If the nurses and midwives of the world cannot become the lead advocates for global goals related to health—especially the health of women, girls and vulnerable infants—who can and who will?" (N. Seth, personal communication, June 25, 2009).

Advocating for the UN MDGs—the 2010 International Year of the Nurse

With this strong encouragement from official leadership inside the UN, NIGH's team followed up to consult with other nursing leaders, some of whom were completing final joint preparations for celebrating the 2010 International Year of the Nurse/Nightingale Centennial, thus honoring Nikhil Seth's recommendation. It was thus established that the "2010 IYNurse"—as it became known—would become a global advocacy strategy to raise awareness among nurses and concerned citizens worldwide and to promote and champion the achievement of all eight UN MDGs (NIGH, 2016j).

To further achieve these ends, NIGH collaborated with *Nursing Spectrum* and *NurseWeek,* of Gannett Publishers, to bring coverage of the 2010 Year, and related webinars, to its 750,000 readers. NIGH's team also cosponsored with STTI the Florence Nightingale Centennial Commemorative Global Service Celebrating Nursing, convened, once again, at the National Cathedral in Washington D.C. In April of 2010, nurses and leaders from across the United States filled this cathedral to overflowing, inspired and informed by nurses who also participated from many parts of the world. During the half hour prior to this service, a series of high-resolution photographs illustrating the eight MDGs was featured on large screens mounted high above both sides of the altar. In ceremony, during this "Evensong" event, the opening and closing featured eight large banners displaying each MDG logo, carried in procession by nursing dignitaries, in the center aisle. Nurses from across the United States regard this event as transformative in the recognition and elaboration of nursing's role in the MDGs and global health and nursing. The five-camera webcast of this event and its keepsake leaflet, featuring the historic Nightingale stained glass window prominent in the cathedral, are still displayed on NIGH's website (NIGH, 2016k).

NIGH's team of presenters were also featured speakers at 2010 events convened across Canada, and in the United States, the United Kingdom, Asia, Africa, and Europe. Further collaborating with STTI, NIGH cosponsored, with STTI's web hosting, a yearlong virtual online celebration at 2010IYNurse.net. (NIGH, 2016j). While live online, this website focused on telling stories about nurses and midwives who were achieving all eight UN MDGs.

During the UN's own MDGs summit convened in New York City in September of 2010, NIGH's team cohosted, with CoNGO, a related *Raise Your Voice* concert, featuring prominent musicians performing at Lincoln Center, to increase aware-ness among the UN delegates attending this summit. Here, a young pianist Shun Yang Lee, studying at the prestigious Bard College Conservatory of Music and also serving CoNGO at its New York office, extended his volunteer work to share his keyboard artistry. Images portraying the MDGs were displayed on a large screen above the grand piano as he performed (NIGH, 2016l). In addition, one of NIGH World's artistic advisors, Maria Knapik, a Polish Canadian operatic soprano, came to New York City with her accompanist Michel Brousseau. Together, they contrib-uted music that "cried" for the plight of people suffering from humanitarian trag-edies highlighted by the MDGs. To address MDG 3—concern for the human rights of women and girls—Maria Knapik sang an aria from Puccini's opera *Tosca*, whose tragic story depicts how women can suffer deeply at the hands of cruel tyrants. To address MDGs 4 and 5—concern for the health of children and mothers—Maria performed a "Lullaby for a Dying Child" from the Polish opera *Halka*. This solo later served as a soundtrack for one of NIGH's online videos, accentuating con-cern for the untimely deaths and suffering of pregnant women and girls and their infants (NIGH, 2016m).

NIGH World also cosponsored 2010 Nightingale events in Canada at national and regional nursing conferences in Toronto and Quebec City and at Anglican, Baptist, and Presbyterian churches across the province of Ontario, including at the governor-general's home church (St. Bartholomew's) in Ottawa. On this latter site, also, Canadian nursing history is continuously honored through display of the Victorian Order of Nurses (VON), established in 1897 by Lady Ishbel Aberdeen, wife of Canada's governor-general from 1893 to 1898. Lady Aberdeen was a close friend and confidant of Florence Nightingale. She deeply understood Nightingale's desire to focus on achieving health through visiting nurses serving on-site at local and "district" levels and advocating concern for the multifactorial determinants of community health (The Governor-General of Canada, 2016; VON, 2016).

During all of these 2010-focused conferences, presentations, meetings, events, articles, and online postings, NIGH's teams focused their mandate, as UN DPI NGOs, to identify and strengthen the connections between the achievements of the world's nurses and midwives and the Goals of the UN, using key messages and multimedia strategies to widely understand and appreciate the value of UN MDGs and the importance of achieving these Goals worldwide. These 2010 proj-ects achieved considerable public appreciation for nurses, and within nurses' ranks, around the globe. These also raised awareness that key UN MDGs still greatly needed worldwide advocacy work, particularly for the goals connected to health and nursing—MDGs 4, 5, and 6—representing billions still at risk.

Daring, Caring, and Sharing as Advocacy for UN MDG 5

Advocacy needs were especially true for the MDG most specific to nursing and midwifery, MDG 5, "To Improve Maternal Health." While the global ratio of mater-nal deaths has declined by 47% since 1990, more than 700 women and girls still die in pregnancy and childbirth each day. This means that one mother still perishes, on average, every 2 minutes—a shocking 280,000 each year. Despite the worldwide challenges of identifying and advocating for the UN MDGs, these continuing trag-edies still require increased public attention and accelerated local intervention, as well as greater social and political support for women and children (WHO, 2014).

And, as nurses know, these actions must include strategies to strengthen health care delivery, particularly the services of nurses and midwives in rural and marginalized areas (WHO, 2015).

Thus, NIGH's team is always asking, "How would Nightingale have dealt with these concerns?" In fact, she acted and advocated for approaches that included more and better training for birth attendants, as well as education for young women and girls about their own reproductive health. Her answers and action would also mobilize public opinion, raise awareness of such needs, and increase commitment to improved health outcomes worldwide.

Starting in 2012, through 2014, NIGH's team thus worked on advocating for greater global achievement of UN MDG 5 by mounting a campaign for "Daring, Caring & Sharing to Save Mothers' Lives" to increase public awareness—engaging nurses and midwives in daring and caring to share stories that could turn the prevailing tide from apathy to action. In Manhattan, at St. Bart's Episcopal Church on Park Avenue, and sited close to the UN, leading nurse educators and students, who served in and around the city, gathered to launch this campaign. Speakers and ceremony focused on telling this oft-untold story and championed the needs and deeds of those nurses and midwives who are already making a difference to maternal health worldwide. Over the next 24 months, this campaign's online postings and social media outreach online analytics totaled 3.5 million recorded hits from more than 90,000 unique visitors online in 146 nations (NIGH, 2016n).

ONE NURSE MAKING A DIFFERENCE: A CASE STUDY

Holly K. Shaw, PhD, RN, is an associate professor at Adelphi University College of Nursing and Public Health in Garden City, New York, where she became the first nursing faculty member to serve as this university's UN DPI-NGO representative. She also serves as an advanced practice clinical nurse specialist with expertise in crisis, bereavement, and trauma, including refugee trauma, recovery, and global postconflict intervention. As a nurse, Dr. Shaw began to bring nursing's voice and insights to the meetings she attended, on Adelphi's behalf, at UN headquarters. Participating in weekly DPI-NGO briefings, she also facilitated nurses, faculty, and students to be present at the UN and to engage in various campaigns, events, and activities. Since her earliest experiences at the UN, she sought to develop an advocacy role for nurses, worldwide, within the UN family (see Chapter 4 for more on Dr. Shaw's perspectives regarding global nurse citizenship).

In 2009, as STTI's first UN NGO representative, Dr. Shaw connected with NIGH and developed teams of graduate and undergraduate students and faculty to visit UN ambassadors and their staffs to brief these dignitaries about nursing's global advocacy for UN MDGs through the 2010 International Year of the Nurse/ Nightingale Centennial. In 2010 and 2011, she also presented nursing's voice, on NIGH's behalf, at the 63rd International UN DPI-NGO Conference in Melbourne, Australia—as a speaker on an official panel hosted by CoNGO. She also participated in the 64th International UN DPI-NGO Conference in Bonn, Germany (H.K. Shaw, personal communication, September 1, 2011).

In 2012, Dr. Shaw further collaborated with NIGH's team to bring her students to the New York launch of the previously mentioned Daring, Caring & Sharing to Save Mothers' Lives campaign and introduced me to leaders and members of STTI's Eastern New York/New Jersey Region 14. This meeting established the opportunity for two young nurse leaders, Gloria Chan and Hitesh Jani, to serve as NIGH's first UN DPI-NGO youth representatives.

Starting in 2013, Dr. Shaw began serving as NIGH's primary UN DPI-NGO representative, continuing and expanding her nursing advocacy to a wider range of health issues at UN briefings and NGO committee meetings. As NIGH's representative, she was also elected to serve for two terms (4 years) as a director on the executive committee of UN DPI NGOs, collaborating with staff at the UN DPI sited within the complex UN world in New York City. In this leadership role, Dr. Shaw also participated in the planning, preparation, and implementation of the 65th UN DPI-NGO Conference in New York City and the 66th UN DPI-NGO Conference in Gyeongju, Republic of Korea (H.K. Shaw, personal communication, September 1, 2013).

In addition, Dr. Shaw has assumed other elected and appointed leadership positions, serving as an exemplar of the knowledge, expertise, and commitment of nurses worldwide, following in Nightingale's tradition of advocacy for the good of humanity. She participates in the UN Academic Impact (UNAI), a special project of UN Secretary-General Ban Ki Moon. She also provides policy development consultation for the Committee on Teaching About the United Nations (CTAUN) and recruits nursing volunteers to serve on the ground at annual CTAUN conferences. In addition to membership on many UN NGO Committees, Dr. Shaw currently serves as vice-chair of the NGO Committee on Mental Health. From these several vantages, she has provided consultation, expertise, and resources to inform and involve nurses and concerned citizens in UN mandates, also designing, planning, and producing "United Nations Day" events that bring nurses, students, and faculty to the UN headquarters for private tours and briefings to become familiar with UN operative mandates. More than 500 nurses have already participated in these on-site UN programs (H.K. Shaw, personal communication, December 1, 2015).

Tapping these experiences, Dr. Shaw also serves as an ongoing mentor for six successive NIGH DPI-NGO youth representative nurses, further collaborating with Gloria Chan, who, at this writing, also serves as NIGH's UN DPI-NGO representative and as regional coordinator of STTI Region 14 (NIGH, 2016o).

THE UN POST-2015 AGENDA

During this same time, between 2012 and 2014, the overall UN family recognized that although the MDG framework had raised awareness of global advances and increased concern and support for further development, the limited MDG timeframe of only 15 years (2000–2015) was not sufficient to achieve all of the MDG targets.

Thus, the challenge, addressed at the UN Rio+20 summit in 2012, was to devise a fresh plan that would identify and establish a new set of global aims, the Sustainable Development Goals (SDGs), set to be achieved by 2030 (see Introduction for the full list of the 17 SDGs). In addition, to determine what these new SDGs would be, a Post-2015 Agenda was created to encourage global discussions. This agenda reached beyond the limits of UN Member government debates to include participants from global civil society—NGOs, philanthropic organizations, academia, and the private sector (UNDP, 2015).

One of the strategies used to achieve this agenda was a timely UN survey posted and promoted online as "The World We Want". This outreach was developed to increase global civil society interests, input, and dialogue to span the final years of advocacy to achieve the MDGs by 2015 and to gather ideas, from around the world, to better define and determine what the new UN SDGs would need to become.

THE CONTINUED EVOLUTION OF NURSING'S INVOLVEMENT

Getting the UN's Call for Dialogue to the World of Nurses

As all these activities unfolded, the team of nurses participating at the UN headquarters was also evolving. Dr. Shaw, Ms. Chan, and NIGH's then-youth representative David "DJ" Schnabel also collaborated with Raizza Sanchez and Tim Shi, STTI's UN NGO youth representatives. Together, this group of NIGH and STTI reps attended UN briefings and served as volunteers at annual CTAUN and other conferences.

However, this team was not satisfied with simply attending these briefings and meetings as a privileged few. Noting the UN's mandate to generate global civil society discussions beyond such meetings, these nurses wanted to share their briefings more widely with others. As they learned increasingly about the UN and its activities at the Secretariat headquarters in New York—and the working operations of the UN family worldwide—they became determined to establish ways of extending their knowledge to reach nursing colleagues in towns and cities throughout all nations and the world.

Dr. Shaw and I collaborated with this team in April 2014 to convene an all-day workshop, hosted at the New York University Langone Hospital and cosponsored by the STTI Region 14, to familiarize nurses with their relevance to global health issues—specifically to the UN MDGs and to the UN itself. More than 100 nurses and student nurses attended this event. Subsequently, these workshop organizers created a website specific to this increased interest in order to further this work and incorporate the enthusiastic feedback received (NIGH, 2016o).

Then, in response to the UN outreach already mentioned, NIGH's and STTI's UN NGO reps recognized that all nurses—indeed, all nursing activists in global civil society across the world—could also be included in the UN's online dialogue within the Post-2015 Agenda. Hence, this team decided to contribute to "The World We Want" by creating a parallel interactive project called "The World Nurses Want". This plan quickly evolved into creating an online Global Briefing, introducing nurses everywhere to the workings of the UN, to nursing's specific relevance to the UN MDGs, and also to encourage online participation in the UN's "The World We Want" surveys (NIGH, 2016p).

Building on this project and sharing it as an innovative model to increase advocacy for UN mandates, STTI's Raissa Sanchez and Tim Shi and NIGH's Gloria Chan and 'DJ' Schnabel joined Dr. Shaw and me to cohost an official panel presentation themed "The World Nurses Want". This was featured at the 66th International NGO Conference convened at the UN headquarters in New York City (NIGH, 2016p). This opportunity blossomed into further presentations at nearby hospitals and universities, at two STTI International Research Conferences in Hong Kong and Puerto Rico, and at hospitals and related meetings in Shanghai, Singapore, and Cambodia. These presentations were historic in that entry-level nurses, in their first years of professional practice, presented to this elite audience of global nurse leaders (NIGH, 2016q).

Nurses and the UN Commission on the Status of Women

Founded in 1946 and established within UN ECOSOC, the Commission on the Status of Women (CSW) is the UN's principal global body dedicated exclusively to the promotion of gender equality and the empowerment of women and girls. The CSW promotes women's rights, documents the reality of women's lives through-out the world, and shapes global standards on gender equality and the empower-ment of women (UN Women, 2016b). These concerns are also aligned with issues nurses address every day on behalf of patients and within their own ranks, careers, and personal lives.

By UN General Assembly mandate, the CSW convenes an annual 2-week conference, where representatives of UN Member States, NGOs, and UN enti-ties gather at the UN headquarters in New York. Selected NGOs bring updates on long-term issues and recommendations for improvement while UN Member States agree on further actions to accelerate progress and promote women's rights in political, economic, and social fields. The outcomes and recommendations of each session are forwarded to ECOSOC for follow-up (UN Women, 2016b).

In 2015, a milestone was achieved by highlighting the contributions of nurses at this conference. Both NIGH and STTI were awarded the prestigious opportunity to host Parallel Panels at the 59th UN CSW. NIGH's Panel featured the work of Dr. Judith Shamian, ICN's current president, and cohosted a gala reception hon-oring Dr. Shamian during that CSW (NIGH, 2016r; see Chapter 10 for additional information on human resources for health, universal health coverage, and the Sustainable Development Agenda, as discussed by Dr. Shamian and colleagues). STTI's Panel featured ICN's then-CEO David Benton. This was the first time such high-ranking officials from the ICN were featured at the UN in New York City. NIGH's Panel addressed an audience of over 100, featured an introduction to the UN and global nurses' initiatives by Dr. Shaw, and also highlighted a presentation about the status of Indian women and nurses by NIGH board member Phalakshi Manjrekar (NIGH, 2016g). NIGH advisor Heather Maurer introduced the lead-ing-edge work of nurses and midwives at Mother Health International, an NGO establishing safer pregnancy on the remote border of Uganda and South Sudan (MHI, 2016). Dr. Debra Anderson also presented her innovative work achieved, with her colleagues, on global research in cardiology and women's health (Anderson, 2016).

In 2016, NIGH and STTI again hosted official CSW Parallel Sessions. These included the work of Dr. Anderson and her colleagues' cross-cultural findings, from more than 40,000 women, about the risk and protective factors related to reproductive life cycles and cardiovascular health. Another Panel presentation introduced a unique replicable model of collaboration between UN NGO nurse activists and a metropolitan medical center where Dr. Kelly Reilly, director of Nursing Research, Education, and Innovation at Maimonides Medical Center, led nurse leaders to establish changes in nursing practice based on knowledge gained from UN briefings and to develop a standing global health committee to pursue this topic further. In addition, Dr. Cynthia Stuhlmiller presented her work on a student-led health and well-being clinic for an underserved community in Australia (NIGH, 2016s; Stuhmiller & Tolchard, 2015).

Advocating to Achieve the 17 SDGs

With the last months of 2015 passing, the long-awaited MDGs timeline drew to a close. The Post-2015 Agenda, having fostered considerable global debate and dialogue about what to do next, advanced recommendations arising from the 70th session of the UN General Assembly. Therein, 193 UN Member States unanimously ratified the 17 new SDGs to be achieved within 15 years, by 2030. Throughout this book, specific details are developed in 17 chapters devoted to understanding each of these 17 SDGs. The newly adopted Global Goals build upon the many decades of UN agendas, conferences, and collaborative actions as introduced in this chapter. While the MDGs achieved marked improvements in the lives of millions, the world remains with "immense challenges, ranging from widespread poverty, rising inequalities and enormous disparities of opportunity, wealth and power to environmental degradation and the risks posed by climate change." (UN, 2016h).

In addressing these challenges, UN Secretary-General Ban Ki Moon reminded all that the true test of the new SDGs will be the worldwide advocacy and commitments required to implement them.

> We need action from everyone, everywhere. Seventeen Sustainable Development Goals are our guide . . . a to-do list for people and planet and a blueprint for success . . . . an agenda for shared prosperity, peace and partnership [that] conveys the urgency of climate action [and] is rooted in gender equality and respect for the rights of all. Above all, it pledges to leave no one behind. (UN, 2016h. Reprinted with permission.)

Of course, the key UN SDG directly related to nurses is SDG 3, explicitly to "ensure healthy lives and promote well-being for all at all ages" (UN, 2016i). Embedded within this SDG plan is a target identified as Universal Health Coverage (UHC), aimed to "ensure that all people obtain the health services they need without suffering financial hardship when paying for them" (WHO, 2016b).

Anticipating this UHC target, the WHO's Health Workforce Department commissioned me to produce a video featuring the work of nurses and midwives practicing in many environments and addressing the myriad challenges to achieve UHC—*At the Heart of It All*. This video was premiered at the 2014 WHO Global Forum for Government Chief Nursing and Midwifery Officers in Geneva and has since been highlighted at the 2016 Global Forum and shown in student nursing classrooms of WHO Collaborating Centres for Nursing and Midwifery (NIGH, 2016t).

GLOBAL HEALTH—GLOBAL TOOLS AND TASKS

I have often been asked, "How do we practice global nursing?" Here, I return to Florence Nightingale's example. After returning home from her famous achievements during the Crimean War (1854–1856), Nightingale continued for nearly four decades to focus on the global challenges of her time. She analyzed data, wrote statistical reports, and informed politicians, crafting documents that resulted in legislation. She designed hospitals and sought to improve environments in both rural and urban areas, developing collaborative partnerships with others who agreed with her proposed reforms. She met with Queen Victoria, Prince Albert, and other royalty, dignitaries, viceroys, and military officers based in India and from around the world. She changed political will by informing and interacting with government leaders stretching across the worldwide British Empire and beyond (Dossey, 2010).

One of Nightingale's key methods for achieving all this was through her communications skills. She networked constantly through handwritten letters, convened numerous one-on-one briefings, and directly collaborated with media professionals of her time. She also wrote magazine articles herself and was a bestselling author for the general public (Beck, 2010). She called all of these "global" activities "health nursing," broadly defining health as "not only to be well but to use well every power we have" (Nightingale, 1893, p. 289).

Today's nurses are experts in practicing at the hospital bedside. We have a comfort zone within our scope to serve individual patients and their families. Here, we know and identify with our tasks and our tools. But, at the global level, we are not yet widely familiar with the tasks and tools of global health. We have yet to identify protocols to outline a set of global tasks. Nor have we yet identified global tools, such as our familiar syringes and blood pressure cuffs, to deliver health care to the broad scope of humanity. Yet, such a broader scope of nursing practice is emerging beyond our current comfort zones, from UN initiatives and in other global arenas of civil society and continental collaboration (Wilson et al., 2016).

As Nightingale amply demonstrated, global health can be accomplished through determined application of communications at global levels. In the 21st century, the sharing of information is continuing to make a significant impact on the global culture of humanity. To promote health and healthy solutions, nurses can more fully participate in this emerging culture of the global community. Nightingale was a persistently creative and imaginative grassroots-to-global advocate for and about the needs of others, around the world. Sound familiar? Advocacy is traditionally one of nursing's most respected roles. The task of global advocacy is simply a greater widening of our nursing scopes, to share the distinct and unique value of our perspectives and the effectiveness of our practices within a more expansive world. Our global tools are all around us and readily available. These can include communication channels such as websites, radio talk shows, letters to the editor, newspaper human-interest stories, and TV interviews, as well as social media venues such as YouTube. For effective utilization of such media, nurses can be encouraged and trained to become media-skilled health promotion advocates capable of creating, producing, and airing our knowledge relevant to improved health of our communities, our nations, and the whole world.

WHO'S *STRATEGIC DIRECTIONS FOR NURSING AND MIDWIFERY*

The WHO, in September 2015, convened two meetings to strengthen their agenda for nursing and midwifery. The first focused on documenting the rich history of nursing and midwifery involved with WHO to better inform the future of nursing and midwifery, within the context of the multidisciplinary systems of interdependent global health care delivery. The second meeting focused on determining the latest and most relevant strategic directions for nursing and midwifery practice and policy (WHO, 2016c). I was privileged to be one of 45 nursing and midwifery leaders at these meetings, to serve as rapporteur for the first meeting and as a participating observer for the second.

Published in May 2016—at the time of the 60th World Health Assembly in Geneva—the newest *Global Strategic Directions for Strengthening Nursing and Midwifery 2016–2020* is already the principal guiding document for developing these disciplines, worldwide, in all Member States. The foreword of this document notes that the roles of nursing and midwifery "are critical in achieving global mandates such as universal health coverage and the SDGs" (WHO, 2016c, p. 3; see Chapter 2 for the Background, Overview, and Thematic Areas of the WHO's 2016 report).

To achieve these strategic directions, two of this document's themes are fundamental for continuing the involvement of nursing at the UN and in service to our emerging roles in global health, as "global nurses." One of these emerging aims is to "maximize the capacities and potentials of nurses and midwives through intra- and inter-professional collaborative partnerships, education and continuing professional development" (WHO, 2016c, p. 21). Within this mandate, media skills and communications capacities must become a dynamic part of nursing's professional development to impact global health.

A second theme—one that is new to WHO nursing and midwifery publications—is the mobilization of "political will to invest in building effective evidence-based nursing and midwifery workforce development" (WHO, 2016c, p. 23). I ask again, sound familiar? Florence Nightingale invested nearly four decades addressing this very theme, increasing political will by mobilizing public awareness. As a result, she gained a new level of increased public concern for the sick and impoverished people everywhere and sought to identify and remedy the causes of their suffering. Although she faced many barriers, Nightingale stood by her own conviction to advocate for all changes that were necessary. She thereby addressed the global health needs of her time and, indeed, actually anticipated identifying and achieving the UN's 17 SDGs (NIGH, 2016u). In the 1870s, she noted that it would take 150 years for nurses to work in the way she was working to shift public opinion; 150 plus 1870 equals the year 2020!

Today, all nurses can utilize the 17 SDGs as fresh strategic directions, to be our guide. In this chapter, the nurses featured have paved the way for us to consider our roles in global civil society, as NGOs working with the UN across the world, as inheritors of this, our Nightingale legacy. Those referred to here, and others, are demonstrating how nurses can see themselves as global advocates, extending their health and healing worldviews, while also continuing their grassroots actions. Herein, they have revealed distinct global tasks that all nurses can discover and they have begun to establish new roles that each and all can develop. Nurses are, indeed, contributing to the achievement of the aims and mandates established by the UN for the world at large, a collective work contributing to the healthy world community we seek to become, our common future.

WHAT ONE PERSON CAN DO

With every passing day, the world seems smaller and—through mass media's increasing prominence in our lives—global troubles seem much closer to home.

World news headlines almost daily feature an evil "lone wolf" or small clusters of individuals committed to destruction and perpetuating violence upon fellow human beings. This does demonstrate what one or two persons can do to harm and horrify the world.

But we also know that one person such as Florence Nightingale can heal the world, and that small groups of people such as ourselves can change the world (Institute for Intercultural Studies, 2016). Nurses are among these positive people, often ranked among the most respected and trusted professions in the world (Angus Reid Institute, 2016). We each have potential to demonstrate what one person can do. Multiplied by today's estimated 19.3 million nurses and midwives worldwide (WHO, 2011), our potential impact is immense.

This "challenge for change" is reflected in Florence Nightingale's dream for nurses. "May we hope," she said,

> that, when we are dead and gone, leaders will arise who have personally experienced the hard practical work, the difficulties and joys of organizing reforms, and who will lead far beyond anything we have done! High hopes that will not be deceived! (Nightingale, 1893, p. 297)

Ours can become a worldwide advocacy for the health needs of humanity—a most trusted call of care and concern for problems that still need to be solved—a most trusted voice to identify how solutions have been and can be achieved (Dossey, 2016). Nurses have always shared such visions of healing and health with each other. Now, we can and we must also share this vision with everyone seeking to participate in and benefit from a healthy common ground for all humanity through the achievement of the 17 SDGs, planetary health, and beyond.

REFLECTION AND DISCUSSION

- How are the ethical priorities of the UN and those of nursing intertwined?
- What opportunities exist for me to participate in UN initiatives at local and global levels?
- Do I work from the lens of social justice and advocacy role modeled and promoted by Nightingale? Why or why not?
- What are my own "tools" of global health and global nursing?
- Why is a nursing sensibility integral to SDG attainment initiatives worldwide? What unique perspectives do nurses bring to decision-making tables?

REFERENCES

Amnesty International. (2016). We campaign for a world where human rights are enjoyed by all. Retrieved from https://www.amnesty.org/en

Anderson, D. (2016). Why we do what we do: Improving global health one step at a time. Retrieved from http://www.med.monash.edu.au/nursing/academy/docs/danderson-melbourne-presentation-nursing.pdf

Angus Reid Institute. (2016). Nurses, doctors are most respected jobs in Canada, U.S. and Britain. Retrieved from http://angusreid.org/nurses-doctors-are-most-respected-jobs-in-canada-u-s-and-britain

Beck, D.-M. (1996, June 4). In the context of Habitat II: Revisiting Florence Nightingale at Scutari. Keynote address presented at the *International Tribute to Florence Nightingale, United Nations Human Settlements Summit,* Istanbul, Turkey.

Beck, D.-M. (2005). 21st century citizenship for health: "May a better way be opened." In B. M. Dossey, L. Selanders, D.-M. Beck, & A. Attewell (Eds.), *Florence Nightingale today: Healing, leadership, global action* (pp. 177–193). Silver Spring, MD: Nursesbooks.org.

Beck, D.-M. (2010). Remembering Florence Nightingale's panorama: 21st century nursing: At a critical crossroads. *Journal of Holistic Nursing Practice, 28*(4), 291–301.

Beck, D.-M. (2013). Empowering women and girls—empowering nurses: Discovering Florence Nightingale's global citizenship legacy. In S. G. Mijares, A. Rafea, & N. Angha (Eds.), *A force such as the world has never known: Women creating change* (pp. 40–52). Toronto, ON, Canada: Innana Publications.

Beck, D.-M. (2016). Artistic and scientific: Broadening the scope of our 21st-century health advocacy. In W. Rosa (Ed.), *Nurses as leaders: Evolutionary visions of leadership* (pp. 247–263). New York, NY: Springer Publishing.

Beck, D.-M., Dossey, B. M., & Rushton, C. H. (2013). Building the Nightingale initiative for global health—NIGH—Can we engage and empower the public voices of nurses worldwide? *Nursing Science Quarterly, 26*(4), 366–371.

CoNGO. (2016). *Vision, mission and objectives.* Retrieved from http://www.ngocongo.org/who-we-are/vision-mission-and-objectives

Dossey, B. M. (2010). *Florence Nightingale: Mystic, visionary, healer* (Commemorative ed.). Philadelphia, PA: F. A. Davis.

Dossey, B. M. (2016). Integral and whole: Embracing the journey of healing, local to global. In W. Rosa (Ed.), *Nurses as leaders: Evolutionary visions of leadership.* (pp. 61–75). New York, NY: Springer Publishing.

Dossey, B. M., Beck, D.-M., & Rushton, C. H. (2011). Integral nursing and the Nightingale initiative for global health: Florence Nightingale's legacy for the 21st century. *Journal of Integral Theory and Practice, 6*(4), 71–92.

Dossey, B. M., Selanders, L., Beck, D.-M., & Attewell, A. (2005). *Florence Nightingale today: Healing, leadership, global action.* Silver Spring, MD: Nursesbooks.org.

Emmerji, L., Jolly, R., & Weiss, T. J. (2001). *Ahead of the curve? UN ideas and global challenges.* Indianapolis: Indiana University Press.

The Governor General of Canada. (2016). The Earl of Aberdeen 1893–1898. Retrieved from https://www.gg.ca/document.aspx?id=15410&lan=eng

Greenpeace International. (2016). Our story. Retrieved from http://www.greenpeace.org/international/en/about/our-story

Institute for Intercultural Studies. (2016). Frequently asked questions about Mead/Bateson. Retrieved from http://www.interculturalstudies.org/faq.html

International Council of Nurses. (2016). Who we are. Retrieved from http://www.icn.ch/who-we-are/who-we-are

International Federation of Red Cross & Red Crescent Societies. (2016). Who we are. Retrieved from http://www.ifrc.org/en/who-we-are

Keane, J. (2003, November/December). Global civil society? *Foreign Affairs.* Retrieved from https://www.foreignaffairs.com/reviews/capsule-review/2003-11-01/global-civil-society

Manjrekar, P. (2016). Resourceful and unified: Partnering across cultures and worldviews. In W. Rosa (Ed.), *Nurses as leaders: Evolutionary visions of leadership* (pp. 345–358). New York, NY: Springer Publishing.

McDonald, L. (2015). *Florence Nightingale on wars and the war office: Collected works* (Vol. 15, pp. 584–586). Waterloo, ON, Canada: Wilfrid Laurier University Press.

Mother Health International. (2016). With every birth there is a benefit for the world as a whole. Retrieved from http://motherhealth.org

Mwangi, K. (2005). Three decades of NGO activism in international environmental negotiations: Who influences NGOs? In A. Churie-Kallhauge, G. Sjostedt, & E. Corell (Eds.), *Global challenges: Furthering the multilateral process for sustainable development* (pp. 171–183). Saltaire, UK. Greenleaf Publishing.

Nations Encyclopedia. (2016a). Economic and social development—First UN development decade. Retrieved from http://www.nationsencyclopedia.com/United-Nations/Economic-and-Social-Development-FIRST-UN-DEVELOPMENT-DECADE.html

Nations Encyclopedia. (2016b). Economic and social development—Second UN development decade. Retrieved from http://www.nationsencyclopedia.com/United-Nations/Economic-and-Social-Development-SECOND-UN-DEVELOPMENT-DECADE.html

NGO Branch UN Department of Economic and Social Affairs. (2016a). Basic facts about ECOSOC status. Retrieved from http://csonet.org/?menu=100

NGO Branch UN Department of Economic and Social Affairs. (2016b). Introduction to ECOSOC consultative status. Retrieved from http://csonet.org/index.php?menu=30

NGO Global Network. (2016). Definition of NGOs. Retrieved from http://www.ngo.org/ngoinfo/define.html

Nightingale, F. (1860). *Notes on nursing: What it is, and what it is not.* London, UK: Harrison.

Nightingale, F. (1893). Sick-nursing and health-nursing. In B. M. Dossey, L. Selanders, D.-M. Beck, & A. Attewell (Eds.), *Florence Nightingale today: Healing, leadership, global action* (pp. 288–303). Silver Spring, MD: Nursesbooks.org.

Nightingale Initiative for Global Health. (2016a). Wayne Kines, director of communications. Retrieved from http://www.nighvision.net/wayne-kines-director-of-communications.html

Nightingale Initiative for Global Health. (2016b). A United Nations tribute to Florence Nightingale at Scutari barracks. Retrieved from http://www.nighvision.net/nighs-history-mdash-part-1.html

Nightingale Initiative for Global Health. (2016c). How NIGH began? Retrieved from http://www.nighvision.net/how-nigh-began.html

Nightingale Initiative for Global Health. (2016d). NIGH's history: Part 2—Inspire, inform, initiate & involve/1996 to 2006—Shaping the vision. Retrieved from http://www.nighvision.net/nighs-history-mdash-part-2.html

Nightingale Initiative for Global Health. (2016e). Nightingale declaration for a healthy world. Retrieved from http://www.nighvision.net/nightingale-declaration.html

Nightingale Initiative for Global Health. (2016f). NIGH's history: Part 2—Inspire, inform, initiate & involve/2007–2009—Weaving a network. Retrieved from http://www.nighvision.net/nighs-history-mdash-part-2.html

Nightingale Initiative for Global Health. (2016g). Nurses reaching out to the masses: The Indian scenario. Retrieved from http://www.nighvision.net/the-indian-scenario.html

Nightingale Initiative for Global Health. (2016h). Nurses & midwives celebrated via video at WHO's 60th. Retrieved from http://www.nighvision.net/nurses--midwives-at-whos-60th.html

Nightingale Initiative for Global Health. (2016i). How we work. Retrieved from http://www.nighvision.net/how-we-work.html

Nightingale Initiative for Global Health. (2016j). NIGH's history: Part 2—Inspire, inform, initiate & involve/2010 International year of the Nurse/Florence Nightingale centennial. Retrieved from http://www.nighvision.net/nighs-history-mdash-part-2.html

Nightingale Initiative for Global Health. (2016k). Remembering the 2010 International Year of the Nurse/Florence Nightingale Centennial. Retrieved from http://www.nighvision.net/2010-fn-centennial-global-service.html

Nightingale Initiative for Global Health. (2016l). Encore! Pianist highlights the UN MDGs at Lincoln Center in New York City. Retrieved from http://www.nighvision.net/pianist-highlights-un-mdgs.html

Nightingale Initiative for Global Health. (2016m). Crying her song. Retrieved from http://www .nighvision.net/crying-her-song.html

Nightingale Initiative for Global Health. (2016n). Raising awareness for mothers' health—UN MDG # 5. Retrieved from http://www.nighvision.net/raising-awareness-for-mdg-5.html

Nightingale Initiative for Global Health. (2016o). Our team: NIGH's UN DPI NGO Youth Representatives. Retrieved from http://www.nighvision.net/nighs-2014-un-ngo-team .html

Nightingale Initiative for Global Health. (2016p). The world nurses want: Nursing and the United Nations. Retrieved from http://www.nighvision.net/a-global-online-briefing .html

Nightingale Initiative for Global Health. (2016q). NIGH's participation at the United Nations. Retrieved from http://www.nighvision.net/-nighs-united-nations-participation.html

Nightingale Initiative for Global Health. (2016r). ICN's president celebrated at the 2015 UN CSW in New York City! Retrieved from http://www.nighvision.net/icns-president-at-un-csw .html

Nightingale Initiative for Global Health. (2016s). Archives/NIGH Panel Presentation at UN CSW 2016.

Nightingale Initiative for Global Health. (2016t). At the heart of it all: Nurses & midwives for Universal Health Care. Retrieved from http://www.nighvision.net/with-who-mdash-a -video.html

Nightingale Initiative for Global Health. (2016u). NIGH's "2020 vision" & the UN Sustainable Development Goals • SDGs. Retrieved from http://www.nighvision.net/2020-vision --the-un-sdgs.html

Ruhlman, M. (2014). *Who participates in global governance? States, bureaucracies, and NGOs in the United Nations.* Abingdon-on-Thames, UK: Routledge.

Sigma Theta Tau International. (2016). United Nations. Retrieved from http://www .nursingsociety.org/connect-engage/our-global-impact/stti-and-the-united-nations

Stuhmiller, C., & Tolchard, B. (2015). Developing a student-led health and wellbeing clinic in an underserved community: Collaborative learning, health outcomes and cost savings. *BMC Nursing, 14*(1), 32. Retrieved from https://www.researchgate.net/publication/277305374_ Developing_a_student-led_health_and_wellbeing_clinic_in_an_underserved_community _Collaborative_learning_health_outcomes_and_cost_savings

Trained Nurses Association of India. (2016). Homepage. Retrieved from http://www.tnaionline .org

UBUNTU Forum Secretariat. (2009). *Reforming international institutions: Another world is possible.* Abingdon-on-Thames, UK: Routledge.

United Nations. (1988). Report of the world commission on environment and development: Our common future. Retrieved from http://www.un-documents.net/our-common -future.pdf

United Nations. (2011). The millennium development goals report, 2011. Retrieved from http:// www.un.org/millenniumgoals/MDG2011_PRa_EN.pdf

United Nations. (2016a). About the UN. Retrieved from http://www.un.org/en/about-un/ index.html

United Nations. (2016b). History of the United Nations. Retrieved from http://www.un.org/ en/sections/history/history-united-nations

United Nations. (2016c). About DPI. Retrieved from http://www.un.org/en/sections/ department-public-information/about-dpi/index.html

United Nations. (2016d). Consultative status with ECOSOC. Retrieved from http://www .un.org/esa/coordination/ngo/about.htm

United Nations. (2016e). Resolutions adopted by the General Assembly during its twenty-fourth session: Mobilization of public opinion (2567 XXIV). December 13, 1969. Retrieved from http://www.un.org/documents/ga/res/24/ares24.htm

United Nations. (2016f). World conferences: Introduction. Retrieved from http://www.un.org/ geninfo/bp/intro.html

United Nations. (2016g). Historic new sustainable development agenda unanimously adopted by 193 UN Members. Retrieved from http://www.un.org/sustainabledevelopment/blog/2015/09/historic-new-sustainable-development-agenda-unanimously-adopted-by-193-un-members

United Nations. (2016h). The Secretary-General remarks at the summit for the adoption of the post-2015 development agenda. Retrieved from http://www.eg.undp.org/content/egypt/en/home/presscenter/speeches/the-secretary-general----remarks-at-summit-for-the-adoption-of-t.html

United Nations. (2016i). Sustainable Development Goals: 17 goals to transform our world. Retrieved from http://www.un.org/sustainabledevelopment/health

United Nations Centre for Economic and Social Information. (1973). *The case for development; Six studies.* New York, NY: Praeger Publishers.

United Nations Department of Public Information. (2016). Application. Retrieved from https://outreach.un.org/ngorelations/content/application

United Nations Development Programme. (2015). Building the post-2015 development agenda. Retrieved from http://www.undp.org/content/undp/en/home/librarypage/mdg/building-the-post-2015-development-agenda.html

United Nations Development Programme. (2016). Frequently asked questions. Retrieved from http://www.undp.org/content/undp/en/home/operations/about_us/frequently_askedquestions.html

United Nations Economic & Social Council. (2016). About ECOSOC. Retrieved from http://www.un.org/en/ecosoc/about

United Nations Educational, Scientific and Cultural Organization. (2016). Introducing UNESCO. Retrieved from http://en.unesco.org/about-us/introducing-unesco

United Nations High Commissioner for Refugees. (2016). About us. Retrieved from http://www.unhcr.org/about-us.html

United Nations Human Settlements Programme. (2016). History, mandate & role in the UN System. Retrieved from http://unhabitat.org/about-us/history-mandate-role-in-the-un-system

United Nations Institute for Training & Research. (2016). Nikhil Seth became the 8th Executive Director of UNITAR. Retrieved from https://www.unitar.org/nikhil-seth-became-8th-executive-director-unitar

United Nations International Children's Fund. (2016). UNICEF works for a world in which every child has a fair chance in life. Retrieved from http://www.unicef.org/about

United Nations Women. (2016a). About UN women. Retrieved from http://www.unwomen.org/en/about-us/about-un-women

United Nations Women. (2016b). Commission on the Status of Women. Retrieved from http://www.unwomen.org/en/csw

Victorian Order of Nurses. (2016). History. Retrieved from http://von.ca/en/history

Wilson, L., Costa Mendes, I. A., Klopper, H., Catrombone, C., Al-Maaitah, R., Norton, M. E., & Hill, M. (2016). "Global health" and "global nursing": Proposed definitions from the Global Advisory Panel on the Future of Nursing. *Journal of Advanced Nursing, 72*(7), 1529–1540.

World Health Organization. (2006). *Report of the forum for government chief nurses and midwives.* Geneva, Switzerland: WHO Department of Human Resources for Health.

World Health Organization. (2011). *World health statistics report 2011.* Retrieved from http://www.who.int/whosis/whostat/2011/en

World Health Organization. (2014). MDG 5: Improve maternal health. Retrieved from http://www.who.int/topics/millennium_development_goals/maternal_health/en

World Health Organization. (2015). *WHO nursing & midwifery progress report 2008 to 2012.* Geneva, Switzerland: Author. Retrieved from http://www.who.int/hrh/nursing_midwifery/progress_report/en

World Health Organization. (2016a). *Nursing and midwifery: WHO strategic directions for strengthening nursing and midwifery 2016–2020.* Geneva, Switzerland: Author. Retrieved from http://www.who.int/hrh/nursing_midwifery/global-strategic-midwifery2016-2020.pdf

World Health Organization. (2016b). What is universal health coverage? Retrieved from http://www.who.int/features/qa/universal_health_coverage/en

World Health Organization. (2016c). *Global strategic directions for nursing & midwifery.* Geneva, Switzerland: Author. Retrieved from http://www.who.int/hrh/nursing_midwifery/global-strategy-midwifery-2016-2020/en

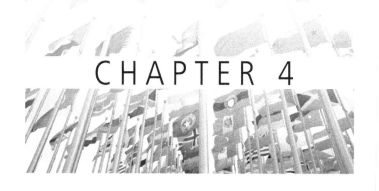

CHAPTER 4

Global Nurse Citizenship: Toward a Safe and Inclusive Civil Society

William Rosa and Holly K. Shaw

[Global citizenship] is a way of living that recognizes our world is an increasingly complex web of connections and interdependencies. One in which our choices and actions may have repercussions for people and communities locally, nationally or internationally. . . . Global citizenship nurtures personal respect and respect for others, wherever they live. It encourages individuals to think deeply and critically about what is equitable and just, and what will minimize harm to our planet. (IDEAS for Global Citizenship, n.d.)

The growing emphasis on globalization highlights the issues of global health for consideration among health professions practitioners, students, faculty, and policy makers (Wilson et al., 2016). A global nurse is not necessarily one who travels or leaves his or her country of origin, but rather practices from a global perspective and cares for patients, families, and communities from that stance. Our work as global nurses may call us to engage with populations across nations and continents, but more than anything, it requires a shift in our consciousness. It requires us to develop an understanding of others as interconnected to our shared humanity and to value health care as a human right. Global health asks us to examine how we are leading. It beckons us to reflect and hone in on exactly what we are striving for and the intentions driving our actions: Are we aiming for others to experience health and vitality as we understand it from our lens, or are we promoting their experience of well-being from their subjective worldview? Do we lead initiatives based on individual moral codes or do we accept that ethical considerations adjust according to the cultural paradigms, norms, and value systems in which we find ourselves? Ultimately, global citizenship is about allowing ourselves to evolve past self-limiting definitions and embrace partnerships that nurture health and wellness for all involved.

EMBRACING GLOBAL CITIZENSHIP

It has become necessary to expand and elucidate the concept of *global health* from the previous reference to *international health* in order to more accurately reflect contemporary paradigms (Wilson et al., 2016). This shift from international to global health is characterized by a shift from concerns regarding the management of infectious disease, global epidemics, and health disparities among lesser resourced populations to a concern for universal health as a human right for all, regardless of place, social status, or resources (Janes & Corbett, 2009). Nursing leaders have proposed new definitions of global health that focus on the priority of universal health equity and social justice, and the development of sustainable health systems that promote planetary health, which includes ecological, environmental, as well as traditional views of human and animal health (Wilson et al., 2016; see Chapter 2 for these updated definitions; see Chapter 33 for more on planetary health).

Global health concerns are based on the proposition that all behaviors are comprehensible within the context in which they originate and manifest. Global nursing refers to an enhanced awareness of issues and determinants of health that underlie evidence-based nursing processes to promote planetary health and equity, including individual- and population-level direct care, as well as leadership, research, education, and policy initiatives. Global nurses play a key role in implementing and supporting programs that create and sustain access to quality care throughout the global village (Nicholas & Breaky, 2015).

This approach requires an openness to the integration of context into how care is conceived, described, and delivered. Globalized health concepts mandate that there is no "one way" of doing things, no "right path" to addressing disparities, and no "correct approach" to any problem. There is only context, communication, compromise, and collaboration. We must embrace the ethical concepts of human rights and dignity as well as skills in flexibility, understanding, empathy, patience, and deep listening. A global citizen lens used to guide our perceptions and assessments provides the opportunity to appreciate the human story behind the data, the individual implications beneath the collective circumstances. If we are able to nurture effective collaboration and partnerships rooted in bidirectional communication and mutual understanding among communities and providers, the goal of compassionate and culturally sensitive health care becomes possible (Benjamin, 2012; Wilson et al., 2016). Traditionally, nurses have made immeasurable contributions to global health and are currently considered to play critical roles in the achievement of contemporary global health goals (Jamison et al., 2013; World Health Organization [WHO], 2006).

While addressing universal global health issues, the relationship between global and local health remains an important consideration, whereby the differences and variances between national and multinational factors influence and shape the local context (Janes & Corbett, 2009). "Glocal" approaches refer to the interdependence of populations and posits that the reciprocal relationship of enhancing local health systems and populations leads to the achievement of improved global health (Beck, Dossey, & Rushton, 2013; Janes & Cobett, 2009). Contemporary nurses are encouraged to become authentic advocates, be transparent about the unique contributions of the nursing profession, and think and act both locally and globally in addressing critical issues (Beck et al., 2013).

Appropriate questions for self-reflection might include the following: How do I define or identify myself? Is it by my profession, my ethnicity, my religion? Do I limit myself as a "man" or a "woman," as a "PhD" or "MPH"? How might I expand this self-definition to extend beyond these traditional narrow parameters? It is helpful to remember that the inherent limitations of rigid labels, categories, and classifications can prevent authentic, culturally humble, and appropriate interactions. Expanding one's self-concept toward the ideals of global citizenship has much to offer both the profession of nursing and global health at large. Hugh Evans, cofounder of Global Citizen (2012–2016), an international community striving to end extreme poverty and inequality worldwide, defines a "global citizen" as "someone who identifies first and foremost not as a member of a state, tribe or nation, but instead as a member of the human race," and he emphasizes that "[w]hen you make global citizenship your mission you suddenly find yourself with extraordinary allies" (Evans, 2016). And who among us doesn't need more allies in the processes of integrating context and relationship?

Global citizenship is a mindset that can guide global nurses in working toward the goals and targets of leading transnational health organizations. WHO (2016a) recently released the *Global Strategic Directions for Strengthening Nursing and Midwifery, 2016–2020* report, which states this vision: "Accessible, available, acceptable, quality and cost-effective nursing and midwifery care for all, in support of universal health coverage and the Sustainable Development Goals" (p. 13). WHO (2016a) proposes that through ethical action, relevance, ownership, partnership, and quality, nursing and midwifery can be effective coleaders in raising the caliber of health for all countries and regions throughout the global village (see Chapter 2 to read sections 2, 3, and 4 of the report in their entirety). The thematic areas identified by WHO's (2016a) report are:

1. Ensuring an educated, competent and motivated nursing and midwifery workforce within effective and responsive health systems at all levels and in different settings
2. Optimizing policy development, effective leadership, management, and governance
3. Working together to maximize the capacities and potentials of nurses and midwives through intra- and interprofessional collaborative partnerships, education, and continuing professional development
4. Mobilizing political will to invest in building effective evidence-based nursing and midwifery workforce development

The aforementioned vision and associated themes are in alignment with the *Global Strategy on Human Resources for Health: Workforce 2030* (WHO, 2016b) report that was compiled by WHO's Global Health Workforce Alliance in 2015, and was recently presented and unanimously adopted by Member States of the 69th World Health Assembly on May 27, 2016, in Geneva, Switzerland (WHO, 2016c).

From practice to policy, throughout research and education, global citizenship must be an ideal that is at the root of professionalism and ethical engagement. International associations of nursing, such as the Honor Society of Nursing, Sigma Theta Tau International (STTI, n.d., 2005, 2016), and the International Council of

Nurses (ICN; Shamian, 2015a, 2015b), actively continue to foster and promote it. Nursing education must prepare professional nurses to embrace global citizenship by elucidating the values of human dignity, respect, and social justice that underlie it, integrating global health competencies into curricula, procuring multinational clinical placements to promote a global perspective, and providing authentic online learning and advocacy opportunities to nurture global perspectives when overseas student experiences are not possible (Burgess, Reimer-Kirkham, & Astle, 2014; Strickland, Adamson, McInally, Tiittannen, & Metcalfe, 2013; Visovsky, McGhee, Jordan, Dominic, & Morrison-Beedy, 2016).

Globally conscious nurses must be empowered to engage the world with critical literacy regarding this complex concept of global citizenship. At the core of education for global citizenship is the engagement in complex local/global processes and diverse perspectives to examine the origins and implications of one's own and others' assumptions, negotiate change, transform relationships, think interdependently, and make responsible and conscious choices about our own lives and understand how those choices affect others (Dobson, 2005).

Andreotti (2006) analytically compared and contrasted "soft" global citizenship education with "critical" global citizenship education to make a case for critical literacy. Soft global citizenship, while potentially appropriate for the context at hand and potentially an improvement based on an alternative of limited global exposure, carries with it the danger of promoting a colonialist-type view of saving or civilizing the world (Andreotti, 2006). However, critical global citizenship and literacy assume "that all knowledge is partial and incomplete, constructed in our contexts, cultures and experiences" and that "we lack the knowledge constructed in other contexts, cultures and experiences" (Andreotti, 2006, p. 49). This "critical" element encourages students to ask questions, surrender assumptions, and take cross-culturally informed and sensitive action. In short, soft global citizenship is rooted in a sense of beneficence and moral obligation, whereas critical global citizenship is realized by a more thorough immersion into sociopolitical, economic, and historical determinants, as well as a culturally relevant context of social justice (Burgess et al., 2014). Table 4.1 offers a comparison of soft versus critical citizenship education (see Chapter 32 for competencies related to global citizenship).

As global citizens, we must know where the communities we serve have been so that we might be of relevant value in moving them forward with respect to their self-identified targets. The most well-known and unprecedented transnational initiatives for global health were born out of the 2000 United Nations (UN) Millennium Summit and are known as the Millennium Development Goals (MDGs; UN Millennium Project, 2006). The MDGs were designed as a 15-year plan to improve global economic, social, and environmental well-being (see Chapter 2 for a full list of the MDGs). While global nurses have played notable key roles in furthering Goals 4, 5, and 6 (Beck, 2016; Nightingale Initiative for Global Health [NIGH], 2016), these authors contend that we, as a transnational profession, have influenced each of them in our sustained efforts to promote and procure worldwide holistic health for every man, woman, and child on the planet.

The 2015 *Millennium Development Goals Report* demonstrates that the collaborative efforts implemented to realize the MDGs have saved millions of lives and exacted dramatic improvements in even the poorest of countries (UN, 2015). However, there is much more work to be done. Considerable worldwide attention has focused on global health goals as the multinational UN community shifts

Table 4.1 Soft Versus Critical Citizenship Education

	Soft Global Citizenship Education	Critical Global Citizenship Education
Problem	Poverty, helplessness	Inequality, injustice
Nature of the problem	Lack of "development," education, resources, skills, culture, technology, etc.	Complex structures, systems, assumptions, power relations and attitudes that create and maintain exploitation and enforced disempowerment and tend to eliminate difference.
Justification for positions of privilege	"Development," "history," education, harder work, better organisation, better use of resources, technology.	Benefit from and control over unjust and violent systems and structures.
Basis for caring	Common humanity/being good/sharing and caring. Responsibility *FOR* the other (or *to teach* the other).	Justice/complicity in harm. Responsibility *TOWARDS* the other (or to *learn with* the other) – accountability.
Grounds for acting	Humanitarian/moral (based on normative principles for thought and action).	Political/ethical (based on normative principles for relationships).
Understanding of interdependence	We are all equally interconnected, we all want the same thing, we can all do the same thing.	Asymmetrical globalisation, unequal power relations, . . . elites imposing own assumptions as universal.
What needs to change	Structures, institutions and individuals that are a barrier to development.	Structures, (belief) systems, institutions, assumptions, cultures, individuals, relationships.
What for	So that everyone achieves development, harmony, tolerance and equality.	So that injustices are addressed, more equal grounds for dialogue are created, and people can have more autonomy to define their own development.
Role of "ordinary" individuals	Some individuals are part of the problem, but ordinary people are part of the solution as they can create pressure to change structures.	We are all a part of the problem and part of the solution.
How does change happen	From the outside to the inside (imposed change).	From the inside to the outside.
Basic principle for change	Universalism (non-negotiable vision of how everyone should live [and] what everyone should want or should be).	Reflexivity, dialogue, contingency and an ethical relation to difference (radical alterity).
Goal of global citizenship education	Empower individuals to act (or become active citizens) according to what has been defined for them as a good life or ideal world.	Empower individuals to reflect critically on the legacies and processes of their cultures, to imagine different futures and to take responsibility for decisions and actions.

(continued)

Table 4.1 Soft Versus Critical Citizenship Education (*continued*)

	Soft Global Citizenship Education	Critical Global Citizenship Education
Strategies for global citizenship education	Raising awareness of global issues and promoting campaigns.	Promoting engagement with global issues and perspectives and an ethical relationship to difference, addressing complexity and power relations.
Potential benefits of global citizenship education	Greater awareness of some of the problems, support for campaigns, greater motivation to help/do something, feel good factor.	Independent/critical thinking and more informed, responsible and ethical action.
Potential problems	Feeling of self-importance and self-righteousness and/or cultural supremacy, reinforcement of colonial assumptions and relations, reinforcement of privilege, partial alienation, uncritical action.	Guilt, internal conflict and paralysis, critical disengagement, feeling of helplessness.

Source: Reprinted with permission from Andreotti (2006).

from UN MDGs to the Post-2015 Agenda. With the 2015 United Nations General Assembly adoption of the Sustainable Development Goals (SDGs), endorsed by 193 world leaders, nations across the globe will collaborate over the remaining 13 years to "build on the success of the MDGs . . . end all forms of poverty, fight inequalities and tackle climate change, while ensuring that no one is left behind" (UN Sustainable Development, 2016). This corresponds to the upcoming 2020 Nightingale Bicentennial and an interest in global health among nurses everywhere.

Nurses worldwide will continue to have major roles in the development, design, and implementation of policies, resources, and services related to the attainment of the SDGs. Myriad approaches will emerge to engage nurses as leaders and global citizens to impact the lives of individuals, populations, and the planet. The nursing profession is well suited to provide direction for a productive trajectory in meeting the challenging global agenda. A sound conceptual foundation for developing global citizenship action plans is articulated in *The ICN Code of Ethics for Nurses* (ICN, 2012) and the AACN (American Association of Colleges of Nursing) elucidation of the core values of professional nursing integrated into baccalaureate nursing education and clinical practice, including human dignity, integrity, autonomy, altruism, and social justice (AACN, 2008).

Building on ethical standards, core professional values, and concepts of global citizenship, specific strategies can be developed for local/global intervention. Methodologies involve a variety of approaches and creative role adaptations, such as collaborators in meeting global health needs and as global health diplomats forging global relationships and partnerships (Beck et al., 2013; Upvall et al., 2014). Baumann (2013) encourages equality in affiliations and partnerships and avoiding any disparity in power or self-determination, merging respect for human dignity, human rights, and human universality. Adopting a premise with which to embody the ideals of global citizenship prepares nurses to be effective contributors in their partnerships and global health endeavors.

MORAL IMAGINATION: AN ETHICAL PREMISE FOR THE GLOBAL NURSE CITIZEN

Global nurse citizenship integrates the ideals mentioned in the preceding text with the core values of professional nursing. It requires a strong ethical rooting that promotes and procures human dignity as foundational to health and healing (see Chapter 6 for a more detailed discussion on traditional ethical principles in relation to global health). "Moral imagination" is an ethical premise for human engagement that has been employed in creating healthy and respectful cross-cultural collaborations (Novogratz, 2009). It has been defined as "the humility to accept things as they are and the audacity to see things as they could be" (Acumen, 2016). It implies a willingness to be present to people, places, and circumstances in their respective contexts so that, through globally relevant partnerships, quality of life can be improved for all involved. As both starting and ending point for relationships, moral imagination asks that one place oneself in the shoes of another human being and establish meaning, intention, and purpose from that worldview (Novogratz, 2010).

Current Ethical Perspectives in Nursing and Moral Imagination

Nursing, as a human healing art and science, must be rooted in a strong moral/ethical foundation in order to be effective as a service to humankind (Rosa, 2016a). As the largest health care professional sector worldwide, the collectivity of ethically based practices—or the lack thereof—wields the influence to powerfully impact outcomes, systems, and global infrastructures. There must be an intentionality that creates the necessary environments for healing to take place and a commitment to live and embody those values that are representative of dignity. Countless nurse leaders over time have articulated their views on which morals and ethics constitute such a practice. A summary of such perspectives can be found in Table 4.2.

Holistic advocates for the nursing profession suggest an integral perspective of human beings and relationships (Dossey & Keegan, 2016; Kreitzer & Koithan, 2014). This notion describes the interconnectedness that exists not only between mind, body, and spirit but also between and among human beings and their environments. In this sense, a loss of integrity in any aspect of well-being may have negative consequences on the well-being of the whole person and the global community at large. Levinas (1969/2000) shared this perspective in his seminal work, noting that all people inherently hold a collective and first ethic of *belonging* to the common thread of humanity before *being* as an individual entity. It has also been referred to as the *transpersonal*: the spirit facet of each being that is universal and sacred (Quinn, 2016; Schaub & Schaub, 2013). This holistic paradigm depicts humanity as a shared experience, promotes the evolution of awareness and self-knowledge, and honors the healing possible when human dignity is protected and maintained.

Moral imagination provides an avenue to translate these theories into action. It suggests *how* we can evolve personal–professional applications and practices

Table 4.2 Moral/Ethical Foundations for Practice Proposed by Nurse Leaders

Author	Moral/Ethical Foundation	Brief Explanation
Cowling (2016)	Unitary appreciation	Human beings are inherently whole and each has a subjective lived experience that is both true and valid
Fitzgerald (2016)	Equality	Equal care to all populations without stratification of delivery due to socioeconomic status, age, gender, sexual orientation, race, ethnicity, disability, etc.
Giovannoni (2016)	Heart-centered wisdom	Supports the conscious cultivation of loving kindness toward self and others as a way to become more *biogenic* or life-giving
Goldin (2016)	Love	Identifies nurse caring as love in action
McClure (2016)	Safety	Commits to safety in hiring practices, effective checks and balances systems, a "just culture" in attending to clinical errors, and rewarding integrity in practice
Pesut (2016)	Self-knowledge	Knowledge of one's strengths and weaknesses allows for the translation of virtue ethics into practice
Rosa (2016b)	Compassion	Celebrates demonstrations of compassionate caring as the soul work of nursing through kindness, generosity, patience, empathy, etc.
Schaub (2016)	Transpersonal awareness	Honors the dormant transpersonal nature of each person and healing as a unique process of self-awareness
Vonfrolio (2016)	Moral courage	A fearless commitment to advocate for one's ethical beliefs and values
Watson (2016)	Human caring science	Recognizes caring-healing presence and actions that procure human dignity as central to nursing's identity

to become influential leaders of ethical character. By listening deeply, being generous of self, reflecting on biases, and continuing to develop a vision of possibility that motivates actions and guides decisions, moral imagination becomes a compass noting the direction of interpersonal integrity and dignified relationships (Novogratz, 2016). It has the power to translate notions of shared humanity into measurable forces for healing and transformation. Figure 4.1 illustrates how moral imagination, through the actions mentioned previously, offers one potential mechanism to translate theories and concepts, such as holism, love, and caring, into interpersonal integrity and dignified relationships. For example, one who adopts compassion as a moral/ethical foundation for practice uses moral imagination to engage others, offering both self-compassion in facing one's own biases and in developing a vision, and compassion for others through deep listening and practicing generosity. This compassionate ethic becomes compassionate practice, informing the development of integrity between persons and the procurement of dignity within relationships.

| Figure 4.1 | The framework of moral imagination in translating theory to action. |

Expanding the Concept of Moral Imagination

In order to translate moral imagination into meaningful outcomes, the concept must be expanded upon to adequately explore its myriad implications. Acumen (2016), in its Manifesto, further describes the texture of moral imagination through its commitment to ethically rooted leadership: It involves listening to clients who frequently go ignored or overlooked, focusing on potential and hope amid cynicism and despair, admitting failure and recommitting to the vision at stake, and, ultimately, "building a world based on dignity." It is not just about how one sees the world, but remaining deliberate regarding one's ethical agenda to improve the quality of life for all human beings and demonstrating actions that align with such principles.

Box 4.1 lists Assumptions of Moral Imagination identified by these authors. These assumptions honor the ideals of moral imagination as a premise for ethical

| Box 4.1 | Assumptions of Moral Imagination |

Moral imagination:

- Implies a shared humanity between individuals, communities, and nations.

- Requires the promotion, protection, and procurement of human dignity as a priority and ethical starting point.

- Identifies authentic interpersonal relationships as foundational to the change process.

- Warrants a holistic perspective on the mental-emotional-spiritual-physical health of both individuals and populations at large.

- Calls for a consciousness of cultural and interpersonal humility.

- Fosters the acceptance of people, places, and circumstances as they are.

- Acknowledges another's lived experience as truth and uses his or her subjective context as a premise for collaboration.

- Demands both moral courage and moral empathy to create systems changes that are sustainable and humane.

- Compels partners in the change process to create and consistently refine a vision for the future that considers the well-being of all stakeholders.

- Measures outcomes related to financial and organizational ventures in terms of quality of life advancement.

Source: Based on Acumen (2016).

engagement between individuals and stakeholders, communities, nations: all strata of the global village. They suggest that true healing partnerships are not possible without ideals and practices of acceptance, authenticity, respectful communication, humility, and a holistic understanding of people and processes. The Assumptions of Moral Imagination call the profession and all concerned global citizens to social justice (Nickitas, 2016) and offer a continuing opportunity to more deeply understand and apply moral imagination in a host of settings.

Requisites of Moral Imagination: Self-Awareness and Self-Reflection

Self-awareness and self-reflection are not only required aspects of moral leadership and moral imagination (Novogratz, 2016) but are also very much related to personal–professional growth, renewal, individual wellness, and organizational well-being (Pesut, 2016; Sherwood & Horton-Deutsch, 2012, 2015). Reflective inventories provide an opportunity for heightening self-awareness and practicing self-reflection. They have been used in nursing to assess self-care needs, observe institutional practices related to dignified care, promote interpersonal relationships in the workplace milieu, and identify flexibility and resilience related to change (Rosa, 2014a, 2014b, 2017; Rosa, Estes, & Watson, 2017; Rosa & Santos, 2016).

Related to the assumptions of moral imagination discussed previously, Table 4.3 provides a Moral Imagination Reflective Inventory for the benefit of reader awareness and reflection. The left-hand column restates the Assumptions of Moral Imagination found in Box 4.1, and the right-hand column poses questions for further introspection. This inventory may assist to assess one's relationship to the ideals of moral imagination, as well as identify barriers, judgments,

Table 4.3 Moral Imagination Reflective Inventory

Assumptions of Moral Imagination Moral Imagination	Reflective Inventory Questions Based on Moral Imagination Assumptions Reflect Upon the Following
Implies a shared humanity between individuals, communities, and nations.	*Do I believe we are all in this together? Am I committed to the belief that all men, women, and children are created equal?*
Requires the promotion, protection, and procurement of human dignity as a priority and ethical starting point.	*How is my commitment to human dignity translated into action? Do I base my ideas and interventions on a premise of shared humanity?*
Identifies authentic interpersonal relationships as foundational to the change process.	*What is the quality of my relationships with others? Am I authentic in my presence, deep listening, and communication or do I withhold myself?*
Warrants a holistic perspective on the mental-emotional-spiritual-physical health of both individuals and populations at large.	*In what ways do I integrate a holistic perspective of the other into my partnerships? Am I considerate of the nonphysical obstacles and barriers others experience?*
Calls for a consciousness of cultural and interpersonal humility.	*Where and how do I demonstrate cultural arrogance? In what ways am I able to surrender outdated personal frameworks and adapt to what the context requires?*
Fosters the acceptance of people, places, and circumstances as they are.	*Do I resist "what is"?* *How can I release the need to fix, change, or adjust?*
Acknowledges another's lived experience as truth and uses his or her subjective context as a premise for collaboration.	*Do I strive to hear another's story from his or her perspective and worldview? How can I make another's needs, hopes, and concerns a priority for my planning and practice?*
Demands both moral courage and moral empathy to create systems changes that are sustainable and humane.	*Do I consider what is "right" from an understanding of cultural norms and values? Do I hold the space and demonstrate empathy for another?*
Compels partners in the change process to create and consistently communicate a vision for the future that considers the well-being of all stakeholders.	*Have I enrolled others to cocreate a vision for a mutually beneficial and globally conscious future? Do I share and communicate that vision in a way others can understand and receive it?*
Measures outcomes related to financial and organizational ventures in terms of quality of life advancement.	*How do I measure "quality of life"? Do I hold an improved quality of life as the primary goal throughout my collaborations with others?*

and opportunities for personal–professional development. The inventory may be employed by individuals or groups, as a basis for open discussion or private contemplation, and as either a preparatory tool to foster dignified relationships or a debriefing instrument postengagement. The questions may be altered based on the needs of the user and are offered merely as a tool to deepen one's personal experience of moral imagination.

Moral imagination is not merely a theoretical perspective or paradigm; it is a tangible and ethical precept for human betterment. It has shown real-word benefits to improved quality of life and it deepens the authenticity of human relationships. Moral imagination invokes the possibility of collaborative, caring–healing relationships rooted in dignity and is reflective of an evolved and global consciousness. It offers just one path for ethical behavior and personal–professional progress in global health, global nursing, and global citizenship.

GLOBAL NURSE CITIZENSHIP AND THE UN

Moral imagination and professional nursing's core values of human dignity, altruism, autonomy, integrity, and social justice (AACN, 2008) may be applied in problem solving, decision making, clinical practice, and nursing education. Participation in the United Nations System and nongovernmental organization (NGO) community offers an emerging opportunity for worldwide nursing to have an impact on global health and social policy advocacy. The UN Department of Public Information (DPI) establishes working relationships with NGOs and provides them with information about the UN and global issues of concern. The UN DPI/NGO at the New York City (NYC) headquarters organizes informational briefings, materials, and programs that are disseminated among the 1,500 officially accredited NGOs within the UN System.

An annual NGO/DPI conference is mandated by the UN charter to afford NGOs the opportunity to collaborate and share information and resources helpful in meeting the myriad needs of the "Peoples of the World" (United Nations, 2013). The conference, convened in 2016 in the Republic of Korea, was attended by more than 3,000 global NGO representatives and provides a valuable forum for participants both in person and virtually. Throughout the year, NGO representatives meet in committees and working groups to educate, advocate for there respective vested interests, and collaborate with NGO colleagues and UN staff and diplomats. Imbued with knowledge, skills, wisdom, and commitment, nursing NGOs can provide guidance and leadership in addressing many contemporary issues affecting the world's population.

Attaining official accreditation by which NGOs request affiliation with the UN is a formal process available to not-for-profit, nongovernment, nonmunicipal organizations (www.un.org) throughout the world (see Chapter 3 for a brief history of the UN, including the work of NGOs and global civil society). The Nightingale Initiative for Global Health (NIGH) contends that increasing the number of professional nursing associations in the UN NGO community will have a powerful influence on issues of global concern and have a goal of facilitating 200 NGO UN affiliations by 2020 (see Chapters 3 and 7 for more details on NIGH's global citizenship work). Please refer to the following UN websites for information about affiliation:

- General information: www.un.org
- Affiliation with the Department of Public Information (DPI/NGO): http://csonet.org/index.php?menu=17
- Accreditation Economic and Social Council (ECOSOC): United Nations http://esango.un.org/civilsociety/displayDPISearch.do?method= search&sessionCheck=false
- For questions, recommendations, and guidance: nurseunorg@gmail .com or drhollyshaw@aol.com

CONTEMORARY EXEMPLARS OF GLOBAL NURSE CITIZENSHIP

Global nurse citizenship challenges us as professionals to bring the sensibilities and ethical priorities of the nursing collective to our global citizenship endeavors. While this book provides countless real-world examples of global nurses leading change and influencing global health with a nursing sensibility, each of the following four exemplars demonstrates the key attributes of global nurse citizen advocacy and activism: an egalitarian, collegial partnership based on mutually assessed and determined goals and the core professional values of altruism, autonomy, human dignity, integrity, and social justice (AACN, 2008), as well as reliance on skills like communication, compromise, collaboration, and flexibility. Each originated from a vision and the knowledge, passion, and hope to make it happen. These dedicated nurses were seeking to enhance their contribution of utilizing multiple and varied resources and collaborators to create a pathway to excellence and contribution, receiving inspiration, inspiring others, identifying gaps, and envisioning ways to fill them. Each exemplar also includes a "right now" opportunity for readers to become involved themselves and make a global difference by contributing time, energy, awareness promotion, or funding, as an individual nurse citizen or as a member of a professional group or social network.

Exemplar 1: Nurses Day at the UN

In nursing domains worldwide, discussions are taking place regarding emerging 21st-century global health issues and policy considerations affecting the lives of people and their communities. Through discussions and collaboration, the nurse's role as global citizen and nurse advocate influences change across the spectrum— locally and globally. Nurses' impact on the determinants of health behaviors and outcomes, which include, but are not limited to, reducing disease burden, lowering risk factors, promoting health and wellness, and developing a sustainable health and nursing workforce are particularly important when considering the most marginalized, vulnerable, and underrepresented citizens of the world.

Nurse activists at the UN participate in a variety of global, regional, and local nursing programs, and work to disseminate information and share anecdotal experiences and unique perspectives of an insider's view of establishing a role for nurse advocates within the UN System and as leaders in the global NGO community. Because the preponderance of impact comes from beyond the walls of the UN with the affiliated NGOs and concerned citizens, we promote discussions to explore ways for nurses to be involved in civil society. Whether a nurse who practices in a large urban hospital, a nurse who cares for a village of rural farmers, a nursing student, or a nurse who has retired from active practice, all can make a difference and contribute to the critical conversations in the global health and nursing arena.

NIGH representative Dr. Shaw developed a unique project with Maimonides Medical Center (MMC) Nursing Department, Brooklyn, New York, to honor the Nightingale legacy through education, advocacy, and clinical application of contemporary information regarding critical global health and nursing issues. This occurred in conjunction with the MMC's Second Annual Nursing Research Conference, *Advancing Nursing Science Across the Globe: Are We Ready?* focusing on nursing's contribution to global and population health. Based on interest generated at the conference, Dr. Shaw and Dr. Kelly Reilly, Director of Nursing Education, Research, and Innovation, designed Maimonides Nurses Day at the UN to provide conference follow-up and offer a special recognition for nurse leaders and staff in honor of International Nurses Day. This collaboration reflected the synergy between nurses with diverse backgrounds, skills, and interests, committed to the noble aspirations of the Charter of the UN and the equally noble Nightingale legacy. The goals of the program were:

1. To provide a specialized, focused program for MMC nurses
2. To honor MMC nurse leaders with a special program focusing on stated interests
3. To provide information to MMC RNs, leaders, and advanced practice nurses regarding

   a. United Nations: history and relevance

   b. Contemporary global health issues: Ebola and human trafficking

   c. Emerging, innovative role for nurses at UN

   d. Opportunities for engagement and official UN affiliation for nurse citizen groups

With the support and encouragement of the nursing administration, which planned the event to honor nurse leaders and staff for International Nurses Day, we planned private tours of the UN, a special luncheon in the delegates' dining room, and two private briefings by UN staff, including an excellent presentation on "Human Trafficking: Implications for Nurses." The state-of-the-art material presented was so relevant and informative, the nurse leaders formed a hospital committee and revised policies and procedures regarding screening, assessment, and intervention related to trafficked persons presenting to the hospital. Physicians soon became interested and formed their own committee, leading to a hospital-wide conference addressing the issue. Drs. Shaw and Reilly made a formal presentation of the program to an audience of 150 at the 66th Session of the UN Commission on the Status of Women, and they are collaborating with the *American Journal of Nursing* on a journal article. This project serves as an exemplar of global nurse citizenship with "glocal" implications for education, research, policy, and service.

Nursing organizations, associations, and schools can contact Dr. Shaw to design a customized UN experience by contacting nurseunorg@gmail.com or drhollyshaw@aol.com.

Exemplar 2: Middle Eastern Nurses and Partners Uniting in Human Caring: Honoring Our Shared Humanity

We build a caring community through outreach, education, and research. As Middle Eastern nurses, we are faced daily with the threat of harm—harm to our communities, our families, and ourselves. We stand together to advocate for healthier communities through care, compassion, and understanding. Centered in West and East Jerusalem, we reach out to all the Middle East to join us in our fight for tolerance and respect. (Middle Eastern Nurses, 2015. Reprinted with permission.)

Following a Palestinian truck driver's 3-month hospitalization and extended rehab, his Israeli nurses at Hadassah Hospital Medical Center, Ein Kerem, Israel, formulated a basic discharge plan so that he could continue to heal from a crushed pelvis, abdominal hemorrhage, and a left-foot amputation in a location close to his home in Hebron. While the implementation of a smooth, comfortable, and productive transition is a task accomplished routinely by nurses throughout the world, it was impossible for Nurses in the Middle East (NME) cofounder, Julie Benbenishty, and colleagues due to a lack of communication and collaboration by health professionals caught in the political and social conflict in the Middle East. In 2011, Ms. Benbenishty reached out to medical colleagues and NGOs, but despite being less than 100 kilometers from each other, she could not identify a single nurse "on the ground" to whom she could communicate the patient information.

The imperative of open, professional, collaborative communication between Israeli and Palestinian nurses in the service of optimal patient care served as the foundation for creating a network of nurses dedicated to "health care diplomacy," which they envisioned would bridge the formidable and complex sociopolitical barriers to comprehensive, compassionate care. Collaborating with scholar Dr. Jean Watson and Watson Caring Science Institute, the Middle Eastern Nurses United in Human Caring promotes the practice and application of Human Caring Science, translating theory into concrete, ethically grounded, evidence-based approaches, encouraging nurses to be ambassadors of caring, and through patient care, to create communities of compassion and understanding, ensuring that care has no boundaries and carries no identification card (middleastnurses .squarespace.com).

In only 5 years, these exemplary global nurse leaders, educators, clinicians, and administrators have transcended the powerful regional and local disparities, and through collaborative outreach, education, and research, have created avenues of communication throughout their region and the world, supporting the holistic health of individuals and communities. Meeting monthly in neutral and mutually convenient settings, cofounders Julie Benbenishty, RN, MA, and Naela Hayek, RN, MA, report that they are developing a growing relationship with the UN and have assembled a West/East Jerusalem Board of Directors to advise joint projects and research on a range of topics including nurse burnout, infant injuries, and hope in the Middle East. Collaborative learning opportunities and West/East nurse/student exchanges facilitate comfort and a think tank to develop standards of practice for mass casualty situations.

Supported by Watson Caring Science Institute, their largest project is the annual Middle Eastern Nurses and Partners Uniting in Human Caring international conference, focusing on nursing care in the region and offering an unprecedented opportunity for Middle Eastern nurses' networking, collaborative learning, and scholarly presentation. Held annually during February in Jordan, the attendance has quadrupled since the first conference and results in abstract publication in the *International Journal of Healing and Caring* and consensus papers authored by nurse participants from more than a dozen countries, including the United States, South Africa, the Philippines, Bahrain, Iraq, Afghanistan, Switzerland, and China. The registration fee is intentionally low ($50), as are the conference accommodations to allow for maximum participation by colleagues with limited resources.

Amid ongoing turmoil and often escalating conflict, this story of global nurse citizenship stands as a spectacular model of professional accomplishment based on the values of caring, respect, integrity, and determination. A remarkable aspect of this group of Israeli and Arab nurses is that their mission is not to modify their own political or nationalistic views, but to transcend them in the service of their patients and their communities. They exemplify the most noble and caring vision: to utilize their skills, knowledge, and expertise to serve others and humanity, regardless of national origin, political, racial, religious, or ethnic orientation. Nurses from throughout the world can support this noble and challenging endeavor by raising international awareness among colleagues and contributing to important programming. Share this hopeful and inspiring story with friends and colleagues! (See Chapter 11 for more information on this initiative, as well as position statements from Nurses in the Middle East. Please visit middleast nurses.squarespace.com and www.facebook.com/middleastnurses/?fref=ts or e-mail partnerscaring@gmail.com)

Exemplar 3: Promoting Health in Haiti: Supporting Sustainability and Haitian Nursing Education

Mission: *To improve health and wellness for the citizens of Haiti by educating highly skilled nurses* through collaboration between North American and Haitian nursing educators (nursesforhaiti.webs.com).

As in many underresourced countries besieged by poverty, illness, and lack of adequate health care, nurses in Haiti are at the core of the health care system. They are frequently the only health care providers available and often provide health service beyond basic nursing care. Already strained by the demands of an impoverished, needy population, the 2010 earthquake was particularly devastating for nursing. The nursing school in Port-au-Prince was leveled, killing students and faculty and leaving no structures for class except makeshift tents. While the health care needs of the country have increased, the basic preparation of nurses is at the diploma level, leaving gaps in education and service. Nurses are often called upon to provide much more specialized models of care than those for which they have been educated: primary care, prenatal care, and complex levels of care. This dire situation has resulted in significant gaps in education and service, and an urgent need for a much more highly trained workforce prevails.

Promoting Health in Haiti (PHH), a nonprofit organization, was founded by Hunter College nursing professors Carol Roye, EdD, RN, Steven Baumann, PhD, RN, Joanna Hofmann, EdD, RN, and Hunter Alumna Carmelle Bellefleur, PhD, RN, in cooperation with Lucille Charles, past-president of the Haitian Nurses Association, and Yolande Nazaire, the head of the School of Nursing in

Port-au-Prince. The organization's goal is to create collaborations between North American and Haitian schools of nursing in order to cultivate baccalaureate and graduate-level nursing education.

The team has focused on the development of the family nurse practitioner (FNP) role as a newly developing, major component of the health care system, which they assessed would provide the greatest benefit to the health of the Haitian population. Collaboration was necessary between PHH and government officials to secure the role of FNP in Haiti and to ensure that the FNP role would be recognized.

Last year, the Haitian government signed a memorandum of understanding establishing the FNP role as an official profession. According to Dr. Roye, this represents a significant milestone for Haitian nurses, who had access only to a diploma education when PHH was formed; they now have access to graduate education. This demonstrates the government's recognition that Haiti desperately needs primary care providers, the beneficiaries of which will be the people of Haiti (C. Roye, personal communication, August 20, 2016).

Student nurses in the program study in Haiti and in the United States. Currently, students have completed the clinical courses, including pathophysiology, pharmacology, primary pare of infants and children, women's health, and adult health and are preparing to engage in placements for the clinical experience necessary to complete graduation requirements by January 2017.

Advocating for women's health is a prime concern for PHH. Dr. Roye indicates that although cervical cancer is preventable, Haitian women die of the disease at far greater numbers than women in the rest of the world, due to lack of access to gynecologists and the routine procedures and resources leading to early diagnosis and treatment (C. Roye, personal communication, August 20, 2016). PHH and their students have become leaders among providers addressing the cervical cancer crisis by providing cancer screening in resource-poor areas of Haiti (C. Roye, personal communication, August 20, 2016).

PHH nurse leaders have been so successful in educating Haitian government officials regarding the vital role of FNPs that Haitian leaders not only recognize and support advanced practice nursing in primary care but have also requested PHH to develop an FNP program at the University of Haiti (UEH). An agreement with UEH and the Ministry of Health established a two-part program at UEH that educates Haitian nurses at the bachelor's degree level and prepares them to enroll in the FNP master's degree program. The first group of 20 students began their FNP studies in the spring of 2016. The Ministry of Health supports them so they can devote 1 week a month to their education with pay. This program and its advancement of nursing education and the nursing profession represent an enormous accomplishment, which will be life altering for the people of Haiti and for which Drs. Roye, Baumann, Hoffman, and Bellefleur have risen to authentic, altruistic global citizenship.

Exemplar 4: Cambodia Nurses Council: Creating Professional Nursing Standards of Practice, Regulation, and Registration

Each of the previous exemplars has involved a unique collaboration of global nurse citizen activists reaching out to colleagues in resource-challenged settings to share ideas and resources to enhance the competence and resilience of nursing and health systems. The Cambodian Council of Nurses (CCN)/Cambodian Caring Professional Society (CPS) exemplar involves nurse leaders from Cambodia coming together to refine, elaborate, and develop the profession of nursing by reaching out to international colleagues for supportive input. Three decades of war and internal armed conflict in Cambodia were followed by severe, extreme oppression by Pol Pot, resulting in millions of Khmer people enslaved and tortured, and over 3 million massacred in the 1970s (McGrew, 1990). Anyone who was even minimally educated, or presumed to be educated simply because of using glasses as an optical device, were among the first to be executed. Many who were not killed were forced to leave their comfortable homes to work and live in rice paddies and farms, suffering from malnutrition, exhaustion, and disease. Infrastructures and health and educational systems were destroyed, as were the individuals who worked in the professions. Survivors have disclosed that there was no safe haven, even among families and communities. Secret police sought to capture and exterminate anyone suspected of being an enemy, leading to neighbor turned against neighbor, child against parent.

After the demise of the Pol Pot regime in 1979, health resources were nearly nonexistent, with fewer than 50 physicians in the entire country in 1990 (McGrew, 1990) and a population almost universally suffering from conditions associated with starvation, malnutrition, infectious disease, and chronic illness. Nearly all Khmer had been subjected to traumatic conditions of horror and helplessness, crisis, and bereavement, making the pathway to healing and recovery arduous and tenuous (Challay, personal communication, 2016).

A fragile, fledgling government was called on to provide for people who had no resources or abilities to care for themselves or others. It was in this milieu of distress and deprivation that many of the current nursing workforce were developed and became committed to lifelong calling in service to their people. These noble, heroic nurses aim to rebuild their country as well as the health and spirits of their elders, forced to endure more than most believe possible.

The current Cambodian nursing profession is in a state of active, energetic development, led by trailblazers who have stimulated and inspired this generation of health professionals. Ms. Manila Prak, RN, BSN, president of the CPS (pmanila@angkorhosital.org) and her colleague Mr. Virya Koy, RN, SNA, MNSc, MHPEd, president of the CCN (virya2403koy@gmail.com), which serves as the professional body responsible for collaboration with the government to develop, approve, and implement regulatory standards, along with the support and input from international colleagues, organizations, and agencies are transforming the nursing profession and health care policy, practice, and education.

Ms. Prak is effusive in her description of being highly influenced by her mentor, John Morgan, RN, a brilliant, passionate, visionary expat nurse from Rhode Island, United States, executive director of the Angkor Hospital for Children (AHC; 1998–2006). Ms. Prak was Nursing Education Coordinator and later director of External Programs Department, AHC, and is now director of Quality Health Services for the United States Agency for International Development (USAID) and member of the International Board of Directors, AHC. Ms. Prak sought to promote the value of the nursing contribution that Mr. Morgan promulgated. She became passionate about the opportunity to develop nursing skills beyond simply "following physician orders," which were limiting and constraining, to feeling empowered by learning strategies to help and comfort patients through implementing the nursing process, thus developing and refining the delivery of nursing care. She transformed inspiration into action and, as a leader in Cambodia nursing education and practice, has implemented the integration of the nursing process as fundamental to professional practice.

In her role as president of the CPS, a professional association developed to promote and provide for the professional development of future nurse leaders in Cambodia, she has provided advanced training for nurse leaders and faculty as well as student placements to learn and practice the nursing process. Ms. Prak and Mr. Koy are partners in the endeavor to introduce contemporary standards of professional nursing, enhance the role and responsibilities of professional nursing practice, and meet the ongoing educational and support needs of nurses in Cambodia within the context of national history and experience, cultural views, and imperatives and challenged professional and societal resources. Mr. Koy, Ms. Prak, and colleagues worked with government officials, including H. E. Prof. Thi Kruy, Secretary of State, Ministry of Health, U.S. consultant/volunteer at AHC, Richard Henker, PhD, CRNA, FAAN, University of Pittsburgh, and Ms. Kyoko Koto, Japan International Cooperation Agency (JICA), and developed comprehensive standards, policies, and cornerstone documents for Cambodian nurses including the *Nursing Process Framework, Code of Ethics for Nurses*, and *Scope of Practice and Standards of Care for Cambodian Nurses* (Henker, Prak, & Koy, 2015).

This altruistic work, demonstrating concern for their country, its citizens, and professionals, is shaped by the values of human dignity and social justice, addressing disparities and social determinants of health while increasing access to and enhancing quality of health services to rural as well as urban inhabitants. Ms. Prak and Mr. Koy have highlighted integrity and autonomy in their multiple collaborations with government officials as well as international nurse consultants to shift nursing practice from task-oriented roles to those involving critical thinking and autonomous professional identity and standards and scope of practice. Ms. Prak is pursuing a master's degree at Chulalongkorn University in Bangkok, Thailand, and Mr. Koy, a nurse anesthetist, is pursuing a PhD at Chulalongkorn University. The next steps include ongoing collaboration with NIGH and Dr. Shaw regarding a series of professional development seminars and research initiatives that will connect Cambodian nurses with international colleagues and global health issues.

CONCLUSION

Each exemplar demonstrates an innovative and contextually appreciative approach to global nurse citizenship and conveys a model for nurses worldwide to engage in their own aspirations for global leadership and advocacy. As the world prepares for engagement with the SDGs, nurse activists can take action to support this global endeavor by educating themselves and others about the SDGs and ways in which all people everywhere can support and attain them. All nurse citizens must hold governments accountable to the Global Goals they endorsed in partnership with the UN in September 2015. Accountability mechanisms should be addressed so that civil society can monitor and assess plans and progress. Exploring the UN website and its myriad resources can provide a basis for self-education and programing for staff development and organizational meetings. Stakeholders should be involved in determining which of the SDGs hold the greatest priority for their communities, which can be disseminated through the use of social media and public relations departments of hospitals, universities, and private organizations. Direct outreach efforts to the exemplars included in this chapter could form the basis for satisfying, mutually beneficial relationships. Financial assistance is a currency that matters greatly and funding support is always an essential element of successful program development. Exploring personal philanthropy as well as community fund-raising projects should be considered. Volunteering to help with grant writing, publicizing, and other efforts to share information can be helpful to both local and global initiatives. Joining and participating in professional associations that support the Global Goals is meaningful for new nurses as well as those more experienced. "Reconstituting ourselves for the transformation of the world" is necessary for global citizenry to be meaningful (Bautista, 2011, p. 9).

Attaining official affiliation with the UN System and helping others to do so will be a powerful and enduring action, ensuring that Nightingale's approach to advocacy, activism, and civil engagement can continue to inspire commitment and contribute to a global milieu in which all humans can heal, grow, and thrive.

REFLECTION AND DISCUSSION

- How do I define my role as a global citizen and how does this role impact my nursing role?
- What part do the concepts of communication, compromise, collaboration, and flexibility play in my global nursing work?
- How has soft education for global citizenship impacted my global perspectives?
- What are the connections between the MDGs and the Post-2015 Agenda?
- What are my preconceptions about nursing's responsibilities to ending poverty, fighting inequalities, and tackling climate change so that no one is left behind?
- What are my most ambitious and optimistic goals for engagement in "glocal" nursing/citizen endeavors?
- How can all nurses, not only nurse educators, ensure that nurses are educated as global nurse citizens?

REFERENCES

Acumen. (2016). Manifesto. Retrieved from http://acumen.org/manifesto

American Association of Colleges of Nursing. (2008). Essentials of baccalaureate education for professional nursing practice. Washington, DC: American Association College of Nursing.

Andreotti, V. (2006). Soft versus critical global citizenship education. Policy and Practice: A development Education Review, 3, 40–51.

Baumann, S. L. (2013). Global health nursing: Toward a human science-based approach. Nursing Science Quarterly, 26(4), 365. doi:10.1177/0894318413500404

Bautista, L. C. (2011, February 25). Peace education and women's empowerment: A reprise of old themes and recurrent concerns. Presented to Taipei Economic and Cultural Office in New York at a

Forum on Peace Education and Women's Empowerment held on the occasion of the 55th Session of the United Nations Commission on the Status of Women.

Beck, D.-M. (2016). Artistic and scientific: Broadening the scope of our 21st century advocacy. In W. Rosa (Ed.), *Nurses as leaders: Evolutionary visions of leadership* (pp. 247–263). New York, NY: Springer Publishing.

Beck, D.-M., Dossey, B. M., & Rushton, C. H. (2013). Building the Nightingale Initiative for Global Health-NIGH: Can we engage and empower the public voices of nurses worldwide? *Nursing Science Quarterly, 26*(4), 366–371. doi:10.1177/0894318413500403

Benjamin, B. A. (2012). Building relationships and engaging communities through collaboration. In A. L. C. Curley & P. A. Vitale (Eds.), *Population-based nursing: Concepts and competencies for advanced practice* (pp. 211–238). New York, NY: Springer Publishing.

Burgess, C. A., Reimer-Kirkham, S., & Astle, B. (2014). Motivation and international clinical placements: Shifting nursing students to a global citizenship perspective. *International Journal of Nursing Education Scholarship, 11*(1), 1–8.

Cowling, W. R., III. (2016). Unitary and appreciative: Nourishing and supporting the human spirit. In W. Rosa (Ed.), *Nurses as leaders: Evolutionary visions of leadership* (pp. 49–60). New York, NY: Springer Publishing.

Dobson, A. (2005). Globalisation, cosmopolitanism, and the environment. *International Relations, 26*, 1005–1020.

Dossey, B. M., & Keegan, L. (2016). *Holistic nursing: A handbook for practice* (7th ed.). Burlington, MA: Jones & Bartlett.

Evans, H. (2016). What does it mean to be a citizen of the world? Retrieved from http://www.ted.com/talks/hugh_evans_what_does_it_mean_to_be_a_citizen_of_the_world?language=en

Fitzgerald, M. A. (2016). Powerful and beneficent: Seizing opportunity in practice and equality in health care. In W. Rosa (Ed.), *Nurses as leaders: Evolutionary visions of leadership* (pp. 77–86). New York, NY: Springer Publishing.

Giovannoni, J. (2016). Egoless and interconnected: Suspending judgment to embrace heart-centered health care. In W. Rosa (Ed.), *Nurses as leaders: Evolutionary visions of leadership* (pp. 265–277). New York, NY: Springer Publishing.

Global Citizen. (2012–2016). Who we are. Retrieved from https://www.globalcitizen.org/en/about/who-we-are

Goldin, M. (2016). Empathic and unselfish: Redefining nurse caring as love in action. In W. Rosa (Ed.), *Nurses as leaders: Evolutionary visions of leadership* (pp. 279–291). New York, NY: Springer Publishing.

Henker, R., Prak, M., & Koy, V. (2015). Development and implementation of cornerstone documents to support nursing practice in Cambodia. *The Online Journal of Issues in Nursing, 20*(2), Manuscript 5.

Honor Society of Nursing, Sigma Theta Tau International. (n.d.). "Global" health policy position statement. Retrieved from http://www.nursingsociety.org/docs/default-source/position-papers/stti-global-health-policy-position_final.pdf?sfvrsn=4

Honor Society of Nursing, Sigma Theta Tau International. (2005). Resource paper on global health and nursing research priorities. Retrieved from http://www.nursingsociety.org/docs/default-source/position-papers/position_ghnrprp-(1).pdf?sfvrsn=4

Honor Society of Nursing, Sigma Theta Tau International. (2016). Connect & engage: Global. Retrieved from http://www.nursingsociety.org/connect-engage/our-global-impact

IDEAS for Global Citizenship. (n.d.). What is global citizenship? Retrieved from http://www.ideas-forum.org.uk/about-us/global-citizenship

International Council of Nurses. (2012). The ICN Code of Ethics for Nurses. Retrieved from http://www.icn.ch/images/stories/documents/about/icncode_english.pdf

Jamison, D. T., Summers, L. H., Alleyne, G., Arrow, K. J., Berkley, S., Bingwaho, A., . . . Yamey, G. (2013). Global health 2035: A world converging within a generation. *Lancet, 382*, 1898–1955. doi:10.1016/s0140-6736(13)62105-4

Janes, C. R., & Corbett K. K. (2009). Anthropology and global health. *Annual Reviews of Anthropology, 38*, 167–183. doi:10.1146/annurev-anthro-091908-164314

Kreitzer, M. J., & Koithan, M. (Eds.). (2014). *Integrative nursing*. New York, NY: Oxford University Press.

Levinas, E. (1969/2000). *Totality and infinity* (14th ed.). Pittsburgh, PA: Duquesne University.

McClure, M. L. (2016). Accountable and interprofessional: Owning the breadth of the nursing role. In W. Rosa (Ed.), *Nurses as leaders: Evolutionary visions of leadership* (pp. 137–148). New York, NY: Springer Publishing.

McGrew, L. (1990). Health care in Cambodia. *Cultrual Survival Quarterly, 14(3)*. Retrieved from https://www.culturalsurvival.org/publications/cultural-survival-quarterly/health-care-cambodia

Middle Eastern Nurses. (2015). Home. Retrieved from http://middleastnurses.squarespace.com

Nicholas, P. K., & Breakey, S. (2015). Global health and global nursing. In S. Breakey, I. B. Corless, N. L. Meedzan, & P. K. Nicholas (Eds.), *Global health nursing in the 21st century* (pp. 3–24). New York, NY: Springer Publishing.

Nickitas, D. M. (2016). Ethical and economical: Calling the profession to social justice. In W. Rosa (Ed.), *Nurses as leaders: Evolutionary visions of leadership* (pp. 149–163). New York, NY: Springer Publishing.

Nightingale Initiative for Global Health. (2016). Raising awareness for mothers' health. Retrieved from http://www.nighvision.net/raising-awareness-for-mdg-5.html

Novogratz, J. (2009). *The blue sweater: Bridging the gap between rich and poor in an interconnected world*. New York, NY: Rodale.

Novogratz, J. (2010). Inspiring a life of immersion. Retrieved from https://www.ted.com/talks/jacqueline_novogratz_inspiring_a_life_of_immersion?language=en

Novogratz, J. (2016). What it takes to move the world: 5 traits of moral leaders. Retrieved from https://medium.com/acumen-ideas/what-it-takes-to-move-the-world-41ababbe10f9#.q8qrb1ett

Pesut, D. J. (2016). Transformed and in service: Creating the future through renewal. In W. Rosa (Ed.), *Nurses as leaders: Evolutionary visions of leadership* (pp. 165–178). New York, NY: Springer Publishing.

Quinn, J. (2016). Transpersonal human caring and healing. In B. M. Dossey & L. Keegan (Eds.), *Holistic nursing: A handbook for practice* (7th ed., pp. 101–110). Burlington, MA: Jones & Bartlett.

Rosa, W. (2017). Change agent. In P. Dickerson (Ed.), *Nursing professional development core curriculum* (5th ed., pp. 211–222). Chicago, IL: Association for Nurses in Professional Development.

Rosa, W. (2014a). Caring science and compassion fatigue: Reflective inventory for the individual processes of self-healing. *Beginnings, 34(4)*, 18–20.

Rosa, W. (2014b). Conscious dying and cultural emergence: Reflective systems inventory for the collective processes of global healing. *Beginnings, 34(5)*, 20–22.

Rosa, W. (Ed.). (2016a). *Nurses as leaders: Evolutionary visions of leadership*. New York, NY: Springer Publishing.

Rosa, W. (2016b). Awakened and conscious: Reclaiming lost power and intraprofessional identity. In W. Rosa (Ed.), *Nurses as leaders: Evolutionary visions of leadership* (pp. 359–376). New York, NY: Springer Publishing.

Rosa, W., Estes, T., & Watson, J. (2017). Caring science conscious dying: An emerging meta-paradigm. *Nursing Science Quarterly, 30(1)*. doi:10.1177/0894318416680538

Rosa, W., & Santos, S. (2016). Introducing the Engaged Feedback Reflective Inventory in a preceptor training program. *Journal for Nurses in Professional Development, 32(4)*, E1–E7.

Schaub, B. G. (2016). Vulnerable and spiritual: Utilizing the process of transpersonal nurse coaching. In W. Rosa (Ed.), *Nurses as leaders: Evolutionary visions of leadership* (pp. 377–392). New York, NY: Springer Publishing.

Schaub, R., & Schaub, B. G. (2013). *Transpersonal development: Cultivating the human resources of peace, wisdom, purpose and oneness*. Huntington, NY: Florence Press.

Shamian, J. (2015a). Global voice, strategic leadership and policy impact: Global citizens, global nursing. *International Nursing Review, 62(1)*, 435–436.

Shamian, J. (2015b). Strong nursing presence is vital to global health. *International Nursing Review, 62(4)*, 435–436.

Sherwood, G., & Horton-Deutsch, S. (Eds.). (2012). *Reflective practice: Transforming education and improving outcomes*. Indianapolis, IN: Sigma Theta Tau International.

Sherwood, G., & Horton-Deutsch, S. (Eds.). (2015). *Reflective organizations: On the frontline of QSEN and reflective practice implementation*. Indianapolis, IN: Sigma Theta Tau International.

Strickland, K., Adamson, E., McInally, W., Tiittenen, H., & Metcalfe, S. (2013). Developing global citizenship online: An authentic alternative to overseas clinical placement. *Nurse Education Today, 33*, 1160–1165.

United Nations. (2013). *United Nations at a glance*. New York, NY: Author.

United Nations. (2015). The Millennium Development Goals report: 2015. Retrieved from http://www.un.org/millenniumgoals/2015_MDG_Report/pdf/MDG%202015%20 rev%20(July%201).pdf

United Nations Millennium Project. (2006). What they are. Retrieved from http://www .unmillenniumproject.org/goals

United Nations Sustainable Development. (2016). The sustainable development agenda. Retrieved from http://www.un.org/sustainabledevelopment/development-agenda

Upvall, M. J., & Leffers, J. M. (Eds.). (2014). *Global health nursing: Building and sustaining partnerships*. New York, NY: Springer Publishing.

Visovsky, C., McGhee, S., Jordan, E., Dominic, S., & Morrison-Beedy, D. (2016). Planning and executing a global health experience for undergraduate nursing students: A comprehensive guide to creating global citizens. *Nurse Education Today, 40*, 29–32.

Vonfrolio, L. G. (2016). Unafraid and confident: Empowering the staff nurse with fearless moral courage. In W. Rosa (Ed.), *Nurses as leaders: Evolutionary visions of leadership* (pp. 209–219). New York, NY: Springer Publishing.

Watson, J. (2016). Caring and compassionate: Unveiling the heart of humanity. In W. Rosa (Ed.), *Nurses as leaders: Evolutionary visions of leadership* (pp. 221–229). New York, NY: Springer Publishing.

Wilson, L., Mendes, I. A. C., Klopper, H., Catrambone, C., Al-Maaitah, R., Norton, M. E., & Hill, M. (2016). "Global health" and "global nursing": Proposed definitions from, The Global Advisory Panel on the Future of Nursing. *Journal of Advanced Nursing, 72*(7), 1529–1540.

World Health Organization. (2006). *The world health report 2006—Working together for health*. Geneva, Switzerland: Author. Retrieved from http://www.who.int/whr/2006/whr06_ en.pdf

World Health Organization. (2016a). *Global strategic directions for strengthening nursing and midwifery, 2016–2020*. Geneva, Switzerland: Author. Retrieved from http://www.who .int/hrh/nursing_midwifery/global-strategic-midwifery2016-2020.pdf?ua=1

World Health Organization. (2016b). *Global strategy on human resources for health: Workforce 2030*. Geneva, Switzerland: Author. Retrieved from http://apps.who.int/iris/bitstre am/10665/250368/1/9789241511131-eng.pdf

World Health Organization. (2016c). Global momentum for human resources for health at the sixty-ninth World Health Assembly. Retrieved from http://www.who.int/ workforcealliance/media/news/2016/ghwa_wha16_global-momentum/en

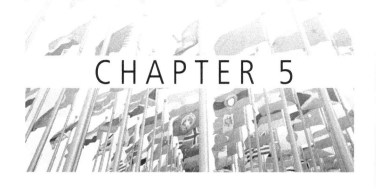

CHAPTER 5

Transforming Our World by 2030: Leadership Requisites to Guide the Global Village

William Rosa and Karen H. Morin

There is one assumption to embrace: Everyone is a leader. This means that every nurse, whether holding a formal leadership title or not, has a responsibility to influence the advancement of the . . . profession. . . . [We must not] underestimate the compelling value proposition of nursing as being a prime contributor of healthcare transformation. (Andrus & Shanahan, 2016, p. 597)

Global nurses have the potential to transform health care, not only at the point of delivery but also in the creation, direction, and implementation of systemwide advances that increase access to and delivery of quality care across nations. Transformation is not possible until nurses understand their potential as leaders. We must each foster the development of powerful leaders at all levels of nursing and global health in order to realize the vision of health equity, a safe and inclusive society, and the collaborative interprofessional partnerships called for by the United Nations 2030 Agenda for Sustainable Development (see the Appendix to view the Agenda in its entirety).

Global nursing and a global consciousness have been cornerstones of the profession we know today since its inception. Starting with Nightingale's transnational advocacy work, and demonstrated repeatedly by exemplary nurse leaders over time, the global impact of nursing's contributions is a part of our disciplinary heritage; it is in our blood, so to speak (Forrester, 2016). It is a history that directly informs our collective identity and guides us in carrying out the ideals and ethical foundations of the profession (Dossey, Selanders, Beck, & Attewell, 2005). Global nurses must maximize their leadership potential through all avenues available to them and capitalize on both formal and informal opportunities for growth (Sullivan, 2013). For the purposes of global health and the unknown future of the 2030 Agenda, one cannot underestimate the importance of creating and continuing to develop a vision for leadership and influence. Through self-reflection and allowing for creative expression related to personal–professional development, one must become aware of opportunities to clarify one's future leadership vision, act deliberately to integrate strategies that will help implement it, and identify potential obstacles (Grossman & Valiga, 2013); in short, "think positively, speak in possibilities, and [don't] give up" (p. 89).

The socially just, healthy, and peaceful society sought by the Sustainable Development Goals (SDGs) mirrors the longstanding priorities, targets, and ethical values inherent to nursing. The SDGs are not new for us, and yet, we do not currently play widely recognized leadership roles in their implementation processes. It is up to global nurses to be clear about the greater calling of the profession beyond technical competencies and scope limitations, the expertise we possess in local and international arenas, and the contributions we are prepared, equipped, and determined to make as global health leaders.

EVOLUTIONARY LEADERSHIP: A FOUNDATION FOR GLOBAL NURSING

In *Nurses as Leaders: Evolutionary Visions of Leadership* (Rosa, 2016a), more than 30 of the profession's most accomplished clinicians, nurse educators, deans, chief nursing officers, executives, acclaimed authors, global advocates, policy experts, holistic guides, nurse coaches, editors in chief, organizational presidents, nongovernmental organization (NGO) founders, spiritual practitioners, and administrators provide their unique perspectives on what constitutes leadership and how nurses can learn to embody it. *Evolutionary leadership*

> . . . merges all corners of the discipline into a cohesive force for health and well-being; . . . fully embraces the art and strategically engages the science of nursing; . . . [provides] historical context and . . . foresight; and [seeks] to unveil and awaken the inherent leader dwelling within each nurse, regardless of position, title, credentials, or specialty. (Rosa, 2016b, p. xxiii)

It is not enough to have a vision for leadership; it must be translated into action, both locally and globally, through an ongoing commitment to advocacy. Global action was a vital agenda item for Nightingale in her times. The increasing globalization of the world and health care require nursing's ongoing and reinforced commitment to such leadership sensibilities.

Several themes emerged from the contributions of the authors in the preceding text regarding evolutionary leadership. They painted leadership in a humanistic and caring light guided by the ideals of social justice and the emerging advances of science: a true nursing paradigm. These themes were renamed the Evolutionary Leadership Assumptions (ELAs; Rosa, 2016c) and are listed in Box 5.1.

Box 5.1	Evolutionary Leadership Assumptions

- Evolutionary leadership calls for a state of openness and self-awareness.
- Evolutionary leadership requires self-renewal and self-reflection.
- Evolutionary leadership implies a willingness to mature in ways of being, doing, thinking, seeing, and knowing.
- Evolutionary leadership acknowledges the difference between striving and perfectionism.
- Evolutionary leadership is "both/and" and not "either/or."
- Evolutionary leadership respects all voices in the room.
- Evolutionary leaders rehumanize work environments to promote ethical engagement and meaningful partnerships.
- Evolutionary leaders work to unveil and promote the truth.
- Evolutionary leaders allow for the transformation of self and systems.

Source: Reprinted from Rosa (2016c).

These principles may assist the global nurse in creating healing relationships and environments that will promote the values inherent to the SDGs and in accomplishing the related targets. They are discussed in greater depth in the following text.

Evolutionary Leadership Assumptions[1]

Evolutionary Leadership Embraces Vulnerability

Brown (2012) defines "vulnerability" as "uncertainty, risk, and emotional exposure" and acknowledges it as "the birthplace of love, belonging, joy, courage, empathy, and creativity . . . the source of hope . . . , accountability, and authenticity . . . [and the way to gain] greater clarity in our purpose . . . and more meaningful . . . lives" (p. 34). Brown (2012) writes that to "dare greatly" is to meet the fear of vulnerability head-on and to muster the strength to be our fully expressed selves in environments that do not give any guarantees. Ultimately, she goes on to say, "Vulnerability sounds like truth and feels like courage" (p. 37).

If a nurse is going to own and demonstrate behaviors representative of leadership, such as questioning the tasks presented, forming individual opinions, taking risks, building relationships, showing excitement about work, creating adventure, providing something to believe in, and inspiring others (Taffinder, 2006), then learning to navigate and embrace vulnerability is essential. Having the courage to embrace and relate to one's own vulnerability and that of another contributes to developing a compassionate practice and the ethical formation of nursing care (Curtis, 2014; Thorup, Rundqvist, Roberts, & Delmar, 2012). In fact, it has been

---

[1] *Source:* Reprinted from Rosa (2016c).

noted that in environments where nurses' vulnerability is acknowledged and their whole person is honored and celebrated, beyond the limitations of their technical skills and abilities, human flourishing for both nurses and those for whom they care is possible (Sumner, 2013).

Evolutionary Leadership Calls for a State of Openness and Self-Awareness

As a leader, as one whose actions will impact those around him or her either through influence or direct action, it is vital to maintain an attitude of openness. Openness requires suspending preconceived judgments and being willing to see things from another's point of view. It can also be thought of as "coming from nothing" or surrendering the automatic labels and meanings we tend to place on anything and everything that hinder our abilities to grow and consider life from a different perspective (DiMaggio, 2011a).

> The nothing that's available for us to experience is not nothing as a negation of self . . . [but the ability] to create, design, and live with a freedom that's not available when we create from something . . . a clearing that frees [us] from [our] own self-imposed restrictions. (DiMaggio, 2011a, p. 18)

We can also think of the application of openness as the concept of the beginner's mind in Zen practice (Suzuki, 1983), or unknowing, releasing previously held beliefs as a way of experiencing a phenomenon in nursing practice (Munhall, 1993). Coming from nothing, employing a beginner's mind, and applying unknowing are all forms of openness that allow for a clean slate in the teaching–learning process and create space for new possibilities to emerge that are inaccessible when coming from something, employing an expert's lens, and honoring previously held knowing as fact.

Maturing in self-awareness and taking action to improve upon observed growth opportunities increase the nurse's capacity to provide caring and healing to self and others (Thornton & Mariano, 2016). As it pertains to the learning process and the work milieu, self-awareness can alert us when we are clinging to outdated beliefs and patterns that prevent us from being open and available to the concepts presented. Self-awareness may assist us in identifying and acknowledging those areas where we are resistant to growth and evolution and may also engender the willingness necessary to surrender those self-imposed limitations that no longer serve us.

Evolutionary Leadership Requires Self-Renewal and Self-Reflection

Nurse leaders "reflect on action to become aware of values, feelings, perceptions, and judgments that may affect actions, and they also reflect on their experiences to obtain insight for future practice" (Mariano, 2016, p. 66). These reflections are just one component of the self-renewal work needed to meet the anticipated demands of effective leadership. This ELA is deeply related to increasing self-awareness and helping one to remain open to what is available in the moment, as mentioned earlier, but maintains further implications in the development and application of leadership-based ethics. While the questions offered at the end of each chapter provide one avenue for ongoing and progressive introspection, self-renewal and self-reflection work can also take the form of journaling, storytelling, meditation, creative expression, and other mindfulness practices. These outlets allow the nurse leader to process the events and people around him or her, reframe experiences from a different perspective, reconnect and recommit to inner purpose and intention, and come to know the self at a deeper level. Quite simply: "Reflection is a means of renewal" (Pesut, 2005, p.1). Responsibility for self-renewal is necessary for the individual mental, emotional, and spiritual well-being of nurses who are committed to the delivery of humane, quality care (Pesut, 2012). Reflective practice, while shown to improve individual performance outcomes, can also elevate organizational consciousness when applied at a systems level (Sherwood & Horton-Deutsch, 2012, 2015).

Evolutionary Leadership Implies a Willingness to Mature in Ways of Being, Doing, Thinking, Seeing, and Knowing

"Willingness" suggests one who is flexible and adaptive, tolerant and mindful, in touch with one's inner wisdom, and appreciative and stable in one's sense of self (Schaub & Schaub, 1997). All ways of being, doing, thinking, seeing, and knowing are invited to expand and mature throughout this book journey. It is not a task you are asked to complete. Rather, it is an offering that implores you to acknowledge and personalize that which is beneficial to your journey as a nurse leader from the wealth of the authors' lived experiences. As you read and reflect upon the histories of these nurse leaders, continue to ask yourself important questions such as: Who am I being? Does that way of being support me in realizing my highest potential as a nurse leader? Would doing things in a new way contribute toward the betterment of myself or another? How can I think about my leadership from a different vantage point? Would it benefit me to release what I know in order to relearn and reconsider? Leadership becomes stagnant without a willingness to unravel previously held, long-standing beliefs and emerge into a way of being-doing-thinking-seeing-knowing you may never have considered before.

Evolutionary Leadership Acknowledges the Difference Between Striving and Perfectionism

Brown (2010) states that the quest for perfectionism is very different from healthy striving and a desire to be one's best:

> Perfectionism is not about healthy achievement and growth. Perfectionism is the belief that if we live perfect, . . . we can minimize or avoid the pain of blame, judgment, and shame. . . . Perfectionism is not self-improvement. . . . Healthy striving is self-focused—How can I improve? Perfectionism is other focused—What will they think? (pp. 94–95)

Healthy striving keeps our contributions as unique individuals and our journeys of self-growth, self-realization, and self-expression rooted in personal integrity. The process of striving helps us to understand that leadership is not about perfection and that the idea of perfect outcomes of any kind is a drain on our energy and interpersonal resources. In fact, the nurse leader who can acknowledge mistakes, ask for help, take risks, and share creative ideas without fear of others' judgments or opinions is living authentically (Brown, 2012). Striving is an inherent aspect of the human experience (Watson, 2012); the quest to become more evolved and grounded in who we are; the unyielding motivation to improve upon ourselves mentally, emotionally, and spiritually; and the desire to reconnect with our inner and highest wisdom. Striving calls for the authentic integration of the personal and professional; in other words, fostering the integrity of a unified self. Inversely, the path of perfectionism further compartmentalizes how we see ourselves, our lives, and our contributions. It is in our commitment to healthy striving and releasing the need for perfectionism that we find the freedom to embrace our individualism as nurse leaders.

Evolutionary Leadership Is "Both/And" and Not "Either/Or"

There is no need for inner fragmentation, for a mental–emotional separation of our personal–professional life, as previously noted, or for the self-limitations that keep us from experiencing a reality of inclusivity. Nurse leaders do not have to choose between leadership methodologies: between being holistic or not, incorporating nurse theories or not, believing in caring as the essence of nursing or not. Leadership is an adventure into "both/and." As intelligent and accountable nurse leaders, we have the opportunity to select the concepts, ideas, and inquiries that will support us in becoming an effective force for positive change, as we are, with what we have to contribute, at this point in time. Pressuring ourselves to choose between "either/or" diminishes the integrity of our innate human complexities and creates barriers to our wholeness. Living an undivided life and reading the pages that follow from a perspective of "both/and" can help in learning how to shape an integral experience, derive meaning and value in community, teach and learn for transformation, and understand how to influence valuable and peaceful social change (Palmer, 2004).

Evolutionary Leadership Respects All Voices in the Room

As a nurse who was licensed and educated in the United States, the largest representative organization advocating and promoting professional rights is the American Nurses Association (ANA). Their ethical standards prepared and continued to guide me in my work at local and global levels. Provision 1 of the ANA's (2015) *Code of Ethics for Nurses With Interpretive Statements* is clear that "the nurse practices with compassion and respect for the inherent dignity, worth, and unique attributes of every person" (p. 1). Attention to this provision ensures that human dignity is preserved in all interactions and that people feel heard and acknowledged. As you read, you may see statements or opinions with which you disagree or doubt. Feel free to reflect upon any resistance you encounter, but do your best to respect each chapter as an expression of an author's lived experience and as what the author knows to be true. Consider the context from which the insight was offered, glean what you can, and remain open to what it can teach you.

Provision 5 of the ANA (2015) *Code of Ethics* states that "the nurse owes the same duties to self as to others, including the responsibility to promote health and safety, preserve wholeness of character and integrity, maintain competence, and continue personal and professional growth" (p. 19). This means that self-respect is integral to this journey of learning and expansion. Strive to cultivate self-respect as you challenge yourself, explore new perspectives, and engage in self-development.

Evolutionary Leaders Rehumanize Work Environments to Promote Ethical Engagement and Meaningful Partnerships

Leaders and those with whom they partner thrive in environments where creativity is valued, vulnerabilities are embraced, and people are respected for who they are and what they bring to the table. Brown (2012) points out in the "Daring Greatly Leadership Manifesto":

> When learning and working are dehumanized—when you no longer see us and encourage our daring, or when you only see what we produce or how we perform—we disengage and turn away from the very things the world needs from us: our talent, our ideas, and our passion. (p. 212)

It is no secret that many health care environments have become dehumanized by succumbing to bureaucratic dictates (Watson, 2005, 2008) that focus on employee output, patient outcomes, insurance reimbursement, regulatory standards, and the adage "Do more with less." Nursing has witnessed the submergence of its humanistic core values—its own dehumanization of value and purpose (Watson, 2012).

This fact is not something to resist or resent but something to acknowledge in one's evolving nurse–leader journey. The business of health care is a reality that must be considered and included in nurse leadership dialogue at this time. All nurses need to be educated to understand and respect the places and spaces where business and nursing merge. The altruistic ethics of nursing are vital for the preservation of dignity wherever it is threatened,

> but empathy is only our starting point. It must be combined with focus and conviction, the toughness to know what needs to get done and the courage to follow through. . . . We will only succeed if we fuse a very hardheaded analysis with an equally soft heart. (Novogratz, 2009, p. 284)

In rehumanizing our learning experience, in coming to value both the experiential wisdom of others and our own individual uniqueness, we create new possibilities for our understanding of both nursing and leadership.

Evolutionary Leaders Work to Unveil and Promote the Truth

When nurses are taught how to complete a thorough pain assessment, they are reminded about the subjective truth of the patient: "Pain is whatever the patient says it is." It is with the same nonjudgmental and available approach that the nurse leader seeks out the subjective truth of the populations and communities they serve. Ethical commitments to beneficence and social justice guide our leadership on a truth-seeking journey to ensure the equitable access to and delivery of services. It is this mission to engage, acknowledge, and understand the truth of another that allows the nurse leader to be sure he or she is acting from a place of moral and ethical integrity. Quality, dignified health care is a human right and it is the nurse–leader's role to honor and procure this truth.

Evolutionary Leaders Allow for the Transformation of Self and Systems

"Transformation" may be simply defined herein as allowing for the positive and reflective growth of self so that we are never the same. It is a bold action—a commitment to learning new ways of interacting with the surrounding world, exploring previously untapped parts of ourselves, and teaching-learning-role modeling with consideration to "what is" while believing in "what could be."

> Transformation has the power to upset the status quo, to unseat us from business as usual—it gives us a platform for being all we can . . . to live consistent with what we know is possible. . . . Transformation carries with it . . . a knowing that we have a choice about who we are. (Dimaggio, 2011b, p. 49)

Transformation of self and systems go hand in hand. As individuals transform how they engage with health care, the infrastructures they create and sustain will come to reflect their heightened ethics and values. Individual transformation on a mass scale advances systems toward the ideals of a caring society.

In order to become evolutionary nurse leaders in the service of global health, we must start where we are. We can begin by expanding how we think of our current role in the broader global context.

TOWARD GLOBAL LEADERSHIP[2]

The ELAs provide a wonderful foundation upon which to consider leadership in a global context. After all, leadership is about having a solid understanding of our current and future abilities, as well as the critical role self-development plays relative to those abilities. That said, considerable work has been undertaken in the past decade to help us be more effective leaders in the global arena (Black & Morrison, 2014; Gundling, Hogan, & Cvitkovich, 2011; Mendenhall et al., 2013). Although many of these authors are grounded in business and management, nurses can learn much from their work, as can be seen in the following paragraphs.

No discussion of global leaders can start without being clear about who global leaders are. They are

> individuals who effect change in organizations by building communities through the development of trust and the arrangement of organizational structures and processes in a context involving multiple cross-boundary stakeholders, multiple sources of external cross-boundary authority, and multiple cultures under conditions of temporal, geographical, and cultural complexity. (Mendenhall et al., 2013, p. 20)

Being a global leader, then, requires us to appreciate the inherent complexity that is "global." This complexity calls for the expansion of some of the ELAs and the development of others.

What, then, are attributes of global leaders? One of the key attributes is that of having a global mindset (Cabrera & Unruh, 2012). A person with a global mindset

---

[2] *Source:* Adapted from Morin (2011, 2015).

can "perceive, analyze, and decode behaviors and situations in multiple *cultural* contexts and understand the dynamics of the interactions between multiple cultures" (p. 39). Having a global mindset means that we have to think outside our typical reference points, an activity that is not easily undertaken, as we tend to constantly compare what is happening to that which is the most familiar to us. Take for example, the case of how women give birth around the globe. U.S. nurses may consider they provide the best care; however, this assumption can be challenged by nurse colleagues from countries where childbirth has been less medicalized but shows better birth outcomes. As global leaders, it is important to assess what our mindset is. Cabrera and Unruh (2012) have developed an instrument based on their research to assess global mindset. A sample of the instrument can be found at globalmindset.thunderbird.edu/home/global-mindset-inventory/sample-survey. We encourage you to explore this link and the site.

Other attributes offered by Gundling, Hogan, and Cvitkovich (2011) include being able to

- See differences: Leaders who see differences are *culturally aware* and invite the unexpected. Global leaders appreciate that their world is *not* the center of the world; they appreciate that what worked in one situation may not work in another culture; and they experience differences frequently and willingly. They *invite the unexpected* by demonstrating a readiness to learn, refining language skills, asking questions, and having outstanding listening skills.

- Close the gap: Leaders close the gap by respecting the critical role *relationship*s play in global interactions, acknowledging interdependence, and recognizing the contributions a cultural guide can make to their understanding of culture influences. They develop the ability to "frameshift," an activity that "requires cognitive and behavioral agility to alter both one's leadership style and strategic approach" (p. 62).

- Open the system: Leaders who open the system *expand ownership*; that is, leaders "create a sense of engagement in a shared process and accountability for setting and achieving targets with both global and local significance" (p. 79). In addition, they *develop future leaders*.

- Preserve balance: In order to preserve balance, global leaders must be able to *adapt and add value*. Thus, they must be sensitive to local circumstances as they "demonstrate an ability to make a valuable contribution" (p. 99). Equally important is the leader's ability to identify his or her core values, that is, those key values that may need to be defended during global interactions.

- Establish solutions: Leaders who are able to establish solutions *influence across borders* by acknowledging their role can be similar to that of an ambassador or diplomat. Thus, they need "sufficient political acumen to be cognizant of corporate governance and confidentiality concerns" (p. 115). When addressing solutions, global leaders "bracket previous ideas and practices, relate to build trust across differences, inquire for mutual learning and insight, cocreate solutions and/or options, and commit to implementation" (p. 120). Consistency and transparency are also important behaviors.

It is important to be culturally self-aware, establish solid relationships, help develop future leaders, add value to conversations, and think of solutions that cross boundaries. Gundling and colleagues also have an instrument to help develop as a global leader. It can be found at http://www.aperianglobal.com/learning-solutions/online-learning-tools/globesmart-profile-2. This instrument is particularly helpful as it can help you gain an understanding of how your behavior and beliefs mesh with other cultures. For example, having completed the instrument, I learned that my communication style was more indirect than direct and that I valued relationships more than tasks when compared with the reference group I selected—Healthcare/Hospitals. This information is invaluable as I interact with health care colleagues from other countries; I now craft my messages so that they are more explicit and, when appropriate, acknowledge the importance of tasks.

Other attributes considered important to global leaders include being inquisitive, having a perspective that embraces uncertainty and appreciates balancing tension, possessing the critical character attributes of integrity and emotional connectedness, and having organizational savoir faire (Black & Morrison, 2014). To find out where you stand, ask yourself questions such as: Do [I] love to travel to new parts of the world? (p. 74; reflects how inquisitive you are), [Am I] comfortable with uncertainty? (p. 74; reflects your perspective), and How well do [I] understand [my] health care organization or system compared with that of another country? (p. 74; reflects your savoir faire).

As is evident, there are many approaches to global leadership. All require an openness to the unfamiliar, tremendous humility, a willingness to learn, and a comfort with uncertainty. These are not attributes with which nurses are typically most familiar—other than humility—yet they are essential to our ability to serve as global leaders. What is most exciting is that we have the abilities to excel as global leaders, as our focus is always on how best to improve the health of those for whom we provide health care.

Lessons Learned

As a president of Sigma Theta Tau International (STTI) during 2009–2011, I was privileged to interact with nurse leaders from around the globe. I learned several important lessons along the way. Interestingly, as I reflected on my journey, I found my lessons were comparable to those of other leaders (Kouzes & Posner, 2010). Five are highlighted.

Humility

The first lesson I learned was how very critical humility is in fostering relationships. By "humility," I mean being sensitive to cultural practices, intellectual contributions, and being open to different perspectives and norms. I was struck by how nurses in other parts of the world are much more hospitable than in the United States. For example, when I traveled to Korea, my hostess made a point of assigning at least two doctoral students to serve as my interpreter and guide. When I traveled to Saudi Arabia, I was confident that there would be someone to greet me at the airport. These simple acts reminded me how we, in the United States, often expect our colleagues from outside the country to make their way on their own to our functions. How different would their experience be if we employed some of their practices?

I also gained a much better understanding of and appreciation for the knowledge colleagues in other parts of the world are generating that truly has an impact on patient outcomes. For example, colleagues in other countries had a more comprehensive perspective of primary health care and were pursuing studies that highlighted the critical role nurses play in primary health care (note, I am speaking about primary *health* care, not primary care). These investigators, and their work, challenged me to reconsider how health care was provided in my country of residence and how nurses are addressing solutions.

Self-Development

Leadership, as a journey, involves being willing to develop. Over the course of my time with STTI, I have spent considerable time identifying my strengths and using those strengths to invite members to join the organization's mission and vision. I also had the opportunity to observe nurse leaders, such as Dr. Wipada Kunaviktikul, dean of Chiang Mai School of Nursing in Thailand, as she and others helped nurses appreciate the contribution a chapter of STTI could make to the development of nurses and leaders in that county. Interaction with nurse leaders from around the globe helped expand my understanding of what constitutes a global mindset, appreciate differences, and become more comfortable with uncertainty.

Individuals Make a Difference

Interacting with STTI members, as well as members of other professions, reinforced the fact that each one of us is the most important leader (Kouzes & Posner, 2010). When you believe "in yourself and in your capacity to lead, you open yourself up to hearing the call. You open yourself up to making a difference in the world" (p. 14). Being open leads to opportunities by which to have an impact. This point was reinforced during interactions with participants in the STTI and Johnson & Johnson pilot of the Maternal–Child Health Nurse Leadership Academy in South Africa. One participant, in particular, stands out. She was a staff nurse employed in a public hospital. Interestingly, staff nurses in public hospitals are not well respected in South Africa, so she was not undertaking her project from a position of strength. Nonetheless, she was committed to improving care to childbearing women, particularly in terms of prevention of postpartum hemorrhage. She knew that the current institutional practice did not reflect best practice, so she developed and offered an all-day workshop to address knowledge gaps. Although her institution did not provide any support for the workshop, she obtained external funding to support the workshop, which was an outstanding success. More than 200 participants from her institution, as well as other institutions, attended. Given the response to her workshop, her hospital committed resources to holding an annual workshop. Her impact extended beyond her immediate sphere of influence. *She* made a difference!

Appreciate Values

Amazingly, nurses around the globe have similar values. We want to provide the best care that is based on evidence, with adequate materials and supplies, in an environment that is safe. We want leaders who are transparent in their decision making, who are approachable, and who support the work that we do. It does not matter where you are in the world—these values surface consistently.

Passion Counts

Nurse leaders with whom I have interacted all were passionate about improving health for their patients: They spoke their passion and they lived their passion. Nurse leaders were also passionate about developing the next generation of leaders. Alina Kushkyan, MD, PhD, director, Yerevan State Armenian American medical college, Erebouni, and chief nursing specialist of the Ministry of Health of the Republic of Armenia, is a wonderful example of passion and of what passion can accomplish. Although not a nurse, her passion for the nursing profession is exceptional. As a physician, not only does she understand the critical role nurses play in enhancing the health of a nation's people, but she also understands the importance of having an educated nurse workforce and of having that workforce connect with colleagues from around the globe. She has been instrumental in orchestrating biannual nursing conferences that draw participants from former USSR countries, the United States, Turkey, South Africa, and England. It is her passion that excited people to share and learn. Truly, she exemplifies: "Being a leader brings with it a responsibility to do something of significance that makes families, communities, work organizations, nations, the environment, and the world better places than they are today" (Kouzes & Posner, 2010, p. 13).

As is evident, global nurse leaders possess the characteristics and abilities consistent with leaders in other disciplines. Moreover, interacting with them highlights how they have taken advantage of opportunities present at the local, regional, national, and global levels to strengthen abilities to enhance the contribution nurses can make to the health of people.

A WORD ON CULTURAL HUMILITY

> In a multicultural world where power imbalances exist, . . . achieving cultural humility [results in] mutual empowerment, respect, partnerships, optimal care, and lifelong learning. . . . Cultural humility involves a change in overall perspective and way of life. [It] is a way of being . . . [and] should be employed daily with all individuals in the basic interest of kindness [and] civility. (Foronda, Baptiste, Reinholdt, & Ousman, 2016, pp. 213–214)

The global nurse leader is both a leader and advocate in service to the greater good. All too often, health care workers (HCWs), whether nurses or other interprofessional partners, can get caught up in their subjective perceptions of idealistic care, inadvertently overlooking the client's unique health goals and the culture in which he or she lives and experiences health. There is, at times, an inherent arrogance in the care delivered to differing cultures of race, ethnicity, religious affiliation, sexual orientation, gender identification, socioeconomic standing, and age. This arrogance can be observed again and again in health care when HCWs believe, as the "experts" in the field, that the information they possess is of greater importance or holds more validity than the client's experiential values, norms, and traditions. HCWs may subtly and unknowingly adopt a "greater than, less than" approach to engagement, where "we," as experts, are "greater than" in resources and evidence, and "they" are "less than" in their limited scope of education related to health, nursing, or medicine.

Who is to say that HCWs' science and evidence trumps clients' self-knowledge and cultural expertise? After all, clients, whether they be individuals, identified populations, or countries, know far more about their health goals, needs, beliefs, and ethics than an outsider could ever understand. Though many HCWs receive significant training in cross-cultural communication or competency training, many still find it difficult to establish positive and effective rapport with clients across the cultural divide (Hook & Watkins, 2015).

The term "cultural humility" was first coined by Tervalon and Murray-Garcia (1998) during research that looked at how to train medical students in their responses to culturally diverse clientele. Tervalon and Murray-Garcia (1998) suggested the attainment of "cultural competence" is a misnomer. They skillfully explain that there is no end point or goal of "competence" in learning to authentically and respectfully navigate the depth and dimension of another culture. In fact, they proposed that cultural humility is a process requiring:

- Self-reflection and lifelong learning in order to accept, understand, and incorporate differing beliefs and health practices;
- Patient-focused interviewing and care that replaces power imbalances seen in paternalistic provider–patient dyads;
- Community-based care and advocacy that leads to mutually beneficial partnerships for both providers and recipients of health care services.

Emphasis should be placed on the idea that cultural humility is, indeed, a *process*. Isaacson (2014) provided a glimpse of the individual's journey toward an experience of cultural humility. She described three themes: "seeing with closed eyes" or confronting cultural assumptions and preconceived notions; "seeing through a fused horizon" or merging personal worldviews with new meanings through cultural immersion; and "disruption to reshaping" or the vulnerability that is experienced with being open to cross-cultural populations and present to the power inequities that exist (Isaacson, 2014, pp. 254–256). HCWs' practice of cultural humility has been shown to be very important to clients in their experience of being acknowledged; it improves the strength of the HCW–client working alliance and helps to prevent HCWs from making cross-cultural assumptions or overvaluing their personal meanings and perspectives within the context of the client relationship (Hook, Davis, Owen, Worthington, & Utsey, 2013).

Foronda and colleagues (2016) identify two antecedents to cultural humility—diversity and power imbalances—and suggest several attributes that can be honed and applied in a host of settings. Table 5.1 lists the attributes of cultural humility with brief definitions.

Through awareness, engagement, and application, these attributes can be fostered to deepen the relational domains of cultural competence—the intrapersonal, interpersonal, system/organization, and global—toward an emerging praxis of cultural humility (Soulé, 2014a, 2014b).

It is vital for global nurse leaders to examine preconceived beliefs and values about their role and how those beliefs and values are communicated to clients. As the nurse begins to explore his or her willingness, or lack thereof, to remain flexible and open to other cultures and how health is perceived through their lenses,

Table 5.1 Attributes of Cultural Humility With Definitions

Attribute	Definition
Openness	• "Possessing an attitude that is willing to explore new ideas . . . one of the initial steps in the process of cultural humility" (p. 211)
Self-awareness	• "Being aware of one's strengths, limitations, values, beliefs, behavior, and appearance to others. The exact terms of awareness and self-awareness [are] noted repeatedly throughout the literature" (p. 211)
Egoless	• "Require[s] humbleness or throwing away ego. Descriptive terms [include] requiring modesty . . . , down to earth, having neutrality, having humble attitude, being equitable . . . , approach (others) as equals, and lack of superiority" (p. 212)
Supportive interactions	• "Intersections of existence among individuals that result in positive human exchanges. The actions that fall under this heading include . . . interaction, intersectionality, sharing, taking responsibility for interactions with others . . . , engaging, and engaged/active" (p. 212)
Self-reflection and critique	• "A critical process of reflection on one's thoughts, feelings, and actions. Terms used [include] . . . self-reflection and discovery, self-questioning and critique . . . , self-reflective process, knowledge acquisition and reflective practice, reflective openness and introspection" (p. 212)

Source: Identified by Foronda et al. (2016).

he or she may begin to discover the places where he or she has become personally and professionally stagnant. Through this self-reflection, global nurse leaders bear witness to longstanding prejudices, opinions, and aversions. Cultural humility requires ongoing attention to cultural issues and reflection on personal experiences over time; it is a method of personal–professional growth and development that gradually illuminates the beauty of diversity and reveals the hidden areas where thought and action are delivered with unconscious judgment (Schuessler, Wilder, & Byrd, 2012). Cultural humility requires both self-confrontation and a gentle honesty in order to unveil the many cross-cultural and unchallenged assumptions to which "we" have become mindlessly habituated over time. Some important questions to ask oneself might be:

- Am I emotionally available and respectful to clients when they share their traditional health beliefs, practices, and rituals? Am I considerate and inclusive of their beliefs, practices, and rituals in the plan of care?
- Do I believe that the nursing care and knowledge I provide is better for clients than what they believe is most important for themselves?
- Do I see myself as the expert and the client as the novice?
- Whom else do I consider in my interactions with the client?
- Do I view my role as a teacher who imparts knowledge or as a coach who assists the client in his or her journey of self-discovery?
- In my opinion, are mutually beneficial client partnerships a gateway to growth and optimal care or a nuisance requiring time and energy?

Be honest and understand that your answer may not be a black or white response; it will most likely occur on a spectrum. If you can spot your own arrogance, simply recognize it, acknowledge how it hinders your ability to be fully present to another person, and identify ways to surrender that outdated belief pattern to create a new one rooted in humility. Shedding light on the corners where arrogance lingers has the power to return global nurse leaders to a context of shared humanity and an ethical obligation to procure dignified human-centered care.

Soulé (2016) writes,

> Humility . . . can be thought of as an accurate assessment of oneself, an ability to recognize and acknowledge limitations, and a willingness to be influenced by alternate values and worldviews. Humility . . . may actually be perceived as antithetical to competence, professionalism, and professional practice. (p. 425)

If the global nurse leader is to impact change, lead improvements in global health care access and delivery, and advocate for health equity for every man, woman, and child on the planet, self-awareness must be cultivated regarding how one sees the world. The ideals that guide the practice of cultural humility are powerful instruments in repairing and rerouting subpar or undignified care, particularly in settings where the stress of resource constraints may lead to care encounters that are rushed, impersonal, insensitive, and at times, disrespectful (Kools, Chimwaza, & Macha, 2015). Rather than walking blindly, global nurse leaders should be encouraged to face the fear that accompanies self-knowledge and self-truth and confront themselves with both compassion and courage. Humility reconnects global nurse leaders to their deeper intention, purpose, and motivation.

CONCLUSION

If you are a bedside nurse caring for patients at the individual level, start to consider how you impact an entire community through the intimacy of your one-on-one nurse–patient relationship. Through the care you give, education you provide, and advocacy you demonstrate, your efforts impact an entire family, block, neighborhood, and population. That service transcends borders and boundaries. Bedside nurses are global nurse leaders.

If you are an educator, consider how your beliefs about health and well-being inspire entire classrooms of students, who take your expertise back to their colleagues, patients, and families. *What* you teach and *how* you teach it maintains far-reaching effects. It lives in the minds and spirits of those to whom you impart your wisdom. Educators are global nurse leaders.

And if you are an administrator, just take a moment to acknowledge how the policies and protocols you promote, the safety you procure, and the quality outcomes you strive for elevate the very health of a city, state, or country, impacting people from around the world and with global networks each day. Without a doubt, administrators are global nurse leaders.

Our roles as leaders are deeply personal, textured, and varied. Maintaining a holistic view of leadership reminds us that we may mean different things to different people and be called upon to fulfill purposes and drive meaningful efforts we had not necessarily anticipated. Andrus and Shanahan (2016) describe such a leader as a multifaceted and skilled practitioner who fulfills roles related to being a

- Visionary
- Inspirational presence
- Role model
- Mentor
- Champion for clinical excellence
- Courageous advocate
- Cultural transformational agent

With time and practice, these roles become fluid and deeply interrelated. They are, after all, inherently characteristic of our quest for human betterment on a global scale. Indeed, the global nurse leader is charged with ushering in a higher level of transformed and transformational consciousness: one that nudges us to consider global problems as our own personal duties; take accountability for how we personally contribute to economic disparities; confront power imbalances and the systems we support that keep those inequities in play; support those human beings who challenge outdated worldviews in the hopes for peaceful and inspiring possibilities; and maximize our change agent and global citizen contributions across nations (Sharma, 2006).

As you move forward through this textbook, you will begin to explore the links that connect us, regardless of our current position or title, to global health systems and international health goals worldwide. Global nursing is a service to the well-being of humanity, a process of striving to honor cultural differences while redefining what it means to be a global citizen.

You are a global nurse. You are a global leader.

Carry on.

REFLECTION AND DISCUSSION

- How do I represent the great lineage of nurse leadership each day?
- How am I called to grow in order to become an evolutionary leader?
- What do I see as possible in the future as a result of my leadership and global influence?
- In what ways can I empower myself to remain committed to your goals?
- How do I embody a global and interconnected sensibility on an ongoing basis?
- How will I use this information to refine my global leadership abilities?

REFERENCES

American Nurses Association. (2015). *Code of ethics for nurses with interpretive statements.* Washington, DC: Author.

Andrus, V. L., & Shanahan, M. M. (2016). Holistic leadership. In B. M. Dossey & L. Keegan (Eds.), *Holistic nursing: A handbook for practice* (7th ed., pp. 591–607). Burlington, MA: Jones & Bartlett.

Black, J. S., & Morrison, A. J. (2014). *The global leadership challenge.* New York, NY: Routledge.

Brown, B. (2010). *The gifts of imperfections: Letting go of who we think we should be and embracing who we are.* Center City, MN: Hazelden.

Brown, B. (2012). *Daring greatly: How the courage to be vulnerable transforms the way we live, love, parent, and lead.* New York, NY: Gotham.

Cabrera, A., & Unruh, G. (2012). *Being global. How to think, act and lead in a transformed world.* Boston, MA: Harvard Business Review Press.

Curtis, K. (2014). Learning the requirements for compassionate practice: Student vulnerability and courage. *Nursing Ethics, 21*(2), 210–223.

DiMaggio, J. (2011a). Something about nothing. In J. DiMaggio & N. Zapolski, *Conversations that matter: Insights & distinctions: Landmark essays* (Vol. 1, pp. 13–18). San Francisco, CA: Landmark Worldwide.

DiMaggio, J. (2011b). Big shoes to fill—There's no going back. In J. DiMaggio & N. Zapolski, *Conversations that matter: Insights & distinctions: Landmark essays* (Vol. 1, pp. 45–49). San Francisco, CA: Landmark Worldwide.

Dossey, B. M., Selanders, L., Beck, D.-M., & Attewell, A. (2005). *Florence Nightingale today: Healing, leadership, global action.* Silver Spring, MD: Nursesbooks.org.

Foronda, C., Baptiste, D.-L., Reinholdt, M. M., & Ousman, K. (2016). Cultural humility: A concept analysis. *Journal of Transcultural Nursing, 27*(3), 210–217.

Forrester, D. A. (2016). *Nursing's greatest leaders: A history of activism.* New York, NY: Springer Publishing.

Grossman, S. C., & Valiga, T. M. (2013). *The new leadership challenge: Creating the future of nursing* (4th ed.). Philadelphia, PA: F. A. Davis.

Gundling, E., Hogan, T., & Cvitkovich, K. (2011). *What is global leadership? 10 behaviors that define great global leaders.* Boston, MA: Nicholas Brealey Publishing.

Hook, J. N., Davis, D. E., Owen, J., Worthington, E. L., Jr., & Utsey, S. O. (2013). Cultural humility: Measuring openness to culturally diverse clients. *Journal of Counseling Psychology, 60*(3), 353–366.

Hook, J. N., & Watkins, C. E., Jr. (2015). Cultural humility: The cornerstone of positive contact with culturally different individuals and groups? *American Psychologist, 70*(7), 661–662.

Isaacson, M. (2014). Clarifying concepts: Cultural humility or competency. *Journal of Professional Nursing, 30*(3), 251–258.

Kools, S., Chimwaza, A., & Macha, S. (2015). Cultural humility and working with marginalized populations in developing countries. *Global Health Promotion, 22*(1), 52–59.

Kouzes, J. M., & Posner, B. J. (2010). *The truth about leadership.* San Francisco, CA: Jossey-Bass.

Mariano, C. (2016). Holistic nursing: Scope and standards of practice. In B. M. Dossey & L. Keegan (Eds.), *Holistic nursing: A handbook for practice* (7th ed., pp. 53–76). Burlington, MA: Jones & Bartlett.

Mendenhall, M. E., Osland, J. S., Bird, A., Oddou, G. R., Maznevski, M. L., Stevens, M. J., & Stahl, G. K. (2013). *Global leadership: Research, practice, and development* (2nd ed.). New York, NY: Routledge.

Morin, K. H. (2011, November 21). *Lessons learned: Leadership in a global world,* Pinnacle Lecture, Boston College School of Nursing, Newton, MA.

Morin, K. H. (2015, March 5). *Using evidence-informed leadership strategies to influence health in the global village.* Parry Lectureship, Texas Women's University-Houston, Houston, TX.

Munhall, P. (1993). "Unknowing": Toward another pattern of knowing in nursing. *Nursing Outlook, 41*(3), 125–128.

Novogratz, J. (2009). *The blue sweater: Bridging the gap between rich and poor in an interconnected world.* New York, NY: Rodale.

Palmer, P. (2004). *A hidden wholeness: The journey toward an undivided life: Welcoming the soul and weaving community in a wounded world.* San Francisco, CA: Jossey-Bass.

Pesut, D. (2005). Foreword to the scholarship of reflective practice [Resource paper]. Retrieved from https://www.nursingsociety.org/docs/default-source/position-papers/resource_reflective.pdf?sfvrsn=4

Pesut, D. (2012). Self-renewal. In H. R. Feldman, R. Alexander, M. J. Greenberg, M. Jaffee-Ruiz, A. McBride, M. McClure, & T. D. Smith (Eds.), *Nursing leadership: A concise encyclopedia* (2nd ed., pp. 337–338). New York, NY: Springer Publishing.

Rosa, W. (Ed.). (2016a). *Nurses as leaders: Evolutionary visions of leadership.* New York, NY: Springer Publishing.

Rosa, W. (Ed.). (2016b). Preface. In W. Rosa (Ed.), *Nurses as leaders: Evolutionary visions of leadership* (pp. xxiii–xxvii). New York, NY: Springer Publishing.

Rosa, W. (Ed.). (2016c). Nurse as leader: A journey of privilege. In W. Rosa (Ed.), *Nurses as leaders: Evolutionary visions of leadership* (pp. 1–14). New York, NY: Springer Publishing.

Schaub, B., & Schaub, R. (1997). *Healing addictions: The vulnerability model of recovery.* Albany, NY: Delmar.

Schuessler, J. B., Wilder, B., & Byrd, L. W. (2012). Reflective journaling and development of cultural humility in students. *Nursing Education Perspectives, 33*(2), 96–99.

Sharma, M. (2006). Conscious leadership at the crossroads of change. *Shift: At the Frontiers of Consciousness, 12,* 16–21.

Sherwood, G., & Horton-Deutsch, S. (Eds.). (2012). *Reflective practice: Transforming education and improving outcomes.* Indianapolis, IN: Sigma Theta Tau International.

Sherwood, G., & Horton-Deutsch, S. (Eds.). (2015). *Reflective organizations: On the frontlines of QSEN and reflective practice implementation.* Indianapolis, IN: Sigma Theta Tau International.

Soulé, I. (2014a). Cultural competence in health care: An emerging theory. *Advances in Nursing Science, 37*(1), 48–60.

Soulé, I. (2014b). Exploring the meaning of cultural competence. *Advances in Nursing Science Blog.* Retrieved from http://ansjournalblog.com/2014/03/20/exploring-the-meaning-of-cultural-competence

Soulé, I. (2016). Flexible & responsive: Applying the wisdom of 'It Depends.' In W. Rosa (Ed.), *Nurses as leaders: Evolutionary visions of leadership* (pp. 417–430). New York, NY: Springer Publishing.

Sullivan, E. J. (2013). *Effective leadership and management in nursing* (8th ed.). Upper Saddle River, NJ: Pearson.

Sumner, J. (2013). Human flourishing and the vulnerable nurse. *International Journal for Human Caring, 17*(4), 20–27.

Suzuki, S. (1983). *Zen mind, beginner's mind.* New York, NY: Weatherhill.

Taffinder, P. (2006). *The leadership crash course: How to create personal leadership value* (2nd ed.). Philadelphia, PA: Kogan Page.

Tervalon, M., & Murray-Garcia, J. (1998). Cultural humility versus cultural competence: A critical distinction in defining physician training outcomes in multicultural education. *Journal of Health Care for the Poor and Underserved, 9*(2), 117–125.

Thornton, L., & Mariano, C. (2016). Evolving from therapeutic to holistic communication. In B. M. Dossey & L. Keegan (Eds.), *Holistic nursing: A handbook for practice* (7th ed., pp. 465–478). Burlington, MA: Jones & Bartlett.

Thorup, C. B., Rundqvist, E., Roberts, C., & Delmar, C. (2012). Care as a matter of courage: Vulnerability, suffering and ethical formation in nursing care. *Scandinavian Journal of Caring Sciences, 26*(3), 427–435.

Watson, J. (2005). *Caring science as sacred science.* Philadelphia, PA: F. A. Davis.

Watson, J. (2008). *Nursing: The philosophy and science of caring* (Rev. ed.). Boulder: University Press of Colorado.

Watson, J. (2012). *Human caring science: A theory of nursing* (2nd ed.). Sudbury, MA: Jones & Bartlett.

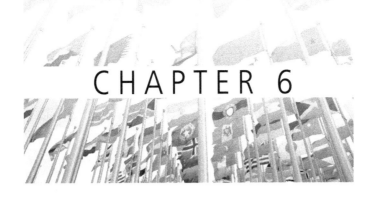

CHAPTER 6

Global Health Ethics[1]

Suellen Breakey and Linda A. Evans

Let there be justice for all. Let there be peace for all. Let there be work, bread, water, and salt for all. Let each know that, for each, the body, the mind, and the soul have been freed to fulfill themselves. The sun shall never set on so glorious a human achievement. (Mandela, 1994)

WHAT IS GLOBAL HEALTH?

Global health has been defined as "an area for study, research, and practice that places a priority on improving health and achieving equity in health for all people worldwide" (Koplan et al., 2008, p. 1995; see Chapter 2 for the most recent definitions of *global health* and *global nursing* according to the Sigma Theta Tau International Global Advisory Panel on the Future of Nursing). Working toward these goals is a challenging endeavor. Progress is slowly being made, but the factors that constrain these efforts are complex and extend beyond the limits of health care into economic, social, and political spheres. Millum and Emanuel (2012) observe that only recently have bioethicists begun to shift from a domestic to a global focus. They also point out that the complexity of the issues surrounding global health has necessitated that ethicists expand their areas of concern from the traditional (e.g., issues that occur within patient–provider relationships) to other areas such as health policy as well as political and economic theory (Millum & Emanuel, 2012). In this chapter, we examine the effects that social determinants and economic globalization have had on the health of the world's people, particularly in low- and middle-income countries (LMICs). We also explore the concept of global health ethics and discuss how it is distinct from traditional ethics. Finally, we discuss frameworks that can be used to examine the complex global issues at the population health level.

---

[1] *Source:* This chapter has been adapted from Breakey and Evans (2015).

INFLUENCE OF GLOBALIZATION ON GLOBAL HEALTH

According to Parekh and Wilcox (2014), "globalization" is the "economic, social, cultural, and political processes of integration that result from the expansion of transnational economic production, migration, communications, and technologies" (para. 1). This definition implies that these processes are being integrated and shared equally. Sen (1999) contends that the process of integration has been unequal and that globalization has led to increased Westernization of the world as opposed to a more equal diffusion of these processes. One potential consequence of an increasingly Westernized world is the potential for Western values and beliefs to become the dominant view at the expense of local cultural values, beliefs, and traditions.

The current global political economy is based on neoliberal ideology. The policies derived from neoliberal thought support trade liberalization, deregulation, privatization of public assets, including natural resources such as minerals and forests, elimination of social welfare programs, and restrictions on immigration (Parekh & Wilcox, 2014). Specifically, economic integration, removing regulatory constraints such as tariffs and restrictions on investments, leads to freer movement of goods and, thus, economic growth (Shah, 2010). Proponents of the current global economy argue that the effects of these policies have created employment opportunities for people worldwide, particularly in developing countries, moving them out of poverty, while opponents disagree.

In addition to enhanced economic growth *for some*, the benefits of globalization include rapid advances in scientific and technological innovation, improved health and life expectancy *for some*, and expanded access to communication. These advances have increased our ability to generate new knowledge and to share knowledge among a larger global audience that has led to what Roland Robertson refers to as the "compression of the world." As Benatar, Gill, and Bakker (2011) point out, the minority who benefit in the current global political economy are large investors and transnational corporations, resulting in a widening gap between the wealthy and the poor both between and within countries. For instance, in order to satisfy the conditions of World Bank or International Monetary Fund loans, some countries must prioritize profit making over the interest and well-being of its citizens (Falk-Rafael, 2006).

For the sick living in poor countries, or to borrow Paul Farmer's term "the destitute sick," economic integration has an even more direct effect on health. Tighter intellectual property rights protection, for example, which maximizes profits for wealthy companies by granting them exclusive rights, keeps the prices of goods high, which disadvantages poor countries (Haynes et al., 2013). In the case of pharmaceutical companies, such arrangements limit access to essential life-saving medications that may be cost prohibitive for either governments in poor countries or individuals to purchase. Although globalization was predicted to be "the rising tide that would lift all boats" (World Health Organization [WHO], 2012a, p. vii), LMICs continue to bear a significant burden of poverty and, as a result, disease.

Extreme Poverty and the Global Burden of Disease

The total number of people living in extreme poverty may be decreasing, but the numbers are still devastatingly high. The gap between the wealthy and poor continues to widen. Over 3 billion people live on less than US $2.50 per day (Shah, 2013), and the relationship between poverty and health is clear. When it comes to health, WHO statistics from 2012 indicate that people living in LMICs fare far worse than those in high-income countries (WHO, 2014). Case in point, in 2012, the overall global life expectancy at birth was 70 years. When aggregated and compared according to level of income, however, the disparities become evident; those in high-income countries had a life expectancy of 79 years versus a life expectancy of 62 years for those living in low-income countries (WHO 2014). This trend was similar for infant mortality and mortality by age 5 years. Likewise, when comparing the incidence and prevalence of infectious diseases, both the incidence and prevalence of disease (e.g., malaria, HIV/AIDS, and tuberculosis) were consistently higher in low-income countries than the global measure and much lower than the global measure in high-income countries (WHO, 2014). African countries, in particular, fare worse in all areas compared to low-income countries on the whole (Table 6.1; WHO, 2014). In addition to the economic strain placed on poor countries as a result of a disproportionate amount of disease—both from the loss of productivity and the cost of illness—individuals and families are also directly affected financially leading to further expansion of the wealth–poverty gap.

The conditions that contribute to poor health and premature death of individuals worldwide, and in poor countries in particular, are preventable. The most basic resources, such as access to clean water and sanitation, are critical for survival and freedom from preventable disease. Yet, 780 million people lack access to clean water. Moreover, greater than 3.4 million deaths each year, 99% of which occur in the developing world, are water, sanitation, and hygiene related (Pruss-Ustun, Bos, Gore, & Bartram, 2008). In many cases, the reason for lack of access to these most basic resources is not due to a lack of availability of the actual resource, for example, water. Instead, it is an economic issue at either the individual level, the government level, or both. Poor countries may lack the financial resources needed to create effective infrastructures that will protect its citizens, such as systems to provide access to clean water or health care systems to treat waterborne diseases.

Table 6.1 Impact of Wealth on the Occurrence of Selected Health Indicators (2012 Data)

	Global	High Income	Low Income	African
Life expectancy at birth (years)	70	79	62	58
Infant mortality by age 1 (1/1000)	35	5	56	63
Mortality by age 5 (1/1000)	48	6	82	95
Malaria (incidence per 100,000)	3752	0	11,165	18,579
HIV/AIDS (incidence per 100,000)	33	16	89	176
HIV/AIDS (prevalence per 100,000)	511	265	1788	3203
Tuberculosis (incidence per 100,000)	122	23	246	255
Tuberculosis (prevalence per 100,000)	169	31	352	303

Source: WHO (2014).

Even when appropriate infrastructures exist within low- or middle-income countries, many individuals are too poor to access these services and die a preventable death as a result.

The widening gap between the wealthy and the poor is a moral issue. Pogge (2010) identifies three facts that support the contention that global poverty is morally troubling. First, the growing disparity occurs in the face of unprecedented global affluence. He estimates that a 2% shift in the global household income would be sufficient to eradicate severe poverty. Second, global poverty continues to increase, and finally, as stated previously, the world is shaped by international interactions including the development of treaties, conventions, and economic policies that benefit the wealthy disproportionately. Therefore, those who contribute to global economic inequality, the severe poverty it perpetuates, and the resultant detriments to health are morally implicated (Pogge, 2010).

Social Determinants of Health

Social determinants of health are the conditions into which people are born and live and are shaped by the distribution of power, money, and resources (WHO, 2008). Examples of such conditions include level of education, occupation, income, gender, ethnicity, and race. In all countries, regardless of income, health and illness follow a social gradient—the lower one's socioeconomic status, the poorer one's health (WHO, 2008). Further, much of the global burden of disease is in fact avoidable and is a result of a "toxic combination of poor social policies and programmes, unfair economic arrangements, and bad politics" (WHO, 2008, p. 1). As such, many have contended that working to improve social determinants cannot be successful within the health sector alone (WHO, 2012a). It follows then, that if health is in part socially constructed, it is necessary to protect and promote not only the civil and political rights of all people but also economic, social, and cultural rights.

Human Rights and Health

> In short, we live in a world where inequalities in health and economic development continue to pervade our development trajectory and where exclusion from social systems remains the most fundamental obstacle to realizing human potential worldwide. (London, 2008, p. 66)

Forman and Nixon (2013) contend that human rights, in and of themselves, are also determinants of health. Human rights are those basic rights to which all persons are entitled; they are considered indivisible, interrelated, and interdependent. *The Universal Declaration of Human Rights* (UDHR) was adopted by the United Nations (UN) General Assembly in December 1948 following the atrocities of World War II and is considered to be the foundation for international human rights law. The purpose of the document is to make explicit those inalienable rights that are necessary for freedom, justice, and peace. Subsequently, the *International Covenant on Civil and Political Rights* (ICCPR) and the *International Covenant on Economic, Social and Cultural Rights* (ICESCR) were derived from the UDHR and adopted in 1976. These international covenants serve as a means to hold those Member States that ratify them accountable under the law for promoting and observing the rights of their people. Together, these documents are known as the International Bill of Human Rights.

Article 25 (1) of the UDHR specifically addresses the right to health in the context of an adequate standard of living:

> Everyone has the right to a standard of living adequate for the health and well-being of himself and of his family, including food, clothing, housing, and medical care and necessary social services, and the right to security in the event of unemployment, sickness, disability, widowhood, old age or other lack of livelihood in circumstances beyond his control. (United Nations General Assembly [UNGA], 1948)

In addition, Article 12 (1) of the ICESCR states that "the States Parties to the present Covenant recognize the right of everyone to the enjoyment of the highest attainable standard of physical and mental health" (UNGA, 1976). This treaty has been ratified by many Member States of the UN. However, the United States has yet to ratify the ICESCR. Finally, the *Declaration of Alma-Ata*, developed at the International Conference on Primary Health Care in 1978, elaborated on the notion that health is a fundamental human right by recognizing that health inequalities exist between those in developed and developing countries and that attainment of health is a "world-wide social goal whose realization requires the action of many other social and economic sectors in addition to the health sector" (WHO, 1978).

Jonathan Mann, whom some have characterized as the founder of the health and human rights movement, and his colleagues (1994) were the first to describe a provisional framework connecting health and human rights. Their framework is based on the following assumptions: Health policies impact human rights; human rights violations impact physical, mental, and social well-being; and human rights and health are fundamentally and inextricably linked (Mann et al., 1994). The link between human rights and health is exemplified in the following ways. First, certain human rights violations have a direct negative effect on health such as in the case of torture or slavery. Second, violations that impact economic, social, and cultural rights (e.g., the right to education, food and nutrition, and water) lead to an increased vulnerability to illness. And finally, the development of programs that either do not consider individuals' rights or violate those rights altogether may be discriminatory or violate a person or group's right to privacy (WHO, n.d.).

Mann and colleagues argued that using public health research methodology, education, and fieldwork expertise could not only advance our understanding of the health impacts resulting from human rights violations but also "give voice" to and possibly expedite actions to address these issues (Mann et al., 1994). While the links between human rights and health are complex, over the past 20 years their thesis has provided the basis for examining and understanding the effects that ignoring or violating certain human rights has had on health. Examples include violence against women, certain traditional practices within cultures such as female genital mutilation, and slavery.

CAN TRADITIONAL ETHICAL PRINCIPLES BE APPLIED TO GLOBAL HEALTH?

The challenges to promoting and defending human rights to achieve the highest standard of health and well-being and to eradicate inequities—in essence, creating a socially just society—are complex. The traditional ethical principles, autonomy, beneficence, nonmaleficence, and justice, are useful but not sufficient to examine global health issues. A global ethics framework is needed.

Respect for Autonomy

In the Western tradition, *autonomy* refers to one's right to self-determination, free from controlling influences or limitations (Beauchamp & Childress, 2012). Two general conditions must be met in order for a person to act autonomously: liberty and agency. *Liberty* refers to the ability to be free from controlling influences, and *agency* refers to the capacity for intentional action (Beauchamp & Childress, 2012). When we have full autonomy, that is, the ability to reason and to make choices based on our beliefs, values, and wishes, then one element necessary to achieve well-being has been satisfied.

Provision 1.4 of the American Nurses Association (ANA, 2001) *Code of Ethics for Nurses With Interpretive Statements* addresses the nurse's ethical responsibility to respect individual autonomy and the right to self-determination. From a traditional Western bioethical perspective, respect for autonomy is regarded as the ethical principle that underlies the concept of informed consent, the patient's right to make decisions based on accurate information regarding the nature of the treatment, as well as the risks, benefits, and alternatives to that treatment. *The Code of Ethics for Nurses* (International Council of Nurses [ICN], 2006) addresses the nurse's duty to respect autonomy from a broader perspective stating that "in providing care, the nurse promotes an environment in which the human rights, values, customs and spiritual beliefs of the individual, family and community are respected" (p. 2).

Autonomy in social and political philosophy is used as the ideal against which unjust, or oppressive, social conditions are critiqued (Christman, 2003). To acknowledge an individual as an autonomous agent is to recognize and respect the right of that individual to have personal values and beliefs as well as her or his right to make choices and act on her or his values and beliefs. Conditions that interfere with an individual's or group's ability to exercise autonomy are considered oppressive.

Threats to Autonomy From a Global Ethics Perspective

As the ANA *Code of Ethics* (2001) for nurses suggests, nurses working in wealthy countries often consider the principle of autonomy from the perspective of an individual's right to self-determination in decision making and care. In clinical settings, a nurse's role in protecting and respecting autonomy is often related to the patient's decision-making capacity and the extent to which it is affected by illness or the presence of comorbid conditions. In this way, the concern is often one of agency, the capacity to make informed decisions, and to a lesser extent, liberty, freedom from forces that constrain decision making. On the other hand, from a global ethics perspective, a focus on liberty and on efforts to remove constraining forces, for example, poverty, lack of access to clean water and sanitation, or gender inequality, is often the central moral issue impacting health.

Crigger (2008) refers to autonomy as "the ethics of affluence" (p. 22). She argues that our Westernized view of autonomy, which places great importance on personal autonomy and individual rights, is not transferrable to all settings, particularly resource-challenged settings where poverty and a lack of material resources have a devastating impact on health (Crigger, 2008). These settings often differ in many ways from Western culture. Often, the social and economic welfare of the family is reliant on the joint efforts of each family member. Because of this dependency, family members are often key stakeholders in the decision-making process, and less emphasis is placed on the individual. Autonomy, then, would be understood differently in settings where this is true. Therefore, understanding relevant cultural values, beliefs, and norms that may shape one's definition of autonomy is essential. Using a global ethics perspective to understand threats to autonomy in global health necessitates a broader, deeper view, one which incorporates knowledge of the social, economic, and political constraints to achieving health and well-being and knowledge of the specific culture.

To illustrate the distinction between a traditional and global ethics framework, consider the concept of informed consent. In order to ensure informed consent in a global health setting, one must first acknowledge that despite the social circumstances of an individual (e.g., poverty, illiteracy), the obligation to engage in the process of informed consent remains. In the case of HIV testing, an issue where people are particularly vulnerable to stigmatization and discrimination, WHO (2012b) made explicit the steps to ensure basic human rights protection and optimal treatment of people living with HIV. Informed consent is a central concern as well as maintaining confidentiality, offering counseling, ensuring correct results and connection to care.

However, results from Madhivanan and colleagues' (2014) study in India to understand women's experiences and perceptions of HIV testing during antenatal care illustrate instances where these steps are violated. They found that informed consent was not obtained for either the antenatal care the women received or HIV testing. Moreover, the participants' right to privacy and confidentiality were routinely violated during visits when the women were informed of their positive test results. And while told they needed to be on medication, they were not given any further information and were not referred for counseling; clearly the WHO guidelines were not practiced. In fact, although these private providers had the necessary resources to continue to care for these HIV-positive women, the women's care was transferred to either governmental facilities or nongovernmental organizations (NGOs; Madhivanan et al., 2014). Within a Western framework, autonomy was clearly violated. Informed consent was not obtained and the participants' right to privacy and confidentiality were violated. Solutions based on this analysis would be based primarily in the health care setting and include such things as educating providers on the elements and significance of informed consent, restructuring practices to adhere to the WHO guidelines, and holding individual providers accountable for their breaches in practice.

Examination of the study from a broader global ethics perspective uncovers morally significant sociopolitical factors—poverty and gender inequality—that must be factored into an ethical solution to the problem. The moral issue, then, of violating individual women's right to autonomy by disregarding the process of informed consent is raised to a societal level taking into account the constraining effects of poverty and women's inequality on autonomy. Considering the issue this way takes into account not only actors at the local level (the physicians and nurses) but also the government and other institutions that permit or perpetuate these practices and fail to protect its citizens, in this case, poor women. Therefore, the focus shifts from violations of informed consent and threats to individual autonomy to violations rooted in social inequity, thereby necessitating examination from a perspective of justice.

Beneficence

The principle of "beneficence" refers to a moral obligation *to act* for the good of others to help further their interests, often by preventing or removing harm (Beauchamp, 2013). Some have argued that this *positive obligation* to act for the good of others is too demanding, an ideal rather than an obligation, and that we are not morally obligated to benefit others even if we are so able. Anderson and colleagues (2009) point to a lack of concern for "distant and different others" (p. 282), and Wolff (2012) discusses a diffusion of responsibility as a possible reason why individuals disregard a humanitarian duty to assist those in need. But some, notably Singer (2009) and Pogge (2010), as discussed previously, dispute the contention that beneficence is an ideal and argue that individuals living in wealthy countries have a duty to assist those living in poverty.

Singer (2009) uses a hypothetical situation to state his case. He begins by first begging the question: If you were walking to work, wearing expensive shoes, and encountered a girl drowning in a shallow pond, would you save her? He asserts that people would choose to wade into the pond to save the girl because the girl's life is more important than the loss of the expensive shoes and the resulting inconveniences of getting wet, having to go home to change, and being late for work, for example. However, most people do not feel the same moral obligation to save the lives of poor children in Africa, even though we could through charitable giving. His analogy provides support for Anderson and colleagues' (2009) notion that we feel more of a moral obligation to those in close proximity than for the distant and different other. Further, Singer (2009) argues that we do indeed have a duty to help the thousands of children whom we know are dying from poverty-related, preventable diseases daily, and this duty is as morally significant as our duty to save the drowning girl from a preventable death. He proposes that individuals give 1% of their income to the poor as a means to promote a culture of giving (Singer, 2009).

Yet, while there may be a wide consensus that those in middle-income or poor countries are entitled to basic human rights that are essential for health and well-being, a consensus has not been reached whether humans have a positive right to assistance or to what extent we are obligated to assist. Beauchamp (2013) suggests that beneficence exists on a continuum starting with strict obligation (core norms of beneficence in ordinary morality) and ending with high-level supererogatory, or heroic, acts of self-sacrifice. As Beauchamp (2013) points out, the debate lies in where obligation ends and supererogation begins. While our individual duties to act for the good of others remain unclear, our professional responsibilities are well articulated; Provision 8 of the *Code of Ethics for Nurses* (ANA, 2001) states that the nurse has a responsibility to promote health at the community, national, and international levels. Provision 8 also informs nurses of the responsibility to be aware of the "broader health concerns such as world hunger, environmental pollution, lack of access to health care, violation of human rights, and inequitable distribution of nursing and health care resources" (p. 13).

Nonmaleficence

Simply put, "nonmaleficence" refers to our moral obligation to not inflict harm on others. Whereas beneficence requires an action to promote good, nonmaleficence requires that we intentionally refrain from actions that cause harm to another (Beauchamp & Childress, 2012). Harm may take the form of physical or mental injury or danger, but may also include setbacks to other interests held by an individual or party (Beauchamp & Childress, 2001). Examples of moral rules that are supported by this principle include: Do not kill; Do not incapacitate; and Do not deprive others of the goods of life (Beauchamp & Childress, 2001).

To view this principle from a global ethics perspective, refer back to the earlier example related to intellectual property rights protections. International laws and agreements that favor pharmaceutical companies and the protection of their right to intellectual property could be considered a violation of the principle of nonmaleficence since the link between poor health and poverty is well established. If a company is allowed to continue to hold exclusive rights to a drug that could save lives, it prohibits the manufacture and distribution of generic drugs that would be cheaper and more accessible to the poor. Such policies or arrangements that knowingly perpetuate a lack of access to life-saving resources in order to financially benefit a large wealthy company inflict harm on the potential beneficiaries whose lives could be saved and violate the principle of nonmaleficence. While violations of nonmaleficence do occur, it should also be noted that many pharmaceutical companies include statements of social responsibility in their mission and contribute to humanitarian efforts. For example, in 2013, Janssen Pharmaceuticals, a pharmaceutical company of Johnson & Johnson in the United States, developed a drug donation program for HIV treatment–experienced children who are in need of new treatment options (Johnson & Johnson, 2013).

Threats to Doing More Harm Than Good

There is an increasing number of nurses interested in engaging in global health work, either by providing direct care or by partnering with NGOs or governments to provide and develop education or to assist in developing programs to address specific health issues. In fact, nurses are perfectly suited to undertake this work but need a broader global ethics view to enhance their understanding of how autonomy may be viewed differently depending on needs, priorities, and traditions in the setting in which they are working. It is equally important to view the principles of beneficence and nonmaleficence from a global ethics perspective in order to avoid unintentionally doing more harm than good.

Fuller (2012) describes cultural imperialism as providing care or services in such a way that it forces potential recipients of those services to choose between accessing the care being offered, which would be unavailable otherwise but that violates traditional norms and practices, and not receiving assistance (Fuller, 2012). Clearly, those who work in global health settings do not set out to cause harm. However, the recipient of care may be harmed if the care or assistance being offered does not cohere with the norms, values, or traditions that are important to the individual and community. The end result may be that the potential beneficiary of the assistance is forced to make the difficult decision to abandon those values and opt for the care from which she or he may benefit, which, under normal circumstances, would not be available. This decision may have devastating social implications for the individual and her or his family. One important aspect in preventing such harm is the provision of culturally competent care, or what some call "cultural humility." The recently published document *Guidelines for Implementing Culturally Competent Nursing Care* (Douglas et al., 2014), which was endorsed by the ICN, provides recommendations that can assist nurses working globally. These provisions are listed in Box 6.1.

Box 6.1 Guidelines for Implementing Culturally Competent Nursing Care

Guideline	Description
1. Knowledge of Cultures	Nurses shall gain an understanding of the perspectives, traditions, values, practices, and family systems of culturally diverse individuals, families, communities, and populations they care for, as well as knowledge of the complex variables that affect the achievement of health and well being.
2. Education and Training in Culturally Competent Care	Nurses shall be educationally prepared to provide culturally congruent health care. Knowledge and skills necessary for assuring that nursing care is culturally congruent shall be included in global health care agendas that mandate formal education and training, as well as required ongoing continuing education for all practicing nurses.
3. Critical Reflections	Nurses shall engage in critical reflection of their own values, beliefs, and cultural heritage in order to have an awareness of how these qualities and issues can impact culturally congruent nursing care.
4. Cross-Cultural Communication	Nurses shall use culturally competent verbal and nonverbal communication skills to identity client's values, beliefs, practices, perceptions, and unique health care needs.
5. Culturally Competent Practice	Nurses shall utilize cross-cultural knowledge and culturally sensitive skills in implementing culturally congruent nursing care.
6. Cultural Competence in Health Care Systems and Organizations	Health care organizations should provide the structure and resources necessary to evaluate and meet the cultural and language needs of their diverse clients.
7. Patient Advocacy and Empowerment	Nurses shall recognize the effect of health care policies, delivery systems, and resources on their patient populations, and shall empower and advocate for their patients as indicated. Nurses shall advocate for the inclusion of their patients' cultural beliefs and practices in all dimensions of their health care.
8. Multicultural Workforce	Nurses shall actively engage in the effort to ensure a multicultural workforce in health care settings. One measure to achieve a multicultural workforce is through strengthening of recruitment and retention efforts in the hospitals, clinics, and academic settings.
9. Cross-Cultural Leadership	Nurses shall have the ability to influence individuals, groups, and systems to achieve outcomes of culturally competent care for diverse populations. Nurses shall have the knowledge and skills to work with public and private organizations, professional associations, and communities to establish policies and guidelines for comprehensive implementation and evaluation of culturally competent care.
10. Evidence-Based Practice and Research	Nurses shall base their practice on interventions that have been systematically tested and shown to be the most effective for the culturally diverse populations that they serve. In areas where there is a lack of evidence of efficacy, nurse researchers shall investigate and test interventions that may be the most effective in reducing the disparities in health outcomes.

Source: Douglas et al. (2014). Reprinted with permission from Sage Publishing Company.

Anderson and colleagues (2009), along with Douglas and colleagues (2014), recommend that nurses working in global health settings should engage in critical self-reflection. Critical self-reflection takes into account not only the economic, cultural, and political context in which health inequities exist, but also the potential consequences of the power differentials behind the inequities. For instance, those providing assistance are often from wealthy countries while recipients of care live in poverty. Critical self-reflection can lessen the risk of nurses' objectifying the experience of those who are disadvantaged and marginalized, which can lead unintentionally to feelings of moral superiority or knowing "what's best" (Anderson et al., 2009). As Crigger (2008) points out, the risk of doing more harm than good may be realized if the focus of global health efforts does not match the needs and goals of the beneficiaries of the assistance. Moreover, when decisions to do "what's best" are made without regard for the local culture, traditions, or insights from stakeholders living in the local setting, the end result is paternalism.

Using a global ethics lens to design care, education, or assistance programs can mitigate this potential for harm. Fuller (2012) offers the following suggestions that, in addition to critical self-reflection, are particularly useful for global health nurses. Recommendations include engaging key local stakeholders in the work; focusing care or development efforts on the needs that are identified by the local experts; ensuring that the assistance being provided does not violate moral or religious beliefs that are central to those who live in the setting; and having a good understanding of the local cultural practices and incorporating them appropriately into the assistance being provided. Similarly, Murphy and colleagues (2013) outline elements of successful global health research partnerships. Although they discuss these in the context of international research, the elements they discuss can be applied to all types of global partnerships—whether aimed at capacity development, health programs and policies, clinical services, or educational partnerships. Included are the importance of mutual trust and respect among global partners, shared decision making, and national ownership (Murphy et al., 2013); the presence of these characteristics indicates a true partnership rather than a paternalistic relationship.

Justice

The principle of justice is a fundamental consideration when examining possible solutions to address the inequities that impact global health. Theories of justice are complex; bioethicists as well as social and political philosophers have been and continue to be engaged in extensive discussions about the nature and scope of this concept. The overview of justice presented here provides a basic understanding of its importance in global health discussions.

Distributive justice refers to fair, equitable, and appropriate distribution of material goods and services such as income, wealth, health care, and jobs (Lamont & Flavor, 2013). The concept of distributive justice is very closely linked to the economic framework of each society, since it is that framework, comprising its laws, policies, and institutions, that influences how both economic benefits and burdens are distributed to individuals (Lamont & Favor, 2013). In other words, who will reap the benefits, and who will be placed at an economic, political, or social disadvantage? An *institution* refers to an organization or practice that holds an important place in a society. Examples of institutions include health care, religion, industry, law and the legal system, and the military. Principles of justice provide societies with a moral framework to determine the political processes and structures that affect the distribution of economic benefits and burdens (Lamont & Favor, 2013). Beauchamp and Childress (2001) define specific material principles of justice as those principles that specify the characteristics of equal treatment and help to guide distribution of resources.

1. To each person an equal share;
2. To each person according to need;
3. To each person according to effort;
4. To each person according to contribution;
5. To each person according to merit;
6. To each person according to free-market exchanges (p. 228).

Principles of justice, therefore, have the potential for practical application if used to help shape the laws and policies that govern the distribution of economic benefits and burdens. There is, however, an ongoing discussion and a lack of consensus regarding the nature of equality—what goods and resources are we obligated to share equally? An equal need for certain resources does not necessarily exist universally, but consideration should be given to fair distribution. It is clear that there may be inherent conflicts of interest that would influence the determination of how resources ought to be distributed fairly. Realistically, there is no one pure theory, rather a host of principles that help shape decision making and attempt to address the questions: How do we distribute burdens and benefits fairly? And how do we define "fair or equal"? The four traditional theories of justice include egalitarianism, utilitarianism, libertarianism, and communitarianism (Beauchamp & Childress, 2012). What follows is a general description of each.

Theories of Justice

The belief that people are created as equals and have equal moral status underlies egalitarian theories of justice. Egalitarians, therefore, hold the belief that all people should be treated equally (Beauchamp & Childress, 2012). In this way, equality is central to justice, and there exists certain absolute humanitarian principles such as autonomy, freedom, and human dignity (Gordon, 2006). John Rawls's (1971) theory of justice as fairness has significantly shaped, informed, and influenced discussions related to justice. In his account, individuals are free and possess equal basic rights; the principal task of government is "to distribute fairly the liberties and economic resources individuals need to lead freely chosen lives" (Bell, 2012, para. 1).

Utilitarians believe that the morally right action in a situation is the action that produces the most good or maximizes value (Driver, 2009). Utilitarianism falls into the category of consequentialism. Broadly, consequentialists believe that determination of whether an act is morally right depends only on the consequences of that act (Sinnott-Armstrong, 2011). As such, all other morally relevant factors are disregarded since it is the consequence or outcome that is morally significant.

Libertarian theories place significant emphasis on individual rights as opposed to social or economic liberty (Beauchamp & Childress, 2012). In this view, individuals have full self-ownership; a just society provides protection for individual rights, for example, property and liberty (Vallentyne & van der Vossen, 2014). All persons should have the freedom to improve their circumstances on their own initiative (Beauchamp & Childress, 2012). Determination of just acts from a libertarian viewpoint centers on whether people have been justly treated and whether their individual rights have been respected and not on the outcome or consequences of that act (Vallentyne & van der Vossen, 2014).

Unlike libertarianism, communitarian theories of justice derive conceptions of good as those that are created in moral communities, and dismiss theories of justice based on individual rights (Beauchamp & Childress, 2012). Communities can take on several forms. They may be based on geographical location, for example, the place where one calls home; they may be based on memory, for example, strangers who share a morally significant history; or they may be psychological communities, for example, families (Bell, 2012).

The Scope of Justice: Cosmopolitanism Versus Statism

Another question that is asked when issues of justice are examined is: How far do our responsibilities extend? How ethicists and political philosophers answer this question depends on whether they take a cosmopolitan or statist view. A cosmopolitan view suggests that all human beings are citizens of one community and that our collective duties to each other extend beyond national borders (Kleingeld & Brown, 2013). As Emanuel (2012) contends, where a person is born or lives is arbitrary from a moral perspective and should not factor in the determination of entitlement to basic rights, opportunities, or resources. In other words, regardless of how far we live from those who lack access to basic resources, for example, food, water, and health care, we have a collective duty to assist. This duty is based on the idea that those suffering from these burdens, many of whom live in low-income countries, have the same right to health as those living in wealthy countries. Singer's (2009) argument related to our individual duties to the poor is based not only on our obligation of beneficence, but also on a cosmopolitan view of justice.

On the other hand, the statist view, put forth primarily by Rawls, is concerned not with the well-being of individuals, but with creating just institutions within a society (Emanuel, 2012). Statists acknowledge the existence of states that experience abject poverty, but the primary concern lies not in the existence of economic insecurity, but with the inability of those nation states to develop and establish just social and political institutions. There is, therefore, a duty to assist these states to allow them to reach a minimal level of economic security so that just institutions may be established, but there is not an ongoing obligation of justice (Emanuel, 2012). As one can see, justice as a duty to others and what we owe to others who have less than we have is complicated and influenced deeply not only by our individual values and beliefs but also by the moral and social norms that shape our communities and nations.

Emerging Theories of Justice: The Capability Approach

One responsibility of the society in which we live is to provide a "social minimum," defined by White (2004) as "the bundle of resources that a person needs in order to lead a minimally decent life in their society" (para. 2). However, the fairness of this definition has been challenged since the idea of a minimally decent life will look different depending on one's circumstances. One born into deprivation may have different expectations and adapt to a lack of resources that will in turn affect her or his definition of a "minimally decent life" (White, 2004). Therefore, the bundle of resources will be different depending on whether one lives in a poor or wealthy country. For the poor, a minimally decent life may mean access to food, water, or education. For those living in wealthy countries, a minimally decent life will extend beyond these basic needs; some have argued that the social minimum in wealthy societies is more costly (White, 2004).

A set of theories of justice, "capabilities theories," has emerged over the past few decades that represents a departure from the traditional theories of justice and is particularly promising to address global issues, such as health inequities that have arisen from globalization. A capability approach may in some ways also address the inconsistencies with the social minimum. This approach was first developed by Sen (1999) as a means of making cross-cultural judgments regarding quality of life and was further explicated by Nussbaum and others. Capability theory is more normative than explanatory and takes into consideration what people are able to realistically be and do (Kleist, 2010). Beings and doings described by Sen (1992),

> can vary from such elementary things as being adequately nourished, being in good health, avoiding escapable morbidity and premature mortality, etc., to more complex achievements such as being happy, having self-respect, taking part in the life of the community, and so on. (p. 39, as cited in White, 2004)

Within this approach, poverty is not merely the lack of material resources required for survival but is viewed as deprivation of the capability to live a good life, the quality of which is defined by the individual. As such, capabilities theories extend beyond traditional theories of justice; while basic needs are required for good health and well-being, the goal is to achieve human flourishing, or optimal well-being.

One of the difficulties with this theory is determining universally what capabilities are absolutely necessary to allow one to flourish, since conceptions will surely be influenced by what is culturally accepted within a particular society. However, there are some basic needs that ought to be considered urgent moral and political priorities—capabilities that most would agree are required, for example, education, nutrition, shelter, and, importantly, health. Development and the distribution of resources, therefore, are focused on expanding capabilities (Wells, 2012).

Sen and Nussbaum have differing accounts of capability theory. For instance, Sen's account emphasizes freedom, while an important aspect of Nussbaum's theory is the concept that human dignity is necessary for human flourishing (Wells, 2012). But the central tenet of the theories is similar: certain capabilities—those that are realistic and achievable—and various accompanying forms of freedom are essential for a flourishing life of the kind we have reason to value (Beauchamp & Childress, 2012).

While Sen is reticent to make a list of essential capabilities (Wells, 2012), Nussbaum (2000) has identified 10 capabilities that are necessary for a full life. They are: life; bodily health; bodily integrity; senses, imagination, and thought; emotions; practical reason; affiliation; relationship with other species; play; and control over one's environment (both political and material; Nussbaum, 2000). Nussbaum emphasizes two of the 10 capabilities that constitute a truly human pursuit, one that is self-constructed and in which one is not just following or being shaped by others. The first, practical reason, is the ability to form a conception of and critically reflect on the notion of the good. The second is affiliation, which focuses on the ability to live with and show concern for others and the ability to have self-respect and be treated with dignity and self-worth (Kleist, 2010). Moreover, the capabilities approach shows promise for use in assessing individual well-being, evaluating and assessing social arrangements, and designing policies related to addressing inequities (Robeyns, 2011).

FRAMEWORKS FOR THE APPLICATION OF A GLOBAL HEALTH ETHIC TO ISSUES IN GLOBAL HEALTH

Examining the four traditional ethical principles, autonomy, beneficence, nonmaleficence, and justice, with respect to global health and reconceptualizing them through a global ethics lens serves as a guide for individuals to understand global health inequities and for ethical practice in global health. In addition, global health experts are engaged in serious discussions centered on developing viable population level solutions to address the global health crisis. Three frameworks that have particular merit are advanced here: Ford's Global Health Advocacy framework, a rights-based framework, and the more recently proposed Framework Convention on Global Health (FCGH).

An Ethical Framework for the Common Good: Global Health Advocacy

Ford (2013) describes "global health advocacy" as "people in one part of the world advocating for the improved health of people in another part of the world" (p. 136), clearly a cosmopolitan view of justice. This term and Ford's definition of it suggest an approach to global health that is rooted in normative ethics—what ought to be done. However, Ford (2013) also acknowledges that global health has a political context and, therefore, should have a political solution. His framework is useful for addressing global health issues affecting large numbers of people as a result of health inequities. He also notes that, while policy change is not a linear process, it is useful to have clear, logical, stepwise process to ensure a comprehensive approach to the issue at hand. The steps of his Global Advocacy framework are outlined in the following text.

- *Define the problem* and determine if it is important to overcome.
- *Gather the evidence* in a way to be sure all aspects of the health problem—sociopolitical, cultural, and economic—are being addressed. This step may include, for example, gathering epidemiologic data, information on current effective standards of care related to the health issue being addressed, relevant health policy information, as well as any existing financial barriers to prevention or treatment.
- *Formulate and propose a possible solution.*
- *Build alliances* with people who have expertise related to all aspects of the issue to strengthen the case.
- *Challenge the status quo.*

- *Seize opportunities* that may arise that will strengthen or increase public awareness of the global health issue.
- *Build consensus.*
- *Support implementation.* (Ford, 2013)

This framework is particularly useful for addressing specific global health problems.

A Rights-Based Framework to Global Health

A tension exists between advances in science and technology and the ability of current social policies to meet the basic needs of the world's people such that technological innovation adds to health inequities since expensive technologies are not available to those are who unable to pay for them (Crigger, 2008; London, 2008). Crigger (2008) also notes that the ethical issues created from these cutting-edge technologies, for instance, ethical issues related to genetic mapping, face transplantation, or the development of an artificial heart, seem more relevant or interesting to some than issues such as dire poverty and lack of access to clean water and sanitation—all of which impact health negatively. To those living in wealthy countries, this second set of problems seems far removed from our everyday lives—or as Anderson and colleagues (2009) would suggest, problems of the distant and different other. Yet, at the core of all of these issues is the basic right to health.

Since the right to health is protected under international law through the International Bill of Human Rights, governments who have ratified the ICESCR owe a duty to promote and protect the health of their citizens, and this duty is legally binding (Forman & Nixon, 2013). This requirement applies mainly to governments, however, and much less so to the duties of organizations or transnational corporations to uphold the right to health (Forman & Nixon, 2013). Further, while forward progress toward achieving a right to health is occurring, particularly through the work of the UN-appointed rapporteur, a more robust attempt to hold nation-state and nonstate actors accountable to their legal and ethical duties presents a challenge, particularly to economically disadvantaged countries where achievement of the right to health is difficult (Forman & Nixon, 2013).

Civil and political rights are indivisible from economic, social, and political rights. Therefore, health and social policies need to be developed that address obligations to fulfill the human right to health (London, 2008). Integrating a human rights approach to health and social policies can offer new opportunities for addressing global health challenges. In addition to providing standards for states' conduct as emphasized by Forman and Nixon (2013) voice must be given to those whose rights are being violated, by including them in the decision-making process. London (2008) specifically addresses the responsibilities of health workers in working to advance health as a human right by proposing that professional codes of conduct use stronger human rights language to make them a more effective means for self-regulation. Reliance on ethical frameworks, he argues, to guide professional behavior have limited effect. London admits that a human rights framework may not be successful in achieving the right to health but, at the very least, it will mobilize civil society to action, which he believes is necessary for social change. *Social mobilization*, increasing society's awareness of the government's legal obligation to facilitate the right to health, will empower rights holders, particularly those whose rights to health are being violated, to make rights-based claims to health (Friedman, Gostin, & Buse, 2013; Haynes et al., 2013; London, 2008).

Framework Convention on Global Health

More recently, Gostin and colleagues (2013) have advanced a more formalized concept of a rights-based approach to health that they believe will increase accountability at both the domestic and international level. They point out that since the concept of a right to health is vague, it has had limited use in efforts to hold responsible parties accountable (Gostin et al., 2013). They propose an FCGH that will "dramatically reduce the health disadvantages experienced by the marginalized and the poor, both within countries and between them, while reducing health injustices across the socioeconomic gradient" (Gostin et al., 2013, p. 790). The authors of this proposal note that, while progress toward global health has been made through the implementation of the UN Millennium Development Goals, the health gap still exists; they contend that this is in part due to the lack of existing health and social policies that are equally as robust as current international trade and investment policies (Gostin et al., 2013). Therefore, to achieve global justice, the focus must extend beyond achieving health to include achieving equity (Gostin et al., 2013). The FCGH, as proposed, provides strategies for action to achieve equity by including interventions focused in the economic, social, and political domains. Specifically, the FCGH would ensure three conditions essential for a healthy life: well-functioning health systems that have the ability to provide quality care; a full range of public services such as the access to nutritious food, clean water, and healthy environments; and access to economic and social determinants for good health such as employment, housing, income support, and gender equality (Gostin et al., 2013). These conditions would be met through a global governance structure and new international law that would establish a health financing network with clear obligations and lines of accountability in addition to standards for monitoring and enforcement (Haynes et al., 2013).

The FCGH would also include actions against what they call "drivers" of health disparities such as intellectual property rules, migration policies that encourage health worker migration, and policies that fail to address the harmful health effects of climate change and environmental hazards (Friedman et al., 2013; Gostin et al., 2013). Social mobilization underlies the proposed FCGH by not only promoting awareness among individuals regarding the right to health but also enlisting others engaged in global health such as women's rights organizations, human rights groups, and environmental advocacy groups (Gostin et al., 2013). While some criticisms to the FCGH exist, the answers to which warrant further consideration (Hoffman & Rottingen, 2013), it is a promising practical approach to advancing global health.

CONCLUSION

Globalization has benefitted civil society in many ways. Yet with those benefits have come great consequences that have been experienced disproportionately by the poor.

The profession of nursing has a long history of attending to and advocating for the world's most vulnerable. Our work continues in this effort, and new problems continue to arise. Grootjans and Newman (2013) identify three essential attributes for nursing practice in a globalized world that complement the global ethics perspective presented in this chapter. First, the nurse must understand the environment including environmental determinants as well as physical and socially constructed determinants of health; second, the nurse must make health promotion a priority where promotion of health is taken to mean not just the absence of disease but the promotion of well-being; and finally, the nurse practicing in a globalized world must consider how actions at the local level impact the health of others on a global level (Grootjans & Newman, 2013). These recommendations cohere with the notion that incorporating a global ethics perspective, one that leads us to examine the larger societal factors and their impact on an individual's potential to realize optimal health and well-being, can serve as a guide for action as we continue our important role in helping the world's people to flourish.

"Addressing injustice and enhancing global health is a matter of practical action. It requires careful thinking, initiative and a willingness to experiment with new approaches. Most importantly, it requires that we think ethically and then act ethically" (Orbinski, 2013, p. x).

REFLECTION AND DISCUSSION

- In what ways do I witness the disparities between global poverty and global affluence in my own home environment? How do these disparities impact health and well-being?

- What actions do I take each day in my current role to defend and advocate for health as a human right?

- Reflecting on the past, what threats to doing more harm than good can I now identify in my cross-cultural relationships and while working in contextually diverse settings?

- What are my own theories and views on social justice and its role in global nursing?

- How can I more effectively integrate advocacy for social policy equity into the global health conversation and the Sustainable Development Agenda?

REFERENCES

American Nurses Association. (2001). Code of ethics with interpretive statements. Retrieved from http://www.nursingworld.org/MainMenuCategories/EthicsStandards/CodeofEthics forNurses/Code-of-Ethics.pdf

Anderson, J. M., Rodney, P., Reimer-Kirkham, S., Browne, A. J., Khan, K. B., & Lynam, M. J. (2009). Inequities in health and healthcare viewed through the ethical lens of critical social justice: A contextual knowledge for the global priorities ahead. *Advances in Nursing Science, 32*(4), 282–294.

Beauchamp, T. (2013). The principle of beneficence in applied ethics. *Stanford Encyclopedia of Philosophy.* Retrieved from http://plato.stanford.edu/entries/principle-beneficence

Beauchamp, T., & Childress, J. F. (2001). *Principles of biomedical ethics* (5th ed.). New York, NY: Oxford University Press.

Beauchamp, T., & Childress, J. F. (2012). *Principles of biomedical ethics* (7th ed.). New York, NY: Oxford University Press.

Bell, D. (2012). Communitarianism. *Stanford Encyclopedia of Philosophy*. Retrieved from http://plato.stanford.edu/entries/communitarianism

Benatar, S. R., Gill, S., & Bakker, L. (2011). Global health and the global economic crisis. *American Journal of Public Health, 101*(4), 646–653.

Breakey, S., & Evans, L. A. (2015). Global health ethics. In S. Breakey, I. B. Corless, N. L. Meedzan, & P. K. Nicholas (Eds.), *Global health nursing in the 21st century* (pp. 49–71). New York, NY: Springer Publishing.

Christman, J. (2003). Autonomy in moral and political philosophy. *Stanford Encyclopedia of Philosophy*. Retrieved from http://plato.stanford.edu/entries/autonomy-moral

Crigger, N. J. (2008). Towards a viable and just global nursing ethics. *Nursing Ethics, 15*(1), 17–27.

Douglas, M. K., Rosenkoetter, M., Pacquiao, D. F., Clark Callister, L., Hattar-Pollara, M., Lauderdale, J., . . . Purnell, L. (2014). Guidelines for implementing culturally competent nursing care. *Journal of Transcultural Nursing, 25*(2), 109–121.

Driver, J. (2009). The history of utilitarianism. *Stanford Encyclopedia of Philosophy*. Retrieved from http://plato.stanford.edu/entries/utilitarianism-history

Emanuel, E. J. (2012). Global justice and the "standard of care" debates. In E. Emanuel & J. Millum (Eds.), *Global justice and bioethics* (pp. 181–212). New York, NY: Oxford University Press.

Falk-Rafael, A. (2006). Globalization and global health: Towards nursing praxis in the global community. *Advances in Nursing Science, 29*(1), 2–14.

Ford, N. (2013). The political context of global health and advocacy. In A. D. Pinto & R. E. G. Upsher (Eds.), *An introduction to global health ethics* (pp. 136–147). New York, NY: Routledge.

Forman, L., & Nixon, S. (2013). Human rights discourse within global health ethics. In A. D. Pinto & R. E. G. Upsher (Eds.), *An introduction to global health ethics* (pp. 47–57). New York, NY: Routledge.

Friedman, E. A., Gostin, L. O., & Buse, K. (2013). Advancing the right to health through global organizations: The potential role of a framework convention on global health. *Health and Human Rights, 15*(1), 71–86.

Fuller, L. (2012). International NGO health programs in a non-ideal world: Imperialism, respect, and procedural justice. In E. Emanuel & J. Millum (Eds.), *Global justice and bioethics* (pp. 213–240). New York, NY: Oxford University Press.

Gordon, G. S. (2006). Moral egalitarianism. *Internet Encyclopedia of Philosophy*. Retrieved from http://www.iep.utm.edu/moral-eg

Gostin, L. O., Friedman, E. A., Buse, K., Waris, A., Mulumba, M., Joel, M., . . . Sridhar, D. (2013). Towards a framework convention on global health. *Bulletin of the World Health Organization, 91*, 790–793.

Grootjans, J., & Newman, S. (2013). The relevance of globalization to nursing: A concept analysis. *International Nursing Review, 60*, 78–85.

Haynes, L., Legge, D., London, L., McCoy, D., Sanders, D., & Schuftan, C. (2013). Will the struggle for health equity and social justice be best served by a Framework Convention on Global Health? *Health and Human Rights, 15*(1), 111–116.

Hoffman, S. J., & Rottingen, J. (2013). Dark sides of the proposed framework convention on global health's many virtues: A systematic review and critical analysis. *Health and Human Rights, 15*(1), 117–134.

International Council of Nurses. (2006). *The ICN code of ethics for nurses*. Geneva, Switzerland: Author.

Johnson & Johnson. (2013). Janssen, the pharmaceutical companies of Johnson & Johnson, announces first-of-its-kind drug donation program for HIV treatment-experienced children. Retrieved from http://www.jnj.com/news/all/Janssen-the-Pharmaceutical-Companies-of-Johnson-Johnson-Announces-First-of-its-Kind-Drug-Donation-Program-for-HIV-Treatment-Experienced-Children

Kleingeld, P., & Brown, E. (2013). Cosmopolitanism. *Stanford Encyclopedia of Philosophy*. Retrieved from http://plato.stanford.edu/search/searcher.py?query=cosmopolitanism

Kleist, C. (2010). Global ethics: Capabilities approach. *Internet Encyclopedia of Philosophy*. Retrieved from http://www.ep.utm.edu/ge-capab

Koplan, J. P., Bond, T. C., Merson, M. H., Reddy, K. S., Rodriguez, M. H., Sewankambo, N. K., & Wasserheit, J. N. (2008). Towards a definition of global health. *The Lancet, 373*, 1993–1995.

Lamont, K., & Favor, C. (2013). Distributive justice. *Stanford Encyclopedia of Philosophy*. Retrieved from http://plato.stanford.edu/entries/justice-distributive

London, L. (2008). What is a human rights-based approach to health and does it matter? *Health and Human Rights Journal, 10*(1), 65–80.

Madhivanan, P., Krupp, K., Kulkarni, V., Kulkarni, S., Vaidya, N., Shaheen, R., . . . Fisher, C. (2014). HIV testing among pregnant women living with HIV in India: Are private healthcare providers routinely violating women's human rights? *BMC International Health and Human Rights, 14*, 7. Retrieved from http://www.biomedcentral.com/1472-698X/14/7

Mandela, N. R. (1994). Statement of the President of the African National Congress at his inauguration as president of the Democratic Republic of South Africa. Retrieved from https://www.africa.upenn.edu/Articles_Gen/Inaugural_Speech_17984.htm

Mann, J., Gostin, L., Gruskin, S., Brennan, T., Lazzarini, Z., & Fineberg, H. V. (1994). Health and human rights, *Health and Human Rights, 1*(1), 7–23.

Millum, J., & Emanuel, E. J. (2012). Introduction: Global justice and bioethics. In J. Millum & E. J. Emanuel (Eds.), *Global justice and bioethics* (pp. 1–14). New York, NY: Oxford University Press.

Murphy, J., Neufeld, V. R., Habte, D., Asseffa, A., Afsana, K., Kumar, A., . . . Hatfield, J. (2013). Ethical considerations of global health partnerships. In A. D. Pinto & R. E. G. Upsher (Eds.), *An introduction to global health ethics* (pp. 117–128). New York, NY: Routledge.

Nussbaum, M. (2000). *Women and human development: The capabilities approach.* Cambridge, MA: Cambridge University Press.

Orbkinski, J. (2013). Foreword. In A. D. Pinto & R. E. G. Upshur (Eds.), *An introduction to global health ethics* (p. x). New York, NY: Routledge.

Parekh, S., & Wilcox, S. (2014). Feminist perspectives on globalization. *Stanford Encyclopedia of Philosophy*. Retrieved from http://plato.stanford.edu/entries/feminism-globalization

Pogge, T. W. (2010). *Politics as usual: What lies behind the pro-poor rhetoric.* Cambridge, UK: Polity Press.

Pruss-Ustun, A., Bos, R., Gore, F., & Bartram, J. (2008). *Safer water, better health: Costs, benefits, and sustainability of interventions to protect and promote health.* Geneva, Switzerland: World Health Organization.

Rawls, J. (1971). *A theory of justice.* Cambridge, MA: Harvard University Press.

Robeyns, I. (2011). The capability approach. *Stanford Encyclopedia of Philosophy*. Retrieved from http://plato.stanford.edu/entries/capability-approach

Sen, A. (1992). *Inequality reexamined.* Oxford, UK: Blackwell.

Sen, A. (1999). *Development as freedom.* New York, NY: Anchor Books.

Shah, A. (2010). A primer on neoliberalism. *Global Issues*. Retrieved from http://www.globalissues.org/article/39/a-primer-on-neoliberalism

Shah, A. (2013). Poverty facts and stats. *Global Issues*. Retrieved from http://www.globalissues.org/article/26/poverty-facts-and-stats

Singer, P. (2009). *The life you can save: Acting now to end world poverty.* New York, NY: Random House.

Sinnott-Armstrong, W. (2011). Consequentialism. *Stanford Encyclopedia of Philosophy*. Retrieved from http://www.plato.stanford.edu/entries/consequentialism

United Nations General Assembly. (1948). Universal declaration of human rights. Retrieved from http://www.un.org/en/documents/udhr/index.shtml

United Nations General Assembly. (1976). International covenant on economic, social, and cultural rights. Retrieved from http://www.ohchr.org/EN/ProfessionalInterest/Pages/CESCR.aspx

Vallentyne, P., & van der Vossen, B. (2014). Libertarianism. *Stanford Encyclopedia of Philosophy*. Retrieved from http://plato.stanford.edu/entries/libertarianism

Wells, T. (2012). Sen's capability approach. *Internet Encyclopedia of Philosophy*. Retrieved from http://www.iep.utm.edu/sen-cap

White, S. (2004). Social minimum. *Stanford Encyclopedia of Philosophy*. Retrieved from http://plato.stanford.edu/entries/social-minimum

Wolff, J. (2012). Global justice and health: The basis of the global health duty. In E. Emanuel & J. Millum (Eds.), *Global justice and bioethics* (pp. 78–101) New York, NY: Oxford University Press.

World Health Organization. (n.d.). Linkages between health and human rights. Retrieved from http://www.who.int/hhr/HHR%20linkages.pdf?ua=1

World Health Organization. (1978). Declaration of Alma-Ata. Retrieved from http://www.euro.who.int/__data/assets/pdf_file/0009/113877/E93944.pdf?ua=1

World Health Organization. (2008). *Closing the gap in a generation: Health equity through action on the social determinants of health*. Geneva, Switzerland: Author.

World Health Organization. (2012a). *All for equity: World conference on social determinants of health*. Geneva, Switzerland: Author.

World Health Organization. (2012b). *Service delivery approaches to HIV testing and counseling (HTC): A service policy framework*. Geneva, Switzerland: Author.

World Health Organization. (2014). *World Health Statistics 2014*. Geneva, Switzerland: Author.

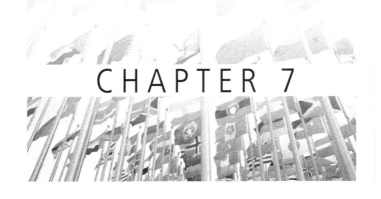

CHAPTER 7

Florence Nightingale's Legacy: The Rationale for an Integral Worldview in Achieving the Sustainable Development Goals

Barbara Montgomery Dossey, Deva-Marie Beck, Sarah Oerther, and Phalakshi Manjrekar

Health is not only to be well, but to use well every power we have. (Florence Nightingale, 1893, p. 289)

Florence Nightingale (1820–1910), the founder of modern secular nursing and the first nurse theorist, began to write in the 1870s that it would take 100 to 150 years for the kind of nurses and nursing she envisioned (Dossey, 2010a). She left us—as 21st-century Nightingales—with an expansive worldview of how to carry forward her vision of health, including what we would today call "health determinants"—as depicted in the "Word Cloud" (Figure 7.1) (McDonald, 2001–2011; Nightingale, 1860, 1893). She identified "environmental health determinants," such as clean air, water, food, houses, and so forth, as well as "social health determinants," such as poverty, education, family relationships, and employment—local to global. Nightingale foresaw the complex global problems and challenges and anticipated the 17 United Nations (UN) Sustainable Development Goals (SDGs; UN, 2016).

"Health" is the central common thread running through all 17 UN SDGs and they point directly back to the work Nightingale had achieved in her time (Beck, 2005, 2010). These SDGs are clearly related to nurses themselves, as they are working to achieve them today, at grassroots levels, everywhere. Her legacy provides a model for effective voices calling for and demonstrating the healing, leadership, and global activism required to address the challenges in these troubled times—local to global.

| Figure 7.1 | Florence Nightingale's "health determinants." |

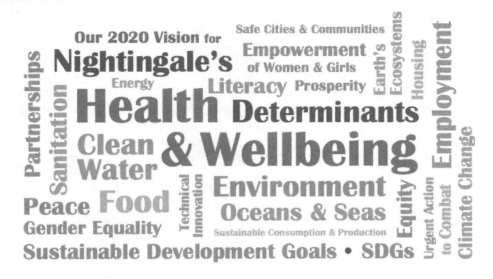

Source: Used with permission of the NIGH (2015).

This chapter explores Nightingale's legacy, the Theory of Integral Nursing, the application of this theory with the work of the Nightingale Initiative for Global Health (NIGH), and how nurse coaching empowers this vision. Two case studies are included as examples of the translation of NIGH's integral lens, mission, and vision into action.

NIGHTINGALE INITIATIVE FOR GLOBAL HEALTH (NIGH)

In 2001, Nightingale scholars Deva-Marie Beck, Barbara Dossey, and Louise Selanders entered into reflective dialogues to create an innovative, transformational nursing approach that would encourage people to move—beyond their often-limited view of Florence Nightingale—to new wider lenses to see Nightingale in a 21st-century context (Beck, 2016; Dossey, Selanders, Beck, & Attewell, 2005; NIGH, 2016a).

As Nightingale scholars and educators, we saw that Nightingale's own wider individual and collective "interior and exterior" work and insights involved many approaches that could certainly be relevant to today's 20.7 million nurses and midwives working across the world (Sarna, Wolf, & Bialous, 2012). We pondered the possibilities of an evolution of nursing and health in and beyond our time (Dossey et al., 2005).

In 2003, we brought our Nightingale scholarship into dialogue with three interprofessional colleagues and together established the NIGH—as a catalytic, integrally informed, grassroots-to-global movement to honor and extend Nightingale's legacy (Beck, Dossey, & Rushton, 2013, 2014; NIGH, 2016a). NIGH's interrelated twin purposes are (a) to increase public concern for global health issues; and (b) to inform, engage, and empower nurses, midwives, and concerned citizens to participate in this advocacy.

During NIGH's early development, the Theory of Integral Nursing (Dossey, 2008a, 2015, 2016a) informed our work, as discussed next. We asked: How might we—through the development of NIGH as a global outreach—encourage individuals to become such "agents of transformation," following in Nightingale's footsteps? Our deep reflection guided us to write a basic *individual interior* experience with the *Nightingale Declaration for A Healthy World* (Nightingale Declaration for A Healthy World, 2007) for local *individual and collective exterior* commitments (see Beck's Chapter 3 for more on NIGH's endeavors). Now, in 2017, the NIGH team continues to take a deep dive exploring how Nightingale's legacy can assist us to advocate for and achieve the 17 SDGs—to promote the health of humanity by 2030 (NIGH, 2016b).

How would Nightingale have demonstrated nursing's capacities—local to global—with collaborative projects using smartphones, the Internet, YouTube, Facebook, Twitter, Skype, conference calls, webinars, apps, and other emerging technologies? Within NIGH, our aim is to initiate new approaches by empowering both individuals and groups to see through an integral nursing lens and to revisit the integral approach to Nightingale's legacy in 21st-century terms. In the next section, we explore the Theory of Integral Nursing and how it has helped NIGH shape its global mission and vision.

NIGH AND THE THEORY OF INTEGRAL NURSING

Following Nightingale's legacy, our NIGH team asked: How might we—with nurse colleagues and other stakeholders—expand our identities beyond "me" (egocentric) to "us" (ethnocentric) to "all of us" (world-centric)? To map and guide NIGH projects and endeavors for theory-guided, evidence-based practices, Barbara Dossey's grand nursing theory, the Theory of Integral Nursing, was identified to assist us with NIGH's integral vision and integral mapping (see Dossey, 2015, 2016a for a detailed discussion).

The Theory of Integral Nursing is a grand nursing theory—informed by an in-depth study of Nightingale's life and insights—to develop relevant evolutionary growth processes, stages, and levels of human development and consciousness, moving the nursing world toward a comprehensive integral philosophy and understanding. The Theory of Integral Nursing assists nurses to map human capacities—beginning with healing and evolving transpersonal self and connection with "divine energies"—however defined or identified—and, thus, to support nursing's collective endeavors to create a healthier world (see Dossey, 2010a, 2010b for an in-depth discussion of Nightingale's mysticism).

Integral and Integral Dialogue Defined

"Integral" can be defined as a comprehensive way to organize multiple phenomena of human experience related to four perspectives of reality:

- The individual interior "I" (personal/intentional)
- The individual exterior "It" (physiology/behavioral)
- The collective interior "We" (shared/cultural)
- The collective exterior "Its" (systems/structures)

By understanding an integral perspective, nurses are able to enter into integral dialogues to map and translate their work at a deeper level of integration.

| Figure 7.2 | Integral quadrants. |

Integral model

Upper left		Upper right
Individual interior (intentional/personal)		**Individual exterior** (behavioral/biological)

"I" space includes self and consciousness (self-care, fears, feelings, beliefs, values, esteem, cognitive capacity, emotional maturity, moral development, spiritual maturity, personal communication skills, etc.) | "It" space that includes brain and organisms (physiology, pathophysiology [cells, molecules, limbic system, neurotransmitters, physical sensations], biochemistry, chemistry, physics, behaviors [skill development in health, nutrition, exercise, etc.])

- Subjective
- Interpretive
- Qualitative

I   It

We   Its

- Objective
- Observable
- Quantitative

Collective interior (cultural/shared)	**Collective exterior** (systems/structures)

"We" space includes the relationship to each other and the culture and worldview (shared understanding, shared vision, shared meaning, shared leadership and other values, integral dialogues and communication/morale, etc.)

"Its" space includes the relation to social systems and environment, organizational structures and systems (in health care—financial and billing systems), educational systems, information technology, mechanical structures and transportation, regulatory structures (environmental and governmental policies, etc.)

Lower left   Lower right

Source: Wilber (2000) with permission from Ken Wilber by Barbara Dossey ©2007.

An *integral dialogue* can be defined as the transformative and visionary exploration of ideas and possibilities—across disciplines—where the individual interior (personal/intentional), individual exterior (physiology/behavioral), collective interior (shared/cultural), and collective exterior (structures/systems) are considered as equally important to understanding exchanges and outcomes. Take a moment to explore Figure 7.2, which illustrates this *individual interior and exterior and the collective interior and exterior.*

A brief overview of the Theory of Integral Nursing is explored next (see Dossey, 2016a for details).

Theory of Integral Nursing Intentions

The Theory of Integral Nursing has three intentions:

1. To embrace both the unitary whole person and the complexities of the nursing profession and health care

2. To explore the direct application of integral processes and worldviews to include four perspectives of realities—the individual interior and exterior and the collective interior and exterior

3. To expand nurses' capacities—as 21st-century Nightingales—to extend relevant practice roles for nurses as health diplomats, health communicators, and as integral/integrative nurse coaches who are coaching to achieve a healthier humanity based on integral perspectives— at both local and global levels (Dossey, 2016a)

Theory of Integral Nursing Content

The content of a nursing theory includes the subject matter and building blocks that give a theory its form, as seen in Figures 7.3A through 7.3F.

It comprises the stable elements that are acted on or that take the action. In the Theory of Integral Nursing, the subject matter and building blocks are as follows:

- Healing (Figure 7.3A)

- The meta-paradigm of nursing (Figure 7.3B)

- The patterns of knowing (Figure 7.3C)

- The four quadrants that are adapted from Wilber's Integral Theory: individual interior "I" (subjective, personal/intentional), individual exterior "It" (objective, behavioral), collective interior "We" (intersubjective, cultural), and collective exterior "Its" (interobjective, systems/structures; Figure 7.3D)

- Wilber's "AQAL—all quadrants, all levels, all lines, all states, all types" (Figure 7.3E; Wilber, 2000; see Dossey, 2016a for details)

All content components are represented together as an overlay that creates a mandala to symbolize wholeness (Figure 7.3F).

NIGH'S INTEGRAL MAPPING

Across her lifetime, Nightingale achieved her own global *collective interior and exterior* communications health promotion strategies. These included her proactive contribution to many forms of print journalism such as her *Notes on Nursing: What It Is, and What It Is Not* (Nightingale, 1860a). This textbook was written first for the general public and became an immediate popular bestseller upon first printing. Later, it was expanded as the first nursing textbook. Nightingale also consciously cultivated her connections with the journalists and media professionals of her time, making sure they understood, communicated, and shared her messages. This was her outreach to the general public and to widely influence political will. Her writing continued for 40 years with more than 14,000 letters and 200 publications, culminating with her last great essay "Sick-Nursing and Health-Nursing" that was presented for her at the 1893 Chicago's World Fair (Beck, 2005; Dossey et al., 2005; Dossey, 2010a; Nightingale, 1893).

Our NIGH team understood that this global communications capacity—which Nightingale demonstrated across decades of her own work—is still far beyond what most nurses and many citizens—who work mainly from *individual interior* and *exterior* mindsets—are achieving, even today (Dossey, Beck, & Rushton, 2011). We saw that understanding and applying this broader Nightingale approach could indeed be useful to today's problems, certainly to those problems related

Figure 7.3 **Theory of Integral Nursing. (A) Healing; (B) Healing Metaparadigm in Nursing Theory; (C) Healing and Patterns of Knowing in Nursing; (D) Healing and Four Quadrants; (E) Healing, AQAL; (F) Healing, Metaparadigm in Nursing, Patterns of Knowing in Nursing, Four Quadrants, AQAL.**

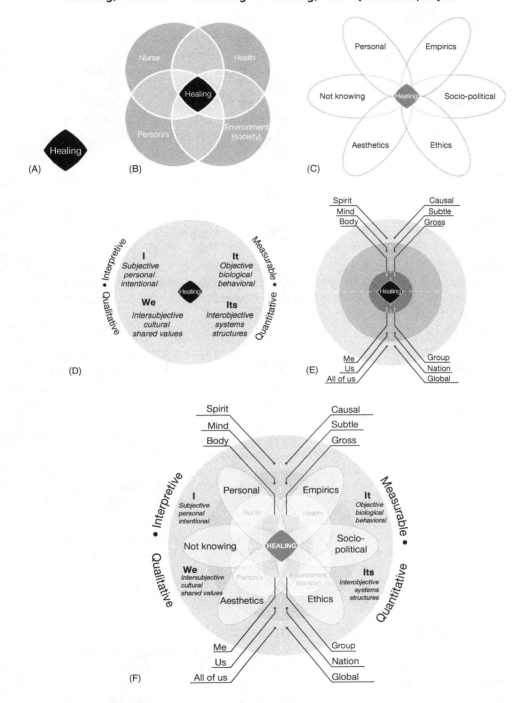

Source: Used with permission ©2007 Barbara Dossey. (C) Adapted from Carper (1978); (D, E) Adapted from Wilber (2000); (F) Adapted from Dossey (2008b).

to nursing and to health, and particularly in the context of the UN Sustainable Development Agenda.

Exploring Events Through "I," "We," "It," "Its" Lens

Our NIGH team saw that the four integral quadrants can illustrate that any event can be interpreted from a first-person perspective "I"—*how I personally see and feel about an event*. We also saw the second-person perspective "We"—*how others see the event*—and a third-person perspective "It" or "Its"—*the objective or interobjective view of the event*. These interrelated views provide us with the most perspectives possible. Integrating this four-quadrant approach, we can explore our understanding of health and our ability to serve health—by connecting the dots from each perspective as seen in the following bullets:

- Without focusing on strengthening and sustaining individuals, groups of individuals cannot thrive (*individual and collective interior*).
- Without focusing on the worldviews underlying all situations in any society, the structures within which we live and work cannot be properly understood and sustained (*individual and collective exterior*).
- Without first populating an understanding of the nature of these worldviews—with real people in real groups with real needs in mind—structures can quickly become limited, and related narrow worldviews become irrelevant.
- Without understanding the value of envisioning and proposing structures from worldviews that can make a difference in the world, people and groups tend to drift away from purposeful efforts to actually ever make a difference.

Holon and Increasing Complexity

Wilber uses the word *holon* to describe anything that is both a whole and a part of another whole, thus creating structures of increasing complexity (Wilber, 2000). Persons are individual holons, whereas groups are social holons. (A full description of these distinctions is beyond this discussion.) For example, the individuals whom we placed in the upper left (UL) quadrant are really holons of all four quadrants as discussed in the next section. Based on our own life experiences within and beyond nursing, we understood what Wilber meant when he noted that omitting the focus of any one of the integral quadrants would cause *hemorrhaging* in attempts to achieve work represented by the other three integral quadrants. Our NIGH projects thus explore the complex dynamics of integral theory organization at first, second, and third levels of complexity (Wilber, 2000).

NIGH's Jigsaw Puzzle Metaphor—Integral Model A

As Nightingale scholars, we were already *integral* thinkers, seeing parts of NIGH's development puzzle as a whole. We knew that each *puzzle piece* already had a *relationship* to our overall whole picture. We knew that choosing *just one* piece, now, would not work because just one activity or project could not be effectively achieved without the other pieces in place—just as a jigsaw puzzle cannot be *solved* with only one piece. Each jigsaw puzzle piece is a tiny yet critical fraction of an entire puzzle picture.

Thus, we chose this jigsaw puzzle metaphor to illustrate these four quadrants (Figure 7.4A) as follows—the upper left (UL) "I" quadrant named "among Individuals"; the lower left (LL) "We" quadrant named "within Groups"; the upper right (UR) "It" quadrant named "at Grassroots Levels"; and the lower right (LR) "Its" quadrant named "at Global Levels."

NIGH's online tagline became—INFORM, INSPIRE, INITIATE, & INVOLVE—and developed within the framework of the NIGH's Integral Models—identifying our four key interconnected approaches. Next, we explore our four NIGH Models as follows:

- Identify four interrelated problems—Integral Model B (Figure 7.4B).
- Propose four synthesis solutions—Integral Model C (Figure 7.4C).
- Implement four integral initiatives—Integral Model D (Figure 7.4D).
- Articulate four anticipated outcomes—Integral Model E (Figure 7.4E).

NIGH's Four Interrelated Problems Identified—Integral Model B

NIGH has identified four interrelated problems illustrated together in NIGH Integral Model B (Figure 7.4B). At NIGH, we believe that our Integral approach—to increase public concern for solving these problems—will assist with this global effort. As examples, our NIGH teams will develop themes on SDG 3—Health and Well-Being, SDG 4—Quality Education, SDG 5—Gender Equality, and SDG 6—Clean Water and Sanitation.

- **Problem 1**: NIGH's subject focus—as noted in the *LR At Global Levels quadrant of Model B* (Figure 7.4B)—is the challenge of achieving the UN SDGs.
- **Problem 2**: NIGH's team has identified several interrelated and related challenges—as represented in the *UL Among Individuals quadrant of Model B* (Figure 7.4B). Among individuals—there has been a marked lack of public concern for and informed public involvement to meet these critical global health issues. The worldwide scope of this challenge seems beyond what individuals believe they can consider or do.
- **Problem 3**: As represented by the *UR At Grassroots quadrant of Model B* (Figure 7.4B)—is directly related to the second.
- **Problem 4**: Is identified in the *LL Within Groups quadrant of Model B* (Figure 7.4B). The chronic yet continually critical global nursing shortage is one of the key factors in this silent struggle.

NIGH's Four New Synthesis Solutions—Integral Model C

Today's NIGH team is developing and implementing four solutions synthesized to create new levels of societal understanding—to initiate new grassroots structures and to further establish ways in which more people can effectively respond to these and other global health challenges. These four synthesis solutions are as follows as seen in Figure 7.4C.

- **Synthesis Solution 1**: *At Grassroots Levels UR quadrant of Model C* (Figure 7.4C)—NIGH is using a broader view of health—beyond the absence of

Figure 7.4 NIGH Integral Model. (A) Jigsaw Puzzle Metaphor, (B) Interrelated Problems, (C) Synthesis Solutions, (D) Interrelated Initiatives, (E) Outcomes—Strength Upon Strength.

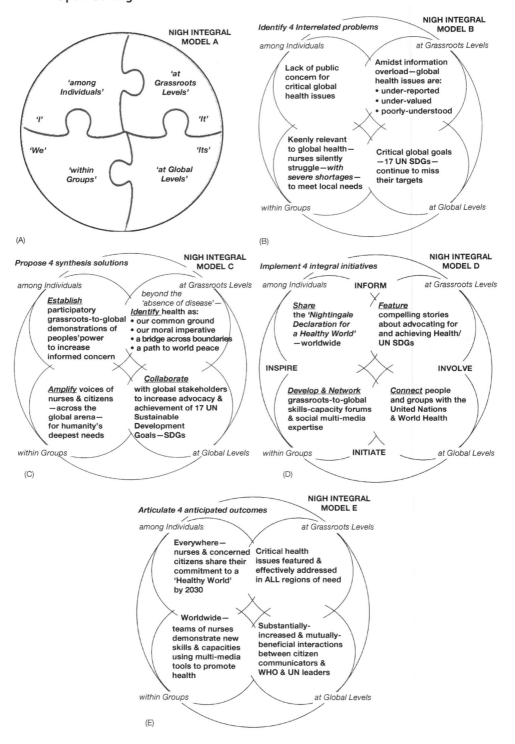

Source: Used with permission of the Nightingale Initiative for Global Health (2016b) © NIGH.

disease—as a common ground between all 7+ billion people who live on earth. Each of us wants health for ourselves and for our families. If I know that my health depends on your health, I am more likely to care about your health and the health of others. In this way, health becomes a moral imperative for everyone.

- **Synthesis Solution 2**: *Among Individuals UL quadrant of Model C* (Figure 7.4C)—as we collaborate with people across the world, we are using the Internet, Facebook, Twitter, and other online tools to establish new ways to demonstrate individual grassroots-to-global participation and to increase public concern for health. As we further develop the use of these tools, the UL of *individuals* will be better informed and increasingly concerned.

- **Synthesis Solution 3**: *Within Groups LL quadrant of Model C* (Figure 7.4C)—NIGH's team seeks to amplify the voices of nurses, midwives, and community health workers—and, indeed, groups of citizen stakeholders concerned with the health of humanity. Nurses and midwives are most often "on location" in these places. They can develop new groups of effective online voices, sharing what the world needs to know. They can also become the knowledgeable eyes, ears, and voices to broadcast the solutions that can be found and replicated elsewhere.

- **Synthesis Solution 4**: *At Global Levels LR quadrant of Model C* (Figure 7.4C)—NIGH's team is specifically collaborating with key global officials—particularly within UN agencies, including WHO—to communicate global health concerns at grassroots levels.

NIGH's Four Interrelated Initiatives—Integral Model D

Building upon this new synthesis of solutions—working among Individuals and within Groups at Grassroots and Global Levels—NIGH's team is establishing four sets of initiatives as outlined in Figure 7.4D.

From our integral, holistic, and integrative nursing perspectives, we have found that employing four quadrants together will be more effective than using only one or two approaches in isolation from the others.

- **Interrelated Initiative 1**: In the *UL Among Individuals quadrant of Model D* (Figure 7.4D), NIGH's initial work established the *Nightingale Declaration for A Healthy World*—available to sign online at www.nighvision.net/nightingale-declaration.html—where individual nurses and concerned citizens are participating from across the world (see Chapter 3, Figure 3.1). Over the next months and years, NIGH's growing team will encourage many thousands more to sign, asking their networks to do the same, creating a ripple effect of participation and concern. This foundational NIGH project continues to establish ways to inspire individual people, worldwide, to newly see what they are already achieving and ponder what else they can do and share.

- **Interrelated Initiative 2**: In the *LL Within Groups quadrant of Model D* (Figure 7.4D), NIGH's team has also developed an initial series of group workshops to build skill sets around media and related communication capacities. These sessions have become quite popular, now desired across the world. They include ways to assist nurses to tell their stories—as described in the two case studies that follow—and how to incorporate nurse coaching skills that are discussed after these case studies.

- **Interrelated Initiative 3:** In the *UR Grassroots quadrant of Model D* (Figure 7.4D), with NIGH's current website—www.NIGHvision.net—and by developing NIGH's wider "Global Internet Portal" in the coming months and years, we are establishing the online venue of sharing nurses' and midwives' stories from around the world. These online stories are needed to further involve many groups of nurses, midwives, students, and others to develop and network their grassroots-to-global skills in social multimedia outreach—for the promotion of health.

- **Interrelated Initiative 4**: In the *LR Global quadrant of Model D* (Figure 7.4D), the NIGH team has already participated in many meetings at the UN in New York City, as well as at WHO headquarters in Geneva and at WHO and UN regional offices in Asia, Africa, Europe, the Americas, and Australia. Through these activities, NIGH's team has confirmed that we can indeed connect proactive grassroots people and groups with friends and colleagues working at global levels. This approach can well assist global health leaders to better reach a worldwide grassroots audience. It can also encourage, support, and sustain grassroots voices to therefore initiate projects that commit to what they deeply care about—to be truly heard, understood, and valued.

NIGH's Four Outcomes to Build Strength Upon Strength—Integral E

In keeping with four integral approaches to NIGH's work as illustrated in NIGH Integral Model E (Figure 7.4E), we are anticipating a synthesis of successes as outcomes to these plans. NIGH's team has learned that our pioneering pilot projects have already made strong, significant contributions to nursing and health across the world, as demonstrated in two case studies.

- **Outcome 1**: As in the *UL Among Individuals quadrant of Model E* (Figure 7.4E), and in response to broadening the global outreach of the *Nightingale Declaration for A Healthy World*—we expect that a growing number of individual nurses and concerned citizens everywhere will continue keen to share their commitment to achieving a "Healthy World by 2020"—the Bicentennial year of Nightingale's birth.

- **Outcome 2**: As in the *UR Grassroots quadrant of Model E* (Figure 7.4E), we know this outreach can drive online traffic and build continuing interest in learning more about health problems—particularly of vulnerable children and women—worldwide. We look forward to the day when our collaborative stories, features, and "news" will significantly increase grassroots public concern to make a key difference.

- **Outcome 3**: As in the *LL Groups quadrant of Model E* (Figure 7.4E), we envision well-received teams of collaborators focused on demonstrating their new skills and capacities—using multimedia tools. "News" crafted by groups from the world of nursing—for the rest of the world to read— can go a long way toward achieving a better understanding of global health. This will be of interest, as many are concerned about their own health, the health of their families, as well as the suffering of humanity. These new multimedia endeavors will reinforce how nurses are now regarded among the most trusted professionals in the world.

- **Outcome 4**: As in the *LR Global Levels quadrant of Model E* (Figure 7.4E), NIGH's team is already looking to substantially increase many mutually beneficial interactions between grassroots-based nurses, concerned citizen stakeholders, and global health leaders and communicators. Through these efforts, we are working within the family of 193 Member States of the UN and with UN organizations and agencies, including the WHO.

In the next section, we explore NIGH's developing journey through partnerships and "six lines of development."

NIGH'S DEVELOPING JOURNEY

NIGH's partnerships and relationships have been an exciting and evolving cocreated lived story leading healthy individuals, stakeholders, communities, and nations to impact all domains of our global village. This has included both *relational knowing* and *embodied knowing* (Wright & Brajtman, 2011). "Relational knowing" is coming to know individuals and groups through narratives that start with *autonomy*—respecting both individual and collective integral dialogues. "Embodied knowing" is the recognition of every person as living in her/his body in the world—a way of coming to know self to self and self to others. "Autonomy," as a lived experience, is relational and involves both independence and interdependence.

From our beginnings, NIGH's integral mapping and planning have focused on wholeness—physical-mental-emotional-social-spiritual-cultural-environmental—and the interconnectedness of individuals and groups (Beck, Dossey, & Rushton, 2014). This has required a commitment to self-reflection and self-awareness, as well as a "shift in consciousness" to our own interiority. As Sharma reminds us, this is remembering to source from our deepest personal wisdom (Sharma, 2004, 2007). In our NIGH integral mission, we consciously touch six lines of development, described in Table 7.1, and do so in relation to our individual selves, to others, and to the natural world, where we can find new ways to deepen our integral and holistic understanding each day (Dossey, 2016a, p. 29).

In the next section, we explore NIGH's journey with global colleagues and the translation of the Theory of Integral Nursing into action through two case studies.

NIGH'S JOURNEY WITH GLOBAL COLLEAGUES: TWO CASE STUDIES

Low- and middle-income countries (LMICs) enjoy a steady stream of energetic and highly educated college student volunteers, expending time, talent, and treasure in hopes of improving standards of living in poor communities. The challenge is to ensure that the good intentions of volunteers are channeled effectively into endeavors that generate locally acceptable, sustainable improvements in health. An application of the Integral Theory allows researchers and students to explore multiple phenomena of such human experience—offering a balanced view of conditions

Table 7.1 Six Lines of Development

Cognitive—"Awareness of What Is"	Capacity to make observations from different perspectives in a coherent manner; an awareness of what leads to new understanding related to possibilities, insights, action steps, breakdowns, and resistance to change.
Emotional—"Awareness to Spectrum of Emotions"	Capacity to skillfully recognize our own emotional (present, past, future) and what life conditions are related; recognizing what situations evoke various emotions (challenges, difficulties, disappointments, joy, fears, anger, etc.); ability to enter into the present moment and energy field with another person to listen deeply, noticing your own intuition to any emotional state/s that the person does not recognize.
Somatic—"Awareness of Body/Mind"	Capacity to feel, notice, and respond to your body sensations (tired, tight, open, energized) and to connect these sensations with the present moment; ability to skillfully access one's personal innate wisdom and make subtle shifts.
Interpersonal—"Awareness of How I Relate to Others"	Capacity to be engaged socially with others from different perspectives (I/We/It) and to listen deeply to others' intentions, goals, and desires, and to offer appropriate support.
Spiritual—"Awareness of Ultimate Issues"	Capacity to explore feelings, thoughts, experiences, and behaviors that arise from a search for meaning around ultimate issues, questions, and concerns: "Who am I?" "What is my soul's purpose?" "How am I part of the interconnected web of life?" (includes from "me" to "us" to "all of us").
Moral—"Awareness of What to Do"	Capacity to reach a decision about a choice about what is the right thing to do and to enact chosen behavior/s and action/s (includes from "me" to "us" to "all of us").

Source: Dossey (2016a).

that affect health, including subjective experiences, cultural worldviews, physiological manifestations of diseases, and social systems (Dossey, 2008a, 2015).

For example, this theory offers a balanced view for those seeking to address maternal health issues because it includes wider range perspectives on a pregnant woman's condition. These include past pregnancies, psychological concerns, cultural concerns, access to care, and insurance coverage, as well as her physical environment and financial situation (Azaiza & Cohen, 2006; Luna, 1994; Mubeen, Mansoor, Hussain, & Qadir, 2012; Tsianaksa & Liamputtong, 2002).

Practice–Academe Innovative Collaboration

In 2009, a partnership was formed between the University of Cincinnati (UC), Ohio, and NM Sadguru (a nongovernmental organization [NGO] based within India). Initially, the UC team worked across the disciplines of engineering, business, science, and design to consider interventions to improve economic opportunity within the context of a rural, agricultural setting in India. In addition, as part of the UC team, nurses offered a critical perspective that health should be used as an important lens to evaluate the effectiveness of these interventions. Improved economic opportunity should result in healthier people.

This project initially began as a collaboration to allow interdisciplinary study-abroad students—from engineering, business, science, and design—to focus on gaining experience to develop projects that improved livelihoods in rural villages within India. The project expanded to include a critical need to engage with the nursing profession within India to gain local, cultural knowledge, as well as nursing skills. Through a series of interactions, the importance of considering health was expanded to align with the Theory of Integral Nursing.

A Multidisciplinary Approach Including Nursing Clinical Practice and Research

The original team, led by Project Managers Professor Dr. Daniel Oerther and nurse educator Sarah Oerther, from UC and NM Sadguru, reached out to collaborate with NIGH to include practicing nurses from an urban setting within India. This intentional choice—inviting practicing nurses from an urban setting—allowed the team to explore both cross-cultural and cross-disciplinary collaborations, as well as the opportunity for practicing nurses within India to experience the gradient of cultural and socioeconomic status from urban to rural settings. This was a unique educational experiment because some of the students were from the United States and some of the nurses came from Indian institutions. All were working across disciplinary boundaries. And—in terms of socioeconomic status—all were working outside the comforts of their past experience.

This intentional choice was critical because individuals from the same cultural background cannot always articulate the practices they perform in everyday life. An individual's cultural knowledge relies on tacit assumptions that can be invisible to themselves—even to those who come from a similar Indian cultural environment but from a different socioeconomic status (Crossley, 2001; Rhynas, 2005). Therefore, the collaboration employed a team approach to more effectively assess development conditions for rural villages as seen in Figure 7.5.

Figure 7.5   **Engineering students from the United States, engineering students from India, and staff nurses from the P. D. Hinduja National Hospital getting ready to board a train to the rural villages.**

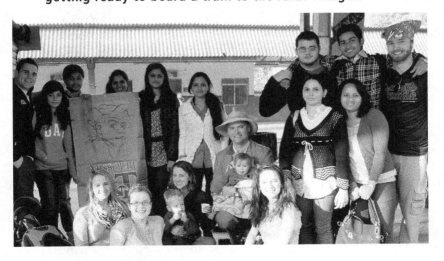

Source: Photographer: Sarah Oerther. Used with permission.

| Figure 7.6 | A nurse (right) from Mumbai's P. D. Hinduja National Hospital interviews a recently pregnant mother to discover needs for improved maternal health. |

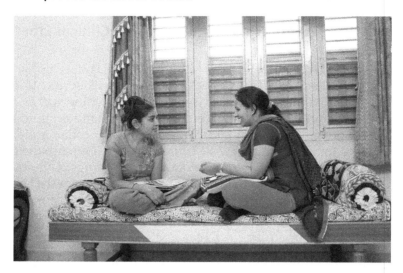

Source: Photographer: Sarah Oerther. Used with permission.

The format of this collaboration allowed for sharing in two ways:

1. Through interdisciplinary means
2. Using cross-culture competence including the rural-to-urban divide present within India

This collaboration has helped to create a sustainable nursing workforce at the P. D. Hinduja National Hospital (PD HNH) and Medical Research Centre (MRC) in Mumbai, India, and to extend the impacts within India, five additional nursing schools have been recruited to be part of this project. Figure 7.6 illustrates one of the nurses and patients involved.

Case Study 1

Background

The UC developed a term-long honors seminar class that focused on the development of sustainable technologies for sanitation, potable water, cooking, and agriculture in LMICs. The UC honors students—a multidisciplinary group of business, engineering, and industrial design majors—specifically focused on the development of a drip irrigation system that would allow farmers to grow cash crops. Figures 7.7 through 7.9 show testing of the water for this system in different settings.

This thereby improved their economic opportunity—allowing farmers with increased financial resources to better care for their families. Design efforts of the drip irrigation system focused on affordability and acceptability for the Gujarati

Figure 7.7 **Missouri University of Science and Technology student tests water quality.**

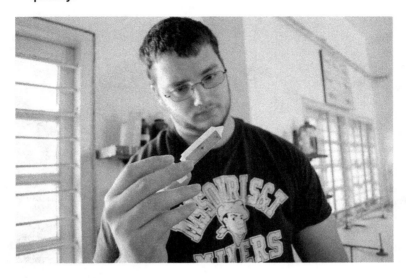

Source: Photographer: Sarah Oerther. Used with permission.

Figure 7.8 **Nurse testing water for nitrate. The level for this community was greater than 50 mg nitrate-nitrogen per liter. In the United States, if the level is over 10 mg/L, everything is shut down. Elevated levels of nitrate in drinking water can cause blue baby syndrome in infants.**

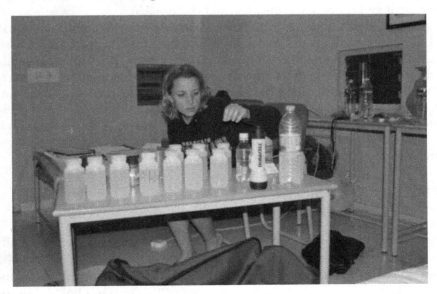

Source: Photographer: Sarah Oerther. Used with permission.

Figure 7.9 Missouri University of Science and Technology student tests water quality.

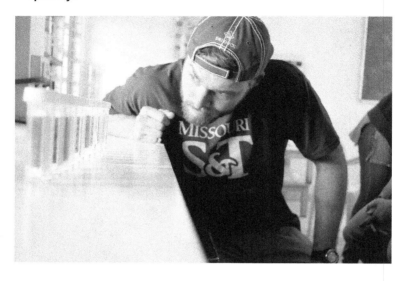

Source: Photographer: Sarah Oerther. Used with permission.

people. The class worked with NM Sadguru, a local nonprofit NGO located in the Dahod District of Gujarat.

Sadguru's mandate focuses on watershed management, rural development, organic farming, agroforestry, indigenous rights, and women's rights. At the end of the 10-week term in the United States, a team of 10 students traveled to Gujarat to implement and refine what they learned (Figure 7.5).

Meanwhile, two nurses from India were provided scholarships to work with these UC honors students in Dahod. In return, the nurses were asked to assist the UC students to implement their course knowledge using principles of sustainability and focusing on local environmental conditions. Creators of the course hoped that—within this community of indigenous people—the nurses would be able to equip the UC students to address a comprehensive range of social and biological determinants of health. In addition, practicing nurses—from within an urban Indian context—were selected to afford their opportunity to work across the socioeconomic gradient from urban to rural India.

Reflections

At the end of the 2-week-long experience, Nurse Shweta reflected,

> In innumerable ways, I benefited personally as well as professionally from this trip. We conducted household surveys including the health and agricultural aspect of the villagers. We did water testing from the lake, hand pumps, and wells. We educated villagers about health aspects of water and sanitation and also about drip irrigation and composting. Anthropometric measurements were performed on schoolchildren to

assess their nutritional status. We presented the health aspects of the project to the community leaders of the village.

Our best experience of the trip was when we informed the community about elevated nitrate levels in one drinking water well (Figure 7.10)

Nitrate is a common contaminant often found in wells in agricultural areas. Major sources of nitrate contamination can be from fertilizers. Elevated levels of nitrate in drinking water can cause blue baby syndrome in infants. The level for this community was greater than 50 mg nitrate-nitrogen per liter. In the United States, if the level is over 10 mg, everything is shut down and alternative water supplies are identified to protect the health of infants. We helped inform the community of the health risks, and the community responded by immediately discontinuing use of the well. The local NGO will start to work on educating this community about the risk of disposing of fertilizers near wells. It was very encouraging to work with UC students and we were surprised with their friendly and extremely warm welcoming behavior. We have learned lots of things while working with the other disciplines, especially that it creates innovative ideas, which can't be created if people from the same base of knowledge work

---

Figure 7.10 Three nurses at a community water well that they identified as having elevated nitrate levels at a village pump. The level for this community was greater than 50 mg nitrate-nitrogen per liter. In the United States, if the level is over 10 mg/L, everything is shut down. Elevated levels of nitrate in drinking water can cause blue baby syndrome in infants.

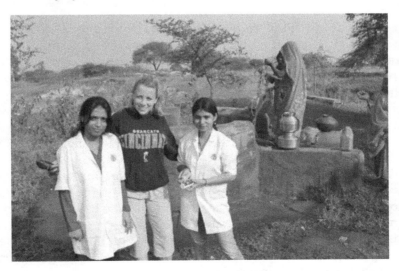

Source: Photographer: Sarah Oerther. Used with permission.

on a problem. Also, it gives ideas about the way a person from different disciplines addresses a problem. For example, the way of looking at a problem a business student is different from the engineering student.

Nurse Ancy agreed and said,

> I have been into serving patients in the hospital in various departments. This trip has helped to improve my interaction to a greater extent and it has helped me update myself with health and sanitation problems in the villages. I appreciated learning about village life within India.

The UC students from the class all said the best part of the trip was their interactions with these two nurses from India—because the nurses were able to provide cultural insight into the project and to explain health from an Indian's point of view.

Proof of Sustainability

Nurse leaders continued to work with NIGH and plans were developed for a related new course to be offered at Missouri University of Science and Technology (MST). Recognizing that the addition of the two practicing Indian nurses had substantially improved the overall experience for American students—also resulting in positive patient outcomes—it was decided that additional activities would be undertaken.

First, a curriculum to contribute a series of workshops and lectures was developed by the partners. Second, the inclusion of additional nurses from India was planned to help accelerate the cross-cultural training. Third, while the original focus was on improving rural villages, it was decided that it would be important to link the rural village experience with the urban experience. This was a component that had been envisioned specifically to improve urban patient outcomes for PDHNH.

Case Study 2

Background

A related series of workshops and lectures was delivered to 50 staff and student nurses at PDHNH, where the programs were hosted and visiting faculty from MST were welcomed (Figure 7.11).

Example program titles included "Research Methods in Community Nursing and Public Health." The goals of these programs included empowering NIGH's global team to continue their efforts to build a sustainable nursing workforce within India. NIGH further coordinated efforts to bring more than 150 students, faculty, and clinical nurses to two additional sessions, hosting and offering a collaborative networking lunch.

Then, PDHNH staff nurses and students—collaborating with the multidisciplinary engineering, business, and design students from the United States—conducted home health assessments to identify women who had recently given birth. Working with translators through oral interviews, a questionnaire was administered and data were collected covering a wide range of maternal and infant experiences, also noting demographic data of maternal attitudes and behaviors before, during, and shortly after pregnancy (Figure 7.12).

The collaborative aim of this project was to more fully integrate electronic medicine and digital peer–peer and nurse coaching into the rural and urban Indian

Figure 7.11   **Nurses perform anthropometric measurements on schoolchildren to assess their nutritional status.**

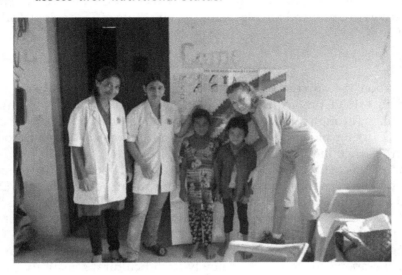

Source: Photographer: Daniel Oerther. Used with permission.

Figure 7.12   **A nurse (right) from Mumbai's Hinduja Hospital, records a recently pregnant mother's story about her concerns for her health and her baby's health.**

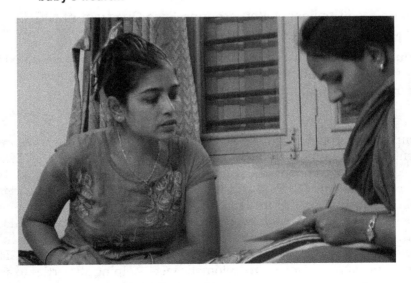

Source: Photographer: Sarah Oerther. Used with permission.

maternal health arena. International nursing teams from the United States and India analyzed the data. The results were published after peer review and presentation at the First International Humanitarian Technology Conference sponsored by Harvard University and the Massachusetts Institute of Technology (MIT) in the spring of 2014.

Expansion

Building upon the success of this expanded field study, a program was then designed to extend this experience to positively impact upon continuing staff development. Through a collaboration that included PDHNH and five additional colleges of nursing, at least 700 nurses in urban Mumbai have been introduced to the lessons learned in this case study.

As part of this collaboration, the rural–urban divide between the communities targeted for intervention—versus the regular patient population of PDHNH—provided a lens through which the "urban nurses" of PDHNH became sensitized and more fully aware of the unique and common challenges to health care among the rural poor of India.

Through field practicums and classroom lectures, staff nurses and nursing students were empowered to use their newly found cultural sensitivity to improve the care of the "urban poor"—especially those who were regular patients at the free clinics operated by PDHNH. By working across the rural–urban divide, these staff nurses and nursing students became better at caring for patients from diverse socioeconomic backgrounds. The PDHNH nurses and students took turns to care for patients below the poverty line who were presenting with health care needs at the free clinic. According to Ms. Phalakshi Manjrekar—PDHNH's Director of Nursing and member of Hinduja's Board of Management—improved patient outcomes were clearly identified (Figure 7.13).

Four Interrelated Challenges Representing Each Quadrant of NIGH's Integral Model

While much was accomplished over almost a decade of work represented in these two case studies, these efforts to forge a strong and lasting collaboration did face a number of obstacles and tipping points.

Among Peoples

An example of a tipping point was on December 25, 2012, two days before a team of students arrived in India from the United States. One of the nurses, Liza—who was scheduled to accompany the team—lost her husband who was killed tragically in a car accident. PDHNH and NIGH quickly provided, *among individuals,* an excellent substitute nurse leader, Nidhi, for the project. No money was lost. No student time was lost. And, everything moved forward. Also, NIGH negotiated with PDHNH for paid time off for the nurses to participate in the collaboration—even as Liza took leave for her grieving. Through this process, NIGH's team members demonstrated *individual* diplomatic tact—helping all parties to adhere to their agreements—fostering an equitable exchange of time and resources among the diverse partners, from the United States and urban and rural India, across multiple socioeconomic gradients.

Figure 7.13 **Daniel Oerther, Director of the Ohio Center of Excellence in Advanced Energy, and Sarah Oerther, Adjunct Instructor of Nursing at Xavier University, and their children, Barney and Emmalise, beside P. D. Hinduja National Hospital Director of Nursing and NIGH World Director, Phalakshi Manjekar (center).**

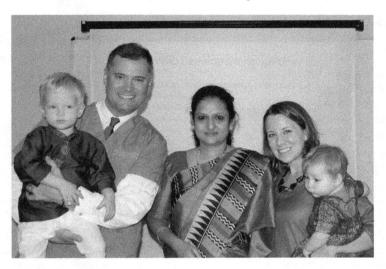

Source: Photographer: Bhavna Nayak. Used with permission.

Within Groups

Academic partners from engineering, business, and design disciplines had to be sensitized to the value of including professional nurses and their art of caring and evidence-based nursing. As well, the medical staff of PDHNH had to be convinced of the value of providing nursing staff to participate in these programs, also with paid leave. But, when these *group* challenges were addressed, new reflections on the value of *group* interactions emerged. While these initiatives needed to form multidisciplinary teams, the nurses participating also needed to understand and form their own roles as core members in this *group*. As it happened in this case, experience—involving numerous experts and students from varied fields—provided participating nurses with a first-hand opportunity to see what personnel from other fields can contribute to their own work. If it had not been for their interactions within the multidisciplinary team, these nurses—who collaborated, for the first time, with people from other fields—would not have gained this team's new "among groups" experience.

Darrell, an engineering student from the United States, also reflected on a similar outcome:

> I feel that through the research and working in a team atmosphere (with me being the only American in the group) helped me grow as a professional. Yes, I have worked in teams before, but not in a team of all Indians and me! At first, my team and I were on two different tracks with the research,

especially me trying to understand fully what their goals were, but after taking the afternoon off and grabbing ice cream and brownies just to create team chemistry, we were able to achieve a common goal! I know that after this semester I am excited to take these skills I learned, while in India, to my internship in Kansas City this summer.

At Grassroots Levels

Bridging cultural barriers was difficult, at times, both for the Indian nurses and for the students from the United States. To address this challenge, again *at the grassroots*, NIGH's team helped all parties to navigate the complex day-to-day hurdles of language barriers, cultural cues, ambiguity in goals, and work–rest balance. Everyone learned the importance of meeting both the American professional service objectives and the Indian research objectives of evidence-based nursing practice. NIGH's team provided phone/e-mail contact nearly every day, even when the Indian nurses were overwhelmed with the students' lack of cultural understanding. This allowed the nurses to debrief and share the stress. This became a collaboration between the participating nurses and senior PDHNH nurses who helped to mentor the younger nurses through their experience.

The critical *grassroots* tipping point that moved the collaboration in a positive direction was the ability to build trust among all the collaborators and to thus bridge cultural understanding. Katelyn, an engineering student, reflected,

> The language barrier while working with farmers also presented a challenge. It taught me a lot of patience and trust in the rest of my group as we worked to get surveys answered and questions conveyed correctly (Figure 7.14).

> Questions needed to be asked in different ways to make sure everything was understood and nothing was accidentally left out. As there were several different backgrounds within the group (nursing, engineering, and science), it was an inspiring and informative experience to see each of us present new ideas or questions that were unique to each of our field (Figure 7.15).

> Having a well-rounded group helped me to learn more and I think helped to broaden the views that each of us brought individually.

At the Global Level

The planners of this partnership were challenged to recruit collaborative partners, identify funding sources, negotiate contracts, and assure the safety of all participants. This included seeing to the overall welfare of the faculty and students from the United States, of staff nurses and nursing students from PDHNH, and of the communities and patients who were part of the work. This challenge required and demonstrated everyone's creativity, leadership, and tenacity.

While the WHO (2016) identifies strategic global directions for nurses, most nurses work at hands-on levels and have difficulty seeing themselves and their work related to global aims. This endeavor that focused on rural issues in India also reflected the WHO's goals for populations. Participation in this project provided

Figure 7.14 Indian nurse working with an engineering student to more fully integrate electronic medicine and digital peer-to-peer and nurse coaching with a villager in rural India.

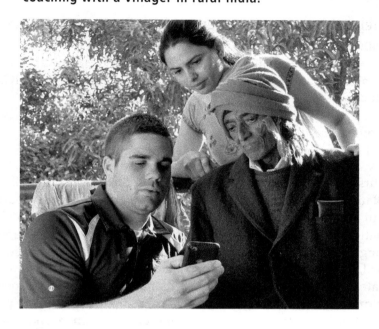

Source: Photographer: Sarah Oerther. Used with permission.

Figure 7.15 Engineering student participates in a meeting with farmers in India.

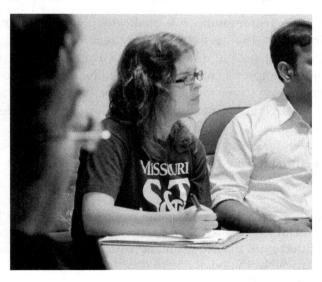

Source: Photographer: Sarah Oerther. Used with permission.

the participating nurses with the experience of contributing to global health goals. During their participation, the nurses came to more fully appreciate the significance of their work as required to achieve global health goals.

Four Interrelated Successes Representing Each Quadrant of NIGH's Integral Model

These two case studies also illustrate the value of appreciation for success within each integral quadrant and the integration that occurs across NIGH's whole Integral Model.

Among Peoples

As PDHNH's Director of Nursing, Phalakshi Manjrekar reflected,

> The nursing culture that is supported here in this hospital directly led to this planning and achieving this initiative. Planners understood that— without the opportunity to experience the lifestyle *among the peoples* and populations of rural India—it would not be possible to conceptualize assisting them in any way. With the success of this project and hence forward, PDHNH's nursing department continues to encourage and facilitate any program that can allow its nurses to gain this experience. While many are not able to take up this hardship, those who are positive and can do so, however, receive all possible encouragement and assistance to achieve their goals. Thus success happened *among the peoples* working at PDHNH. When a few nurses decided to go ahead and take this challenge, they received all the support and the success was multiplied.

Amanda, an engineering student, reflected:

> I learned an immense amount while on the trip. Diving into a new culture is great fun, but is also an exercise in patience, trust, and confidence. Collaborating with people of vastly different cultures and disciplines was a chance to improve communication skills. This collaboration was excellent preparation for working in a globally connected world. Our agriculture research group was composed of a nurse, two scientists, and two engineers, all from different regions of India and the USA. It was neat to see how each team member's unique skills, personality, training, and outlook benefitted the project.

Within Groups

A series of workshops and lectures was developed and delivered by visiting faculty from UC and MST. Fifty staff and student nurses at PDHNH (Manjrekar, 2016) thus benefitted from the program and from learning with each other. First, as mentioned previously, the NIGH team coordinated efforts to bring more than 150 Indian students, faculty, and clinical nurses to two sessions—also hosting and offering collaborative networking lunch. This project expanded into continued staff development—further implemented for 700 nurses within PDHNH's staff and then expanded to include five other colleges of nursing. In this way, NIGH's team was able—*within all these groups*—to continue their efforts to enhance the sustainable nursing workforce in India (D. B. Oerther, Oerther, & Manjrekar, 2013).

At Grassroots Levels

Improved patient outcomes were achieved in the form of reduced exposure to life-threatening nitrate in ground water supplies used for drinking water in rural India. This success is an example of the kinds of opportunities upon which NIGH's team is focusing.

NIGH is founded on Florence Nightingale's philosophy and practices, where she took nursing, beyond the sick bedside, to focus on improving environments *at grassroots levels*. Although these case studies are very small initiatives in comparison with her mammoth contribution to global nursing, these demonstrate her philosophy of starting small and building big over time. We build a foundation by starting at the base of the pyramid, as emphasized herein. Hence, nurses—who witnessed a very minuscule detail related to the presence of unwanted chemicals in basic drinking water and came to understand how this small detail affected such a large population—benefitted immensely from such an opportunity to work at this grassroots base.

At Global Levels

In late 2013 and throughout 2014—the overall successes of these interrelated projects received further recognition. An expanded analysis of the results collected over the winter break of 2012/2013 was performed. With these further outcomes, additional presentations were featured and publications were well received at the Humanitarian Technology Conference—sponsored by Harvard University and MIT—in the spring of 2014 (S. E. Oerther, Manjrekar, & Oerther, 2014).

The examples of partnership as demonstrated in these case studies specifically address Goal 4—reduce child mortality—and Goal 5—improve maternal health—that were present in the UN MDGs that directed development from 2000 through 2015. But perhaps even more significantly, the partnerships documented in these case studies point forward toward Goal 17 of the UN SDGs—strengthen the means of implementation and revitalize the global partnership for sustainable development. Partnerships—among government, nongovernment, and the private sector and among disciplines—among the rural-to-urban divide—are a key aspect of the approach to development from 2015 through 2030. And these case studies document some of the benefits and some of the challenges of creating and sustaining complex partnerships aimed at achieving the interrelated nature of the UN SDGs. Further, as noted earlier, these case studies demonstrate how interrelated outcomes improve when seen through the lens of integral theories. When considering what it will take to accomplish the Global Partnership Outcomes of SDG 17, in projects both large and small, these case studies clearly point to the value of integral lenses and integral approaches toward achieving this key aim to progress in human development.

In the next section, we explore how the earlier two case studies demonstrate effective nurse coaching approaches and interactions that will be foundational to our continued mission with the SDGs through 2030 and beyond.

NIGH AND NURSE COACHING

NIGH's mission and vision engages our NIGH team and colleagues with integrative, integral, and holistic approaches to explore the root cause(s) of a problem. In the earlier case studies, we have also witnessed a nurse coaching approach that was built upon the individual and community strengths rather than attempting to "fix" weaknesses (Dossey, Luck, & Schaub, 2015; Hess et al., 2013; International Nurse Coach Association, n.d.). These nurses and their interprofessional team were able to engage in a cocreative process with clients, families, communities, and colleagues using both individual and group sessions, as well as interprofessional collaboration. They created a safe space for integral dialogues and were sensitive to individual issues of trust and vulnerability. This cocreating partnership process allowed for reflecting upon and addressing challenges—where a heightened degree of awareness, choice, imagination, creativity, and healthy lifestyle behaviors emerged.

Professional nurse coaching is a skilled, purposeful, results-oriented, and structured relationship-centered interaction with clients provided by registered nurses for the purpose of promoting achievement of client goals (Hess et al., 2013). It also includes partnerships and collaboration with the interprofessional team members and community. A nurse coach establishes a cocreative partnership with a client— where the client is the expert and identifies her or his own priorities and areas needing change. Goals thus originate from clarifying and identifying a client's own "coaching" agenda. The change process is grounded in an awareness that effective change evolves from within—before it can be manifested and maintained externally (Integrative Nurse Coach Certificate Program, n.d.).

This coaching approach and process enhances potentials for health and well-being that may lead to decreased illness and injuries, and significantly decreases chronic disease epidemics. With the focus on the whole person, we use principles and modalities that integrate all the bio-psycho-social-spiritual-cultural-environmental dimensions toward human flourishing (Dossey, 2016b). See Chapter 28 for more information on how to use nurse coaching strategies to build sustainable and mutually beneficial partnerships.

CONCLUSION

NIGH's mission and vision engage Nightingale's legacy and the values and wisdom of millions of nurses, midwives, and concerned citizen stakeholders to act as catalysts for the transformation of individuals, communities, and society—toward the achievement of a healthy world. Our inclusive, collaborative, and synergistic initiatives continue to give nurses a voice and to create new opportunities for them to discover possibilities for their unique contributions toward health and well-being for all—local to global.

We are now focused on the application of nursing's endeavors to advocate for and achieve the SDGs—thus continuing to contribute to the global health agenda. The Theory of Integral Nursing continues to illuminate our work—to increase our integral awareness, our healing and wholeness, and to strengthen our personal and professional capacities to be more fully open to the mysteries of life's journey—the wondrous stages of self-discovery, for ourselves and others. The nurse coaching approach assists us to achieve a deeper level of partnerships with many—to engage all to come from our deepest wisdom.

Our times demand new paradigms and a new language—where we integrate the best of what we know in the science and art of nursing—including holistic, integrative, integral, and human caring theories and modalities. Our NIGH integral approach and worldview places us in a better position to share the depth of nurses' knowledge, expertise, critical-thinking capacities, and skills for assisting others to create health through stories of healing—local to global. Only by paying close attention to the sacred heart of nursing—the words "sacred" and "heart" reflecting common meanings—can we generate the vision, courage, and hope required to unite nursing in achieving all that we envision for a truly healthy world.

REFLECTION AND DISCUSSION

- How can I use nursing theory to inform my practice? In what ways do I already engage an integral approach to my clinical and scholarly work?

- How do I describe "healing" in my own words? How do the goals of nursing, at both local and global levels, further the healing of individuals and the human collective?

- In what ways can I improve the delivery of nursing care in relation to the SDGs in partnership with individuals, among peoples, and at grassroots and global levels?

- Case Study 1 chronicles the collaborative initiative between the University of Cincinnati, United States, and NM Sadguru in India. What other opportunities can I identify for practice and academe to join forces in the procurement of health and well-being outcomes?

- Why is it important to cocreate a partnership with a client, where the client is the expert and self-identifies his or her own areas that require change or improvement? In what ways do I already embrace a professional nurse coaching lens?

REFERENCES

Azaiza, F., & Cohen, M. (2006). Health beliefs and rates of breast cancer screening among Arab women. *Journal of Women's Health, 15*(5), 520–530.

Beck, D.-M. (2005). 21st century citizenship for health: 'May a better way be opened.' In B. M. Dossey, L. Selanders, D.-M. Beck, & A. Attewell (Eds.), *Florence Nightingale today: Healing, leadership, global action* (pp. 177–193). Silver Spring, MD: Nursesbooks.org.

Beck, D.-M. (2010). Remembering Florence Nightingale's panorama: 21st century nursing: At a critical crossroads. *Journal of Holistic Nursing Practice, 28*(4), 291–301.

Beck, D.-M. (2016). Artistic and scientific: Broadening the scope of our 21st-century health advocacy. In W. Rosa (Ed.), *Nurses as leaders: Evolutionary visions of leadership* (pp. 247–263). New York, NY: Springer Publishing.

Beck, D.-M. (2017). A brief history of the United Nations and nursing: A healthy world is our common future. In W. Rosa (Ed.), *Global health: Global nursing: Our contributions to the sustainable development goals* (pp. 55–81). New York, NY: Springer Publishing.

Beck, D.-M., Dossey B. M., & Rushton C. H. (2013). Building the Nightingale Initiative for Global Health—NIGH: Can we engage and empower the public voices of nurses worldwide? *Nursing Science Quarterly, 26*, 366–371. doi:10.1177/0894318413500403

Beck, D.-M., Dossey, B. M., & Rushton, C. H. (2014). Global activism, advocacy, and transformation: Florence Nightingale's legacy for the twenty-first-century. In M. J. Kreitzer & M. Koithan (Eds.), *Integrative nursing* (pp. 526–537). New York, NY: Oxford University Press.

Carper, B. A. (1978). Fundamental patterns of knowing in nursing. *Advances in Nursing Science, 1*(1), 13–23.

Crossley, N. (2001). The phenomenological habitus and its construction. *Theory and Society, 30*(1), 81–120.

Dossey, B. M. (2008a). Theory of integral nursing. *Advances in Nursing Science, 31*(1), E52–E73.

Dossey, B. M. (2008b). Integral and holistic nursing: Local to global. In B. M. Dossey & L. Keegan (Eds.), *Holistic nursing: A handbook for practice* (5th ed., pp. 3–46). Sudbury, MA: Jones & Bartlett.

Dossey, B. M. (2010a). *Florence Nightingale: Mystic, visionary, healer* (Commemorative ed.). Philadelphia, PA: F. A. Davis.

Dossey, B. M. (2010b). Florence Nightingale: A 19th-century mystic. *Journal of Holistic Nursing, 28*(1), 10–35.

Dossey, B. M. (2015). Theory of integral nursing. In M. C. Smith & M. E. Parker (Eds.), *Nursing theories and nursing practice* (4th ed., pp. 207–234). Philadelphia, PA: F. A. Davis.

Dossey, B. M. (2016a). Nursing: Integral, integrative, and holistic: Local to global. In B. M. Dossey & L. Keegan (Eds.), *Holistic nursing: A handbook for practice* (7th ed., pp. 3–52). Burlington, MA: Jones & Bartlett.

Dossey, B. M. (2016b). Integral and whole: Embracing the journey of healing, local to global. In W. Rosa (Ed.), *Nurses as leaders: Evolutionary visions of leadership* (pp. 61–75). New York, NY: Springer Publishing.

Dossey, B. M., Beck, D.-M., & Rushton, C. H. (2011). Integral nursing and the Nightingale Initiative for Global Health: Florence Nightingale's legacy for the 21st century. *Journal of Integral Theory and Practice, 6*(4), 71–92.

Dossey, B. M., Luck, S., & Schaub, B. G. (2015). *Nurse coaching; Integrative approaches for health and well-being.* North Miami, FL: International Nurse Coach Association.

Dossey, B. M., Selanders, L., Beck, D.-M., & Attewell, A. (2005). *Florence Nightingale today: Healing, leadership, global action.* Silver Spring, MD: Nursesbooks.org.

Hess, D. R., Dossey, B. M., Southard, M. E., Luck, S., Schaub, B. G., & Bark, L. (2013). *The art and science of nurse coaching: A provider's guide to scope and competencies.* Silver Spring, MD: Nursesbooks.org.

Integrative Nurse Coach Certificate Program. (n.d.). Retrieved from http://www.integrativenursecoach.com

International Nurse Coach Association. (n.d.). Retrieved from http://www.inursecoach.com

Luna, L. (1994). Care and cultural context of Lebanese Muslim immigrants: Using Leininger's theory. *Journal of Transcultural Nursing, 5*(2), 12–21.

Manjrekar, P. (2016). Resourceful and unified: Partnering across cultures and worldviews. In W. Rosa (Ed.), *Nurses as leaders: Evolutionary visions of leadership* (pp. 345–358). New York, NY: Springer Publishing.

McDonald, L. (2001–2011). *The collected works of Florence Nightingale* (Vols. 1–16). Waterloo, ON, Canada: Wilfred Laurier University Press. Retrieved from http://www.uoguelph.ca/~cwfn

Mubeen, S., Mansoor, S., Hussain, A., & Qadir, S. (2012). Perceptions and practices of fasting in Ramadan during pregnancy in Pakistan. *Iranian Journal of Nursing and Midwifery Research, 17*(7), 467–471.

Nightingale, F. (1860). *Notes on nursing: What it is and what it is not.* London, UK: Harrison.

Nightingale, F. (1893). Sick-nursing and health-nursing. In B. M. Dossey, L. C. Selanders, D.-M. Beck, & A. Attewell (Eds.), *Florence Nightingale today: Healing, leadership, global action* (pp. 288–303). Silver Spring, MD: Nursesbooks.org.

Nightingale Declaration for a Healthy World. (2007). Retrieved from http://www.nighvision .net/nightingale-declaration.html

Nightingale Initiative for Global Health. (2015). *2020 vision: Working to achieve a healthy world* (PowerPoint slides 11 to 15). Retrieved from http://www.nighvision.net/into-the-former -soviet-union.html

Nightingale Initiative for Global Health. (2016a). NIGH's history, part 2: Inspire, inform, initiate and involve/1996 to 2011. Retrieved from http://www.nighvision.net/nighs-history -mdash-part-2.html

Nightingale Initiative for Global Health. (2016b). *NIGH's "2020 vision" and the UN sustainable development goals*. Retrieved from http://www.nighvision.net/2020-vision--the-un-sdgs .html

Oerther, D. B., Oerther, S., & Manjrekar, P. (2013, November 16–20). *Teaching the MDGs: The role of the nurse in multidisciplinary project based instruction*. Paper presented at STTI 42nd Biennial Convention, Indianapolis, IN.

Oerther, S. E., Manjrekar, P., & Oerther, D. B. (2014). Utilizing mobile health technology at the bottom of the pyramid. *Procedia Engineering, 78*, 143–148.

Rhynas, J. (2005). Bourdieu's theory of practice and its potential in nursing research. *Journal of Advanced Nursing, 50*(2), 179–186.

Sarna, L., Wolf, L., & Bialous, S. A. (2012). Enhancing nursing and midwifery capacity to contribute to the prevention, treatment and management of noncommunicable diseases. *Human Resources for Health Observer*, (12). Retrieved from http://www.who.int/hrh/resources/ observer12.pdf

Sharma, M, (2004). Conscious leadership at the crossroads of change. *Shift: At the Frontiers of Consciousness, 12*, 17–21.

Sharma, M. (2007). World wisdom in action: Personal to planetary transformation. *Kosmos, Fall/ Winter 2007*, 31–35.

Tsianaksa, V., & Liamputtong, P. (2002). What women from an Islamic background in Australia say about care in pregnancy and prenatal testing. *Midwifery, 18*(1), 25–34.

United Nations. (2016). Sustainable development goals: 17 goals to transform our world. Retrieved from http://www.un.org/sustainabledevelopment/sustainable-development- goals

Wilber, K. (2000). *Integral psychology: Consciousness, spirit, psychology, therapy*. Boston, MA: Shambhala.

World Health Organization. (2016). *Global strategic directions for strengthening nursing & midwifery*. Geneva, Switzerland: Author. Retrieved from http://www.who.int/hrh/ nursing_midwifery/global-strategy-midwifery-2016-2020/en

Wright, D., & Brajtman, S. (2011). Relational and embodied knowing: Nursing ethics within the interprofessional team. *Nursing Ethics, 18*, 20–30.

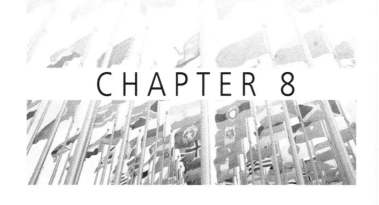

CHAPTER 8

Nursing Education Imperatives and the United Nations 2030 Agenda

Tamara H. McKinnon and Joyce J. Fitzpatrick

Be a global citizen. Act with passion and compassion. Help us make this world safer and more sustainable today and for the generations that will follow us. That is our moral responsibility. (Ki-Moon, 2015)

Nurses are the largest group of health professionals in every country, providing care to individuals, families, and communities everywhere. The increased complexity of our world, including technological advances, global financial challenges, climate changes, natural and human-initiated disasters, and inequities in health within and across nations demand that nurse educators and students are prepared to address the interconnectedness between local and global health challenges. Nurses must be prepared to contribute to the development and implementation of solutions to world challenges, most especially those included in the United Nations (UN) 2030 Agenda for Sustainable Development.

We propose a Knowing, Valuing, and Acting (KVA) framework as the basis for change in nursing curricula to best prepare students as global citizens, equipped to address the UN 2030 Agenda for Sustainable Development and the 17 Sustainable Development Goals (SDGs; see Chapter 4 for more information on global nurse citizenship). Using this KVA framework, we present resources and crucial questions for nurse leaders, educators, and students, and recommendations for curricular innovations.

Integration of content related to SDGs is an ethical imperative and presents a call to action within nursing education. Nurses are global citizens and, as such, have a responsibility for the promotion of health around the corner and across the globe. Schools of nursing, therefore, are faced with the opportunity to integrate SDGs throughout the general and specialist nursing curricula and also specifically within global and community health coursework. Such integration is necessary to prepare professional nurses to take local, national, and global action toward accomplishment of SDGs.

KNOWING, VALUING, AND ACTING

Knowing (Understanding)

> *"The world is really just a village, and the nursing workplace has become the globe"* (Hern, Vaughn, Mason, & Weitkamp, 2005, p. 34).

The UN Sustainable Development Agenda is broad: "This Agenda is a plan of action for people, planet and prosperity" (UN, 2015, p. 1) and has far-reaching implications: "We pledge to foster intercultural understanding, tolerance, mutual respect and an ethic of global citizenship and shared responsibility" (UN, 2015, p. 10). While SDG 3: Ensure healthy lives and promote well-being for all at all ages (UN, 2015, p.16) is the goal most directly related to health and well-being of the world's citizens and the goal that mobilizes and empowers professional nurses to engagement and action, it is important to integrate knowledge of all of the SDGs into nursing curricula.

Academia is cited as a critical partner in operationalizing implementation of the SDGs (UN, 2015, p.11). Nurses not only comprise the majority of health care providers internationally (UN, 2015), they also are the professionals at the direct point of care and service provision throughout the world, in every community and health care organization. Professional nurses are expected to be aware of and respond to the health issues of their communities and the people they serve, in order to achieve the goal of health for all. Further, they are expected to become global citizens. "Becoming global citizens however does not imply that we privilege the global over the local, but that we recognize the interconnectedness between the local and the global" (Mill, Astle, Ogilvie, & Gastaldo, 2010, p. E9).

The following key components of SDG 3 are currently integrated within nursing curricula, yet are often not presented within the global context: maternal mortality; neonatal mortality; epidemics (AIDS, tuberculosis, and malaria); noncommunicable disease mortality; substance abuse; traffic accidents; sexual and reproductive health services; universal health coverage; environmental exposures; tobacco; vaccine and medicine development; and health financing (UN, 2015). Expanding the perspective to include a global lens is the first step in enhancing nurses' knowledge of global health issues and linking nursing work to the SDGs. While this knowledge integration can begin with SDG 3, which is directly related to health and well-being, an expansive view of health as related to economic, sociocultural, political, and environmental components would lead educators to embed knowledge of the additional SDGs into nursing education curricula. Examining the relevance of all SDGs to nursing curricula at all levels is the first step toward knowing and understanding.

Activity #1: Knowing (Understanding)

The following crucial questions provide an opportunity for nurse leaders, educators, and students to assess their understanding of the SDGs and the implications for nursing education. The activity may be performed individually or in a group. Responses lead to a discussion of valuing SDG curricular integration. Using the resources listed at the end of this chapter will assist in developing a more comprehensive response.

Review the SDGs found in the Sustainable Development Agenda in the Appendix of this book and respond to the following questions:

Nurse Leaders

What is nursing's history with SDG development?

Who are the critical stakeholders in the integration of SDGs into nursing curricula?

What have nurse leaders said about integration of SDGs into nursing curricula?

What are the consequences if nursing education does not integrate SDGs into the curriculum?

What resources will you use to increase your knowledge and understanding of this topic?

Nurse Educators

What content areas from SDG 3 are relevant for nursing education?

Does nursing education play a critical role in the preparation of nurses who are equipped to work toward SDG achievement?

What are the educational implications and imperatives?

What happens if nursing education does not integrate SDGs into the curriculum?

Students

Consider a specialty area of nursing in which you may be interested. Do you see that reflected in the SDGs?

On a broader level, what is the relevance of the SDGs to your future career as a nurse?

How are local and global practices reflected in the SDGs?

Valuing (Attitude)

"If the indicators chosen are not sensitive to the work of the largest sector of the health workforce many of the health outcomes (positive or negative) for the country risk invisibility for the 15 years span, 2016–2030" (International Council of Nurses [ICN], 2015, p. 2).

The ultimate goal for all nurse faculty is to prepare nurses as global nurses and global citizens (Dawson, Gakumo, Phillips, & Wilson, 2016). Responses to the crucial questions related to Knowing and Understanding provide perspective for the conversation about Valuing SDG integration into curricula. The value of SDG integration emanates from nursing's core values. These values are reflected in the American Association of Colleges of Nursing (AACN) *Essentials of Baccalaureate Education for Professional Nursing Practice* (AACN, 2008) and in the American Nurses Association (ANA) *Code of Ethics for Nurses With*

Interpretive Statements (ANA, 2015). Both documents support the ethical imperative for nursing education's integration of SDGs into curricula and reflect common themes that include global citizenship, globalization of curricula, and social responsibility.

The AACN *Essentials of Baccalaureate Education for Professional Nursing Practice* includes the following statements that support SDG integration into nursing education curricula:

- "The environments in which professional nurses practice have become more diverse and more global in nature" (AACN, 2008, p. 5).

- "Increasing globalization of healthcare and the diversity of this nation's population mandates an attention to diversity in order to provide safe, high quality care. The professional nurse practices in a multicultural environment and must possess the skills to provide culturally appropriate care" (AACN, 2008, p. 6).

- "Liberal education is critical to the generation of responsible citizens in a global society. In addition, liberal education is needed for the development of intellectual and innovative capacities for current and emergent generalist nursing practice" (AACN, 2008, p. 11).

- "A liberal education for nurses forms the basis for intellectual and practical abilities for nursing practice as well as for engagement with the larger community, both locally and globally" (AACN, 2008, p. 11).

The ANA *Code of Ethics for Nurses With Interpretive Statements* (ANA, 2015) states that "the nurse collaborates with other health professionals and the public to protect human rights, promote health diplomacy, and reduce health disparities" (Provision 8, p. 31) and that "the profession of nursing, collectively through its professional organizations, must articulate nursing values, maintain the integrity of the profession, and integrate principles of social justice into nursing and health policy" (Provision 9, p. 35).

Each country is responsible for knowing about SDG accomplishment within its own nation and can also be expected to respond to the needs of partners abroad (United Nations, 2015). This responsibility highlights the importance of integration of SDG concepts across nursing curricula to prepare nurses to live and work as global citizens. According to Wilson and colleagues (2012), increasing global mobility and technological advances lead to enhanced global interdependence and potential global collaborations.

> These opportunities also present new challenges for health care. It is no longer possible for students in any health discipline to remain focused on local or national health care problems: They must be prepared to face health issues in any setting. (Wilson et al., 2012, p. 213)

Activity #2: Valuing (Attitude)

The following crucial questions provide an opportunity for nurse leaders, educators, and students to explore the value that they place on the SDGs and their implications for nursing education. The activity may be performed individually or in a group. Responses lead to a discussion of actions needed to operationalize

SDG curricular integration. Using the resources listed at the end of this chapter will assist in developing a more comprehensive response.

Review the SDGs found in the Sustainable Development Agenda in the Appendix of this book and respond to the following questions:

Nurse Leaders

Place a copy of the SDGs next to the documents guiding professional nursing practice.

Do the SDGs reflect the core values of the profession of nursing?

What is your opinion about inclusion of SDG-related content in nursing education curricula?

Do you see this as a value upheld by other nurse leaders? Why? Why not?

Nurse Educators

Place a copy of the SDGs next to the mission and vision statement of your school of nursing.

Do the SDGs reflect the mission, vision, and values of your school?

Are you committed to developing experiential learning for students that strengthens their commitment as global citizens?

Students

Think about the trajectory of your career as a nurse.

Do you see yourself having an impact on the achievement of SDGs (locally and/or globally)?

What educational preparation will be required to prepare you to work in a global environment?

How can you view your clinical experiences in alignment with better understanding of the SDGs?

Action

"Between saying and doing, many a pair of shoes is worn out" (Italian proverb).

Curricular innovations required by SDG integration are ambitious and challenging, as well as necessary and possible. Effecting curricular change requires reframing educators' understandings of what they often consider an already "packed" curriculum. Meaningful, sustainable curricular change will vary among schools of nursing but will be driven by both a bottom-up and a top-down approach to change. Academic administrators and professional organizations with an educational mission must commit to the goals of global citizenship. Accrediting bodies could add to the integration goal by requiring the attention to a global perspective in nursing education and direct integration of the SDG content. Educators must make both incremental and substantive overall changes in curricula to ensure sustainable success. Recommended initial steps include the following: Develop an action plan that includes a realistic assessment of available resources; elicit support from all stakeholders; use readily available, open-access resources (refer to the resource section in this and other chapters); form alliances; and seek help from interprofessional colleagues.

As schools of nursing consider integration of SDGs into the curriculum, there is a risk of "pigeonholing" or creating yet another silo in nursing and nursing education by assuming that the SDGs have relevance only for the curricular area of global health. Careful consideration of the SDGs reveals two important facts for nursing:

- Global is local and local is global. The UN 2030 Agenda and call to action is as relevant for nursing practice "around the corner" as "across the globe." SDGs have implications for nurses regardless of geographic boundaries.
- SDG-related concepts can be found throughout the curriculum and must not be relegated solely to coursework pertaining to global health. Examples of relevant concepts and content include, but are not limited to, care of vulnerable persons; care of those from other cultural groups; health inequities; health policy; leadership; evidence-based practice; community health; social determinants of health; interprofessional communication; cultural competency; and global citizenship.

While SDG curricular content is linked to that of global health, the two are not synonymous. SDGs are closely related to social determinants of health, which are increasingly viewed as critical components of nursing curricula. Clark and colleagues conducted a review of the literature related to global health competencies in nursing education and identified 12 categories including "global burden of disease; travel and migration; determinants of health; environmental factors; cultural competency; communication; health systems/delivery; professionalism/ethics; social justice/human rights; partnership/collaboration; management skills; and key players" (Clark, Raffray, Hendricks, & Gagnon, 2016, p. 177). Yet as recently as 2012, a survey of schools of nursing revealed that less than half integrated global health topics throughout the undergraduate curriculum (Wilson et al., 2012, p. 214). This study also indicates that most often, schools of nursing include global health content in the community health curriculum (Wilson et al., 2012).

Integration of these content areas into a nursing education curriculum would provide a platform upon which to begin SDG integration. Yet the fact that not all schools of nursing include this content, along with the fact that SDGs have implications across the curriculum (not solely community health), indicate the need for large-scale curricular innovations. Given the breadth of its scope, SDG content must be integrated across the curriculum. Research on SDG-specific nursing competencies is needed along with clarification of nurses' roles within the interprofessional health care team as it relates to SDG goal attainment.

Activity #3: Action

Knowledge and value precede action. Consider the following questions related to curricular changes necessary to integrate SDGs.

What must be done?

How will it be done?

Who will do it?

How will it be sustained?

Using the resources listed at the end of this chapter will assist in developing a more comprehensive response.

Nurse Leaders

> Whom do you see as the supporters and detractors of curricular innovation related to SDGs?
>
> How will you capitalize on the support and address the critics?
>
> What resources are available to support nursing educators to move forward?
>
> What additional resources are needed?
>
> How can the accrediting and regulatory bodies for nursing education become partners in the quest for integration of SDGs into nursing curricula?

Nurse Educators

> Do you commit to the curricular innovations required to prepare nurses to work toward SDG achievement?
>
> Whom do you see as the supporters and detractors of curricular innovation related to SDGs?
>
> How will you capitalize on the support and address the critics?
>
> How will these be integrated into school of nursing curricula?
>
> Who are the critical stakeholders?
>
> What steps will be taken to move forward?

Students

> You have the power to drive curricular changes that will prepare you to become active participants in the realization of SDGs both locally and globally. How will you act on the call to action for global citizenship?

To enhance the understanding of the call to action for both global citizenship and integration of the SDGs into nursing curricula, we have included commentaries by two key nurse leaders who have championed these curricular changes.

Lynda Wilson, PhD, RN, professor emerita, University of Alabama at Birmingham School of Nursing, comments:

> Twenty-first century nursing educators have a responsibility to prepare students as global citizens who can contribute to the achievement of the

SDGs. Because achieving these goals will require collaboration across disciplines, geographic borders, and socioeconomic divides, it is imperative that students have opportunities for interprofessional and interdisciplinary collaboration, and for exposure to diverse perspectives and challenges. The first strategy for integrating SDGs into nursing curricula is to ensure that students are aware of global developmental challenges and the SDGs that have been proposed to meet those challenges. This content could be introduced during an introductory cross-disciplinary required course for all university students during the freshman year (e.g., Global Citizenship 101). During this course, students could read about the SDGs, develop projects aimed at proposing strategies to address these goals, and perhaps collaborate online with students in other countries and settings to learn about diverse approaches to achieving the goals.

Within the nursing curricula, faculty in each course could be encouraged to integrate one or more SDGs into course assignments. For example, students in a medical surgical nursing course could be asked to identify strategies to achieve target 3.4 (By 2030, reduce by one-third premature mortality from noncommunicable diseases through prevention and treatment and promote mental health and well-being) in a specific country. Students in a maternal-child nursing course might be asked to identify strategies to address target 3.2 (By 2030, end preventable deaths of newborns and children under 5 years of age, with all countries aiming to reduce neonatal mortality to at least as low as 12 per 1,000 live births and under-5 mortality to at least as low as 25 per 1,000 live births; see Appendix for all SDG 3 targets).

To increase awareness about SDGs, schools might consider setting up a display highlighting the SDGs in a prominent location, and inviting students, faculty, staff, and visitors to share their ideas about addressing SDGs on cards that could be posted. They might also organize cross-campus case competitions in which interdisciplinary groups of students are asked to propose innovative solutions to meet one of the SDG targets.

Achieving the SDGs will require innovative and creative strategies and collaboration between educators, policy-makers, and practitioners. Nursing faculty have exciting opportunities to make a difference and to prepare graduates who are global citizens who can make a difference! (L. Wilson, personal communication, August 19, 2016)

Carol Huston, MSN, DPA, FAAN, professor emerita, School of Nursing, California State University, Chico, past president (2007–2009), Sigma Theta Tau International Honor Society of Nursing, comments:

No one country alone has all the answers to the global health care dilemmas we face today, including: hunger; a lack of access to basic sanitation and clean drinking water; gender inequities; preventable communicable and noncommunicable disease; violence and exploitation; and inadequate workforce capacity. In addition, efforts to address social and economic inequality within and among countries and the sustainable use and conservation of precious, finite resources have historically lacked focus and coordination. The 2030 Agenda for Sustainable Development with its 17 SDGs and their associated 169 targets, form a blueprint, however, for addressing these global health care dilemmas.

Professional nurses globally will be challenged to take on key leadership roles in achieving these SDGs. Nursing schools then must prepare graduates who have a global mindset; who understand that global health care issues ultimately impact local, regional, and national health care planning; and that the health threats faced by any one country are ultimately faced by all countries. Ensuring global competence in graduates, however, will require a paradigm shift in nursing education. Global sustainable development, examined from social, economic, and environmental contexts, must become a foundational core of professional nursing curriculums. Only then will professional nurses fully understand the complexity of the goals the UN has laid out for the world and be able to successfully work toward their achievement. (C. Huston, personal communication, August 21, 2016)

RESOURCES FOR CURRICULAR INNOVATION AND INTEGRATION

In addition to the SDGs, there are several resources that can assist nurse educators in initiating curricular innovation and integration of the SDGs throughout the curriculum. While some of these resources are specific to global health (e.g., the Consortium of Universities for Global Health [CUGH]), others more generally address the values inherent in global health (e.g., health as a human right).

The Consortium of Universities for Global Health (www.cugh.org)

CUGH builds interdisciplinary collaborations and facilitates the sharing of knowledge to address global health challenges. It assists members in sharing their expertise across education, research, and service. CUGH is dedicated to creating equity and reducing health disparities everywhere. CUGH promotes mutually beneficial, long-term partnerships between universities in resource-rich and resource-poor countries, developing human capital and strengthening institutions' capabilities to address these challenges. CUGH is committed to translating knowledge into action.

An extensive database is available on the CUGH website. To access links for topic-specific curricular content, follow the links on the home page from Resources to Training Modules.

Global Health Training Module Topic Areas

Non-Communicable Diseases, Injuries, & Related

Infectious, Parasitic and Communicable Diseases

Priority and Vulnerable Populations

Global Child Health (GCHEMP)

Health Systems, Services, Resources, & Programs

Working & Visiting in Low Resource Countries

Global Health: Priorities, Problems, Programs, & Policies

General

Methods, Tools, Skills, & Related

Public Health

Unite for Sight (www.uniteforsight.org), Global Health University: Excellence in Global Health Education

Unite for Sight is a nonprofit organization committed to excellence in global health. Unite for Sight's Global Health University is designed to develop and nurture current and future global health leaders. Global Health University helps to effect widespread innovative change in global health through comprehensive webinars and training workshops, Global Health Certificate Programs, social enterprise consulting, and fellowship and internship opportunities in the United States and abroad. Global Health University offers free webinars with leading experts in global health and social entrepreneurship. More than 20 Online Certificate Programs are also offered. These include a Certificate in Global Health, Certificate in Global Health Research, and Certificate in Responsible NGO Management, among others. More than 70 online courses can also be viewed separately.

Association of American Colleges and Universities (AACU; www.aacu.org), Shared Futures: Global Learning and Social Responsibility

Shared Futures: Global Learning and Social Responsibility is a multiproject, national initiative of AACU. The initiative was built on the assumption that we live in an interdependent but unequal world and that higher education can prepare students to not only thrive in such a world but also creatively and responsibly remedy its inequities and problems. A quality liberal education in the 21st century provides students with opportunities to work collaboratively, to examine the world's human and natural systems from multiple perspectives, and to integrate learning across the curriculum by following the threads in an increasingly complex reality. Such an education, often referred to as "global learning," intentionally wrestles with questions of diversity, identity, citizenship, democracy, power, privilege, sustainability, and ethical action.

By building a network of educators dedicated to this integrative work, Shared Futures facilitates curricular change and faculty development on campuses nationwide. It is the goal of the Shared Futures initiative that these networks of educators lead to collaboration on course design and pedagogy, shared strategies for curricular renewal and globalization of general education, and a fluid, decentralized exchange of resources that opens new opportunities for partnership and learning.

AACU's latest Shared Futures project, General Education for a Global Century, is funded with a generous grant from the Henry Luce Foundation.

Additional Resources

The International Council of Nurses (ICN; www.icn.ch)

ICN is a federation of more than 130 national nurses associations representing the millions of nurses worldwide. Founded in 1899, ICN is the world's first and widest reaching international organization for health professionals. Operated by nurses, and leading nursing internationally, ICN works to ensure quality nursing care for all and sound health policies globally. See Chapter 10 for more information about ICN and their global initiatives.

National League for Nursing (NLN) Center for Diversity and Global Initiatives (www.nln.org)

To increase diversity in nursing, promote global leadership development, and cocreate initiatives, the Center seeks collaborative opportunities with organizations here and abroad. NLN's presence in the global arena includes leadership in the ICN Education Network. The Center will secure funding to advance global health and nursing education, generate publications and research, and support efforts to increase nurse educator and student diversity and inclusivity.

Honor Society of Nursing, Sigma Theta Tau International (STTI; www.nursingsociety.org)

The mission of the Honor Society of Nursing, STTI is advancing world health and celebrating nursing excellence in scholarship, leadership, and service. STTI's vision is to be the global organization of choice for nursing. See Chapter 2 for more information on STTI and the Global Advisory Panel on the Future of Nursing.

The Global Fund (www.theglobalfund.org/en)
United States Agency for International Development (www.usaid.gov)
World Health Organization (www.who.org)
UNICEF (www.unicef.org)

CONCLUSION

This chapter explored the integration of SDGs into schools of nursing curricula through the KVA framework. Critical questions related to these areas allowed the reader to consider his/her role as it relates to each of these areas. Evidence supporting SDG integration as an ethical imperative presents a call to action for nurse leaders, educators, and students. Nurse educators will face obstacles in moving this agenda forward; the changes will not be simple; and they will call upon the innovative spirit of professional nurses from every arena. Greater consequences will be faced if nurses choose to do nothing. We will pass up the opportunity to ensure that every nurse is educated in a way that prepares him or her to work toward achievement of the SDGs. Nursing is ready for this challenge, realizing the changes required will impact nursing and, by extension, will impact the world.

REFLECTION AND DISCUSSION

- How do I see the Sustainable Development Agenda as integral to nursing education and preparation?

- What are my first steps in advocating for nursing education that is inclusive of the SDGs and their related targets?

- In what ways do my responsibilities as a global citizen inform how I know, value, and act?

- How do I believe nursing practice would change at both local and global levels as a result of SDG-informed curricula?

- What are my current obstacles to raising awareness and gaining support for promoting the SDGs as a requisite for nursing education?

REFERENCES

American Association of Colleges of Nursing. (2008). The essentials of baccalaureate education for professional nursing practice. Retrieved from http://www.aacn.nche.edu/education-resources/BaccEssentials08.pdf

American Nurses Association. (2015). Code of ethics for nurses with interpretive statements. Retrieved from http://nursingworld.org/MainMenuCategories/EthicsStandards/Code ofEthicsforNurses/Code-of-Ethics-For-Nurses.html

Clark, M., Raffray, M., Hendricks, K., & Gagnon, A. J. (2016). Global and public health core competencies for nursing education: A systematic review of essential competencies. *Nurse Education Today, 40*, 173–180. doi:10.1016/j.nedt.2016.02.026

Dawson, M., Gakumo, C. A., Phillips, J., & Wilson, L. (2016). Process for mapping global health competencies in undergraduate and graduate nursing curricula. *Nurse Educator, 41*(1), 37–40. doi:10.1097/NNE.0000000000000199

Hern, M. J., Vaughn, G., Mason, D., & Weitkamp, T. (2005). Creating an international nursing practice and education workplace. *Journal of Pediatric Nursing, 20*(1), 34–44. doi:10.1016/j.pedn.2004.12.006

International Council of Nurses. (2015, September 15). The contribution of nursing to the development of a country level plan for meeting the WHO global strategy on human resources for health: Workforce 2030 requirements. Retrieved from http://www.who.int/workforcealliance/knowledge/resources/ICN_PolicyBrief5CountrylevelplansHRH.pdf

Ki-moon, B. (2015). UN Secretary-General's remarks at "Our World, Our Dignity, Our Planet: The Post-2015 Agenda and the Role of Youth" event. Retrieved from http://www.un.org/youthenvoy/2015/05/un-secretary-generals-remarks-world-dignity-planet-post-2015-agenda-role-youth-event

Mill, J., Astle, B. J., Ogilvie, L., & Gastaldo, D. (2010). Linking global citizenship, undergraduate nursing education, and professional nursing: Curricular innovation in the 21st century. *Advances in Nursing Science, 33*(3), E1–E11. doi:10.1097/ANS.0b013e3181eb416f

United Nations. (2015, October 21). Transforming our world: The 2030 agenda for sustainable development. Retrieved from http://www.un.org/ga/search/view_doc.asp?symbol=A/RES/70/1&Lang=E

Wilson, L., Harper, D. C., Tami-Maury, I., Zarate, R., Salas, S., Farley, J., . . . Ventura, C. (2012). Global health competencies for nurses in the Americas. *Journal of Professional Nursing, 28*(4), 213–222. doi:10.1016/j.profnurs.2011.11.021

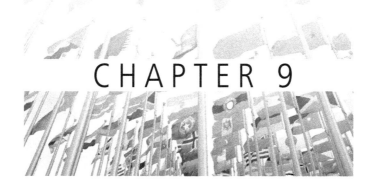

CHAPTER 9

Creating New Knowledge: Nursing- and Midwifery-Led Research to Drive the Global Goals

Allison P. Squires, Sarah Abboud, Melissa T. Ojemeni, and Laura Ridge

For the nursing profession to occupy a forceful role in promoting the aspirations of the Sustainable Development Goals we must see ourselves as partners with our international colleagues, co-creating knowledge and sharing ideas and best practices with a view to seeking innovative solutions to shared health challenges. (Premji & Hatfield, 2016, p. 2)

Nurses and midwives are well positioned to collaborate in research to address global health and achieve better health for all (Premji & Hatfield, 2016). The 21st-century vision for nursing and midwifery involves increased collaboration with international colleagues across research, practice, and policy domains to meet the Sustainable Development Goals (SDGs) by 2030. Nursing- and midwifery-led research (NMLR) has advanced global collective knowledge about health and clients' experiences of wellness and illness. Our joint disciplines are among the few fields of health to consistently incorporate the patient perspective into the design, implementation, and evaluation of research. Our research is frequently incorporated into systematic reviews, including Cochrane studies, thus ensuring our perspectives are integrated into the latest available science.

Despite our contributions to health research, there is a bias in our own work. Most of our research studies have occurred in Western countries where funding for NMLR is strong. Regional funding opportunities, such as those provided by the European Union (EU), have incentivized EU members without strong traditions of NMLR to both develop scholars capable of conducting this work and fund their research projects. This initiative has led to more Eastern European members investing in nursing (and midwifery where the profession exists) research. Language barriers also present a challenge for wider dissemination of NMLR, as the majority of scientific studies are published in English. Not all global regions have the resources to build language capacity and NMLR capacity at the same time, so the works of some low- and middle-income countries (LMICs) are included less often in the literature or rely on colonialist relationships with more industrialized/high-income nations to ensure dissemination of the work.

This chapter seeks to provide a general overview of the state of global NMLR and how our work has contributed and can contribute to meeting the SDGs. We challenge the oft-lamented notion that NMLR does not contribute to Global Goals achievement by attempting to highlight how our work as professionals already influences the programmatic and policy developments pertinent to the SDGs. We then seek to provide a basic foundation regarding how to build capacity for NMLR. We then provide examples of how NMLR has already supported the attainment of SDG targets and where we can make significant future contributions.

GLOBAL GROWTH IN NURSING- AND MIDWIFERY-LED RESEARCH

To understand how the knowledge generated by NMLR research can contribute to the SDGs, it is important to understand the global contributions of NMLR in the early 21st century. This is, at best, a superficial overview and aims to offer a foundation from which we can frame our discussion. When progressing through this chapter, it is important to consider that nursing and midwifery human resources, their state of professionalization, and the resources allocated to them are products of national histories, educational systems, and economic development (Squires et al., 2016). A country's cultural norms around gender and the acceptability of caregiving roles for both sexes will also strongly influence who can obtain research training, what they research, where they can study, how the opportunities emerge, and why NMLR is or is not supported (Kurth, Squires, Shedlin, & Kiarie, 2015).

As we consider the global picture of NMLR in the early 21st century, overall, Asia leads the growth of nursing research worldwide. Middle Eastern countries with strong nursing traditions, such as Jordan and Lebanon, have long developed nursing and midwifery researchers. The Gulf States of the Middle East increasingly invest more in developing nurse researchers. Brazil leads South America with the highest output of nursing research and the largest number of doctoral programs to prepare nurse researchers in the region. The number of countries preparing or sending nursing and midwifery scholars to be prepared to conduct health research is growing annually. Political support from the Pan American Health Organization (PAHO), the Western hemisphere's arm of the World Health Organization (WHO), contributed significantly to this growth and helped break down traditional political barriers that hindered NMLR (Forde, Morrison, Dewailly, Badrie, & Robertson, 2011; Nigenda, Magaña-Valladares, Cooper, & Ruiz-Larios, 2010). Sub-Saharan African (SSA) countries, due in large part to the HIV/AIDS epidemic, have received wide financial support from multinational donors for capacity building around nursing human resources and research training (Lê et al., 2014). Finally, Russia and the former Soviet Union (FSU) states—unless they are part of the European Union—have little capacity for NMLR. Both professions still have the majority of their entry-level education at the high school level and although growing, few nursing bachelor's degree or even technical (associate's degree) programs are available in those countries.

Globally, investments in NMLR are uneven and reflect the resources a country has to support research. In the case of midwifery, the presence of midwives or nurse-midwives conducting research depends on whether or not the country has a tradition of midwifery. In general, fewer midwives, globally, go on for research training than nurses. Consequently, most of the research growth between our two professions comes from nurses. Midwifery, however, has stronger international mobilization for influencing policy and disseminating critical research findings into the policy sphere. *The Lancet* 2014 Midwifery Series (www.thelancet.com/series/midwifery) offered one of the most striking examples of how midwifery-led research can influence both policy and practice. The studies published in that series will have a significant influence on meeting SDG 3, Good health and well-being, which includes maternal child health.

WHAT IS RESEARCH CAPACITY BUILDING?

The term *capacity building* has been historically framed by colonial perspectives and unequal power relationships, but more recently it has been reframed to focus on a collaborative approach of knowledge transfer that is beneficial to all involved (Premji & Hatfield, 2016). "Knowledge transfer promotes access to new knowledge, generally created through research, to those who will use this knowledge" (Premji & Hatfield, 2016, p. 2). Research capacity building has been an important focus within the nursing profession for the past few decades, especially in Western countries. Broadly, *research capacity building* is defined as "enhancing the ability within a discipline or professional group to undertake more high-quality research" (Finch, 2003, p. 427). This is achieved through two components: volume, where more individuals are involved in the production of research, and quality, where the research is conducted using high-quality standards. Capacity building is seen as a process that includes several aspects, such as training nurses to conduct research and lead research programs, educating nurses to understand the value of research in practice and to use it in the clinical setting, developing evidence-based practice (EBP) based on research findings, and fostering nursing environments that are supportive of research and EBP (Bishop & Freshwater, 2003; Finch, 2003; Meyer, Johnson, Proctor, Bryar, & Rosmovtis, 2003).

The literature on building research capacity in nursing is rich; however, the focus has been minimal in LMICs and more deliberate in high-income countries (HICs; Edwards, Webber, Mill, Kahwa, & Roelefs, 2009; Segrott, McIvor, & Green, 2006). In their review of the literature, Segrott and colleagues (2006) found that the majority of the work on research capacity building in nursing has been conducted in the United Kingdom, followed by other Western countries such as Australia, Canada, and the United States.

Research capacity building follows different frameworks and approaches that depend on the setting, the context, and the state of the nursing profession in the partner country, among other factors. It has been developed mostly as part of the academic setting (e.g., see Cooke & Green, 2000; Goeppinger, Miles, Weaver, Campbell, & Roland, 2009; Green et al., 2006); but more recently, research capacity building has been growing in the clinical settings through more structured programs (e.g., see Corchon, Portillo, Watson, & Saracibar, 2011; Jeffs, Smith, Beswick, Maoine, & Ferris, 2013; Moore, Crozier, & Kite, 2012). Many challenges exist in developing, maintaining, and expanding a NMLR program that fosters capacity building (Edwards et al., 2009; Segrott et al., 2006). These include, but are not limited to:

- Limited resources to conduct research and disseminate research findings. This encompasses a shortage of nurses in general, and of nurse researchers in particular. In addition, a shortage of qualified and experienced nurse researchers who can serve as mentors to junior researchers, limited funding opportunities to conduct research, and lack of research infrastructure
- Scarcity of graduate and postgraduate nursing programs that prepare nurses to better use and conduct research
- The profession's historical status and hierarchies of power in the health care systems
- Language barriers for non-English-speaking researchers
- Organizational constraints (high teaching loads, clinical responsibilities, administrative roles, etc.)

WHY RESEARCH CAPACITY BUILDING MATTERS FOR NURSES' AND MIDWIVES' CONTRIBUTIONS TOWARD ACHIEVING THE SDGs

"To achieve a full and healthy life, people require education, nutritious food, clean water, a safe living environment, and at times, medication, various therapies, and social work or case management services" (Shamian, 2016, p. 7). Dr. Judith Shamian, the current president of the International Council of Nurses, has been advocating that nurses need to expand their roles beyond the bedside of individual patient care and collaborate with others at the community, regional, and international levels to promote health for all people in the world (see Chapter 10 for additional thoughts on universal health coverage and human resources for health by Dr. Shamian). She adds that nursing's voice and involvement in achieving the SDGs are very critical in setting global policy. The 17 SDGs and their 169 targets are of significant concern and relevance to all countries around the world. Nurses, making up the largest proportion of the global health care workforce, have ample opportunities to be actively involved in achieving these goals on many different levels.

To enable the profession's contribution to these goals, nurses across multiple settings (hospitals, clinics, communities, schools, etc.) need to be equipped with the adequate knowledge and skills to provide evidence-based health care at the interconnections of health, well-being, and the social determinants of health. Building research capacity in nursing will equip nurses to conduct, disseminate, read, understand, critique, use, and share research to meet the 17 SDGs. Premji and Hatfield (2016) advocate for the concept of "One World, One Health" where nurses embrace a new understanding of their significant contribution to the world's health. Building research capacity that fosters knowledge development and transferability across the globe will contribute to cocreating solutions that will address global health disparities and help meet the 17 SDGs.

HOW DO WE GET THERE?

We have identified four key areas where investments in research capacity building will help nurses and midwives to better contribute to the SDGs and their implementation.

Create Consumers of Research

NMLR has a significant impact on EBP and improving the well-being of patients, families, and communities. It has been well established in the literature that EBP improves patients' outcomes and quality of care and reduces health care costs (Melnyk & Fineout-Overholt, 2011). The one unifying aspect of research that nurses and midwives share is the absolute necessity to become, at a very minimum, consumers of research in order to practice based on the research evidence. A consumer of research is someone who knows how to read research, evaluate its quality, and determine if the results should be applied to clinical practice. EBP ensures that we are working with the most up-to-date information possible.

Historically, research has been led by academic institutions, but in the past few decades, more hospital-based nursing programs have been conducting research by hiring master's- and PhD-prepared nurses to lead and conduct research in clinical settings. These initiatives have been shown to positively influence nurses' perceptions of research and EBP and to develop sustainable nursing research programs (Jeffs et al., 2013).

Yet despite its tremendous benefits, EBP is not the standard of care that is practiced consistently by health care providers, including nurses, around the world. EBP combines the best evidence available from rigorous research studies, clinicians' expertise, and patients' values and preferences. To be effective evidence-based practitioners, nurses need to be key players in research translation into practice. Research translation can be accomplished by changing policies, standards of care, and guidelines to be evidence based.

Thus, research critique skills can help nurses and midwives meet the SDGs by ensuring that only the best quality evidence informs the policies that shape SDG implementation in their home country. These critique skills can also help nurses make the necessary political arguments to advocate for the resources needed for high-quality, cost-effective nursing care—even in limited resource conditions.

Develop Language Skills

Despite English being the third most spoken language in the world, it is considered globally as the universal language for science. Several historical factors (World War II, the birth of the United Nations, the invention of the computer, colonization, growth of science and technology in the United States and other high-income countries, etc.) eased the way to make the English language one of the most widely utilized languages globally (Ammon, 2001).

Nowadays, the majority of funding agencies and peer-reviewed scientific journals require English as the only accepted language. Many high-income countries have either English as their official language or have available resources to assist researchers with either the translation to English or linguistic editorial. LMICs do not usually have this privilege and, consequently, face more challenges when seeking funding or submitting manuscripts for publication. The dominance of the English language in the world of science has provided a production of knowledge that targets mostly individuals, states, and countries that fluently speak and understand English, consequently creating a power differential regarding what and how knowledge is produced, disseminated, and eventually translated into practice.

Having a unified scientific language does facilitate collaborative work across the globe and the attainment of the 17 SDGs. Nonetheless, a unified language also creates many challenges to several parts of the scientific world. We need to not only develop avenues that encourage more translation of the knowledge produced in non-English-speaking countries, but also encourage English-speaking individuals to take on the responsibility to learn additional languages. Fostering collaborations between English- and non-English-speaking researchers helps in decreasing this power differential in knowledge production that is caused by the dominance of the English language.

Finally, a common concern in non-English-speaking countries is that if their nurses and midwives learn English, they will migrate abroad for work and the country will experience "brain drain." The actual risk of this happening, however, is quite low. To become a research consumer, English reading skills are the minimum required, while speaking and writing skills may still be limited (Hull, 2016). The level of English language skills necessary to successfully and safely translate research into practice is significantly higher than just being able to read English. To practice clinically, a nurse needs to demonstrate a sociolinguistic level of competence in speaking, writing, reading, and listening in the language, as measured by a formal assessment mechanism like the Test of English as a Foreign Language (TOEFL; Müller, 2016). Therefore, nurses and midwives can learn to read in English so they can become consumers of research. Reliably accessing evidence to increase consumership of research so we can better inform policies related to the SDGs is an important goal for nurses and midwives, no matter what language they speak.

Integrate Research Training as Professionalization Occurs

Professionalization is a developmental process that structures how an occupational group organizes to advance itself socially, politically, and economically in a country (Squires, 2007). Inherent to professionalization is that the capacity to conduct research related to the profession's customers, workforce, and nature of the work provided by the group be part of the profession's overall occupational structure. Occupational groups that do not produce research or evidence to inform practices, therefore, would not meet the criteria of a profession.

To promote research capacity building, graduate and postgraduate research training is essential. Several opportunities are available for nurses at the doctoral level; however, adequate infrastructure and support need to exist to foster a positive research environment and to develop research careers. Mentoring and supervising doctoral students is greatly needed to prepare the next generation of researchers, especially with an aging nursing workforce, which has been identified mostly in HICs (Sherman, Chiang-Hanisko, & Koszalinski, 2013).

In HICs, doctoral programs are widely available and offer different expertise, funding opportunities, and mentoring to doctoral students. However, in LMICs, doctoral programs are scarcely available. Nurses who seek doctoral education and research careers have limited options and, unfortunately, need to leave their country to join doctoral programs abroad (Edwards et al., 2009; Munjanja, Kibuka, & Dovlo, 2005; Özsoy, 2007). SSA, for example, had doctoral nursing programs in only four countries in 2005 (Kenya, Tanzania, South Africa, and Nigeria), with master's degrees in nursing offered in seven countries (Munjanja, Kibuka, & Dovlo, 2005), though these have expanded significantly in the past few years. Establishing PhD programs is challenging especially in LMICs. Technological advancements in educational program delivery are providing nurses around the world with long-distance educational opportunities. Several doctoral nursing programs in the United States offer online PhD programs where nurses from several parts of the world can receive their education through a distance-learning format. Despite the availability of these online programs, other challenges to research capacity building still exist including availability of funding and scholarships, adequate internet access, fluency in English language, need to travel once or twice a year to meet with the dissertation committee and other researchers, and support in one's country for graduate education and research careers.

Building research capacity in nursing is challenging and takes time, effort, patience, commitment, and resources. Starting with entry-level education is a logical place to begin. Research is best integrated in the educational curriculum as early as possible (secondary school, associate curriculum, and/or undergraduate curriculum) when students would be usually exposed to basic research concepts such as research questions, designs, methods, and EBP. As professionalization in nursing occurs, and in order to develop the passion and enthusiasm for research early on, undergraduate and master's students need to be provided with different opportunities to be actively involved in the research process. Examples include assigning researchers as faculty mentors who can involve students in their research studies, assisting students in turning their classroom assignments into manuscripts and poster presentations, and encouraging students to be involved in professional organizations and research committees (Cleary, Sayers, & Watson, 2016). Nursing students need role models early on in their professional careers and need to be willing to learn, be involved, and use research to support EBP.

A successful example is the Research Enrichment and Apprenticeship Program (REAP), which is an intensive research-mentoring program that was developed to promote opportunities for minority nursing students in the United States to conduct and utilize research in their professional careers (Goeppinger et al., 2009). Despite the many challenges, the program succeeded in promoting a nursing career for these students, which involved graduate education and research. The short-term outcomes of the program included development of community-based research projects that addressed multiple health disparities, dissemination of research findings through poster presentations at conferences, and enrollment in doctoral programs. Overall, a more systematic approach to research capacity building in nursing and midwifery is needed to ensure our ongoing voice in shaping and influencing SDG policies—not to mention their successful implementation on the front lines of health care (where appropriate).

Educational Partnerships to Build Research Capacity

SDG 17, Revitalize global partnerships for sustainable development, identifies partnerships as key to progress in achieving the agenda's goals (see Chapter 32 for more information on building collaborative partnerships). As the importance of research has been more widely recognized, more partnerships have developed to build research capacity where it is needed, primarily in LMICs.

Health-related disciplines, including medicine, nursing, and nutrition, have all utilized partnerships to build research capacity in LMICs. These exchanges can take place between a variety of actors: research institutions, universities, professional interest groups, national health research forums, government agencies, multinational agencies such as the WHO, and health care facilities (Varshney, Atkins,Das, & Diwan, 2016). Frequently, these projects for research capacity building partner an institution from the global North with an institution from the global South, although the number of South–South partnerships is increasing (Airhihenbuwa et al., 2011; Anderson et al., 2014; Lansang & Dennis, 2004).

These partnerships for capacity building can focus on different aspects of the research pipeline. Most are oriented primarily toward developing the research skills of local actors (Birch, Tuck, Malata, & Gagnon, 2013; Sheehan, Comiskey, Williamson, & Mgutshini, 2015). The scope of these programs varies considerably. Partnerships to develop broad research skills have developed master's and doctoral programs, provided fellowships for local actors to gain research skills abroad, and coordinated intracountry mentorship programs, which pair young researchers with established professionals. Other partnerships are relatively narrow, such as those that train particular clinicians on how to conduct research in their clinical specialty area.

Other partnerships have focused on the broader research environment, which must provide meaningful opportunities to conduct research for the benefits of these programs to be realized (Xue Murthy, Tran, & Ghaffar, 2014). Limited infrastructure, insufficient funds, inadequate opportunities for dissemination, and poor leadership can all limit research output. Educational partnerships that seek to address these issues have utilized a number of strategies, including developing health research networks to facilitate collaboration, coupling research to national health priorities to stimulate demand for research, and improving local researchers' access to research tools, such as computational software, via the internet.

Concerns about the quality of these partnerships, the burden they place on host countries, and the possibility that they could reinforce an undesirable power dynamic between well-resourced and poorly resourced participants have led to the development of at least 10 different tools to guide these collaborations. Some of these are specific to certain research modalities, such as participatory research, or particular partners, such as aboriginal peoples, but many are suited for more general use. Guidelines tailored to international partnerships to avoid the challenges inherent in any research relationship, such as issues around data ownership and authorship, have also emerged.

The success of these partnerships in boosting overall research output from LMICs has been mixed. While many individual partnerships report tremendous success, budgetary constraints in LMICs can render some research capacity gains unsustainable or jeopardize local ownership of the research agenda when outside funders step in. Innovative strategies to fund research locally, such as earmarking specified percentages of the national government or national lottery revenues for research, are currently under consideration.

OPPORTUNITIES FOR RESEARCH IMPACT

As we consider the role of NMLR in meeting the SDGs, it is clear that our influence will be limited without stronger research capacity in every country around the globe—but most importantly in LMICs where the impact of the work could be even greater. Table 9.1 provides a geographical overview of where NMLR has historically influenced, is currently influencing, and could in the future influence the policies aimed at realizing the SDGs.

Regarding many aspects of the SDGs, our research has an obvious home, for example, SDG 3, Good health and well-being. We have also historically worked with poverty-stricken individuals and have seen firsthand the consequences of poverty to health and documented them in early descriptive research. For many people in many countries, becoming a nurse can be a way out of poverty and into the middle class—but we lack sufficient research to show the economic benefits

Table 9.1 How Nursing and Midwifery Research Addresses the Sustainable Development Goals

Sustainable Development Goals	Historical	Current	Future
1. No poverty	X	X	X
2. Zero hunger	X	X	X
3. Good health & well-being	X	X	X
4. Quality education	X	X	X
5. Gender equality		X	X
6. Clean water & sanitation	X	X	X
7. Affordable & clean energy			X
8. Decent work & economic growth	X	X	X
9. Industry, innovation, & infrastructure		X	X
10. Reduced inequalities	X	X	X
11. Sustainable cities & communities		X	X
12. Responsible consumption & production		X	X
13. Climate Action		X	X
14. Life below water		X	X
15. Life on land		X	X
16. Peace, justice, & strong institutions		X	X
17. Partnerships for the goals	X	X	X

of pursuing health profession careers (McPake, Squires, Mahat, & Araujo, 2015). Nursing and midwifery workforce researchers and educators have long understood the links between quality education, health, and our own workforce's development. We need a better understanding, however, of the economics behind our educational investments so we can help meet this SDG. Understanding the production mechanisms behind nursing and midwifery human resources, which are strongly linked to education, is also essential (Squires et al., 2016).

SDG 5, Gender equality, presents a mix of opportunities for nurses and midwives. Some would argue that both professions have been strong advocates for gender equality, while others would argue that we have lacked in this area. Some of these efforts may focus on patients, but there is not enough focus on addressing these issues in the workforce. Bringing the nursing perspective to gender equality initiatives should receive more attention through our research.

Success in achieving SDG 5 is also tied to SDG 9, Industry, innovation, and infrastructure. Research shows that when countries have weak institutional infrastructure (e.g., poorly functioning health systems, weak governance mechanisms), there is more gender inequality in a country (Beckfield, Olafsdottir, & Sosnaud, 2013; Owen & You, 2009; Self & Grabowski, 2009). For nurses and midwives, this translates into fewer opportunities. A potential growth area for research in our fields would be to document problems with institutional infrastructure and determine which industry innovations may best address the infrastructure issues.

SDGs 6 and 11 to 13 all have an environmental angle to them. Environmental health–driven research in nursing and midwifery is lacking despite increasing interest in the 21st century. Environmental action by nurses should be more than making sure we do not waste supplies when in practice. Environmental research is community driven, and as more care shifts to the community and out of hospitals, understanding how the environment affects health will become more critical in the future. We lack researchers with the skills in these areas at the moment, so our research will have less impact on these SDGs in the coming years until we have sufficient capacity to address these questions.

For those nursing and midwifery researchers concerned with health disparities and inequalities, SDGs 8 (Decent work and economic growth) and 10 (Reduce inequalities within and among countries) are logical fits for a good portion of our research. Disparities researchers understand that inequalities are driven by social and economic institutions and how those manifest in a country. Research by nurses and midwives in that area has qualified and quantified the impact of those issues on health and well-being and will continue to do so for many years to come.

SDG 8 is important for all nurses, and large international studies like the RN4CAST study—a 15-country pan-European, Chinese, and SSA nursing workforce survey—have helped to demonstrate the importance of decent work environments for nurses and midwives alike. And when nurses and midwives have access to good jobs that pay solid middle-class salaries, they contribute to economic growth. Since nurses represent the majority of health workers in a country, their contributions to economic growth could be substantial. The problem? We currently lack the research to demonstrate the extent of nursing's economic contributions, and the labor market literature is just beginning to quantify it (McPake et al., 2013; McPake, Anthony, & Edoka, 2014). So with SDG 8 (Decent Work and Economic Growth), we have tremendous potential to both train researchers with new skill sets that will help meet both the targets of that SDG and also address a major gap in our own professional literature.

Finally, as we discussed previously, partnerships are key for addressing all of these issues (SDG 17). In the case of research, we have a solid foundation from which to build partnerships that can help meet the SDGs (Kurth et al., 2015). Nonetheless, these partnerships can be complex and often imbalanced in favor of countries with more resources and experience. Ensuring that we value the expertise of all team members and understand the value of local knowledge will go a long way in helping our research contribute to meeting the SDGs and ultimately, help achieve the humanistic targets of SDG 16 (Peace, Justice, and Strong Institutions).

CONCLUSION

As this chapter illustrates, NMLR has the potential to address all of the SDGs and contribute, both directly and indirectly, to meeting their primary aims. Expanding the scope of our research in the areas where we have lacked historical contribution or are underdeveloped in terms of research experience will help ensure that our voices contribute, through research, to meeting the SDGs.

REFLECTION AND DISCUSSION

- Describe the fundamentals of research capacity building. What improvements need to be integrated within my current work environment to promote effective research- and science-building mechanisms?
- How does health research contribute to meeting the SDGs?
- How is NMLR uniquely suited to meet SDG goals and targets?
- In what ways do research capacity building needs change in relation to country income status? What advantages or disadvantages does NMLR in my context experience related to economic status?
- Consider how policy-making processes influence SDG implementation. What are the current opportunities to integrate nursing and midwifery voices into my local, national, and corresponding international policies? What opportunities have yet to be available to nursing and midwifery? How can I lead and inspire the needed changes?

REFERENCES

Airhihenbuwa, C. O., Shisana, O., Zungu, N., BeLue, R., Makofani, D. M., Shefer, T., . . . Simbayi, L. (2011). Research capacity building: A US-South African partnership. *Global Health Promotion, 18*(2), 27–35. doi:10.1177/1757975911404745

Ammon, U. (Ed.). (2001). *The dominance of english as a language of science: Effects on other languages and language communities.* Berlin, Germany: Walter de Gruyter.

Anderson, F., Donkor, P., de Vries, R., Appiah-Denkyira, E., Dakpallah, G. F., Rominski, S., . . . Ayettey, S. (2014). Creating a charter of collaboration for International University Partnerships: The Elmina Declaration for Human Resources for Health. *Academic Medicine, 89*(8), 1125–1132. doi:10.1097/ACM.0000000000000384

Beckfield, J., Olafsdottir, S., & Sosnaud, B. (2013). Healthcare systems in comparative perspective: Classification, convergence, institutions, inequalities, and five missed turns. *Annual Review of Sociology, 39*(1), 127–146. doi:10.1146/annurev-soc-071312-145609

Birch, A. P., Tuck, J., Malata, A., & Gagnon, A. J. (2013). Assessing global partnerships in graduate nursing. *Nurse Education Today, 33*(11), 1288–1294. doi:10.1016/j.nedt.2013.03.014

Bishop, V., & Freshwater, D. (2003). Capacity-building and careers in nursing research: Rationale and context. *Nursing Times Research, 8*(6), 398–406.

Cleary, M., Sayers, J., & Watson, R. (2016). Essentials of building a career in nursing research. *Nurse Researcher, 23*(6), 9–13.

Cooke, A., & Green, B. (2000). Developing the research capacity of departments of nursing and midwifery based in higher education: A review of the literature. *Journal of Advanced Nursing, 32*(1), 57–65. doi:10.1046/j.1365-2648.2000.01447.x

Corchon, S., Portillo, M. C., Watson, R., & Saracíbar, M. (2011). Nursing research capacity building in a Spanish hospital: An intervention study. *Journal of Clinical Nursing, 20*(17–18), 2479–2489.

Edwards, N., Webber, J., Mill, J., Kahwa, E., & Roelofs, S. (2009). Building capacity for nurse-led research. *International Nursing Review, 56*(1), 88–94.

Finch, J. (2003). Commentary: A look at the bigger picture in building research capacity. *Nursing Times Research, 8*(6), 427–428.

Forde, M., Morrison, K., Dewailly, E., Badrie, N., & Robertson, L. (2011). Strengthening integrated research and capacity development within the Caribbean region. *BMC International Health and Human Rights, 11*(2), S7. doi:10.1186/1472-698X-11-S2-S7

Goeppinger, J., Miles, M. S., Weaver, W., Campbell, L., & Roland, E. J. (2009). Building nursing research capacity to address health disparities: Engaging minority baccalaureate and master's students. *Nursing Outlook, 57*(3), 158–165. doi:10.1016/j.outlook.2009.01.005

Green, B., Segrott, J., & Hewitt, J. (2006). Developing nursing and midwifery research capacity in a university department: Case study. *Journal of Advanced Nursing, 56*(3), 302–313. doi:10.1111/j.1365-2648.2006.04022.x

Hull, M. (2016). Medical language proficiency: A discussion of interprofessional language competencies and potential for patient risk. *International Journal of Nursing Studies, 54*, 158–172. doi:10.1016/j.ijnurstu.2015.02.015

Jeffs, L., Smith, O., Beswick, S., Maoine, M., & Ferris, E. (2013). Investing in nursing research in practice settings: A blueprint for building capacity. *Nursing Leadership, 26*(4), 44–59. Retrieved from http://www.ncbi.nlm.nih.gov/pubmed/24377848

Kurth, A. E., Squires, A., Shedlin, M. G., & Kiarie, J. (2015). Interdisciplinary collaborations in global health research. In S. Breakley, I. B. Corless, N. L. Meedzan, & P. K. Nicholas (Eds.), *Global health nursing in the 21st century* (1st ed., pp. 547–563). New York, NY: Springer Publishing.

Lansang, M. A., & Dennis, R. (2004). Building capacity in health research in the developing world. *Bulletin of the World Health Organization, 82*(10), 764–770. Retrieved from http://www.ncbi.nlm.nih.gov/pubmed/15643798

Lê, G., Mirzoev, T., Orgill, M., Erasmus, E., Lehmann, U., Okeyo, S., . . . Gilson, L. (2014). A new methodology for assessing health policy and systems research and analysis capacity in African universities. *Health Research Policy and Systems, 12*(1), 59. doi:10.1186/1478-4505-12-59

McPake, B., Anthony, S., & Edoka, I. (2014). *Analyzing markets for health workers: Insights from labor and health economics.* Washington, DC: The World Bank. doi:10.1596/978-1-4648-0224-9

McPake, B., Maeda, A., Araújo, E. C., Lemiere, C., El Maghraby, A., & Cometto, G. (2013). Why do health labour market forces matter? *Bulletin of the World Health Organization, 91*(11), 841–846. doi:10.2471/BLT.13.118794

McPake, B., Squires, A., Mahat, A., & Araujo, E. C. (2015). *The economics of health professions education and careers: Insights from a literature review.* Washington, DC: The World Bank. doi:10.1596/978-1-4648-0616-2

Meyer, J., Johnson, B., Procter, S., Bryar, R., & Rosmovtis, I. (2003). Practitioner research: Exploring issues in relation to research capacity-building. *Nursing Times Research, 8*, 407–417. doi:10.1177/136140960300800603

Moore, J., Crozier, K., & Kite, K. (2012). An action research approach for developing research and innovation in nursing and midwifery practice: Building research capacity in one NHS foundation trust. *Nurse Education Today, 32*(1), 39–45. doi:10.1016/j.nedt.2011.01.014

Müller, A. (2016). Language proficiency and nursing registration. *International Journal of Nursing Studies, 54*, 132–140. doi:10.1016/j.ijnurstu.2015.01.007

Munjanja, O. K., Kibuka, S., & Dovlo, D. (2005). *The nursing workforce in sub-Saharan Africa.* Retrieved from https://www.ghdonline.org/uploads/The_nursing_workforce_in_sub-Saharan_Africa.pdf

Nigenda, G., Magaña-Valladares, L., Cooper, K., & Ruiz-Larios, J. A. (2010). Recent developments in public health nursing in the Americas. *International Journal of Environmental Research and Public Health, 7*(3), 729–750. doi:10.3390/ijerph7030729

Owen, A. L., & You, R. (2009). Growth, attitudes towards women, and women's welfare. *Review of Development Economics, 13*(1), 134–150. doi:10.1111/j.1467-9361.2008.00466.x

Özsoy, S. A. (2007). The struggle to develop nursing research in Turkey. *International Nursing Review, 54*, 243–248.

Premji, S. S., & Hatfield, J. (2016). Call to action for nurses/nursing. *BioMed Research International, 2016*, 1–5. doi:10.1155/2016/3127543

Segrott, J., McIvor, M., & Green, B. (2006). Challenges and strategies in developing nursing research capacity: A review of the literature. *International Journal of Nursing Studies, 43*, 637–651. doi:10.1016/j.ijnurstu.2005.07.011

Self, S., & Grabowski, R. (2009). Gender development, institutions, and level of economic development. *Review of Development Economics, 13*(2), 319–332.

Shamian, J. (2016). In setting global policy, nursing's voice is needed: It's time to reach beyond the bedside. *American Journal of Nursing, 116*(8), 7.

Sheehan, A., Comiskey, C., Williamson, C., & Mgutshini, T. (2015). Evaluation of the implementation of a PhD capacity-building program for nurses in South Africa. *Nursing Research, 64*(1), 13–23. doi:10.1097/NNR.0000000000000069

Sherman, R. O., Chiang-Hanisko, L., & Koszalinski, R. (2013). The ageing nursing workforce: A global challenge. *Journal of Nursing Management, 21*(7), 899–902. doi:10.1111/jonm.12188

Squires, A., Uyei, S. J., Beltrán-Sánchez, H., Jones, S. A., Anand, S., Bärnighausen, T., . . . Schedler, A. (2016). Examining the influence of country-level and health system factors on nursing and physician personnel production. *Human Resources for Health, 14*(1), 48. doi:10.1186/s12960-016-0145-4

Squires, A. P. (2007). *A case study of the professionalization of Mexican nursing: 1980 to 2005* (Unpublished doctoral dissertation). Yale University, New Haven, CT.

Varshney, D., Atkins, S., Das, A., & Diwan, V. (2016a). Understanding collaboration in a multi-national research capacity-building partnership: A qualitative study. *Health Research Policy and Systems/BioMed Central, 14*(1), 64. doi:10.1186/s12961-016-0132-1

Xue, J., Murthy, B., Tran, N. T., & Ghaffar, A. (2014). Goal setting and knowledge generation through health policy and systems research in low- and middle-income countries. *Health Research Policy and Systems, 12*(1). doi:10.1186/1478-4505-12-39

CHAPTER 10

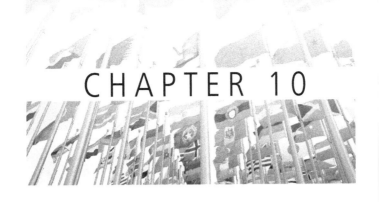

Transnational Nursing Organizations Paving the Way for Global Health: The International Council of Nurses as Exemplar

Elizabeth Holguin, Frances Hughes, and Judith Shamian

I alone cannot change the world, but I can cast a stone across the waters to create many ripples. (Mother Teresa)

Global nursing does not signify only nurses working internationally. As global health professionals, nurses around the world must identify current and future opportunities for engagement; foster professional development and scopes of practice delineation; nurture and build relationships, partnerships, and collaborations; as well as engage in leadership, scholarship, policy, practice, and service roles (Sigma Theta Tau International [STTI], 2016). Doing so will ensure that the nursing profession continues to build upon past successes of building health equity, ameliorating social determinants of health, and achieving universal health coverage (UHC).

As the largest health care profession, nursing has the potential to be a leading powerhouse for positive change and innovation. Nursing, as an integral part of the health care system, encompasses independent and collaborative care of individuals, families, and communities. The nursing profession is comprised of health promotion, disease prevention, and caring for those that are sick or dying. In addition to these tasks, nurses should have roles in advocacy, research, education, and health policy at all levels (International Council of Nurses [ICN], 2002).

PUBLIC HEALTH, INTERNATIONAL HEALTH, AND GLOBAL HEALTH

Public health nursing addresses multiple determinants of health and includes advocacy, policy, development, and social justice issues with a commitment to health equity (American Public Health Association [APHA], 2013). Key elements of practice for public health nurses include focusing on the health needs and inequities of an entire population; population health assessment using a comprehensive, systematic approach; attention to multiple determinants of health; an emphasis on primary prevention; and application of interventions from the individual to the population level within sustainable systems that can impact their health (APHA, 2013, p. 2). The term *international health* has historically signified health work in low-income countries that is focused on infectious and tropical diseases, water and sanitation, malnutrition, and maternal and child health (Brown, Cueto, & Fee, 2006 in Koplan et al., 2009). *Global health* is the most current term and shares characteristics with public health and international health, including:

- Priority on a population-based and preventive focus
- Concentration on poorer, vulnerable, and underserved populations
- Multidisciplinary and interdisciplinary approaches
- Emphasis on health as a public good
- The importance of systems and structures
- Stakeholder participation (Koplan et al., 2009)

(See Chapter 2 for the most recent recommended definitions of *global health* and *global nursing* released by the Global Advisory Panel on the Future of Nursing, STTI.)

Global nursing has long been grounded in service. Nurses and nursing educators have chosen primarily a clinical perspective when incorporating global health into nursing; topics such as the global spread of communicable diseases, necessity of evidence-based nursing interventions, caring for vulnerable populations, and cultural diversity and sensitivity are quite common (Breda, 2012). When global health is viewed through a clinical lens, there is little to no consideration of the underlying economic, social, and political issues (Breda, 2012) that contribute directly to the root cause of many health problems. Therefore, no matter the terminology used to describe our profession, it is imperative to step beyond the clinical realm and incorporate policy, advocacy, and diplomacy into all future efforts.

This chapter features the work of the ICN, which is operated by nurses and leads nurses internationally, while working to support and advance the profession and influence sound health policies on a global scale. First, their mission and strategic vision are outlined. Next, the Sustainable Development Goals (SDGs) are discussed with an in-depth focus on the third goal, health and well-being, in the context of nursing practice and nursing's potential and expected contributions to the achievement of all SDGs. The importance of networking and partnership formation within an ICN framework are described for the reader. Next, there is a discussion on the importance of nurse involvement in policy at all levels. Finally, next steps to accomplish the SDGs are delineated with a special focus on ICN's involvement with the United Nations (UN) High-Level Commission on Health Employment and Economic Growth.

INTERNATIONAL COUNCIL OF NURSES

Founded in 1899, the ICN represents the more than 16 million nurses around the globe. ICN is the world's first and widest reaching forum for health professionals, particularly nurses, and was the first professional organization for women (Bridges, 1967). It comprises a federation of more than 130 national nursing associations (NNAs). ICN is governed by an elected board, members of which come from the seven ICN regions. The ICN board has a president and an executive committee, and a committee structure that sets and monitors policies consistent with the direction set by the council of nursing representatives (CNR). The board also guides the work of the chief executive officer (CEO) and operationalizes the board's agenda; implementing the policies are the responsibilities of the CEO and ICN staff.

The ICN code for nurses is the foundation for ethical nursing practice throughout the world. ICN standards, guidelines, and policies for nursing practice, education, management, research, and socioeconomic welfare are accepted globally as the basis of nursing policy. ICN provides both a regional, as well as a global, focus for its members. ICN forms transnational alliances with nursing and other health care specialty professional groups, nongovernmental organizations (NGOs), businesses and health care associations, university research centers and institutes, as well as other educational and advanced practice organizations.

Mission and Strategic Vision

ICN intends to enhance the health of individuals, populations, and societies by championing the contribution and image of nurses worldwide; advocating for nurses at all levels; advancing the nursing profession; and influencing health, social, economic, and educational policy. ICN's core values are built upon visionary leadership, innovativeness, solidarity, accountability, and social justice. These values are described in greater detail in Table 10.1.

ICN has four strategic priorities for 2014–2018: global voice, strategic leadership, policy impact, and diversification. ICN has identified these priorities to most effectively represent nurses and their involvement in the global health agenda at the highest levels of policy making. In this way, global nurses can foster solidarity and cooperation with stakeholders; empower discerning advocacy by and for nurses,

Table 10.1 ICN's Core Values

Visionary leadership	To sustain and advance the nursing profession, health, and policy through creativity, ingenuity, dedication, and determination
Innovativeness	To establish nurses in nontraditional nursing roles in order to bring a nursing perspective to health problems related to education, economics, and policy
Solidarity	To elevate nurses to key roles to foster partnerships and collaboration on public policy design and implementation
Accountability	Reinforcing informed decision making and reporting to maintain a transparent and accessible path to information
Social justice	To achieve equity and equality for both those in the nursing profession and for society as a whole

ICN, International Council of Nurses.

nursing, and health; influence design and implementation of health and public policy; and procure and diversify revenue generating opportunities to continue to support the goals of ICN, its NNA members, and global nurses everywhere.

The current global agenda takes precedence for heads of states, international agencies, and global donors and funders grounded in building and maintaining strong health care and social systems in order to have better functioning and increasingly productive societies. The global agendas of UHC (Vega, 2013), people-centered care (World Health Organization [WHO], 2015), and the SDGs (United Nations Development Programme [UNDP], 2016) are core foci for each individual country to achieve global advancement. In each of these agendas, nursing is a central and essential player. To reach and care for all populations in a safe and inclusive manner, the world needs nurses and more of them; nurses with the right knowledge, competencies, and proper geographical distribution (Shamian, Tomblin-Murphy, Rose, & Jeffs, 2015a, 2015b). Nursing is an integral part of the solutions for a growing health care workforce gap, economic growth, climate change, and achieving UHC. While there is a growing appreciation of the importance of nurses as frontline clinicians and system managers, there is limited understanding of the place nursing can and should hold, both at the policy table and at the evidence-informed arena for system transformation, while building cost-effective and accountable systems.

THE SDGs

The SDGs will impact global health and global nursing in a way that the Millennium Development Goals (MDGs) did not have the opportunity to. The MDGs were eight time-bound (2000–2015) and quantifiable targets created in 2000 at the UN Millennium Summit, where world leaders adopted the UN Millennium Declaration. The MDGs were meant to address extreme poverty in all aspects including income, hunger, disease, lack of adequate shelter, and exclusion, while also promoting gender equality, education, environmental sustainability, and basic human rights (Millennium Project, 2006; see the Appendix for a complete list of the MDGs).

The SDGs are meant for *all* countries, not only low- and middle-income countries (LMICs). The SDGs are a new, universal set of goals, targets, indicators, and metrics that UN Member States adopted in 2015, and will be expected to use to frame their agendas and political policies over the next 15 years (see the Appendix for a complete list of the 17 SDGs). Donors will also be guided by the SDGs in their investments and partnerships. These goals will thus guide both socioeconomic and governmental priorities through 2030. They are more comprehensive than the MDGs, as illustrated by the 169 specific objectives affiliated with the 17 goals, and more clearly incorporate the economic, environmental, and social pillars of sustainable development to end global poverty.

The ICN, Nursing, and the SDGs

Nursing professionals—each individual, as well as the collective—are key stakeholders in promoting health and well-being for clients, communities, and nations. It is critical for nurses to understand the significance and potential impact of the SDGs in relation to nursing, and their role in supporting and furthering SDG advancement. In addition to ICN's mission and strategic vision, the organization's initiatives, through its members and partners, assist in transforming the way health care is provided and support members in achieving their full potential to the best of their ability. The outcomes should significantly improve the health and well-being of populations, reduce health inequalities, strengthen public health, and ensure people-centered health systems that are universal, equitable, and of high quality.

There are numerous drivers that influence how the ICN undertakes its work. Because of the scale, extent, and impact of these drivers, it is important that the ICN understands the issues and prioritizes its work because not all of these can be addressed at the same time. The ICN formulates a response and enacts transformation through its ability to influence change. The core outcomes that will be affected include regulation and education; practice, patient, and people outcomes; and workforce and care environments.

Of the 17 Global Goals, SDG 3 specifically relates to health, but all of the goals have an impact on health. When people are poor, hungry, lacking education, for example, they cannot achieve health. Reducing disparities and socioeconomic inequities is a global and public health goal to which nurses can contribute at every level. The main missive endorsed by heads of state and ministers of health within SDG 3 surrounds UHC as central to the health goal, calling it a "prerequisite for the achievement of all the others [SDGs]" (WHO, 2016b). Because the nursing profession falls mainly under SDG 3, "Ensure healthy lives and promote well-being for all," the next section offers a more in-depth examination of the goal and pertinent targets, but is not meant to be all inclusive.

SDG 3: Good Health and Well-Being: Relevant Targets and Opportunities

SDG 3.1. By 2030, Reduce the Global Maternal Mortality Ratio to Less Than 70 per 100,000 Live Births

The maternal mortality ratio is defined as the number of maternal deaths per 100,000 live births, and was estimated to be at 216 globally as of 2015 (WHO, 2016b). At the 2016 Women Deliver Conference, the African Maternal, Newborn, and Child Health (MNCH) coalition reported that the highest lifetime risk of maternal death is concentrated across Africa. The lack of skilled personnel and shortage of doctors, nurses, and midwives is one of the main causes of maternal mortality (WHO, 2016b); approximately 830 women die every day due to pregnancy and childbirth complications (WHO, 2016b). Key causes of death are hemorrhage, pre-eclampsia and eclampsia, sepsis or other infections, and pre-existing medical conditions that may become exacerbated during pregnancy (WHO, 2016b).

However, home visitation by nurses in the prenatal and infant/toddler stages is a promising means of reducing all-cause mortality in first-born children living in highly disadvantaged settings (Olds et al., 2014), and through care coordination, education, and emotional support, adverse maternal–child outcomes can be significantly diminished (Goyal et al., 2014). The Nurse Family Partnership® (NFP) is a well-known, evidence-based program, rooted in community health, that has had proven effectiveness in the United States for first-time mothers in vulnerable populations. According to NFP, children born to low-income first-time mothers are at the greatest risk for health, educational, and economic disparities (NFP, 2015). Three separate randomized control trials have demonstrated that NFP practices and policies have resulted in improvements in pregnancy outcomes, child health and development, and school readiness and achievement (NFP, 2015, p. 1).

Within the United States, the NFP has served over 31,000 families in 43 states, six tribal organizations, and one territory (NFP, 2015). The program has been adapted to benefit families in Canada with a current randomized control trial underway (Jack et al., 2015); NFP is also being implemented in Australia, Bulgaria, England, Northern Ireland, Norway, Scotland, and The Netherlands. The NFP is already implementing policies recommended by WHO to address inequalities in access to maternal and newborn services, and is strengthening infrastructure and health systems to meet the needs of women while ensuring equity and quality of care. Outside of the NFP, nurses can play a key role in ensuring access to sexual and reproductive health information and services for their patients, and involve themselves in local, state, and national policy to advocate for comprehensive reproductive health care.

In addition to home visitation, other key interventions delineated by the WHO to reduce maternal mortality rates include iron supplementation for maternal anemia (WHO, 2014), prevention and management of postpartum hemorrhage (WHO, 2012), and recognition and treatment of infection or beginning signs of sepsis (Sarna, Wolf, & Bialous, 2016). These interventions can all be handled in community settings by nurses and midwives.

Furthermore, those in public health or community health nursing are in a position to educate women on certain communicable and noncommunicable, absolute or relative contraindications for pregnancy, such as Zika virus or certain heart conditions, and provide them with prevention methods. Community clinics or mobile clinics that provide prenatal care or reproductive health services, and sexual and reproductive education, can be staffed entirely by registered nurses, advanced practice nurses, and nurse midwives.

Community clinics in many nations are also largely supported by community health workers (CHWs) who can partner with nursing staff to deliver such interventions, and who are also able to perform home visits when necessary. In the WHO's widely used definition of a "community health worker," they suggest that a CHW should

> be members of the communities where they work, should be selected by the communities, should be answerable to the communities for their activities, be supported by the health system but not necessarily a part of its organization, and have shorter training than professional workers. (WHO, 2007, p. 1)

This relationship enables the worker to serve as a link between health or social services and the community to facilitate increased access to services while improving the quality and cultural competence of service delivery.

CHWs have a wide range of skills and a diverse profile. In addition to performing home visits, their work contributes toward improvements in environmental sanitation, provision of water supply, first aid, treatment of simple or common ailments, health education, nutrition and surveillance, maternal and child health, family planning activities, tuberculosis (TB), and HIV/AIDS care, malaria control, treatment of acute respiratory infections, communicable disease control, community development activities, referrals, and record keeping and collection of data on vital events (WHO, 2007).

For example, in Kenya, CHWs are helping to expand access to health services and contraceptives in hard-to-reach populations, and performing prenatal home visits. In Malawi, Chad, and Rwanda, CHWs serve as health surveillance assistants to combat malaria in their villages (Jhpiego Corporation, 2015; Kalemba & Bundula, 2015; Morgah et al., 2013). Similar successes have been noted in HIV/AIDS and TB screening and treatment adherence in several African countries including Tanzania, Nigeria, Malawi, Kenya, and Mozambique (Adetiloye, 2011; Brondi, 2011; Jhpiego Corporation, 2016; Mlacha, 2015; Mwaura & Njenga, 2016). CHWs have also begun to implement their skills in the area of noncommunicable diseases (NCDs) to perform basic diagnostic functioning for cardiovascular disease risk assessments in Mexico and South Africa (Abrahams-Gessel, Denman, Gaziano, Levitt, & Puoane, 2016). Nurses should develop collaborative relationships with CHWs focused on skills and knowledge transfer: providing CHWs with additional education and training while receiving further training in local cultural traditions, norms, values, ethics, and health care access/delivery considerations, and building improved interprofessional partnerships at local and global levels to accomplish nursing and health initiatives in alignment with the SDGs.

SDG 3.2. By 2030, End Preventable Deaths of Newborns and Children Under 5 Years of Age

According to WHO, 5.9 million children under the age of 5 died in 2015; the global under-5 mortality rate is 42.5 per 1000 live births (WHO, 2016b). More than half of these deaths are attributable to conditions that are treatable or preventable (prematurity, sepsis, pneumonia, diarrhea, injuries, malaria, etc.) with access to simple and affordable interventions. Safe childbirth and effective neonatal care are essential to prevent these early child deaths. A child's chance of survival increases significantly with delivery in a health facility in the presence of a skilled birth attendant. A "skilled birth attendant" is defined as

> an accredited health professional—such as a midwife, doctor, or nurse—who has been educated and trained to proficiency in the skills needed to manage normal (uncomplicated) pregnancies, childbirth, and the immediate postnatal period, and in the identification, management and referral of complications in women and newborns. (WHO, 2017)

Although globally 73% of births are estimated to be attended by a skilled birth attendant (WHO, 2016b), more than 40% of births in the WHO African region and WHO South-East Asia region are not. A recent study in the United Kingdom found that neonatal units providing one-to-one nursing on a greater proportion of intensive care days demonstrated lower mortality rates, and those with decreased one-to-one nurse–patient ratios were associated with higher inpatient death rates (0.6 in 100 infants receiving intensive care; London, 2016). The WHO calls for improved management of preterm births, inpatient supportive care, and the promotion of kangaroo mother care[1] (WHO, 2016b).

---

[1] Kangaroo mother care refers to skin-to-skin contact between mother and baby, exclusive breastfeeding, and meeting all physical, psychological, and emotional needs of mother and baby without separation.

Nurses also help to prevent sleep-related infant deaths by providing safe sleep recommendations for parents and educating parents on the effects of tobacco use around newborns. For the under-5 population, the most important prevention and treatment strategies include vaccination, appropriate nutrition, exclusive breastfeeding, adequate sanitation, and hygiene and clean water. Nurses are integral to vaccination programs, nutrition education, and can function as lactation consultants. This is especially relevant to populations residing in LMICs. Keith Hansen of the World Bank refers to breastfeeding as a "child's first inoculation against death, disease, and poverty, but also their most enduring investment in physical, cognitive, and social capacity" (Hansen, 2016, p. 416). Breastfeeding reduces morbidity and mortality, reduces malnutrition, increases IQ scores, improves school achievement, and increases adult earnings (Rollins et al., 2016; Victora et al., 2016). Scaling up breastfeeding in LMICs is more important than ever, as the positive benefits of breastfeeding directly align with the SDGs (Hansen, 2016). Vaccines have been proven to be cost effective and an efficient investment (Ozawa, Mirelman, Stack, Walker, & Levine, 2012; Shearer, Walker, Risko, & Levine, 2012). Expanding access to vaccines became a global priority with the advent of the MDGs (Shearer et al., 2012); nurses can be involved in service delivery, policy impacting national immunization programs, education, and access issues.

SDG 3.3. By 2030, End the Epidemics of AIDS, TB, Malaria, and Neglected Tropical Diseases and Combat Hepatitis, Water-Borne Diseases and Other Communicable Diseases

HIV and TB

Although NCDs have now become the leading cause of death, being responsible for 38 million deaths each year, infectious diseases remain a significant contributor to global morbidity and mortality and global health security. ICN recently developed an online vaccination module[2] to:

- Specify how to recognize outcomes associated with failure to obtain vaccinations;
- Highlight common myths associated with vaccinations;
- Guide nurses to identify trends in an aging population at the global level;
- Discern why elders are vulnerable to communicable diseases;
- Identify key barriers and facilitators to vaccination uptake; and
- List appropriate actions the nursing profession may take to promote vaccination of elders.

There are 37 million people worldwide living with HIV, and only half are aware of their HIV-positive status (WHO, 2016b). Although TB is treatable, it remains a major global health burden. There were 9.6 million new cases (133 per 100,000) and 1.5 million deaths in 2014 alone, including 0.4 million among those with HIV (WHO, 2016b). Almost all cases are curable with timely diagnosis and an accurate treatment regimen (WHO, 2016b). Nurses can play a key role in prevention, treatment, and care of both TB and HIV. Essential public health measures include prevention education and counseling, disease screening, and administration of treatment regimens, such as

---

[2] *Source:* ICN Online Vaccination Module.

highly active antiretroviral therapy (HAART) and directly observed therapy (DOT). (Short course DOTs are commonly performed by nurses throughout the world.)

Since 2003, supported and funded by the Eli Lilly and Company Foundation, ICN has worked with the Lilly Multidrug-Resistant Tuberculosis (MDR-TB) Partnership to bring together government leaders, global health organizations, country-level health care providers, community and advocacy organizations, and other stakeholders to increase availability of and access to quality medication used to treat MDR-TB, enhance education for health care professionals in the most vulnerable areas, and raise awareness of the disease among at-risk communities. Experienced HIV and TB nurses train and develop their nursing colleagues and other CHWs to improve patient care delivery and increase treatment adherence.

Malaria

Approximately half of the world's population is at risk for malaria, although 90% of global cases and deaths stem from the sub-Saharan African region (WHO, 2016b). Like TB, malaria is preventable and easily treatable. Nurses can assist with prevention and treatment, and also train CHWs in order to reach a broader population. Key measures include:

1. Distribution of long-lasting insecticidal nets (LLINs)
2. Ensuring *targeted* spraying of insecticides, referred to as "indoor residual spraying"
3. Broad-based distribution of artemisinin-based combination therapies (ACTs), which are now the frontline treatment for malaria (Malaria No More, 2016)

A full one- to three-day course costs around $1 (Malaria No More, 2016). Moreover, nurses involved in policy can devote their efforts toward advocating for a larger portion of foreign aid to be allocated to malaria-endemic countries to further diminish the death counts related to this completely preventable disease. Nurses involved in research may wish to join the collaborative efforts taking place globally to develop a malaria vaccine, and then work to ensure its availability for the populations that need it the most.

SDG 3.4. By 2030, Reduce by One-Third Premature Mortality From Noncommunicable Diseases Through Prevention and Treatment and Promote Mental Health and Well-Being

NCDs kill 38 million people each year, which accounts for about 68% of the deaths in the world (WHO, 2016a)—a staggering figure. The most predominant NCDs include cardiovascular disease, cancer, diabetes, and chronic respiratory disease. The potential for nurses to contribute to the improvement in population health across the world through attention to chronic disease prevention and care has never been greater. There is clear and pervasive evidence (Kavanagh Cimiotti, Abusalem, & Coty, 2012) on the positive and measurable impact of nursing services concerning:

- Decreased length of stay
- Improved clinical outcomes
- Reduced inpatient mortality

- Increased access to care
- Increased productivity and efficiency
- Reduced societal health care costs
- Reduced adverse events

Nurses are involved in provision and coordination of care, chronic care management, and preventive services and have demonstrated provision of equal or better quality of care when compared to physicians in the management of chronic diseases in addition to preventive care and management of common acute illnesses in both inpatient and outpatient settings (Bryant-Lukosius & Martin-Misener, 2016; Stanik-Hutt et al., 2013).

The Global Action Plan for the Prevention and Control of NCDs 2013–2020, outlined and authorized at the May 2013 World Health Assembly, established guidelines for country-level implementation. The plan focuses on risk factors for tobacco use, alcohol consumption, physical inactivity, high sodium intake, obesity, diabetes, and hypertension. It also includes access goals for essential NCD medications, technologies, drug therapy, and counseling for those with existing conditions (WHO, 2016b).

Tobacco control is one such area where nurses can make a strong impact. WHO states that health professionals hold the trust of the population, the media, and opinion leaders, and their messages can potentially be spread across social, economic, and political arenas (WHO, 2005). Nurses can help patients and communities become educated regarding the harms of tobacco use and exposure to second-hand smoke. A Cochrane meta-analysis performed showed a positive effect for structured smoking cessation intervention by nurses, which was more effective than standard care or smoking abstinence (Rice, Hartmann-Boyce, & Stead, 2013). Nurses can begin to involve themselves in policy by promoting smoke-free workplaces and expand tobacco cessation resources at the community and societal levels, as well as contribute to national and global discussions regarding tobacco control efforts (WHO, 2005).

SDG 3.5. Strengthen the Prevention and Treatment of Substance Abuse, Including Narcotic Drug Abuse and Harmful Use of Alcohol

Coupled with tobacco, alcohol is also a large contributor to NCDs. In 2010, data from the Global Burden of Diseases, Injuries, and Risk Factors Study was used to estimate the burden of disease attributable to substance use disorders measured by percentage of disability-adjusted life years (DALYs). Illicit drug disorders accounted for 10.9% DALYs and alcohol use disorders for 9.6% DALYs (Whiteford et al., 2013). Nurses play significant roles in promoting activities to reduce common chronic disease development such as smoking cessation, responsible drinking of alcohol, regular exercise, maintenance of an appropriate weight and a healthy body mass index, and choosing food options that use unsaturated fats to lower disease risk such as vegetable oils, nuts, seeds, and fish, while avoiding trans fats and most saturated fats.

SDG 3.6. By 2020, Halve the Number of Global Deaths and Injuries From Road Traffic Accidents

Accidents and related injuries and deaths most often occur in poorer countries among vulnerable populations; injury and death can further impoverish the victims' families

(WHO, 2013). According to the WHO's *Global Status Report on Road Safety* (2013), helmet laws, seatbelts, child safety harnesses, and alcohol use are the leading global issues leading to decreased road safety. As mentioned previously, nurses can make an impact on alcohol prevention programs. Nurses have long been involved in car seat education for new parents, as well as educators for brain injury prevention programs in elementary schools. The National Injury Prevention Foundation, ThinkFirst© (2015), provides a wide range of injury prevention programs including bicycle and road safety. Founded by neurosurgeons, nurses serve on the board of directors and are customarily chapter leaders, both in the United States and internationally.

SDG 3.7. By 2030, Ensure Universal Access to Sexual and Reproductive Health Care Services, Including for Family Planning, Information and Education, and the Integration of Reproductive Health Into National Strategies and Programs

The NFP discussed earlier is an excellent example of a national strategy. The following section demonstrates how the Girl Child Education Fund (GCEF), an ICN initiative, affects family planning and education in an indirect way. Nurses have the capacity to implement programs such as these both within and beyond their own clinics and communities.

SDG 3.8. Achieve Universal Health Coverage, Including Financial Risk Protection, Access to Quality Essential Health Care Services and Access to Safe, Effective, Quality and Affordable Essential Medicines and Vaccines for All

Please see the section on universal health coverage later in this chapter.

SDG 3.9. By 2030, Substantially Reduce the Number of Deaths and Illnesses From Hazardous Chemicals and Air, Water, and Soil Pollution and Contamination

While this target is not commonly considered to be at the forefront of the nursing agenda, it is essential for nurses to realize the relationship and interconnection of environmental conditions and health. Environmental health is foundational to the values and ethics of nursing and an essential component of integrative—whole-person/whole-people—health and well-being. Nightingale was a staunch environmental activist and was clear about nursing's role (please see the following section, as well as Chapters 17, 23 to 26, and 29 for more details).

Links Between Global Nursing and the Remaining SDGs

Nurses are in a pivotal role to impact the social determinants of health for their patient populations. As defined by *Healthy People 2020*, social determinants of health are "conditions in which people are born, live, learn, work, play, worship, and age that affect a wide range of health, functioning, and quality-of-life outcomes and risks" (ODPHP, 2016). Social determinants included access to educational opportunities, economic opportunities, access to health care services, quality of education and job training, transportation options, public safety, language and literacy, socioeconomic conditions, residential segregation, and culture. Under the domain of physical determinants are things like natural or built environments, worksites, schools, recreational settings, exposure to physical hazards, physical barriers, and so on (ODPHP, 2016).

While it is clear that nurses will do most of their work within the realm of SDG 3, many of the other goals relate to health and will mitigate the effects of the social determinants such as: "SDG 1 No Poverty," "SDG 2 Zero Hunger," "SDG 4 Quality Education," "SDG 5 Gender Equality," "SDG 6 Clean Water and Sanitation," "SDG 8 Decent Work and Economic Growth," and "SDG 10 Reduced Inequalities." These goals are all very much interrelated and cannot easily be discussed as their own independent categories. (All goals are related to the broader domains of nursing, health, and the procurement of human dignity. See Part II of this book for a more in-depth discussion of nursing's involvement with all SDGs.) The WHO has declared poverty to be the single largest determinant of health. In nursing school, we learn that human beings cannot achieve health if they cannot achieve basic needs according to Maslow's hierarchy of needs (Maslow, 1943). We have all witnessed patients choosing between buying food or medicine. Poverty is one of the leading causes of death in the world, and is a major obstacle to social and economic development. Poverty directly affects hunger, education, and clean water. Decent work affects one's level of poverty and societal equality.

EXEMPLARS OF SDG ATTAINMENT PROMOTED BY THE ICN

Girl Child Education Fund

An exemplary illustration of the interconnected relationship among the SDGs, how they affect one another, and the power of the nursing profession can be seen from the remarkable results of the GCEF: an outcome related to the work of the Florence Nightingale International Foundation—the ICN's premier foundation. Due to infectious diseases such as HIV, TB, and malaria, in addition to poverty and natural and man-made disasters, premature death is occurring leaving behind millions of orphaned children, including those of nurses. GCEF works to support the orphaned daughters of nurses living in lower resource countries to go to school. They support the primary and secondary schooling of girls under the age of 18 in LMICs by paying for fees, uniforms, shoes, and books. Partners include NNAs who are members of the ICN to ensure that funds will go directly to pay for education. Each girl in the program is also paired with a nurse volunteer to monitor progress both at school and at home. Currently, 103 girls are being supported in Kenya, Swaziland, Uganda, and Zambia. Over 350 girls have been enrolled since the initiation of the program.

The education of girls saves children's lives, improves maternal health, raises incomes, lowers HIV/AIDS rates, reduces violence, and increases education for the whole family. According to the United Nations Educational, Scientific and Cultural Organization (UNESCO), each additional year that a mother goes to school will reduce the probability of infant mortality by 5% to 10%; and educating girls for 6 years or more drastically improves prenatal and postnatal care, as well as childbirth survival rates (UNESCO, 2011). Moreover, each additional year of education a girl has will delay the age at which a girl marries (Behrman, 2015; UNICEF, 2007) and will reduce the number of children she has (UNICEF, 2007).

Educating girls will raise lifetime incomes for themselves, their families, and their countries through direct or indirect means (Herz & Sperling, 2004; UNAC, 2012), such as increasing literacy rates, which will lead to further opportunities (Behrman, 2015). Girls who have 1 more year of education than their country's national average earn 10% to 20% more, and girls with secondary education have an 18% return in future wages, as compared to 14% for boys (Levine et al., 2009); an educated mother will also be more likely to send her children to school and her education will secure more resources for her entire household (United Nations Population Fund [UNPFA], n.d.). Increased education of girls contributes to increased health. Women with secondary education are five times more likely than illiterate women to be properly informed regarding HIV and AIDS (Vandemoortele & Delamonica, 2000), and a Ugandan study found that enrollment in secondary education significantly increased the likelihood that girls would abstain from sex (Alsan & Cutler, 2013). In addition, educated women are less likely to experience domestic violence, discrimination, and practices, such as female genital mutilation, and more likely to be the recipients of increased educational programs, economic empowerment, and community mobilization efforts (Ellsberg et al., 2015).

Nursing Mobile Library and Wellness Centers

ICN not only advocates for the education of orphaned daughters of nurses, but of nurses themselves. A mobile library was created to bring nursing and health resources to nurses working in remote areas of resource-constrained countries. The nursing mobile library serves to close the gap between the need and availability of health and medical information for nurses; deliver valid and current health care information for those with poor access to information; supplement training programs; promote health and prevent ill health in underserved regions; and foster and sustain lifelong learning for those nursing professionals who serve patients long distances from educational resource centers (ICN, 2015). Partnership with Merck & Co., Inc. provides ongoing funding and Elsevier Publishing oversees the packing and shipping of the libraries in durable trunks, which protects the resources and allows for transport over difficult terrains to individual clinics and wellness centers.

The ICN wellness centers for health care workers (HCWs) was first deployed in sub-Saharan Africa in 2006 as an African, nurse-led response to the hemorrhage of HCWs, especially nurses, due to the HIV pandemic, dysfunctional work environments, and out migration. Today, thanks to the determination and commitment of nurses and NNAs, the wellness centers in Swaziland, Lesotho, and Uganda together serve the needs of thousands of HCWs and their family members. The centers in Zambia, Malawi, and Ethiopia aspire to do the same. These facilities, and the nurses leading and serving them, have opened the door to improved physical and mental health for HCWs and their families, better retention practices, and, perhaps most importantly, a true sense of being valued as HCWs who toil daily on the front lines of fragile systems in Africa.

Additional Programs and Partnerships

The ICN is effective in its transnational initiatives and programs in collaboration with its investment and interprofessional partners for a wide variety of reasons. The clinical and technical expertise of the nursing staff is joined with policy experts to have the ability to advocate for nursing, patient, and health outcome issues on a global level. ICN has an intimate knowledge of global health care systems and is able to draw connections with how local systems can reach their potentials, as well as an understanding of the implementation challenges needing attention to cocreate quality health care system infrastructures. It is also essential to have a working knowledge of the functioning of local health departments, health commissioners, various boards, and hospital systems. The ICN also has access to the largest clinical profession in the world and makes understanding its members' needs a priority.

In addition to the GCEF, Lilly MDR-TB Partnership, and Nursing Mobile Library, the ICN supports a Global Nursing Leadership Institute, clinical skills programs for both HIV/AIDS and TB, wellness centers for HCWs in six different African countries, and an international eHealth work program. ICN has also advocated for safe work environments in conflict zones to reduce danger for HCWs and has joined the "Fight the Fakes" movement, which works to eliminate the distribution of counterfeit medications. The ICN has longstanding relationships with the International Labour Organization (ILO) to promote safe and equal labor conditions for HCWs; the International Council of Midwives (ICM) to collaborate on reducing maternal and child mortality on a global level; and has recently begun building a relationship with Women Deliver, a nonprofit organization dedicated to the rights of women and girls.

THE IMPORTANCE OF NURSE INVOLVEMENT IN POLICY

There are over 19 million nurses and midwives across the globe (Sarna et al., 2012) providing incredible care to the people they serve. While nursing can contribute significantly to the delivery of quality health care, our engagement with health services management, leadership at the local, district, state, national, and global levels is minimal and, often, totally absent. This major gap in the lack of nursing presence, voice, and contribution hinders the attainment of global health, social, and economic goals. Over the last several decades, we have made great progress in our academic education of nurses, the knowledge base we have gathered through research efforts, and the continually expanding implications of improved research capacity. In spite of these great achievements, we do not have the seats we should have at decision-making tables. As nurses, we must secure our seat at the policy table in order to have an impact on health care at the highest levels. We can no longer wait to be invited; we must make our presence known, our knowledge and skills visible, and consistently contribute our scholarly input to the global discussions at hand in equitable partnership with other health professions.

The ICN greatly reinforces the significance of strong relationships and connections with national, regional, and international nursing and non-nursing organizations. The ICN and its member NNAs' various affiliate groups and networks are working tirelessly to take nursing voices to those tables. Continuing to increase networks and creating more expansive and mutually beneficial bonds will place nurses in policy positions both now and in the future. The ICN's work with specialized agencies such as the UN system, in particular the WHO, the ILO, and the World Bank, are important for both nurses and health outcomes in all countries. As outlined earlier, ICN partners with several nongovernmental organizations as well. The ICN joins forces with other professional associations to strengthen the impact of our policy messages. For example, the ICN has joined the World Medical Association to publicly condemn the continued violence against health personnel in Syria and other nations; partnered with Johnson & Johnson and the Chinese Nurses Association to launch a "Leadership for Change" nurse training program in China; and held a joint event with the WHO to launch WHO's (2016e) Strategic Directions for Nursing & Midwifery 2016–2020.

Policy Briefs

Another way to become involved at the state, national, or global level to advocate for issues that are important to nursing, patients, and health care at large is to write and present policy briefs. A *policy brief* is a succinct document used to synthesize a large amount of research and evidence on a particular issue. They may include alternative policy options or an optimal recommendation for policy makers, in addition to policy implications. Policy briefs take on various formats and may include simple graphics, but the main objective is to grab the attention of policy makers who do not have the time to read long documents or research policy issues for themselves.

The ICN publishes several key briefs for various global policy issues, and recently has released many in relation to the *Global Strategy on Human Resources for Health 2030* (WHO, 2016f) and nursing's role within the strategy. They pertain to nursing leadership in primary health care (Tomblin-Murphy & Rose, n.d.) and contributions of nursing and midwifery enterprises in order to achieve the SDGs and *Global Strategy on Human Resources for Health 2030* (Salmon, n.d.); how the nursing workforce affects patient outcomes (Squires, White, & Sermeus, n.d.); and advanced practice nursing and its potential global contribution to sustainable health care (Bryant-Lukosius & Martin-Misener, 2016). With the emergence of the SDGs, nurses will have more opportunity than ever before to branch out into the public policy arena and bring their valuable perspective to areas such as education and the economy, linking these areas back to health.

GLOBAL STRATEGY ON HUMAN RESOURCES FOR HEALTH: WORKFORCE 2030

The ICN has been active in the field of human resources for decades. It is clearly understood that to advance health and social agendas, we need the right number of people at the right place with the right level of education, knowledge, and competencies that are required. More recently, the ICN has been very active in the development of a global strategy that was developed in response to a resolution passed at the 2014 World Health Assembly, which recognized the development of the SDGs and the importance of a global human resources for health (HRH) strategy to support this work. The strategy builds upon global evidence and experience, as well as broad-based consultation in the period 2013–2015 with experts at the regional, national, and global levels, and has been informed by thematic papers, six related global guidelines, policy commitments, and regional strategies and initiatives. The ICN was actively involved throughout this process, participating in the thematic work groups and commenting throughout the drafting of the strategy.

UHC is defined by WHO (2016d) as "ensuring that all people have access to needed promotive, preventive, curative, and rehabilitative health services, of sufficient quality to be effective, while also ensuring that people do not suffer financial hardship when paying for these services" (p. 1). We cannot achieve universal health care access globally without a sufficient health care workforce. The WHO's (2016d) targets to "achieve universal health coverage, including financial risk protection, access to quality essential health care services and access to safe, effective, quality and affordable essential medicines and vaccines for all" (p. 1) and "ensure universal access to sexual and reproductive health care services, including for family planning, information and education, and the integration of reproductive health into national strategies and programs" (p. 1) are especially impacted by the health care workforce. Universal access to sexual and reproductive health care services is key to achieving decreased pregnancy rates, decreased maternal mortality rates, improved adolescent health, and increased educational levels and socioeconomic status of girls globally. For example, although at the global level 76% of women of reproductive age had their family planning needs met with a modern method of contraception, wide disparities exist; 9 out 10 women in the WHO Western Pacific region had their family planning needs met, while less than half of those did in the WHO African region (WHO, 2016b).

High-Level UN Commission on Health Employment and Economic Growth

The global strategy led to the formation of a High-Level UN Commission on Health Employment and Economic Growth. The commission is essentially a political enterprise comprising international agencies and global partners brought together to combine expertise in policy, education, employment, health, labor, technical aspects, research, academia, and foreign affairs. The commission's expertise is needed to lessen the negative implications of a projected shortage of about 18 million health workers for the 40 million health sector jobs that the global economy will create by 2030. The deficit of HRH will be most notable in LMICs. The goals of the commission (WHO, 2016c) are to:

- Recommend multisector responses and institutional reforms to develop health and human resources capacity to achieve the SDGs over the next 15 years;
- Determine innovative financing sources and conditions needed to maximize socioeconomic returns from health and social sector employment investments;
- Analyze risks associated with global and regional imbalances and unequal distribution of health workers and assess the effects of international mobility; and
- Generate political commitment from governmental and other key partners to support the implementation of the commission's proposed action plan (WHO, 2016c).

The ICN is the only health professional group represented on this UN High Commission, which is chaired by the presidents of France and South Africa.

CONCLUSION

As the largest health care profession, nursing is in a powerful position to achieve UHC by impacting access to health care with nurse-led clinics, increasing numbers of nurse practitioners and other advanced practice nurses, and advocating for nurses at all levels to work to the full scope of their knowledge base. The demand for nursing will continue to grow as we look at meeting the demand in not only higher income countries who are members of the Organization for Economic Cooperation and Development (OECD), but especially in LMICs. A nursing education should offer great opportunity for women and youth who want to contribute to the workforce and have a respected, well-paid profession that will help them to lift their families and communities from poverty and offer meaningful service to many.

The strength, resilience, and ongoing success of the ICN is attributed to the fact that it is operated and led by nurses. Using global knowledge and talent, the ICN wields a transnational voice to offer policy solutions and influence health at the local, regional, and global levels. The synergy and partnership that the ICN brings to bear on the global issues, through the commitment and innovation of its members and NNAs, have been deeply influential in bringing about positive widespread change and will continue to yield enormous force. Nurses bring unique attributes to leadership positions owing to their understanding of health, human-centered care, and health systems across the entire spectrum of care. As providers with an influential role in advocating for the health of individuals and communities, nurses are essential and well positioned to lead and promote a healthier world for present and future generations. Further aligning our profession's goals with the SDGs and becoming involved with health and public policy initiatives will advance the overall well-being of our communities, nations, and world.

To achieve our potential contribution and build a healthier planet, we need to understand our roles and responsibilities both at the individual and collective levels. As individual nurses, we need to be aware and informed of the issues relevant to our communities and beyond. As professionals and members of a disciplinary collectivity, we need to do more than deliver great care. We need to advocate and voice our concerns to those who shape and make the decisions. Nurse educators need to broaden their educational focus from disease focus to health, policy, advocacy, and impact. Most nursing programs do not offer much in the field of population/global health, and almost no courses on health policy, politics, and advocacy. To assume our right position in the global arena, we need to educate ourselves differently. Finally, nursing organizations have to demand and advocate for seats at the right tables coupled with evidence-informed policy actions. Nursing organizations should also support nurses to consider careers in politics, policy, and governmental posts. We need to learn to be a forceful player outside of the "nursing bubble" and have a strong presence in the other health and social bubbles, as shown in Figure 10.1.

If we do not insert ourselves into the spheres of decision making beyond the nursing bubble, we will not be able to deliver on our commitment to nursing and health, nor fulfill our potential roles in achieving and realizing the safe and inclusive world called for by the SDGs. The ICN is committed to being a leading-edge voice on the global scene and, together with our national and other nursing partners, we are confident that we will be able to shape future health agendas while elevating the unique contributions and impact of the global nursing profession at large.

| Figure 10.1 | "Bubble theory" and spheres of policy influence: Conceptual elements of an evolving nursing policy model. |

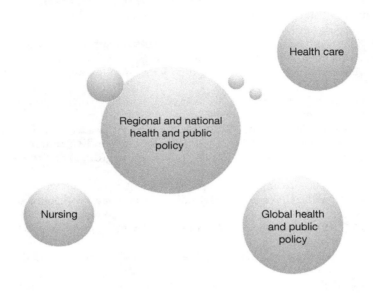

Source: Shamian (2014). Reprinted with permission.

REFLECTION AND DISCUSSION

- How do the SDGs differ from the MDGs? What do these differences change for the nursing profession?
- How does ICN's vision and goals compare and contrast to other international nursing organizations such as Sigma Theta Tau International?
- What are nursing's potential contributions to the achievement of the SDGs? Do contributions differ from high-income to low- to middle-income countries?
- What is a policy brief? What issue would I choose to address given the opportunity to author a brief? Based on my issue, would I address policymakers at the local, state, national, or global level?
- What can I do locally, in my current academic or clinical environment, to promote and participate in global health?

ACKNOWLEDGMENT

The authors would like to acknowledge the ICN staff for their extremely hard work and continued support during the development of this chapter.

REFERENCES

Abrahams-Gessel, S., Denman, C. A., Gaziano, T. A., Levitt, N. S., & Puoane, T. (2016). Challenges facing successful scaling up of effective screening for cardiovascular disease by community health workers in Mexico and South Africa: Policy implications. *Health Systems Policy Research, 3*(1), 26–35.

Adetiloye, O. (2011). Innovative community volunteer program increases follow-up care of HIV/AIDS clients in Nigeria. Retrieved from https://www.jhpiego.org/success-story/innovative-community-volunteer-program-increases-follow-up-care-of-hivaids-clients-in-nigeria

Alsan, M. M., & Cutler, D. M. (2013). Girls' education and HIV risk: Evidence from Uganda. *Journal of Health Economics, 32*(5), 863–872.

American Public Health Association. (2013). *The definition and practice of public health nursing: A statement of the public health nursing section.* Washington, DC: Author. Retrieved from https://www.apha.org/~/media/files/pdf/membergroups/phn/nursingdefinition.ashx

Behrman, J. A. (2015). The effect of increased primary schooling on adult women's HIV status in Malawi and Uganda: Universal primary education as a natural experiment. *Social Science & Medicine, 127*, 108–115.

Breda, K. L. (2012). What is nursing's role in international and global health? *Texto Contexto Enferm, 21*(3), 491–492.

Bridges, D. (1967). *A history of the international council of nurses 1899–1964.* London, UK: Pitman Medical.

Brondi, L. (2011). Fighting TB in Mozambique: Jhpiego offers a comprehensive approach. Retrieved from www.jhpiego.or/success-story/fighting-tb-in-mozambique-jhpiego-offers-a-comprehensive-approach

Brown, T. M., Cueto, M., & Fee, E. (2006). The World Health Organization and the transition from "international" to "global" public health. *American Journal of Public Health, 96*, 62–72.

Bryant-Lukosius, D., & Martin-Misener, R. (2016). *Advanced practice nursing: An essential component of country level human resources for health.* Geneva, Switzerland: ICN Policy Brief.

Ellsberg, M., Arango, D. J., Morton, M., Gennari, F., Kiplesund, S., Contreras, M., & Watts, C. (2015). Prevention of violence against women and girls: What does the evidence say? *Lancet, 385*, 1555–1566.

Goyal, N. K., Hall, E. S., Jones, D. E., Meinzen-Derr, J. K., Short, J. A., Ammerman, R. T., & Van Ginkel, J. B. (2014). Association of maternal and community factors with enrollment in home visiting among at-risk, first-time mothers. *American Journal of Public Health, 104*(Suppl. 1), S144–S151.

Hansen, K. (2016). Breastfeeding: A smart investment in people and in economies. *The Lancet, 387*(10017), 416.

Herz, B., & Sperling, G. B. (2004). *What works in girls' education: Evidence and policies from the developing world.* New York, NY: Council on Foreign Relations.

International Council of Nurses. (2002). Definition of nursing. Retrieved from http://www.icn.ch/who-we-are/icn-definition-of-nursing

International Council of Nurses. (2015). Nursing Mobile Library: Aims and goals. Retrieved from http://www.icn.ch/what-we-do/aim-and-goals

International Council of Nurses Online. (2015). Vaccination module. Retrieved from http://www.icn.ch/images/stories/documents/pillars/Practice/Communicable_Disease/ICN_Vaccination_Module/story_html5.html

Jack, S. M., Catherine, N., Gonzalez, A., MacMillan, H. L., Sheehan, D., & Waddell, C. (2015). Adapting, piloting and evaluating complex public health interventions: Lessons learned from the Nurse-Family Partnership in Canadian public health settings. *Health Promotion and Chronic Disease Prevention in Canada, 35*(8/9), 151–159.

Jhpiego Corporation. (2015). Fighting malaria in pregnancy through community health workers in Rwanda. Retrieved from https://www.jhpiego.org/success-story/fighting-malaria-in-pregnancy-through-community-health-workers-in-rwanda

Jhpiego Corporation. (2016). What to do about tuberculosis in pregnancy. Retrieved from https://www.jhpiego.org/success-story/what-to-do-about-tuberculosis-in-pregnancy

Kalemba, N., & Bundula, M. (2015). You can't fight malaria without community health workers. Retrieved from https://www.jhpiego.org/success-story/you-cant-fight-malaria-without-community-health-workers

Kavanagh, K. T., Cimiotti, J. P., Abusalem, S., & Coty, M. B. (2012). Moving healthcare quality forward with nursing-sensitive value-based purchasing. *Journal of Nursing Scholarship*, 44(4), 385–395.

Koplan, J. P., Bond, T. C., Merson, M. H., Reddy, K. S., Rodriguez, M. H., Sewankambo, N. K., & Wasserheit, J. N. (2009). Towards a common definition of global health. *The Lancet*, 373(9679), 1993–1995.

Levine, R., Lloyd, C. B., Greene, M., & Grown, C. (2008). Girls count: A global investment and action agenda. Washington, DC: The Center for Global Development.

London, J. W. (2016). Fall in 1:1 nursing ratios in neonatal ICUs is linked to higher death rate. *British Medical Journal*, 352, i828. doi:10.1136/bmj.i828

Malaria No More. (2016). The solution: We have the tools to end deaths from malaria. Retrieved from http://www.malarianomore.org/pages/the-solution

Maslow, A. (1943). A theory of human motivation. *Psychological Review, 50*, 370–396.

Millennium Project. (2006). UN Development Group 2002–2006. Retrieved from http://www.unmillenniumproject.org/goals

Mlacha, Z. (2015). Breaking barriers to bring comprehensive HIV services to vulnerable women. Retrieved from https://www.jhpiego.org/success-story/breaking-barriers-to-bring-comprehensive-hiv-services-to-vulnerable-women

Morgah, K., Bonguirada, B., & Gamabe, O. (2013). Community health workers lead activities to defeat malaria in the village of Miandoum in southern Chad. Retrieved from https://www.jhpiego.org.success-story/community-health-workers-lead-activities-to-defeat-malaria-in-the-village-of-miandoum-in-southern-chad

Mwaura, S., & Njenga, S. (2016). Adherence to TB drugs is key to being TB-free. Retrieved from https://www.jhpiego.org/success-story/adherence-tb-drugs-key-tb-free

Nurse Family Partnership. (2015). Public Policy Agenda: 114th Congress, 2nd Session. February 2016. Retrieved from http://www.nursefamilypartnership.org/getattachment/public-policy/2016-NFP-Public-Policy-AgendaNEW.pdf.aspx

Office of Disease Prevention and Health Promotion. (2016). Social determinants of health. Retrieved from http://www.healthypeople.gov/2020/topics-objectives/topic/social-determinant-of-health

Olds, D. L., Kitzman, H., Knudtson, M. D., Anson, E., Smith, J. A., & Cole, R. (2014). Effect of home visiting by nurses on maternal and child mortality: Results of a 2-decade follow-up of a randomized clinical trial. *JAMA Pediatrics*, 168(9), 800–806. doi:10.1001/jamapediatrics.2014.472

Ozawa, S., Mirelman, A., Stack, M. L., Walker, D. G., & Levine, O. S. (2012). Cost-effectiveness and economic benefits of vaccines in low-and middle-income countries: A systematic review. *Vaccine, 31*, 96–108.

Rice, V. H., Hartmann-Boyce, J., & Stead, L. F. (2013). Nursing interventions for smoking cessation. *Cochrane Database of Systematic Reviews*, (8). doi:10.1002/14651858.CD001188.pub4

Rollins, N. C., Bhandari, N., Hajeebhoy, N., Horton, S., Lutter, C. K., Martines, J. C., . . . The Lance Breastfeeding Series Group. (2016). Why invest, and what it will take to improve breastfeeding practices. *The Lancet, 387*, 491–504.

Salmon, M. (n.d.). *Contributions of nursing and midwifery enterprises to achievement of human resources for health targets and sustainable development goals*. Geneva, Switzerland: ICN Policy Brief.

Sarna, L., Wolf, L., & Bialous, S. A. (2012). Enhancing nursing and midwifery capacity to contribute to the prevention, treatment, and management of non-communicable diseases. *Human Resources for Health Observer*, (12). Retrieved from http://www.who.int/hrh/resources/observer12.pdf

Shamian, J. (2014). Global perspectives on nursing and its contribution to healthcare and health policy: Thoughts on an emerging policy model. *Canadian Journal of Nursing Leadership*, 27(4), 44–50.

Shamian, J., Tomblin-Murphy, G., Rose, A. E., & Jeffs, L. P. (2015a). Human resources for health: A new narrative. *The Lancet, 386*(9988), 25–26.

Shamian, J., Tomblin-Murphy, G., Rose, A. E., & Jeffs, L. P. (2015b). No global health without human resources for health (HRH): The nursing lens. *Canadian Journal of Nursing Leadership, 28*(1), 1–5.

Shearer, J. C., Walker, D. G., Risko, N., & Levine, O. S. (2012). The impact of new vaccine introduction on the coverage of existing vaccines: A cross-national, multivariable analysis. *Vaccine, 30*(52), 7582–7587.

Sigma Theta Tau International. (2016). STTI's global initiatives. Retrieved from http://www.nursingsociety.org/connect-engage/our-global-impact/stti's-global-initiatives

Squires, A., White, J., & Sermeus, W. (n.d.). *Quantity, quality, and relevance of the nursing workforce to patient outcomes.* Geneva, Switzerland: ICN Policy Brief.

Stanik-Hutt, J., Newhouse, R. P., White, K. M., Johantgen, M., Bass, E. B., Zangaro, G., . . . Weiner, J. P. (2013). The quality and effectiveness of care provided by nurse practitioners. *Journal of Nurse Practitioners, 9*(8), 492–500.

ThinkFirst. (2015). *ThinkFirst. National Injury Prevention Foundation.* Retrieved from http://thinkfirst.org

Tomblin-Murphy, G., & Rose, A. E. (n.d.). Nursing leadership in primary health care for the achievement of sustainable development goals and human resources for health global strategies. Geneva, Switzerland: ICN Policy Brief.

UNAC. (2012). Why invest in adolescent girls? Retrieved from http://www.clintonglobalinitiative.org/ourmeetings/PDF/actionareas/Why_Invest_in_Adolescent_Girls.pdf

United Nations Development Programme. (2016). UNDP support to the implementation of the 2030 agenda for sustainable development. Retrieved from http://www.undp.org/content/undp/en/home/librarypage/sustainable-development-goals/undp-support-to-the-implementation-of-the-2030-agenda

United Nations Educational, Scientific and Cultural Organization. (2011). *Education counts towards the millennium development goals.* Paris, France: Author.

United Nations International Children's Fund. (2007). *The state of the world's children 2007.* New York, NY: Author.

United Nations Population Fund. (n.d.). The education factor. Retrieved from http://www.unfpa.org/resources/education-factor

Vandemoortele, J., & Delamonica, E. (2000). The "education vaccine" against HIV. *Current Issues in Comparative Education, 3*(1), 6–13.

Vega, J. (2013). Universal health coverage: The post-2015 development agenda. *The Lancet, 381*(9862), 179–180.

Victora, C. G., Bahl, R., Barros, A. J. D., França, G. V., Horton, S., Krasevec, J . . . Rollins, N. C. (2016). Breastfeeding in the 21st century: Epidemiology, mechanisms, and lifelong effects. *The Lancet, 387,* 475–490.

Whiteford, H. A., Degenhardt, L., Rehm, J., Baxter, A. J., Ferrari, A. J., Erskine, H. E., . . . Vos., T. (2013). Global burden of disease attributable to mental and substance use disorders: Findings from the Global Burden of Disease Study 2010. *Lancet, 382,* 1575–1586.

World Health Organization. (2005). *WHO tobacco free initiative: The role of health professionals in tobacco control.* Geneva, Switzerland: Author. Retrieved from http://www.who.int/tobacco/resources/publications/wntd/2005/bookletfinal_20april.pdf

World Health Organization. (2007). *Community health workers: What do we know about them?* (Policy Brief). Geneva, Switzerland: Author. Retrieved from http://www.who.int/hrh/documents/community_health_workers_brief.pdf

World Health Organization. (2012). WHO recommendations on prevention and treatment of postpartum haemorrhage: Highlights and key messages from new 2012 global recommendations. Retrieved from http://apps.who.int/iris/bitstream/10665/120082/1/WHO_RHR_14.20_eng.pdf?ua=1&ua=1

World Health Organization. (2013). *Global status report on road safety 2013: Supporting a decade of action.* Geneva, Switzerland: Author.

World Health Organization. (2014). *WHO Global Nutrition Targets 2025* (Anaemia Policy Brief). Retrieved from http://www.who.int/nutrition/topics/globaltargets_anaemia_policybrief.pdf?ua=1&ua=1

World Health Organization. (2015). *WHO global strategy on people-centred and integrated health services* (Interim report). Retrieved from http://apps.who.in/iris/bitstream/10665/155002/1/WHO_HIS_SDS_2015.6_eng.pdf?ua=1

World Health Organization. (2016a). Regional Office for Europe: Poverty and social determinants. Retrieved from http://www.euro.who.int/en/health-topics/environment-and-health/urban-health/activities/poverty-and-social-determinants

World Health Organization. (2016b). *World Health Statistics 2016: Monitoring health for the SDGs (sustainable development goals)*. Retrieved from http://www.who.int/gho/publications/world_health_statistics/2016/en

World Health Organization. (2016c). Health workforce: High-level commission on health employment and economic growth. Retrieved from http://www.who.int/hrh/com-heeg/en

World Health Organization. (2016d). Health systems: Universal health coverage. Retrieved from http://www.who.int/healthsystems/universal_health_coverage/en

World Health Organization. (2016e). *Global strategic directions for strenghtening nursing and midwifery 2016–2020*. Geneva, Switzerland: Author. Retrieved from http://www.who.int/hrh/nursing_midwifery/global-strategic-midwifery2016-2020.pdf

World Health Organization. (2016f). Global strategy on human resources for health: Workforce 2030. Draft for the 69th World Health Assembly. Retrieved from http://www.who.int/hrh/resources/global_strategy2030en-printversion.pdf?ua=1

World Health Organization. (2017). Maternal, newborn, child, and adolescent health: The case for midwifery. Retrieved from http://www.who.int/maternal_child_adolescent/topics/quality-of-care/midwifery/case-for-midwifery/en

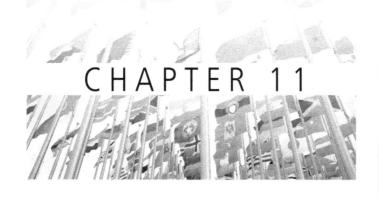

CHAPTER 11

Global Human Caring for a Sustainable World[1]

Jean Watson

While much of political and media discussion on the journey toward more sustainable societies is concerned with technology and policy, there are deeper matters of philosophy and values that we must address.

—Tony Juniper (Kumar, 2015)

NURSING AND THE UNITED NATIONS 2030 AGENDA: GLOBAL HUMAN CARING–HEALING–HEALTH AND PEACE

Nursing is the largest health care profession worldwide. According to World Health Organization's (WHO, 2016) data, there are 20.7 million nurses and midwives in the world. Since the early blueprint of Nightingale, nursing has sustained its mission of compassionate, caring service to humankind, but often unseen, behind the scenes.

At the same time, once uncovered, there are nursing programs and activities occurring worldwide. Nurses are actively, quietly, sometimes often unknowingly, carrying out the United Nations' (UN) vision, mission, and knowledge platform for sustaining Humanity and Planet Earth. The 30-year UN major goals, the Millennium Development Goals (MDGs; 2000–2015) and Sustainable Development Goals (SDGs; 2015–2030), could be substituted for global nursing's timeless actions of sacred human caring–healing services, committed to health care of all.

This chapter focuses on Human Caring and Peace within the context of global nursing embedded in a framework of Caring Science and *Caritas* (Latin word, conveying universal caring and love). Nursing's practice of human caring is an emergent quality of whole systems, making new connections between the unitary energetic patterns of worldwide human caring practices and peace in our world. This relationship between Human Caring and Peace represents a fundamental

---

[1] *Source:* Parts of this chapter have been reprinted with slight modifications by permission of Oxford University Press. From Watson (2016).

path of consciously attending to the pattern of unity and the human–environmental global–universal field of oneness of all.

This unitary relationship with universal, globally informed principles represents what may be referred to as a "quantum world," or even a "quantum cosmology." That is, we now know from science and quantum thinking that the mere act of participating in, or observing a system, causes a system to change its behavior. "Some physicists have postulated that there is something special about (caring) consciousness (and its high vibration), that causes the 'abstract' quantum potentials, described by quantum theory, to 'collapse' into hard physical reality observed in the everyday world" (Vieten, 2012, p. 6). In a quantum world everything is connected: wholeness of all, as discussed in the writings of David Bohm (1980a, 1980b; Bohm & Peat, 1987).

CARING SCIENCE, GLOBAL NURSING, CARING, AND PEACE

Caring Science, as an emerging area of nursing and transdisciplinary study, grounds this expanded, quantum worldview related to global principles and acknowledges a deeper Ethic of "BELONGING" (Levinas, 1969; Watson, 2008) making explicit that we all *belong* to the infinity and universal cosmic energetic (quantum) field of the whole. This core principle becomes a fundamental worldview, or even more encompassing, a cosmology, as a starting point for science, universal values, and, principles, for our global society. Thus, the Ethic of Belonging helps us to understand the universal cocreative relationship between nurses' conscious intentional human caring acts and actions and the emergence of wholeness for all; thus, human caring and peace is one simultaneous individual and global act.

Consistent with this Caring Science ethic phenomenon and line of unitary, quantum thinking, a 2011 research study (on potential for peace between Israelis and Palestinians) affirmed one of the basic Integrative Principles relevant to Unitary and Planetary Health: "Health (and Peace) can be recognized as an ever-changing pattern of creative, adaptive relationships across all dimensions of human experience" (Kreitzer & Koithan, 2011, p.1). That is, this research found that simply teaching Israelis and Palestinians that groups of people are generally capable of change can have a markedly positive effect on their willingness to change and compromise. Indeed, in an Israeli national study, many Israeli Jews,

> believed that groups could change, the more favorable were their attitudes toward Palestinians—and the more willing they were to make major compromises for the sake of peace. These included joint sovereignty over holy places in Jerusalem. . . . When the researchers repeated this study with Palestinians—both within Israel and the West Bank—they found identical results. . . . [The] researchers have already repeated the study in Cyprus— another area with a longstanding political conflict—with promising results). (McClure, 2011)

This line of thinking is congruent with an emergent quality of whole systems within the framework of quantum principles and Caring Science, underpinning the dynamics of Caring and Peace—a truly global paradigm. That is, the consciousness of "believing in change" energetically can affect the quantum field,

resulting in concrete connections between two groups, including a change of attitude for adaptive relationships, acknowledging the fundamental unity within,
and between, all beings and their environments.

The work of David Hawkins, *Power vs Force* (2002), also helps to ground the
Caring Science Ethic of Belonging, along with quantum principles of the power
of Human Spirit and its relationship to the evolution of consciousness. That is,
these unitary principles are related to pure consciousness in the universe, to which
we all Belong, and point toward options for how to access and manifest energetic
(Caring) consciousness patterns that affect the whole. This evolution of higher
(Caring) consciousness is the source of True Power from David Hawkins's work
(2002), in that one is connecting with the universal life force, the infinite energetic field of the cosmos. Thus, in the evolutionary Unitary Caring Science model,
everything is connected energetically; thus, if one holds Love and Caring as their
intentionality and energetic field of consciousness, the one caring is affecting the
whole of humanity, thus contributing subliminally to peace in our world. This is
an example of evolving consciousness for humanity, within a unitary worldview,
a quantum universe and an Ethic of Belonging, underlying Caring Science, which
unites all of humanity and the universe.

This foundational quantum principle of unity and consciousness affects
human–environmental field practices in our world today. The subtle, and not-so-
subtle, connection between Caring and energetic healing, ultimately leads to connections between Caring and Peace. That is, if one is manifesting, energetically
and authentically, a Caring Consciousness, then that person is radiating Love and
Peace into the Unitary field of the whole.

As Hawkins (2002) noted, if we really understood this basic knowledge, the
world as we know it would be irrevocably changed, requiring all practices of politics, war, communications, media, economics, and other fields, including medicine, to transform its consciousness and patterns of practices. That is what Global
and Planetary thinking begins to tap into for our human evolution.

Underlying some of the principles of quantum thinking and Unitary Caring
Science resides Levinas's premise: Ethics (of Belonging) as the first principle of
Science. So, in Unitary Caring Science and the quantum principle model, everything is connected with the infinite universal energetic field of cosmic Love. Basic
human values of Loving–Kindness, Equanimity, Compassion, Forgiveness, and
Tolerance, all messages from wisdom teachers, spiritual leaders and sages across
time, are embedded in the faces of our global community. The global community
to which we all Belong, and to the human caring practices, inform the history and
tradition of nursing and other health and human service professions.

These global and universal messages and values also are embedded in extant
theories, contemporary science, and philosophies guiding human caring and healing for self, other, and our world. For example, the writings of contemporary nursing theorists, such as Martha Rogers, Margaret Newman, Rosemary Parse, Barbara
Dossey, and others (Watson) all converge around some core ontological and episte-
mological unitary transformative principles. They include, for example:

- Unity world views—everything is connected
- Transcendent possibilities for human experiences, while acknowledging
  we are full embodied—(thus immanent and transcendent views of
  humanity)

- Patterns and Processes of relativity of time and space, and one's intentionality
- Evolving Consciousness
- Energetic field of Human–Environment–Cosmos Oneness

Other national U.S. research institutes, such as Fetzer Institute, University of Minnesota Center for Spirituality and Healing, Institute of Notice Sciences, Institute of HeartMath, Cleveland Clinic Heart Brain Institute, The Templeton Foundation, and others are pursuing research models that reside within ontology of a unitary, quantum worldview.

Hawkins (2002) reported that conventional medicine, associated with physical pathology and disease, resides in a lower vibration field and does not allow for evolution of human consciousness to a higher energetic field. Unitary, quantum, human caring connections come from higher vibrational fields, associated with nonlocality, nonphysical domains, such as attitude, one's intentionality, and consciousness of positive, higher vibration emotions, and mental thoughts (e.g., Gratitude, Forgiveness, Grace, Caring, Compassion, Love, and practices of Rituals, Prayer, Spiritual Beliefs of Hope and Faith), all higher consciousness processes and practices that unify physical and nonphysicality as one.

The next turn, perhaps, in unitary nursing principles is to go beyond the dense lower vibrations of exclusive physicality with separation from the energetic–spirit field, to systematically include consciousness, intentionality, and spiritual–energetic nonphysical planes for whole person health, healing, caring, and peace. Unitary nursing principles thus move energetically from human caring to ecocaring, to global universal caring, proclaiming caring and peaceful relations as one way forward, toward honoring all living things in order to evolve, survive, and sustain humanity and Planet Earth.

LOVE, THE HIGHEST LEVEL OF CONSCIOUSNESS: CARITAS (CARING–LOVE) CONSCIOUSNESS FOR PEACE

Margaret Newman, the prominent nursing theorist, who focused on consciousness and quantum patterns as context for healing, titled one of her books, *Health as Expanding Consciousness* (Newman, 1994). So I pose the question for Global Nursing, related to Caring Science, Ethic of Belonging, and Newman's and Hawkins's theories and research: What is the highest level of consciousness?

My answer is LOVE, now considered a higher calibration of unitary consciousness evolution that incorporates Levinas's Ethic of Belonging with the Infinite field of Universal cosmic Love, which unites all.

Ben Okri, the prize winning Nigerian writer, put it this way:

> Individual authenticity lies in what we can find that is worth living for. And the only thing worth living for is love. Love of one another. Love for ourselves. Love of our work. Love of our destiny, whatever it may be. Love for our difficulties. Love of life. The love that could free us from the mysterious cycles of suffering. The love that releases us from our self-imprisonment, from our bitterness, our greed, our madness–engendering

competiveness. The love that can make us breathe again. Love a great and beautiful cause, a wonderful vision. A great love for another, or for the future. The love that reconciles us to ourselves, to our simple joys, and to our undiscovered repletion. A creative love. A love touched with the sublime. (Okri, 1997, pp. 56–57)

Thus, Infinite Love: the highest level of Caritas Consciousness, uniting humanity across continents, worlds, and time, is revealed through a reflective unitary and global nursing context. This relationship, as revealed through heart-centered practices, restores the universality of human tasks and universal connections. Human-to-human, spirit-to-spirit connections, beginning with inner caring and inner peace, radiating out to others, returning us to the heart of healing and peace in our world.

We as nurses practicing unitary global nursing principles know that when we step into the theories and philosophies of human caring, and Caritas (Caring and Unitive Love), we step into a deep ethic and life practice that connects us with the heart of our humanity, of healing the whole; it is here in this connection we touch the mystery of inner and outer peace that unites humanity across time and space around the world. This expanded worldview, indeed evolving cosmology, raises new questions and offers new connections between personal and planetary transformation related to caring, peace, and the power of Love. Such core perspectives from Unitary Caring Science and quantum principles introduce caring as an ethical covenant with humanity.

Within the context of Global Nursing, Caritas Consciousness asks and invites new questions about Caring and Peace:

> What is peace?
>
> What is the origin of peace?
>
> What is inner peace? How do we obtain it?
>
> How do we manifest and sustain human caring and peace in our hearts, minds, and daily acts?
>
> Is there a connection between inner peace and outer peace?

These foundational, yet rhetorical questions reside within philosophical, ethical, and practical ideals from the Latin notion of Caritas and Caring Science. This focus brings together principles and practices that invite us to consider our common tasks as humans on Planet Earth in order to sustain human dignity, basic civility, and humanity itself.

WATSON CARING SCIENCE INSTITUTE AND SELECTED UN SDGs

This chapter uncovers a few specific global nursing and health professional projects, supportive of the UN SDGs. These projects are sponsored by Watson Caring Science Institute (WCSI)—a nonprofit U.S. organization with international projects and programs (www.watsoncaringscience.org). The active programs of WCSI act from a vision of global awakening of humanity, toward Oneness, integrating Caritas (loving caring compassion) with "Communitas" (Oneness of all of humanity—universe)—a Global Moral Community of Caring—Healing and Peace for *all*.

For example, WCSI goals include:

- Transforming the dominant model of medical science to a model of Caring Science by reintroducing the ethic, philosophy, and diverse practices of caring and Love (Caritas–Communitas) necessary for health/healing (SDG 3: Health and well-being);
- Deepening the authentic Caring–Healing relationships between caregiver and patient/family, to restore Love and compassion as the ethical, values foundation of health care. (SDGs 3: Health and well-being; 10: Reduce inequalities; 16: Peace/inclusivity and justice);
- Restoring the profound nature of caring–healing within a unitary caring science framework (SDGs 3: Health and well-being; 4: Inclusive education);
- Being in stewardship to the health care system worldwide, to retain and nurture its most precious resource, caring professional nurses and transdisciplinary care team members (SDGs 4 and 5: Inclusive equitable education—lifelong learning and gender equality; 10: Reduce country inequality; 16: Inclusive institutions at all levels; 17: Partnerships for sustainable development).

Congruent with UN action goals for sustainability, WCSI lives out its mission through specific action programs and projects to deepen and expand Caring Science as an evolved view of Science. Thus, it is guided by timeless core values, philosophies, theories, and ethics, honoring all of humankind via humane practices of Human Caring—between and among nurses, the public, and with all whom each touches, even though "Other" is often perceived as enemy.

WCSI GLOBAL PROGRAMS/PROJECTS ALIGNED WITH UN SUSTAINABLE DEVELOPMENT AGENDA

> "As humanity hangs on a precipice, we need shifts that can be made by each of us, with far reaching implications for the planet and all people." (Vandana Shiva)

While the UN 2030 agenda is a plan of action for People, Planet, and Prosperity, it also seeks connections between broader issues, including health and universal peace. Beyond the SDGs, there is increased recognition about the importance of global health for all health professionals and especially the role and contribution of nurses and midwives in achieving global health goals.

WCSI programs and projects encompass global core values—loving kindness, compassion for self/other, preserving human dignity, creating trusting–caring relationships, honoring unity and diversity of the Whole Person–Health–Healing environments and Planet Earth as One. These WCSI projects, ethically and philosophically led activities in human caring–healing, are cocreating moral communities of caring, contributing to broad UN goals addressing Well-Being, Moral Justice, Equity, Equality, and, ultimately, Peace for a troubled humankind. WSCI's transnational work can be highlighted as exemplars of the specific UN SDGs for 2030.

For example, since the 2008 creation of the nonprofit WCSI, Dr. Jean Watson, founder, and her local/global partners, have held a vision and mission toward serving nurses around the world. It does so through formal intellectual and expe-riential programs, conferences, and workshops in Caring Science theory and practice–research programs. Each WCSI program offers opportunities for nurses to come together to learn more deeply the art and science of human caring and healing. Together they learn to understand the universality of human caring–heal-ing–health that nurses offer to humanity and the world, ultimately living out the Oneness between human caring and peace.

The following WCSI global projects support UN goals as examples:

- I: Middle East Nurses and Partners Uniting in Human Caring
- II: International Global Caritas Consortia: Japan, 2012; South Africa, 2015; China, 2016.
  - 2012 Hiroshima, Japan: WCSI, 2012 International Caring and Peace; 2015 Japan: International Society for Caring and Peace, Tokyo;
  - 2015 South Africa Consortium: Johannesburg *Ubuntu* Universal Caring
  - 2015 China Global Consortium: East Meets West—Soul and Science Unite in Human Caring
  - 2017 Latin America Global Consortium: projected
- III: Watson Caring Science Global Associates: Partnering for global connections worldwide—sharing programs, research, curricula, and faculty–student networking (www.watsoncaringscience.org)

While each of the above global projects and programs are examples of UN goals from the world of nursing and the Watson Caring Science Institute, the one that is perhaps most pressing and important is the Middle Eastern Nurses Project in Human Caring.

UN–WCSI Project: Middle East Nurses and Partners Uniting in Human Caring

WCSI's Middle East Nurses and Partners Uniting in Human Caring consists of a series of conferences that originated in 2012 in Jaffe, Israel at the Peres Peace foundation. It began with a small, private gathering of Palestinian and Israeli nurses who wanted to come together in safe space with Dr. Watson to explore their common unity toward human caring between and among each other, often seen among each other as the "other"—thus the enemy.

However, these nurses came together with a common, courageous, unifying bond and a common commitment of human caring for all their patients, families, and community. These individuals were transcending conflicts, war, and life dif-ferences between them; taking risks, going beyond borders, boundaries, religions, and cultural differences to come together as colleagues and professionals, united in human caring, health, and healing for all.

From this small beginning emerged the WCSI sponsorship of annual International Middle Eastern Conferences held in Jordan since 2013. These are held in partnership with Healing HealthCare, USA (www.healinghealth.com) and Nurses and Partners in the Middle East.

These annual events have created a safe forum and safe passage in Jordan, for all Middle Eastern nurses and health professionals, especially Palestinian nurses, to gather together personally and professionally with Israeli and diverse religious and cultural practices and beliefs. As such, they get to know each other, person to person, nurse to nurse, aligning with shared goals and hopes, uniting in the universality of human caring by transcending separating worldview imprints and dominant political and media views of "Other as Enemy."

This Middle East Nurses Project continues to bring together nurses and health professionals under a shared commitment to offer knowledgeable, compassionate human caring to our global society. For example, this forum is the only professional development forum that allows Palestinian and Israeli nurses to meet safely, face to face, for shared goals, and commitment to better serve both their citizens and diverse people.

As a result of these gatherings, and through the opportunities for this diverse group to unite, a variety of position papers have been developed from the Middle Eastern Nurse Conferences. The position papers identify and propose constructive caring action steps, agreed to by the Middle Eastern Nurses, helping to resolve conflict issues. Thus, these actions of unity are contributing to Peace, at the grassroots level.

See Boxes 11.1 through 11.4 for the Middle Eastern Nursing Uniting in Human Caring position papers. Please note these positions were adopted in 2015 in line with the UN MDGs. However, the positions papers, guided by Human Caring values and philosophies toward humanity, remain current and highly relevant for the current UN 2030 Platform for Sustainable Development. They continue to guide the work of the Nurses in the Middle East and WCSI Middle Eastern Nurses and Partners Uniting in Human Caring.

Box 11.1 Nursing Work in the Global Community: Challenges and Opportunities

In understanding the issues that face our communities globally today, we, as nurses, recognize that we are the Leaders, the Educators, and the Caregivers not only to our local communities, but to the world. By aligning ourselves with the UN Millennium Goals, we recognize the challenges and opportunities that face us in our society today. And it is our hope that through education, leadership, and communication we can transcend the barriers that are presented to us to create a healing environment locally, nationally, and internationally.

In keeping with the UN Millennium Goals, we, the Nurses in the Middle East (NME) of the Watson Caring Science Institute, recognize the following challenges:

- Access to health care is hindered by inadequate delivery systems; cultural and governmental barriers to quality health care; and a worldwide shortage of Qualified Health Care Providers.
- There is an absence of education within the global community, not just of mothers, but of fathers, families, and community and religious leaders to the complications of teenage pregnancies.
- There are insufficient communication channels between health care systems that lead to a delay in communication of critical health care information.

(continued)

| Box 11.1 | Nursing Work in the Global Community: Challenges and Opportunities (*continued*) |

- Extreme poverty, diminished resources, discrimination, health and resource disparities, and restricted access to care hinder the health care process and in turn decrease the quality of care that we are able to provide our patients as a whole.

By recognizing these challenges, we are aware of the following opportunities:

- By increasing awareness and recruitment, we can create Sustainable Nursing Workforces at the local level.
- Early education of mothers, fathers, families, and community and religious leaders can lead to positive outcomes for children and families and the community as a whole.
- Innovative models of care delivery are needed to improve access to resources and availability of services in a culturally appropriate, efficient, cost- and time-effective manner, including community-based primary care, maternal/child health and mental health care.
- Ongoing, frequent multilevel collaboration among government officials, community and tribal leaders, clergy, health care professionals and workers, advocates, and all stakeholders to ensure appropriate, culturally sensitive and relevant care goals, with designated targets and assessment/evaluation processes, are needed.
- Universal primary education for all (girls and boys) and appropriate health education throughout the life cycle, focusing on health promotion and disease prevention, will present opportunities to develop healthy lifestyles for individuals, families, and communities.
- Concerted efforts by governmental and civil organizations are needed to develop and maintain sustainable nursing, health care, and midwife education, and continuous staff development.
- Ongoing interprofessional dialog, particularly among nurses, midwives, and health professionals, is needed to enhance resources and assess areas of greatest need to appropriate allocation of services.
- By utilizing social media—Twitter, Facebook, etc.—we can educate and reach those who otherwise would not have access to education.
- By creating a collaboration between our own local health care systems, governmental systems, and international systems, we can identify barriers and discover creative solutions that will benefit those most vulnerable within our own societies.

Watson Caring Science Institute 3rd Annual Conference of Nurses in the Middle East—Human Caring in a Time of World Crisis: Transcending Culture and Boundaries brought together nurses from across the Middle East—Palestine, Jerusalem, Israel, Bahrain, Iran, Saudi Arabia, and Dubai—and the United States to discuss the issues that face us daily.

(continued)

> **Box 11.1** **Nursing Work in the Global Community: Challenges and Opportunities (*continued*)**
>
> Through our collaboration and exchange of ideas, we recognized that we, the nurses, are the Leaders, the Educators, and the Caregivers of the world.
>
> We understand that as Leaders we can effect change through communication and collaboration at the community, governmental, and international levels.
>
> As Educators, we understand that there are opportunities to provide the knowledge needed to both men and women to prevent teenage pregnancies; the tools to new mothers to ensure safe delivery and care of their newborns; and the resources needed to our communities to raise the level of awareness to the benefit of preventative medicine.
>
> And finally, as Caregivers, we recognize and understand the barriers to care: the lack of qualified caregivers; governmental regulations such as military checkpoints and delay in approval of travel to needed skilled care centers; and cultural bias that can prevent or hinder timely needed care.
>
> *Source:* Watson Caring Science Institute & International *Caritas* Consortium. Nurses in the Middle East & Partners United in Human Caring (n.d.-a). Reprinted with permission.

> **Box 11.2** **Nurses in the Middle East (NME) Position on Safety and Security in the Workplace**
>
> Nurses in the Middle East are committed to providing care to all patients and communities equally without prejudice and with love, dignity, and respect, while at the same time protecting themselves. Governments and health care systems should be required to secure and ensure safe workplace environments where nurses can continue to practice, provide quality patient care without concern, knowing that their own safety and security are protected.
>
> United in caring, we, the Nurses in the Middle East and the Partners United in Caring of the Watson Caring Science Institute, believe:
>
> - Nurses have the right and the duty to learn and empower themselves and demand workplaces that provide safety and security. This empowerment starts in nursing schools and educational systems, and extends to active political participation to represent and have a voice in policies and regulations that affect the settings/environments where nurses practice. Safety and security for all; "all" includes nurses themselves as a start.
> - Systems/facilities/governments are responsible for creating and enforcing policies that ensure environments where nurses can practice while their own safety and security are protected. This translates into securing resources, supplies, training, access to information, continuous education, and physical measurements that enable nurses to practice while feeling safe and secure.

(*continued*)

Box 11.2 **Nurses in the Middle East (NME) Position on Safety and Security in the Workplace (*continued*)**

- We, the Nursing Leaders in the Middle East, are determined to: Create and maintain a culture of safety and quality throughout the (organization); assist our organizations to develop a code of conduct that defines acceptable behavior and behaviors that undermine a culture of safety; help to create and implement a process for managing behaviors that support a culture of safety.

Watson Caring Science Institute 3rd Annual Conference of Nurses in the Middle East—Human Caring in a Time of World Crisis: Transcending Culture and Boundaries brought together nurses from across the Middle East—Palestine, Jerusalem, Israel, Bahrain, Iran, Saudi Arabia, and Dubai—and the United States to discuss the issues that face us daily.

In aligning ourselves with The Joint Commission International, the World Health Organization (WHO), and other leading nursing organizations around the globe, the concept of a "just culture" was discussed—where do the rights of the individual stop and the rights of the other begin?

The American Nurses Association position stated:

A Healthy Work Environment is one that is safe, empowering, and satisfying. Parallel to the World Health Organization's definition of health, it is not merely the absence of real and perceived threats to health, but a place of 'physical, mental, and social well-being,' supporting optimal health and safety. A culture of safety is paramount, in which all leaders, managers, health care workers, and ancillary staff have a responsibility as part of the patient-centered team to perform with a sense of professionalism, accountability, transparency, involvement, efficiency, and effectiveness. All must be mindful of the health and safety for both the patient and the health care worker in any setting providing health care, providing a sense of safety, respect, and empowerment to and for all persons.

It was identified that the threats nurses face daily present a challenge to the profession in their commitments to the ethical principles of beneficence, malfeasance, and self-preservation. Nurses are constantly put on the spot to make quick decisions about their commitments to these principles.

We, the members of NME, recognize that nurses need to be more proactive and become leaders rather than followers when it comes to their own safety and security. We, as nurses, recognize that these threats should be considered seriously in relation to balancing personal and social liberties and personal rights and public rights. And that we, as *nurses*, are dedicated to the prevention of violence in the health care setting by identifying high-risk areas and those who are perpetrators of violence toward our patients.

Source: Watson Caring Science Institute & International *Caritas* Consortium. Nurses in the Middle East & Partners United in Human Caring (n.d.-b). Reprinted with permission.

Box 11.3 Middle East Nurses on Armed Forces in Hospital sanctuaries

Nurses in the Middle East are all in consensus that hospitals are sanctuaries.

While we are aware of the fact that medical facilities have been abused to cover up/ hide terrorist activity, we nonetheless believe that hospitals and other medical facilities (ambulances) need to be a safe environment for any human being, sick or wounded.

Therefore, we strongly believe that armed forces need to adhere to the ethical norms established by the UN.

The UN states, "The UN expects that all peacekeeping armed forces personnel adhere to the highest standards of behavior and conduct themselves in a professional and disciplined manner at all times." Rules of conduct according to the UN:

Dress, think, talk, act, and behave in a manner befitting the dignity of a disciplined, caring, considerate, mature, respected, and trusted soldier, displaying the highest integrity and impartiality. Have pride in your position and do not abuse or misuse your authority.

Respect the law of the land of the host country, its local culture, traditions, customs, and practices.

Treat the inhabitants with respect, courtesy, and consideration. You are there as a guest.

Do not indulge in immoral acts or exploitation of the local population.

Respect and regard the human rights of all. Support and aid the infirm, sick, and weak. Do not act in revenge or with malice, in particular when dealing with prisoners, detainees, or people in your custody.

Show respect for and promote the environment (cdu.unlb.org/UNStandardsof Conduct/TenRulesCodeofPersonalConductForBlueHelmets.aspx).

Source: Watson Caring Science Institute & International Caritas Consortium. Nurses in the Middle East & Partners United in Human Caring (n.d.-c). Reprinted with permission.

Box 11.4 Nurses in the Middle East Uniting in Human Caring: Reframing Violence as a Caritas Nurse

In recognizing that violence in the health care setting is a global issue, we, the Nurses in the Middle East (NME) of the Caring Science Institute, set out to reframe violence in the health care setting. By utilizing our tools as a Caritas Nurse, we aim to see the underlying cause of the troubles and by doing so, deescalate the situation before it reaches a crisis.

Violence in the health care setting is a global concern. Although many nursing organizations and global health organizations have reached out to help define "violence," the support by the infrastructures within the health care community and the governments within whom they are aligned has been minimal. Health care workers around the world are putting their lives on the line just by doing their job.

Violence comes in many forms: criminal intent, patient/family to worker, coworker to coworker and personal relationships outside the workplace that can interfere with our daily routines. By recognizing stages of crisis, nurses can intervene to help minimize violence and alleviate escalating a crisis.

(continued)

Box 11.4 **Nurses in the Middle East Uniting in Human Caring: Reframing Violence as a Caritas Nurse (*continued*)**

- We recognize that all people deserve tolerance, protection, and dignity.
- We believe that through communication, education, and authenticity, we can reach an understanding.
- We believe that by understanding our selves we can promote human-to-human connectedness.
- We recognize that by being nonjudgmental in our thoughts and words we can create a calming environment in which open communication and heart-felt connections can develop.
- We also recognize that regulations must be enabled within our workplace environment and in local and regional governments to protect those most at risk.

Watson Caring Science Institute 3rd Annual Conference of Nurses in the Middle East—Human Caring in a Time of World Crisis: Transcending Culture and Boundaries, brought together nurses from across the region—Palestine, Jerusalem, Israel, Bahrain, Iran, Saudi Arabia, and Dubai—and the United States to discuss the issues that face us daily.

Violence in the health care setting is making headlines around the world. The World Health Organization, Emergency Nurses Association, Joint Commission, and the American Nurses Association are just some of the coalitions that have made strong statements for the protection of the health care workforce and called for legislation to hold accountable those who target them.

The NME of the Caring Science Institute believe strongly in the following Core Concepts of the Human Caring Theory:
- There is a relational caring for self and others.
- There is a moral commitment to protect and enhance human dignity.
- Heart-Centered Encounters with another person can happen.
- There is more than one way of learning and knowing—science, art, personal, cultural, spiritual.
- Through an understanding of self through reflection/meditation, one can have an increasing consciousness of the humanism of one's self and others.
- Caring is inclusive, circular, and expansive.
- And Caring changes self, others, and the culture of groups and environments.

It is through this foundation that we seek to be Leaders, Educators, and frontline Caregivers within our health care organization and our local communities.

Source: Watson Caring Science Institute & International Caritas Consortium. Nurses in the Middle East & Partners United in Human Caring (n.d.-d). Reprinted with permission.

EVOLVING UNITARY HUMAN CARING TASKS: SHARED HUMAN PURSUITS AFFECTING OUR GLOBAL COMMUNITY

A Unitary principle underlying shared human tasks for human evolution is realizing that one person's level of humanity is reflected upon the other; thus, what one does to one's self and what one says to one's self affects others, and the unitary field that unites all (Watson, 2006). More specifically, this concept of shared humanity is identified by Kreitzer and Koithan (2011, p.1) as Integrative principle number 6: "the fundamental unity within and between all beings and their environment."

These shared human tasks related to Caring, Healing, and Peace include, for example: (Watson, 2008, 2012a, 2012b)

- Healing our relationship with Self and Other as the beginning of inner and outer peace; this includes self-acceptance and holding compassion, loving–kindness, forgiveness, and tenderness to self, first, thus opening our hearts with feelings to others, even strangers or so-called enemies; accepting others with loving kindness and compassion;

- Understanding human suffering—our own and others—finding new meanings to live with and transform human suffering, shared as a universal human condition which unites all;

- Finding new depth of meaning and purpose in life and all the vicissitudes of the shared human condition of living, change, loss, grief, death, and dying, honoring the enduring human spirit in the midst of impermanence;

- Finding personal meaning in the life–death cycle and death itself, as part of the larger sacred circle of infinity;

- Coming to terms with our own death and dying;

- "Remembering"—or awakening to the deep nature of life and LOVE; awakening to the Ethic of Belonging and to our infinite field of Universal Love; One Heart/One World—that underneath it all, LOVE is all there is that unites and binds human–Earth—cosmos existence—holding Planet Earth together through the Energy of LOVE.

Unitary Caring Science nursing in this global context is helping to name and awaken us to the shared human tasks of life itself that inform human caring and peaceful actions; such awakening, which if honored today, can help to save succeeding generations from noncaring practices, violence, and untold human sorrow, despair, and destruction of humanity and Planet Earth itself.

This unified focus brings together global principles and human caring practices that invite us to consider our common tasks as humans on Planet Earth—affirming One Heart/One World that holds humanity. It is this consciousness that we seek to sustain human dignity, basic civility, healing our humanity—which is peace in action.

When we engage in Unitary Caritas Consciousness, when we offer our own lives, one person to another, finding more conscious intentional ways to offer/ live gestures of peace within and without, then we become Peace—we are Peace— Living and Speaking Peace from within. Through the simple, yet profound gestures of daily peace, we change the way we live.

The writer, Terry Tempest Williams (2001), reminds us, "the eyes of the future are looking right at us and they are praying for us to see beyond our own time." (www .google.com.mx/#q=quote+Terry+Tempest+Williams+quote+...the+eyes+of+the+ future+are+looking+). There are now 7 billion people on this planet and we have to ask new sacred questions about our survival as humanity and as a planet. The Native American Elders have reminded us across centuries that we have to live to prepare seven generations beyond us in this time.

Our wisdom and traditions from our ancestors and indigenous elders around the world teach us that Peace and Caring come from within the Heart—from the Heart of our humanity, our professions, our connections across cultures, lifetimes, worlds, words, space, and time.

Human cries for Love, for Human Caring and Peace reside within the hearts of Nursing and Health Care professionals, or we would not be here today.

Speaking of Heart—"Caring is a Passage to the Heart."

Did you/we know that:

- The word "heart" is one of the most used words in the world, and in the Bible?
- The heart manifests a radiant field 500 times greater than the brain?
- What we carry in our hearts matters?
- There are new heart–centered approaches being taught related to, for example, "Heart Hypnosis," "Heart Coherence," and "CaritasHeart"?

I share with you some basic premises from Caring Science and Heart Science that underline Unitary views of Human Caring and Peace in a global context:

Did you/we know that:

- The heart is the source for Caring, Compassion, Truth, Beauty, Love, and Caring; the source for sustaining our humanity and our humanness?
- The heart is more than an organ which pumps blood; new research acknowledges that the heart has its own type of intelligence; it produces an electromagnetic field which can be detected several feet around an individual?
- The heart communicates its energetic message nonverbally into the field of our existence at the moment—this energetic message impacts us and our environmental surroundings?
- The heart sends more messages to the brain than the brain sends to the heart?
- "Listening to our hearts" is not just a figure of speech?
- "What we carry in our hearts matters"?
- Love is a form of Unitive energy processed by the heart which brings all of life together; it is referred to as a "fifth force" of subtle energy, which is vital to our life force?
- By connecting and listening to the heart of humanity, we have an inner knowing in our heart of hearts as our inner guide?
- Heart-centered Caritas Practices of Loving Kindness, Compassion, and Forgiveness manifest Peace in our inner and outer world?

- The Heart is the Passage to Caring–Love–Peace?
- This Heart-centered Caritas Consciousness awakening is the Path of Peace?

From this awareness, we now can say that "what we truly love and what we neglect to love affects every aspect in our life." What we carry in our hearts matters.

Love and Peace are inseparable: I have Love, I have Peace, I am Caritas, I am Peace.

As Caritas-conscious and unitary-caring science global nurses, perhaps we have a new role in the world:

> To transform the vision of human health and healing by engaging in service to self and society at a different level, by creating "the energetic field of Caritas," through both overt and subtle practices that transmit and affect the field of the whole. We do this one by one and become part of creating a deeper level of humanity by transforming fundamentally what happens in a given caring moment, in a given situation, by experimenting with "Being in the Integrative *Caritas* Field." This is the truly noble work of nursing and healing that transcends the conventional way of thinking . . . when we proceed and attain this new/old level of wisdom . . . in this line of thinking, there is a connection between Caring (as connecting with, sustaining, and deepening our shared humanity) and Peace in the world. In this noble Integrative Caritas practice we become Bodhisattvas: those who bless others and who become a blessing to self and others. We actively affect the entire universal field of humanity. (Watson, 2008, p. 48, with slight modifications)

These basic Caritas human–heart wisdoms and universal truths are embedded in the FACES of our global community and human caring practices across time. Global Nursing within the context of Caring and Peace, within the framework of Caritas and Caring Science, indeed becomes Sacred Science (Watson, 2006).

Levinas's "Ethics of Belonging and Ethic of Face" reminds us that the only way we can sustain humanity at this very point in time, is through the FACE-to-FACE connection. Whereby, when we look into the face of another person, we are looking into the infinity of human soul, connecting with the infinity of Universal Love, which mirrors back the Infinity of our own soul. And there, in this infinite space of Universal LOVE, we are awakened to our common humanity on this Planet Earth.

As global nursing and nurses, individually and collectively, along with other health and healing practitioners, awaken to our gifts and purpose on the earth plane. We discover through our Global Caritas practices, we are contributing to the quantum evolution of human consciousness; toward a moral community of Caring, Healing, and Peace for our world. It is only such a world that will fully realize the safety, inclusivity, and prosperity for all sought after by the UN 2030 Agenda.

FINAL SECTION: ADDENDUM

This final section includes an International Ethical Charter for Human Caring and Peace located in Box 11.5, introducing basic Unitary–Planetary Caritas principles and processes, consistent with global nursing's future as human caring–healing peacemakers for our turbulent and changing world. You can visit www.watson caringscience.org/the-caritas-path-to-peace/to make your pledge to the Charter.

Box 11.5 | **International Ethical Charter: Human Caring and Peace**©

Presented at First Asian Pacific International Caritas Consortium and International Caring and Peace Conference. Hiroshima, Japan. March 22 to 24, 2012.

Prologue and Basic Premises:

At this time in human history the survival of humanity and Mother Earth is threatened. In order to sustain humanity and Mother Earth the following premises are proclaimed:

- Every human on earth has a right to be treated with respect and dignity, honoring the unity of mind–body–spirit

- Every person in the world has the right to receive humane and compassionate care

- Every human on earth shares and draws upon Mother Earth and all her resources

- Every human is here on Planet Earth for a reason and spirit-filled purpose

- All of humanity is joined in the infinite field of the universe with each other and all living things; all creation is sacred and connected

- Each person's level of humanity reflects upon the whole, allowing for the collective evolution of human consciousness for all of humankind

- Globally, women and children in society carry the predominance of human caring for all of humanity, helping to sustain human caring and humanity for the whole

- The human caring needs of women and children in the world are threatened;

- All humans are entitled to freedom to pursue their dreams and follow their hearts

- All humans Belong to Infinite Source, Life Spirit, the sacred mystery, which unites *all*, before, during, and after the Planet Earth experience.

International Ethical Charter Caring and Peace Processes and Practices for individual and collective–private and public practices:

- Offering Loving–Kindness, Forgiveness, and Equanimity with self–others;

- Being Authentically Present, honoring, and respecting the belief systems and inner life world of self and other;

- Dedicating self to personal caring practices of inner peace for healing our relationships with self, others, and Mother Earth;

- Sustaining a caring–trusting relationship with inner self, other, and universal life Source;

- Allowing for expression of positive and negative feelings in order to listen authentically to another's story and the universal story of our shared humanity;

- Creating intentional conscious acts to guide and develop new solutions toward sustaining caring and peace;

(continued)

Box 11.5	International Ethical Charter: Human Caring and Peace© (*continued*)

- Teaching and coaching each other for evolving consciousness for caring and peace within and without;

- Revisioning of environments for living and sustaining humanity and Mother Earth;

- Assisting others with basic human needs to cooperatively serve others and sustain human dignity;

- Honoring of spiritual, mysterious unknowns of life; allowing for miracles of Peace and Love to prevail on Mother Earth.

Source: Watson (2012c). Reprinted with permission.

REFLECTION AND DISCUSSION

- What is my role in bringing a human caring ethic to the goals and targets of the Sustainable Development Agenda?

- How do the concepts of caring, love, and peace relate to the notion of sustainable health and well-being? Does the language of Caring Science and Caritas Nursing have a place in the creation and implementation of transnational health agendas?

- How does the consideration and application of caring evolve at individual, community, global, planetary, and universal levels?

- What do I carry in my heart? Why does it matter? How does it impact the consciousness of those around me?

- In what ways do the UN SDGs reflect the Unitary–Planetary Caritas principles and practices espoused by the International Ethical Charter for Human Caring and Peace?

REFERENCES

Bohm, D. (1980a). *Quantum theory.* New York, NY: Prentice-Hall.

Bohm, D. (1980b). *Wholeness and the implicate order.* London, UK: Routledge & Kegan Paul.

Bohm, D., & Peat, F. D. (1987). *Science, order, and creativity.* New York, NY: Bantam Books.

Hawkins, D. (2002). *Power vs. Force.* Carlsbad, CA: Hay House.

Institute of Noetic Sciences. (2012). Research roundup. Affirming our potential for peace. *Institute of Notice Science, 3*(2), 5.

Kreitzer, M. J., & Koithan, M. (2011). *Principles of Integrative Nursing Practice. Outline. Integrative Nursing.* Oxford Press Project (unpublished manuscript).

Kumar, S. (2015). *Soil–soul–society.* Lewes, UK: Leaping Hare Press.

Levinas, E. (1969). *Totality & infinity.* Pittsburgh, PA: Duquesne University Press.

McClure, M. (2011). 'People can change' key to Mideast peace. Retrieved from http://www.futurity.org/people-can-change-key-to-mideast-peace

Newman, M. (1994). *Health as expanding consciousness.* Philadelphia, PA: F. A. Davis.

Okri, B. (1997). *A way of being free*. London, UK: Phoenix.

United Nations. (2015). *Transforming our world: The 2030 Agenda for Sustainable Development*. Sustainable Development Knowledge Platform. Retrieved from http://sustainable development.un.org/post2015/transforming our world

Vieten, C. (2012). The noetic post. *Institute of Noetic Sciences, 3*(2), 6.

Watson, J. (2006). *Caring science as sacred science*. Philadelphia, PA: F. A. Davis.

Watson, J. (2008). *Nursing. The philosophy and science of caring*. Boulder: University Press of Colorado

Watson, J (2012a). *Human caring science*. Sudbury, MA: Jones & Bartlett.

Watson, J. (2012b, March 24). *Caritas path of peace*. Paper presented at International Hiroshima Caring and Peace Conference. Hiroshima, Japan.

Watson, J. (2012c). International charter on caring and peace. Retrived from http://www .watsoncaringscience.org

Watson, J. (2015). Middle Eastern nurses uniting in human caring website. Retrieved from https://www.watsoncaringscience.org/middle-eastern-nurses-project

Watson Caring Science Institute. (n.d.). *International ethical charter: Human caring and peace*©. Retrieved from https://www.watsoncaringscience.org/the-caritas-path-to-peace

Watson Caring Science Institute & International Caritas Consortium. Nurses in the Middle East & Partners United in Human Caring. (n.d.-a). Position Paper. Nursing work in the global community: Challenges and opportunities. Retrieved from https://www .watsoncaringscience.org/wp-content/uploads/2016/07/2015-NME-Position-Statement -Nursing-Work-in-the-Global-Community.pdf

Watson Caring Science Institute & International Caritas Consortium. Nurses in the Middle East & Partners United in Human Caring. (n.d.-b). Position Paper. Nurses in the Middle East (NME) position on safety and security in the workplace. Retrieved from https:// www.watsoncaringscience.org/wp-content/uploads/2016/07/july-2015-NME-Position -Statement-Safety-and-Security-in-the-Workplace.pdf

Watson Caring Science Institute & International Caritas Consortium. Nurses in the Middle East & Partners United in Human Caring. (n.d.-c). Position paper. Middle East Nurses on armed forces in hospital setting. Retrieved from https://www.watsoncaringscience .org/wp-content/uploads/2016/07/dec-1-2015-Position-Paper-Middle-East-Nurses-on -Armed-Forces-in-Hospital-setting.pdf

Watson Caring Science Institute & International Caritas Consortium. Nurses in the Middle East & Partners United in Human Caring. (n.d.-d). Position paper. Nurses in the Middle East uniting in human caring: Reframing violence as a caritas nurse. Retrieved from https:// www.watsoncaringscience.org/wp-content/uploads/2016/07/july-2015-NME-Position -Statement-Redefining-Violence-as-a-Caritas-Nurse.pdf

Williams, T. T. (2001). *Red: Passion and patience in the desert*. New York, NY: Pantheon Books. Retrieved from https://www.google.com.mx/#q=quote+Terry+Tempest+Williams+quote +...the+eyes+of+the+future+are+looking+

World Health Organization. (2016). *Global strategic directions for strengthening nursing and midwifery 2016–2020*. Geneva, Switzerland: Author. Retrieved from http://www.who .int/hrh/nursing_midwifery/glob-strategic-midwifery2016-2020

The Sustainable Development Goals: A Primer

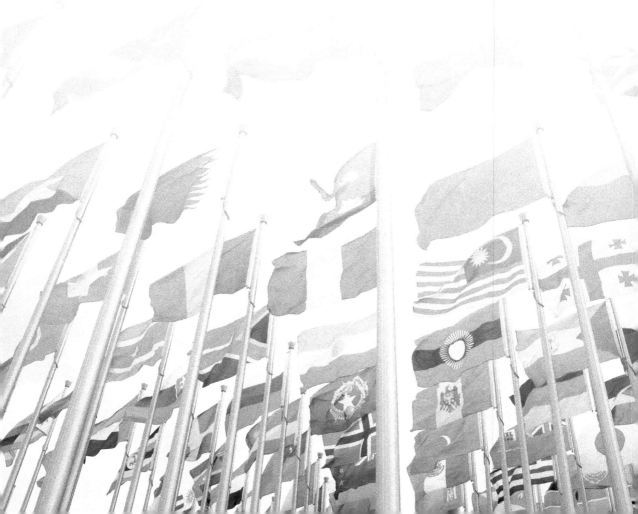

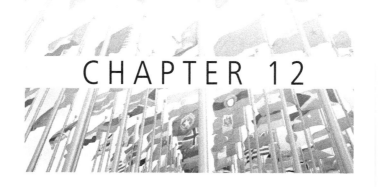

CHAPTER 12

Goal 1. End Poverty in All Its Forms Everywhere

William Rosa

[I]t is all too easy . . . to have low—or no—expectations for low-income people . . . [the poor] are invisible to most. . . . [We need] a philosophy based on human dignity . . . We can end poverty . . . by looking at all human beings as part of a single global community . . . everyone deserves a chance to build a life worth living. (Novogratz, 2009, pp. 212, 273)

With the recent creation and ongoing implementation of the Sustainable Development Goals (SDGs), global nurses play a vital role assisting the United Nations (UN; United Nations Development Program [UNDP], 2016a) in "addressing the root causes of poverty and the universal need for development that works for all people." The SDGs advocate to further address the worldwide antipoverty work initiated by the Millennium Development Goals (MDGs) and improve quality of life for the global community by 2030 (UNDP, 2016b). Global nurses must seek out information about the SDGs and the work being done so they can create opportunities to translate their nursing scope and expertise to each of the goals. The following chapters address how global nursing contributions are essential components of realizing each of the SDGs by 2030.

The first SDG is "End poverty in all its forms everywhere." To be clear, it does not look to simply mitigate the poverty experienced by much of the world's population—it seeks to eliminate it. The targets of SDG 1 are listed in Box 12.1 (see the Appendix to view the Sustainable Development Agenda in its entirety). Extreme poverty throughout the world has been cut in half, from 1.9 billion people in 1990 to 836 million in 2015 (UNDP, 2016c). This means that over 800 million people continue to live on roughly $1.00 per day and have insurmountable barriers to adequate sanitation, clean water, or enough food. Clearly, countries and economies worldwide are not there yet.

Box 12.1 **Sustainable Development Goal 1 and Its Associated Targets**

Goal 1. End poverty in all its forms everywhere

1.1 By 2030, eradicate extreme poverty for all people everywhere, currently measured as people living on less than $1.25 a day.

1.2 By 2030, reduce at least by half the proportion of men, women, and children of all ages living in poverty in all its dimensions according to national definitions.

1.3 Implement nationally appropriate social protection systems and measures for all, including floors, and by 2030 achieve substantial coverage of the poor and the vulnerable.

1.4 By 2030, ensure that all men and women, in particular the poor and the vulnerable, have equal rights to economic resources, as well as access to basic services, ownership, and control over land and other forms of property, inheritance, natural resources, appropriate new technology and financial services, including microfinance.

1.5 By 2030, build the resilience of the poor and those in vulnerable situations and reduce their exposure and vulnerability to climate-related extreme events and other economic, social, and environmental shocks and disasters.

1.a Ensure significant mobilization of resources from a variety of sources, including through enhanced development cooperation, in order to provide adequate and predictable means for developing countries, in particular least developed countries, to implement programs and policies to end poverty in all its dimensions.

1.b Create sound policy frameworks at the national, regional, and international levels, based on pro-poor and gender-sensitive development strategies, to support accelerated investment in poverty eradication actions.

Source: Reprinted with permission from the United Nations (2015).

Farmer (2005) wrote that "the right to survive" is the most basic human right; it "is trampled in an age of great affluence" and "should be considered the most pressing [matter] of our times" (p. 6). Furthermore, he proposed that "anyone who wishes to be considered humane has ample cause to consider what it means to be sick and poor in the era of globalization and scientific advancement" (Farmer, 2005, p. 6). Global nurses are actively improving access to quality services for the "sick poor" around the world. Across the life span and throughout the trajectory of care delivery, global nurses are integral to establishing health care access for impoverished individuals and communities. These nurses are creating referral and information pathways to reduce child poverty in Scotland (Naven & Egan, 2013); increasing cancer-screening rates for low-income and difficult-to-reach populations in Canada (Peart & Crabb, 2016); increasing primary care service utilization for the homeless and marginalized in New Haven,

Connecticut in the United States (Su, Khoshnood, & Forster, 2016); and striving to understand how older adults living in deprived neighborhoods in the Netherlands cope with issues of frailty, care dependency, and other issues related to ageing (Bielderman, Schout, de Greef, & van der Schans, 2015). Diminished or absent access to health care is not a "third-world" issue; it is a complex, and often overlooked, disparity related to social injustice and widespread unawareness and inaction.

If global nurses are to facilitate poverty reduction and, ultimately, end extreme poverty, we need to have all the information: Who are the poor? Where do they live? Where is poverty the deepest? (World Bank, n.d.) Global Finance (2015) shows that of the 25 poorest countries in the world, 21 of them are in Africa, with the poorest nation being the Central African Republic (CAR). With a population of 4.6 million, the country has experienced political instability since its freedom from France in 1960, and in 2013 experienced extreme turmoil as Muslim rebels sought to overthrow the Christian government. Currently, the CAR is under international supervision and being assisted by a UN peacekeeping force while a constitutional referendum and elections hope to stabilize its political status (BBC, 2016).

The link between the political scenario and poverty status in the CAR and the work of every global nurse is clear. Nurses know that health is a human right. But do they realize that the alleviation of economic influences that threaten health—such as poverty—is also a human right (Upvall, Leffers, & Mitchell, 2014)? Poverty and health are intimately related; it becomes an ethical priority of social justice to strive for the identification and eradication of health disparities wherever they may occur (Nickitas, 2016). Global nurses must learn how to articulate the injustices they observe, address the inequities and inefficiencies of health care infrastructures, and clearly delineate how human rights violations, such as extreme poverty, and barriers to health care access and delivery are intertwined (Nickitas, 2008).

Global nurse leaders need to be powerful and informed advocates for equality in health care and understand what it means: equitable care to all populations without compromise (Fitzgerald, 2016). In low- and middle-income countries (LMICs) this can be quite challenging to ensure. For example, nurses in the CAR may be the only provider available throughout rural village areas—the difference between life and death for many—and often go without wages for weeks or months at a time (Jones, 2010). Global nurses must use the power of their voice to hold nongovernmental organizations (NGOs) and program implementation leaders accountable for the appropriate use of funds in improving health care services and investing in sustainable resources (Lindgren, Rankin, & Schell, 2015).

In LMICs, nurses are the agents of change who bring the ideals of health promotion to the doorsteps of those who need care (Manjrekar, 2016). The power of the global nurse as advocate–leader–practitioner cannot be overlooked, particularly when striving to eradicate poverty in the name of social justice and health equity. So if you cannot go to work in the CAR to improve systems, use your voice. If the timing is not right to travel to Africa and facilitate programs that uproot the virus of poverty, take a trip to the resource-constrained areas of your hometown and assess how your skills are needed. Global health–public health–international health: all interconnected and interdependent. Global nurses need not look far to see how their knowledge base and skill set can be aptly utilized.

It is helpful to have an honest understanding of one's beliefs and judgments regarding impoverished people in order to be of true service, free from prejudice and unconscious (or conscious) barriers to partnership. Atherton et al. (1993) originally developed and validated the Attitude Toward Poverty Scale (ATPS) as a reliable tool to aid social workers in identifying students' attitudes toward poor populations and addressing ethical concerns while working in contexts of poverty. The 37-item ATPS, along with the 21-item attitude towards poverty (ATP) short form adapted by Yun and Weaver (2010), have been repeatedly employed to measure nursing and nurse practitioner students' attitudes toward poverty (Kovarna, 2006; Menzel, Willson, & Doolen, 2014; Ritten, Waldrop, & Wink, 2015). The ATP short form (Yun & Weaver, 2010) is provided in Figure 12.1 for reader self-reflection and to foster self-understanding of attitudes, apprehensions, and reservations about working with poor people and in poverty-stricken settings. High scores imply a belief that poverty is caused by structural determinants, while low scores represent a belief that poverty maintains a more individualistic etiology. The assessment explores an individual's beliefs about poverty related to personal deficiency, stigma, and structural perspective. Although the original tool was utilized in the United States and in reference to American social programs for the poor, the questions are globally relevant, and international colleagues can simply replace "welfare" with "governmental financial support" for the purposes of their own self-reflection.

Deva-Marie Beck (2016), international codirector of the Nightingale Initiative for Global Health (NIGH; 2016), asks and answers a pivotal question for our time; it applies to the soup kitchen in Chicago as much as to the city of Bambari in the CAR:

> Global health is accomplished through the application of communications at global levels. It is the worldwide advocacy of the health needs of humanity; the dissemination of care and concern for problems that still need to be solved and the identification of how solutions have been and can be achieved. What are the tasks and tools of global nursing? We are already accomplished advocates. The task of global advocacy is simply the widening of our scopes to share the value of our perspectives and the effectiveness of our practices with the more expansive world. Our tools are all around us. (p. 259)

"End poverty in all its forms everywhere"—the tools are all around you.

REFLECTION AND DISCUSSION

- In what ways does poverty directly impact health?
- Do I consider extreme poverty to be a human rights violation? Why or why not?
- What is the role of social justice in ending poverty? What is my role in procuring social justice?
- How do I define "equality in health care"?
- What are my tools for global advocacy?

| Figure 12.1 | **ATP Short Form.** |

If you strongly agree, please circle SA.
If you agree, please circle A.
If you are neutral on the item, please circle N.
If you disagree, please circle D.
If you strongly disagree, please circle SD.

Poor people are different from the rest of society.	SA	A	N	D	SD
Poor people are dishonest.	SA	A	N	D	SD
Most poor people are dirty.	SA	A	N	D	SD
Poor people act differently.	SA	A	N	D	SD
Children raised on welfare will never amount to anything.	SA	A	N	D	SD
I believe poor people have a different set of values than do other people.	SA	A	N	D	SD
Poor people generally have lower intelligence than nonpoor people.	SA	A	N	D	SD
There is a lot of fraud among welfare recipients.	SA	A	N	D	SD
Some "poor" people live better than I do, considering all their benefits.	SA	A	N	D	SD
Poor people think they deserve to be supported.	SA	A	N	D	SD
Welfare mothers have babies to get more money.	SA	A	N	D	SD
An able-bodied person collecting welfare is ripping off the system.	SA	A	N	D	SD
Unemployed poor people could find jobs if they tried harder.	SA	A	N	D	SD
Welfare makes people lazy. Benefits for poor people consume a major part of the federal budget.	SA	A	N	D	SD
People are poor due to circumstances beyond their control.	SA	A	N	D	SD
I would support a program that resulted in higher taxes to support social programs for poor people.	SA	A	N	D	SD
If I were poor, I would accept welfare benefits.	SA	A	N	D	SD
People who are poor should not be blamed for their misfortune.	SA	A	N	D	SD
Society has the responsibility to help poor people.	SA	A	N	D	SD
Poor people are discriminated against.	SA	A	N	D	SD

Scoring is SA=1, A=2, N=3, D=4, SD=5

ATP, attitude toward poverty.
Source: Yun and Weaver (2010). Reprinted with permission.

REFERENCES

Atherton, C. R., Gemmel, R. J., Haagenstad, S., Holt, D. J., Jensen, L. A., O'Hara, D. F., & Rehner, T. A. (1993). Measuring attitudes toward poverty: A new scale. *Social Work Research & Abstracts, 29*(4), 28–30.

BBC. (2016). Central African Republic country profile. Retrieved from http://www.bbc.com/news/world-africa-13150040

Beck, D.-M. (2016). Artistic and scientific: Broadening the scope of our 21st century health advocacy. In W. Rosa (Ed.), *Nurses as leaders: Evolutionary visions of leadership* (pp. 247–263). New York, NY: Springer Publishing.

Bielderman, A., Schout, G., de Greef, M., & van der Schans, C. (2015). Understanding how older adults living in deprived neighbourhoods address ageing issues. *British Journal of Community Nursing, 20*(8), 394–399.

Farmer, P. (2005). *Pathologies of power: Health, human rights, and the new war on the poor.* Berkeley and Los Angeles: University of California Press.

Fitzgerald, M. A. (2016). Powerful and beneficent: Seizing opportunity in practice and equality in health care. In W. Rosa (Ed.), *Nurses as leaders: Evolutionary visions of leadership* (pp. 77–86). New York, NY: Springer Publishing.

Global Finance. (2015). The poorest countries in the world. Retrieved from https://www.gfmag.com/global-data/economic-data/the-poorest-countries-in-the-world?page=2

Jones, P. (2010). Health workers on the frontline. *British Journal of Healthcare Assistants, 4*(9), 460.

Kovarna, M. (2006, January). *Nursing students' attitudes toward people living in poverty* (Unpublished dissertation).

Lindgren, T., Rankin, S., & Schell, E. (2015). Working globally with faith-based organizations. In S. Breakey, I. B. Corless, N. L. Meedzan, & P. K. Nicholas (Eds.), *Global health nursing in the 21st century* (pp. 453–470). New York, NY: Springer Publishing.

Manjrekar, P. (2016). Resourceful and unified: Partnering across cultures and worldviews. In W. Rosa (Ed.), *Nurses as leaders: Evolutionary visions of leadership* (pp. 345–358). New York, NY: Springer Publishing.

Menzel, N., Willson, L. H., & Doolen, J. (2014). Effectiveness of a poverty simulation in Second Life®: Changing nursing student attitudes toward poor people. *International Journal of Nursing Education Scholarship, 11*(1), 1–7.

Naven, L., & Egan, J. (2013). Addressing child poverty in Scotland: The role of nurses. *Primary Health Care, 23*(5), 16–22.

Nickitas, D. M. (2008). Changing the world with words. *Nursing Economic, 26*(3), 141.

Nickitas, D. M. (2016). Ethical and economical: Calling the profession to social justice. In W. Rosa (Ed.), *Nurses as leaders: Evolutionary visions of leadership* (pp. 149–163). New York, NY: Springer Publishing.

Nightingale Initiative for Global Health. (2016). About. Retrieved from http://www.nighvision.net/about.html

Novogratz, J. (2009). *The blue sweater: Bridging the gap between rich and poor in an interconnected world.* New York, NY: Rodale.

Peart, D., & Crabb, D. (2016). Overcoming barriers to access, one community support at a time. *Canadian Nurse, 112*(3), 24–25.

Ritten, A., Waldrop, J., & Wink, D. (2015). Nurse practitioner students learning from the medically underserved: Impact on attitude toward poverty. *Journal of Nursing Education, 54*(7), 389–393.

Su, Z., Khoshnood, K., & Forster, S. H. (2016). Assessing impact of community health nurses on improving primary care use by homeless/marginally housed persons. *Journal of Community Health Nursing, 32*(3), 161–169.

United Nations. (2015). Transforming our world: The 2030 Agenda for Sustainable Development. Retrieved from https://docs.google.com/gview?url=http://sustainabledevelopment.un.org/content/documents/21252030%20Agenda%20for%20Sustainable%20Development%20web.pdf&embedded=true

United Nations Development Programme. (2016a). Sustainable Development Goals (SDGs). Retrieved from http://www.undp.org/content/undp/en/home/sdgoverview/post -2015-development-agenda.html

United Nations Development Programme. (2016b). World leaders adopt Sustainable Development Goals. Retrieved from http://www.undp.org/content/undp/en/home/ presscenter/pressreleases/2015/09/24/undp-welcomes-adoption-of-sustainable -development-goals-by-world-leaders.html

United Nations Development Programme. (2016c). Goal 1: No poverty. Retrieved from http:// www.undp.org/content/undp/en/home/sdgoverview/post-2015-development-agenda/ goal-1.html

Upvall, M. J., Leffers, J. M., & Mitchell, E. M. (2014). Introduction and perspectives of global health. In M. J. Upvall & J. M. Leffers (Eds.), *Global health nursing: Building and sustaining partnerships* (pp. 1–18). New York, NY: Springer Publishing.

World Bank. (n.d.). The state of the poor: Where are the poor and where are they poorest? Retrieved from http://www.worldbank.org/content/dam/Worldbank/document/ State_of_the_poor_paper_April17.pdf

Yun, S. H., & Weaver, R. D. (2010). Development and validation of a Short Form of the Attitude Toward Poverty Scale. *Advances in Social Work, 11*(2), 174–187.

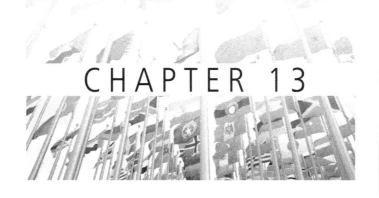

CHAPTER 13

Goal 2. End Hunger, Achieve Food Security and Improved Nutrition, and Promote Sustainable Agriculture

William Rosa

You can't build a peaceful world on empty stomachs and human misery. (Dr. Norman Ernest Borlaug as cited in Beene, 2011, p. 9)

There are people in the world so hungry, that God cannot appear to them except in the form of bread. (Gandhi, n.d.)

This Sustainable Development Goal (SDG) relates not only to hunger, but also to food security and food access, as well as the integrity of food management infrastructures. The need for safe, quality development, and practices regarding nutrition and agricultural/food supply maintenance has never been more crucial to global disease prevention and health promotion. Box 13.1 lists the targets associated with SDG 2 (see the Appendix to view the Sustainable Development Agenda in its entirety).

Why is this goal so important in the modern health scenario? According to United Nations Sustainable Development (UNSD, 2016), roughly 795 million people worldwide (1 in 9 people) are undernourished, poor nutrition causes 45% of deaths in children under the age of 5 each year (3.1 million children per year), and 66 million children are sent to school hungry each day. Furthermore, agriculture provides income and sustenance for up to 40% of the world's population, up to 1.4 billion are at risk for energy poverty (no electricity access), and the global number of hungry people could be reduced by nearly 150 million if women farmers had the same resources as men (UNSD, 2016).

The State of Food Insecurity in the World 2015 report (Food and Agriculture Organization [FAO] of the United Nations, International Fund for Agricultural Development [IFAD], and World Food Programme [WFP], 2015) recently assessed global progress in the progress of nations regarding Millennium Development Goal (MDG) 1c—Halve, between 1990 and 2015, the proportion of people who suffer

| Box 13.1 | Sustainable Development Goal 2 and Its Associated Targets |

Goal 2. End hunger, achieve food security and improved nutrition, and promote sustainable agriculture

2.1 By 2030, end hunger and ensure access by all people, in particular the poor and people in vulnerable situations, including infants, to safe, nutritious, and sufficient food all year round.

2.2 By 2030, end all forms of malnutrition, including achieving, by 2025, the internationally agreed targets on stunting and wasting in children under 5 years of age, and address the nutritional needs of adolescent girls, pregnant and lactating women, and older persons.

2.3 By 2030, double the agricultural productivity and incomes of small-scale food producers, in particular women, indigenous peoples, family farmers, pastoralists, and fishers, including through secure and equal access to land, other productive resources and inputs, knowledge, financial services, markets, and opportunities for value addition and nonfarm employment.

2.4 By 2030, ensure sustainable food production systems and implement resilient agricultural practices that increase productivity and production, that help maintain ecosystems, that strengthen capacity for adaptation to climate change, extreme weather, drought, flooding, and other disasters and that progressively improve land and soil quality.

2.5 By 2020, maintain the genetic diversity of seeds, cultivated plants, and farmed and domesticated animals and their related wild species, including through soundly managed and diversified seed and plant banks at the national, regional, and international levels, and promote access to and fair and equitable sharing of benefits arising from the utilization of genetic resources and associated traditional knowledge, as internationally agreed.

2.a Increase investment, including through enhanced international cooperation, in rural infrastructure, agricultural research and extension services, technology development, and plant and livestock gene banks in order to enhance agricultural productive capacity in developing countries, in particular least-developed countries.

2.b Correct and prevent trade restrictions and distortions in world agricultural markets, including through the parallel elimination of all forms of agricultural export subsidies and all export measures with equivalent effect, in accordance with the mandate of the Doha Development Round.

2.c Adopt measures to ensure the proper functioning of food commodity markets and their derivatives and facilitate timely access to market information, including on food reserves, in order to help limit extreme food-price volatility.

Source: Reprinted with permission from the United Nations (2015).

from hunger—and the more aggressive 1996 World Food Summit's (WFS's) *Rome Declaration on World Food Security* commitment—Eradicate hunger in all countries, with an immediate view to reducing the number of undernourished people to half their present level no later than 2015 (FAO, n.d.; UN, 2006). The progress related to MDG 1c was monitored through two primary indicators: (a) Prevalence of under-weight children under 5 years of age, and (b) proportion of population below min-imum level of dietary energy consumption (UN, 2006). The WFS's target consisted of seven main objectives that pledged economic, political, and social support to create the best conditions for the eradication of hunger and to implement, monitor, and follow up on global advancement toward the goal through 2015 (FAO, n.d.). The key findings from the FAO, IFAD, and WFP (2015) report include:

- About 780 million people—the vast majority of the world's hungry—live in low- and middle-income countries (LMICs), with the prevalence of undernourishment having decreased 44.4% since 1990–1992, currently being measured at roughly 12.9% of the total population.
- By 2015, LMICs reached the MDG 1c hunger target as a whole, but missed the WFS's target by a large margin.
- Wide differences exist across regions: Latin America, eastern and southeastern Asia have reached both MDG1c and WFS targets; Central Asia and northern and western Africa have reached MDG 1c; but the Caribbean, Oceania, Southern Asia, and southern and eastern Africa have progressed too slow to reach MDG 1c.
- About 72 of 129 LMICs have reached the MDG 1c target, 29 of which have also achieved the WFS target.
- Many countries that have reached the international hunger targets witnessed stable political conditions and continued economic growth, with social protection for vulnerable populations.
- Many countries unable to achieve the international hunger targets had experienced natural and man-made disasters, political instability, and/ or economic disparities due to lack of social protections and failure of income redistribution policies.

Furthermore, "the only means to address food insecurity is humanitarian inter-vention . . . hunger eradication can only be pursued if all stakeholders contrib-ute to designing and enacting policies for improving economic opportunities, the protection of vulnerable groups and disaster preparedness" (FAO, IFAD, & WFP, 2015, p. 18). Global nurses must be able to identify food insecurity, partner with organizations that look to mitigate hunger, promote gender equality in food pro-duction and agriculture through social justice initiatives, and educate themselves about the integrity of the food supply.

FOOD INSECURITY

Food insecurity (FI) describes a nonsustainable food system that poses multiple barriers to both self-reliance and social justice; it leads to nutritional inadequacy, unsafe food acquisition and consumption, and dehumanizing coping strategies, such as scavenging and stealing (Kregg-Byers & Schlenk, 2010). FI leads to a host of chronic diseases, impaired cognition, and psychosocial complications related to health and well-being. Global nurses and other health care workers (HCWs) need to become astute at both effectively screening for FI and taking stock of appropriate, accessible referral outlets for clients and communities (Theuri, 2015). Tools such as the FI screen by Hager, Quigg, and Black (2010) allow for a quick and direct assessment of FI across health care and community environments. It asks the client to respond "often true," "sometimes true," or "never true" to two simple statements:

- Within the past 12 months, we worried whether our food would run out before we got money to buy more.
- Within the past 12 months, the food we bought just did not last and we did not have money to get more.

The FI screen is an easily applicable way of identifying individuals and households at risk for FI and its subsequent consequences. Early identification and timely referral/intervention could offset the substantial health care expenditures positively correlated with FI, independent of other social determinants of health (Tarasuk et al., 2015).

Lombe and colleagues (2016) suggest that "[FI] moderate[s] the relationships between knowledge of nutrition and health outcomes with respect to . . . overall health risk," and that "in the absence of food security, the negative effects of vulnerability supersede the protective effects of nutrition education" (p. 454).

FOOD INTEGRITY

The integrity of food, when it is available, sparks broader issues of food production safety and long-term health implications. The National Institute of Environmental Health Sciences (NIEHS, 2010) has shown that chemicals in many everyday products, including the food supply, may interfere with the endocrine system. These "endocrine disruptors" may play a role in improper hormone function, obesity, diabetes, and some cancers (NIEHS, 2010). Similarly, the use of pesticides is an imposing and growing danger to global health. In fact, "There is probably no environmental health topic for which there is a greater level of citizen concern than exposure to pesticides" (Butterfield & Butterfield, 2003, p. 181).

The question of food integrity extends far beyond pesticides and environmental exposures; it a multivariant conversation. It includes genetically modified organisms (GMOs), food irradiation, and the environmental impacts of "slash and burn" agriculture. If individuals are able to access food, low-income communities are still at a dangerous risk of being relegated to highly processed products low in nutrition and high in sugar, salt, and saturated fats: all inductive of their own chronic health sequelae (Stuckler & Nestle, 2012). This is the result of food and beverage companies that monopolize market power across nations and provide low-cost options to the impoverished. Global nurses must continue to be diligent in their attention to dietary guidance and client-specific education regarding nutritional requirements.

INTERVENTIONS UNDERWAY

Supporting organizations have a hand in realizing that SDG 2 is an essential component of health promotion and advocacy. "Stop Hunger Now" (2016) looks to end world hunger by meal packaging for the most vulnerable populations; "The Hunger Project" (n.d.) partners with national and international governing bodies to promote self-reliance in helping men and women end their own hunger; global humanitarian organizations, such as Action Against Hunger/ACF International (2015), seek to battle the hunger pandemic by preventing, detecting, and treating malnutrition; and Heifer International (n.d.) empowers individuals by donating livestock or funding programs that donate livestock. By educating ourselves about these initiatives and the varied worldwide assistance available, global nurses can refer clients to appropriate services that meet their needs and economic criteria.

The Food and Agriculture Organization of the United Nations (FAO, 2009, 2013) confirms that while women make up the majority of the world's rural poor and are primarily charged with meeting the nutritional needs of families and children, they face far more legal and socioeconomic constraints in land ownership and agricultural rights than men. Global nurses have access to country profiles, gender and land-related statistics, and gender-equitable land tenure with the legal assessment tool (LAT) through the Gender and Land Rights Database (GLRD; FAO, 2016). Additionally, the World Bank (2009) provides references such as the *Gender in Agriculture Sourcebook* to help technicians and organizations more effectively implement gender-sensitive responses in the creation and implementation of agricultural initiatives. Intelligently accessing and applying these resources, global nurses are able to identify disparities and coach clients and populations to advocate for needed change and equity initiatives. Social justice and gender equality are clear and present priorities for all nurses, advocates, and leaders striving to overcome the barriers to humane health care and quality of life for all (Nickitas, 2016).

Through the proper assessment of clients and populations, food insecurity, the food choices they make and to which they have access, and the environmental exposure they experience, global nurses can make a great impact in the lives of clients and communities at large by making the connections between food supply and health outcomes. Our leadership roles and responsibilities in realizing SDG 2 require that we must have an increased knowledge of environmental health issues that impact food and agricultural practices, and use our skills in education, advocacy, empowerment, and coaching in order to promote wellness and well-being for all (Luck, 2016). We are each called to procure a culture of safety that prevents malnutrition, ensures equality, preserves the global food supply, and seeks to empower each of us as stewards of exemplary global health. SDG 2 assists us in expanding our global impact, understanding the importance of international resources, and partnering with like-minded organizations invested in the goal of "zero hunger" by 2030.

REFLECTION AND DISCUSSION

- How is ending hunger related to food insecurity, improved nutrition, and sustainable agriculture?

- In what ways will gender equity assist in reaching the targets of SDG 2?
- What is my role in global health education regarding food production, pesticide use, and integrity of the food supply?
- What is my global nursing priority in helping families meet their nutritional needs?
- How do I demonstrate my skills in education, advocacy, and empowerment regarding hunger and access to food?

REFERENCES

Action Against Hunger/ACF International. (2015). Home. Retrieved from http://www .actionagainsthunger.org

Beene, G. (2011). *The seeds we sow: Kindness that fed a hungry world*. Sante Fe, NM: Sunstone Press.

Butterfield, P., & Butterfield, P. (2003). Pesticide exposure. In B. Sattler & J. Lipscomb (Eds.), *Environmental health and nursing practice* (pp. 181–215). New York, NY: Springer Publishing.

Food and Agriculture Organization of the United Nations. (n.d.). Rome declaration on world food security. Retrieved from http://www.fao.org/docrep/003//w3613e/w3613e00.htm

Food and Agriculture Organization of the United Nations. (2009). *Bridging the gap: FAO's programme for gender equality in agriculture and rural development*. Rome, Italy: Author. Retrieved from http://www.fao.org/3/a-i1243e.pdf

Food and Agriculture Organization of the United Nations. (2013). *FAO policy on gender equality: Attaining food security goals in agriculture and rural development*. Rome, Italy: Author. Retrieved from http://www.fao.org/docrep/017/i3205e/i3205e.pdf

Food and Agriculture Organization of the United Nations. (2016). Gender and land rights database. Retrieved from http://www.fao.org/gender-landrights-database/en

Food and Agriculture Organization of the United Nations, International Fund for Agricultural Development, & World Food Programme. (2015). *The state of food insecurity in the world. Meeting the 2015 international hunger targets: Taking stock of uneven progress*. Rome, Italy: Food and Agriculture Organization of the United Nations. Retrieved from http://www .fao.org/3/a-i4646e.pdf

Gandhi, M. (n.d.). BrainyQuote. Retrieved from http://www.brainyquote.com/quotes/quotes/m/mahatmagan103624.html

Hager, E. R., Quigg, M. A., & Black, M. M. (2010). Development and validity of a 2-item screen to identify families at risk for food insecurity. *Pediatrics, 126*, e26–e32.

Heifer International. (n.d.). Home. Retrieved from http://www.heifer.org

The Hunger Project. (n.d.). Home. Retrieved from http://www.thp.org

Kregg-Byers, C. M., & Schlenk, E. A. (2010). Implications of food insecurity on global health policy and nursing practice. *Journal of Nursing Scholarship, 42*(3), 278–285.

Lombe, M., Nebbitt, V. E., Sinha, A., & Reynolds, A. (2016). Examining effects of food insecurity and food choices on health outcomes in households in poverty. *Social Work in Health Care, 55*(6), 440–460.

Luck, S. (2016). Informed and impactful: Stewarding the environmental determinants of health and well-being. In W. Rosa (Ed.), *Nurses as leaders: Evolutionary visions of leadership* (pp. 333–343). New York, NY: Springer Publishing.

National Institute of Environmental Health Sciences. (2010). Endocrine disruptors. Retrieved from https://www.niehs.nih.gov/health/materials/endocrine_disruptors_508.pdf

Nickitas, D. M. (2016). Ethical and economical: Calling the profession to social justice. In W. Rosa (Ed.), *Nurses as leaders: Evolutionary visions of leadership* (pp. 149–163). New York, NY: Springer Publishing.

Stop Hunger Now. (2016). Home. Retrieved from http://www.stophungernow.org

Stuckler, D., & Nestle, M. (2012). Big food, food systems, and global health. *PLOS Medicine, 9*(6), e1001242. doi:10.1371/journal.pmed.1001242

Tarasuk, V., Cheng, J., de Oliveira, C., Dachner, N., Gundersen, C., & Kurdyak, P. (2015). Association between household food insecurity and annual health care costs. *Canadian Medical Association Journal, 187*(14), E429–E436.

Theuri, S. (2015). Diagnosing food insecurity. *Journal for Nurse Practitioners, 11*(8), 834–835.

United Nations. (2006). Millennium Development Goal indicator database. Retrieved from http://unstats.un.org/unsd/mi/mi_goals.asp

United Nations. (2015). Transforming our world: The 2030 agenda for sustainable development. Retrieved from https://docs.google.com/gview?url=http://sustainabledevelopment .un.org/content/documents/21252030%20Agenda%20for%20Sustainable%20 Development%20web.pdf&embedded=true

United Nations Sustainable Development. (2016). Goal 2: End hunger, achieve food security and improved nutrition and promote sustainable agriculture. Retrieved from http://www .un.org/sustainabledevelopment/hunger

World Bank. (2009). *Gender in agriculture sourcebook.* Washington, DC: Author. Retrieved from http://www-wds.worldbank.org/external/default/WDSContentServer/WDSP/IB/ 2008/10/21/000333037_20081021011611/Rendered/PDF/461620PUB0Box3101 OFFICIAL0USE0ONLY1.pdf

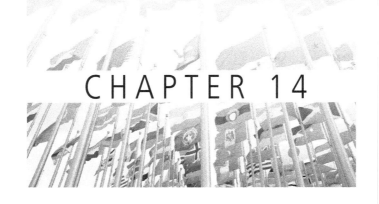

CHAPTER 14

Goal 3. Ensure Healthy Lives and Promote Well-Being for All at All Ages

William Rosa

[N]urses across the globe engage in whole-person health promotion . . .
help individuals, families, and communities find comfort and meaning in
their lives . . . alleviate . . . suffering . . . [and] improve wellbeing . . .
through caring/healing relationships [and the use of] evidence to inform
traditional and emerging interventions that support whole person/whole
systems healing. (Koithan, 2014, pp. 3–4)

Creating environments where health and well-being can flourish is a core responsibility of the nursing profession; a fundamental value rooted in the procurement of human dignity and the protection of human rights. An ongoing commitment to advocacy, social justice, and ethical values makes Sustainable Development Goal (SDG) 3 both a nursing prerogative and priority. Global nurses are at the forefront of this goal, helping to translate the ethic and ethos of human caring to communities and vulnerable populations at large in a way that transforms access to care and provides new possibilities for improved quality of life. Box 14.1 lists the targets associated with SDG 3. (see Appendix to view the Sustainable Development Agenda in its entirety; see Chapter 10 for a more detailed breakdown of the SDG 3 targets and nursing's role in their achievement).

Global nurses play a key role in leading research that decreases the multidimensional impacts of communicable diseases on individuals and nations, guiding policy changes that increase health care coverage for all members of society, and educating the public about the need for medication safety and vaccine scheduling. This global nursing presence is particularly important in low- and middle-income countries (LMICs) that experience the double burden of communicable and noncommunicable diseases (NCDs). Communicable diseases, such as HIV/AIDS, and tuberculosis, continue to reap devastating outcomes throughout the world, remaining a leading cause of morbidity and mortality in LMICs. NCDs—chronic illnesses—such as

Box 14.1 Sustainable Development Goal 3 and Its Associated Targets

Goal 3. Ensure healthy lives and promote well-being for all at all ages

3.1 By 2030, reduce the global maternal mortality ratio to less than 70 per 100,000 live births.

3.2 By 2030, end preventable deaths of newborns and children under 5 years of age, with all countries aiming to reduce neonatal mortality to at least as low as 12 per 1,000 live births and under-5 mortality to at least as low as 25 per 1,000 live births.

3.3 By 2030, end the epidemics of AIDS, tuberculosis, malaria, and neglected tropical diseases, and combat hepatitis, water-borne diseases, and other communicable diseases.

3.4 By 2030, reduce by one-third premature mortality from noncommunicable diseases through prevention and treatment, and promote mental health and well-being.

3.5 Strengthen the prevention and treatment of substance abuse, including narcotic drug abuse and harmful use of alcohol.

3.6 By 2020, halve the number of global deaths and injuries from road traffic accidents.

3.7 By 2030, ensure universal access to sexual and reproductive health care services, including for family planning, information and education, and the integration of reproductive health into national strategies and programs.

3.8 Achieve universal health coverage, including financial risk protection, access to quality essential health care services, and access to safe, effective, quality and affordable essential medicines and vaccines for all.

3.9 By 2030, substantially reduce the number of deaths and illnesses from hazardous chemicals, and air, water, and soil pollution and contamination.

3.a Strengthen the implementation of the WHO (World Health Organization) Framework Convention on Tobacco Control in all countries, as appropriate.

3.b Support the research and development of vaccines and medicines for the communicable and noncommunicable diseases that primarily affect developing countries, provide access to affordable essential medicines and vaccines, in accordance with the Doha Declaration on the Trade-Related Aspects of Intellectual Property Rights (TRIPS) Agreement and Public Health, which affirms the right of developing countries to use to the full the provisions in the agreement on TRIPS regarding flexibilities to protect public health, and, in particular, provide access to medicines for all.

3.c Substantially increase health financing and the recruitment, development, training, and retention of the health workforce in developing countries, especially in least developed countries and small island–developing states.

3.d Strengthen the capacity of all countries, in particular developing countries, for early warning, risk reduction, and management of national and global health risks.

Source: Reprinted with permission from the United Nations (2015).

cardiovascular disease, diabetes, and cancers, in addition to malnutrition, injuries, and exposure to violence, create extreme vulnerability for low-income populations, increasing susceptibility and worsening outcomes related to contracted communicable diseases. This double-burden epidemic was first presented as a global scale priority in the WHO's (WHO, 1999) *World Health Report*, although many researchers, institutions, and previous WHO world health reports had been tracking it for several years earlier (Frenk, Bobadilla, Sepuúlveda, & Cervantes, 1989; Murray & Lopez, 1996; WHO, 1998). In their 1999 report, WHO described the data from many LMICs that showed that NCDs were replacing infectious diseases and malnutrition "as the leading causes of disability and premature death" for the first time in history (p. 14).

The literature has continued to demonstrate that this double burden dilemma is far from over, made more deleterious by the lack of primary care interventions, health care worker shortages, insufficient systems infrastructures, and economically inaccessible or unsustainable treatment plans (Cappuccio & Miller, 2016; Misganaw, Mariam, & Araya, 2012; Ngalesoni, Ruhago, Norheim, & Robberstad, 2015; Iwelunmor et al., 2016). Although most NCDs can be sufficiently controlled by the current medical and public health tools available, the poor—the estimated 800 million who live on less than $1.00 per day—do not likely have access to the innumerable health resources required of effective long-term management (Farmer et al., 2013). Due to the reciprocal and interdependent nature of NCDs and communicable illnesses, global nurses must drive policy that will impact the two simultaneously, rather than advocating to pool already limited funding toward one or the other (Bygbjerg, 2012).

Approaches to global health progress will shift given the particular sociopolitical and economic status of the group, community, or nation. Each country will continue to encounter both unique and shared challenges throughout the SDG implementation processes. For example, Bangladesh faces a paucity of financial and nonfinancial resources, institutional mechanisms for implementation, and lacks nationwide participation and accountability (Bhattacharya, 2015). Pakistan, on the other hand, will need to focus on integrating the global agenda into the national policies, strengthen partnerships between federal and provincial authorities, and build the capacities of local, more regionally centered, governmental structures to deliver enhanced services (Ahmad, 2015). And India, like many LMICs, faces the difficulties of nurse migration, poor rural road infrastructure, and insufficient salaries for nurses, particularly those working outside of major urban areas (Manjrekar, 2016).

Global nurses must continue to build partnerships with governments, nongovernmental organizations (NGOs), donors, and civil societies that lead to collaborative solutions and benefit all involved (Sliney, 2015). In this way, the outcomes and long-term efforts are representative of stakeholders' values and contributions. The health and well-being of any nation depends upon the strength of these partnerships and the willingness of participants to share accountability and refine programs based on evolving needs.

Ultimately, the Sustainable Development Agenda is calling for a global Culture of Health, where the varied needs of diverse populations are reflected in relevant policies, and attended to through a multisector approach to positive change. A "Culture of Health" can be broadly defined as "one in which good health and well-being flourish across geographic, demographic, and social sectors; fostering healthy equitable communities guides public and private decision making; and

> **Box 14.2** **Culture of Health Vision: Underlying Principles (for a global audience)**
>
> 1. Good health flourishes across geographic, demographic, and social sectors, and throughout the global village.
> 2. Attaining the best health possible is valued across cultures and continents.
> 3. Individuals and families have the means and the opportunity to make choices that lead to the healthiest lives possible.
> 4. Businesses, national governments, individuals, and organizations work together to build healthy communities and lifestyles for all men, women, and children.
> 5. Universal health care coverage is accessible and affordable to all because it is essential to maintain, or reclaim, health.
> 6. No one is excluded.
> 7. Health care is efficient and equitable.
> 8. The economy is less burdened by excessive and unwarranted health care spending.
> 9. Keeping everyone as healthy as possible guides public, private, and transnational decision making.
> 10. Global citizens understand that we are all in this together.
>
> *Source:* Adapted from Plough & Chandra (2015). Reprinted with permission from the Robert Wood Johnson Foundation.

everyone has the opportunity to make choices that lead to healthy lifestyles"; it recognizes that such a culture will look different to different people and must be inclusive of varied beliefs, values, and customs (Robert Wood Johnson Foundation [RWJF], n.d.). It requires a commitment on behalf of individuals, communities, and key public and private stakeholders to collaborate toward a healthier society now and for generations to come (Plough & Chandra, 2015). The underlying principles in Box 14.2 have been identified by Plough and Chandra (2015) as foundational to building and sustaining a Culture of Health.

ADVANCED PRACTICE: LEVERAGING THE IMPACT OF NURSING ON HEALTH AND WELL-BEING

SDG 3 holds particular promise for Advanced Practice Registered Nurses (APRNs) to lead and effect measurable change. *APRN* is an umbrella term encompassing certified nurse midwives, certified registered nurse anesthetists, clinical nurse specialists, and nurse practitioners. The International Council of Nurses (ICN; n.d.) recommends a master's degree for entry level as an APRN and defines the role as "a registered nurse who has acquired the expert knowledge base, complex decision-making skills and clinical competencies for expanded practice, the characteristics of which are shaped by the context and/or country in which s/he is credentialed to practice." The APRN role does not exist in all countries worldwide; however, APRN opportunities are expanding internationally and carry with them challenges that must be addressed (Kleinpell et al., 2014). Health care systems that promote APRN practice and nursing- and midwifery-led research have produced notable literature suggesting a positive correlation between appropriate APRN utilization and improved outcomes related to the delivery of high-quality care (Newhouse et al., 2011).

The globally recognized skills of APRNs are transferrable across settings, though regulated by in-country policies, and are essential to SDG 3 target attainment. These skills include the rights to diagnose; prescribe medication and treatment; refer clients to specialists and admit them as needed to hospitals; and guide legislation regarding APRN scope and standards of practice (ICN, 2001-2017). This expanded scope of practice implies an advanced level of education and formal licensure processes. However, in many LMICs, many nurses struggle to clarify scope and standards at the most basic level, and often do not have access to additional education for a host of reasons. There are additional challenges to the APRN role in the global arena, such as limited access to and poorly structured nursing education programs; a system-wide focus on the medical model; lack of knowledge regarding the APRN role; absence of regard for nursing as a profession; dominance of medicine or physician-led systems; and multifactorial issues that complicate credentialing (Pulcini, Jelic, Gul, & Loke, 2010). Ultimately, APRNs can become viable change agents by communicating about the APRN role and value of APRN-delivered care to stakeholders; instituting media campaigns to raise awareness; lobbying for progress in policy development; implementing models that leverage the APRN contribution to health care; educating global partners at all levels of government and health about APRN practice and contributions; and disseminating knowledge related to collaborative models of health care inclusive of APRNs (Brassard & Smolenski, 2011; Kleinpell et al., 2014; RWJF, 2013).

The American Association of Nurse Practitioners (AANP) is just one organization that helps to guide the future of APRNs. The AANP (2012-2017) promotes core values of integrity, excellence, professionalism, leadership, and service to assist nurse practitioners specifically in obtaining their purpose of high-quality health care for all. These core values are guideposts for all APRNs that choose to take pioneering leads in the globalization of the APRN role and ensure good health and well-being for all peoples everywhere, as guided by SDG 3. The APRN is truly a transformational advocate in implementing these core values and leading populations toward healthier lives (Rosa & Lubansky, 2016).

PALLIATIVE AND END-OF-LIFE CARE

While palliative care is not expressly stated as a component of the Sustainable Development Agenda, as global nurses, we cannot ignore the deeply complex experiences faced by human beings amid advanced serious illness and at the end of life. So whether addressing maternal, neonatal, and infant mortality (targets 3.1 and 3.2); AIDS, tuberculosis, and malaria (target 3.3); or the diseases secondary to the use of hazardous chemicals and air, water, and soil pollution (target 3.9), global nurses must lobby and drive the local and global policies that determine the access to and delivery of equitable, quality palliative care. Palliative care is defined by the WHO (2017) as "an approach that improves the quality of life of patients and their families facing the problems associated with life-threatening illness, through the prevention and relief of suffering by means of early identification and impeccable assessment and treatment of pain and other problems, physical, psychosocial, and spiritual." Palliative care can be given in conjunction with curative treatment or with an exclusive focus on comfort and aggressive symptom management. Palliative care has been identified as a human right (Brennan et al., 2015), its ideals are being furthered through countless international initiatives worldwide (Connor, 2015), and it is considered an altruistic and essential component of human-centered care, even in the face of scarce resources, mass casualty events, and situations of conflict (Cherny, 2015; Wilkinson & Matzo, 2015). Ultimately, palliative care strives to maximize quality of life while minimizing distressing disease-related symptoms, align care planning with the patient's values and wishes, and ensure that the whole person needs of the patient—mental, emotional, social, physiological, and spiritual—are attended to. While "palliative care" is often used interchangeably with "end-of-life care," palliative care can be initiated at any point along the trajectory of advanced serious illness, and its scope is not limited to the patient at end of life. However, there are an estimated 20.4 million people globally in need of palliative care at the end of life, the vast majority of whom live in LMICs (Worldwide Palliative Care Alliance, 2014).

Global nurses have an obligation to usher in increased consciousness and sensitivity regarding not only the quality of people's living and lives, but also that of their dying and deaths. Nurses do this by creating healing environments that respect patients as whole human beings in the sacred process of dying (Rosa & Estes, 2016; Rosa, Estes, & Watson, 2017), strategizing end-of-life care that promotes patient–family togetherness and quiet spaces for reflection and patient dignity (Keegan & Drick, 2011, 2013), and providing opportunities for peace and peaceful presence (Keegan & Drick, 2016). We have an obligation to constantly evaluate our systems and practices to maintain ethical integrity in how patients' dying is supported and guided (Rosa, 2014). This must be accomplished in culturally sensitive ways that respect both personal feelings of all involved and professional and ethical obligations.

Reflective practice is particularly useful to nurses working in end-of-life settings as a way to make sense of difficult emotions and support ongoing personal and professional well-being (see Chapter 30 for more on reflective practice). The article that follows, reprinted in full from Rosa (2016), is an example of such a reflection; an expression that moves from self-doubt and judgment of other toward an emerging personal–professional paradigm of acceptance and unity.

Dying and Caring in a Rwandan Intensive Care Unit

I hold Uwimana as she nears the end of her life. Uwimana translates as "daughter of God" and I think to myself that she is my sister. And so we must share this Parent; this origin, this spirit space. I try to be of service while attempting to employ what one of my modern-day heroines, Jacqueline Novogratz, calls "moral imagination"; the humility to see things as they are and the audacity to imagine them as they could be (Acumen Fund, 2016). This fine line of caring calls me to surrender in acceptance and yet strive for possibility; to respect the cross-cultural exchange and yet honor my individual ethical code; to understand setbacks while striving for balance and a dignified dying and death.

Uwimana was admitted to intensive care when it became clear the internal medicine wards were unable to provide the palliative measures required to relieve the symptomatic distress of her end-stage illness. Here in Rwanda, the socioeconomic notion that money buys everything is a solid reality; if you don't have the cash, you don't get the bed. Administration was assured that compensation was not a problem and she was wheeled in.

I looked at Uwimana and took a momentary assessment. Mental status: unresponsive. Vital signs: alarming. Her face: somehow peaceful. I asked the intensive care unit (ICU) physician if we were expected to resuscitate in the event of a cardiac arrest and received a shoulder shrug accompanied by an obligatory, "If the family wants."

Rwanda's referral hospital ICU demographic is dependent upon a severely resource-constrained medical system. Most patients are initially treated at district hospitals outside the major city of Kigali. Patients undergo surgical interventions from general practitioners; physicians who have been trained in medical school for 5 years and then afterward serve a 1-year multispecialty internship are then expected to be versatile practitioners.

They are placed in the distressful position of attending to village populations and providing myriad procedures for which they do not possess the training required. As a consequence, patients very often become septic or progress in illness without appropriate medical treatment. By the time they are transferred to a referral hospital, their disease process is nearly impossible to curtail.

The professional–cultural response to death has become habituated to frequent experience with loss. Interdisciplinary teams in low-income countries like Rwanda have become accustomed to high rates of patient mortality, and end-of-life care does not receive any distinctive sensitivity or attention. Here, patients die on a regular basis from what high-income countries would consider highly preventable conditions. In the face of these repetitive and emotionally complex circumstances, what is the cost of caring? This is a question that remains unaddressed largely because it goes unasked.

Consider also a national history of genocide: Just under one generation ago, approximately 1 million Rwandans were killed as a result of ethnically divisive crimes against humanity. While there has been progress and healing and evolution, undercurrents of resentment and anger still linger. Maybe human caring is too much to strive for when so many have settled for mere survival. When one is just trying to get through the day, there is little room to thrive or give of oneself in ways above what is required.

Uwimana's dying has become just another event during just another day. I try to see this systemic reality for what it is. I try to imagine it as it could be and watch my fellow Rwandan nurses grieve for their patients. I see how deeply they care underneath their efforts to be strong. Their caring is expressed in the disappointment of "another patient lost." The nurses don't have the resources to do enough for their patients, to care for their patients well enough, or to make it all happen quickly enough. And so they feel insufficient as healers. It is as if they shy away from demonstrations of caring so they don't have to face the pain staring back at them. They focus on the tasks to be completed so they can leave their hearts alone.

Amid this cultural dilemma, there is an opportunity to care for Uwimana in her need. She is now labeled "comfort care," but it is not "comfort" as I know it. I wince as adrenalin is primed and intubation is debated. I dig deep to muster responses of patience and support for my Rwandan nursing family; the same patience and support they lovingly cultivate for me on a daily basis. But I speak my heart; I ask for what I think she would ask for and for what I see she needs. They listen and try to make room for my opinions in the room.

My Western-oriented mental rant has its go at me: Where is the clinical management of her pain? Shouldn't comfort be what I think it should be? Shouldn't the unfolding of dying and death be honored as sacred and an opportunity for healing?

I find out later that my Rwandan colleagues are seeing me with the same perplexed perspectives. They have been thinking: Let her die in peace. Allow the dying process to be as it is. Let us not interfere. There is nothing for us to do; this is for her to do on her own. We are two cultures, shoulder to shoulder, with the same concern but completely different approaches to achieving it.

It is all very foreign to me, this yearning to accept conditions and circumstances about which I remain so confused. I let go of the need to have it look like what I want it to look like. I am merely a guest; a visitor who searches for the lens required to understand. There is a universality to death that affects us all, and extends across diverse societal norms and socioeconomic strata, and I know death: I've seen death. I've witnessed it. I've held it.

The unfolding moments now call for my caring sensibilities. They urge me to embrace a new way of being that is one of presence and deep listening; a more decisive way of doing with attention and authenticity, and particularly heightened ways of knowing that suspend judgment and invite transpersonal acceptance.

I stand next to Uwimana as she lies with eyes closed, unresponsive to my voice, the uncertainty of a next breath somehow weighing on her chest. She moves through her dying. I place one hand on her head and one on her heart—it feels like the right thing to do. I stay with her until her end. The ICU physician has assured me no resuscitation will take place and that intubation is off the table. He's even surprised me with his order for morphine to ease her struggle to breathe.

I share with the nurses how to be with a dying person at this time. They share with me how to let a dying person be. I attune myself to her fluctuating breaths. In that moment I learn the most precious of lessons once again. By my actions, not my words, I influence humanity, for this blessed moment at least. In choosing to listen to another, I've been granted the gift of being heard. In that space, all is as it should be.

In this quiet labyrinth I reflect on whom I've really nursed. Was I easing my pain or hers? I welcome a moment of clarity: Here lies a 98-year-old Rwandan woman who has seen countless family members die, who has lived through several genocides and ethnic pogroms, and who has been through all of that most likely without the contributions of narcotics or technology or even medical involvement. Most likely too, she already knew how to be present with dying and death and was prepared. Maybe she didn't need my help at all.

In the end Uwimana ceases to be Rwandan or a woman or rich or poor. She transitions while being honored and cared for among nurses who are learning to grow and evolve, myself included. She does not die alone. She is given a sacred passage defined by loving kindness. It is the sacred passage of one, through the awakening of caring, compassion, and connection that lights a path of self-illumination for all of us.

Source: This copy is reprinted from Rosa (2016), with permission of the *Journal of Art and Aesthetics in Nursing and Health Sciences* © 2016.

SELF-CARE

The tenets of good health and well-being also apply to our individual wellness journeys. Global nurses are called to be role models of self-care and health consciousness as vanguards of an inclusive future where no one is left behind; this includes ourselves. An ongoing commitment to the process of self-development—the reflective and restorative practices that bring renewal and self-knowledge over time—is an ethical cornerstone and foundational component of bringing about a peaceful and caring society (Pesut, 2016; Shields & Stout-Shaffer, 2016). The first steps toward good health and well-being begin now, with what we have and what we know, acknowledging how we feel and what we think, and creating a vision of where we want to be and what is needed to get us there.

An integrative approach can aid us in identifying and assessing the broad spectrum of contributors to overall health and well-being. The Integrative Health and Wellness Assessment (IHWA; Dossey, Luck, & Schaub, 2015) considers the following life areas of the human being in our journey toward wholeness and optimal health:

- Life balance and satisfaction
- Relationships
- Spirituality
- Mental
- Emotional
- Physical (nutrition, exercise, weight management)
- Environmental
- Health responsibility

The IHWA "assists people in becoming aware of their human potential in each of these categories, identifying strengths and weaknesses, and considering and creating new health goals" (Dossey & Luck, 2016, p. 705) and the categories that compose it are illustrated by the IHWA wheel (Figure 14.1).

Figure 14.1 | **Integrative Health and Wellness Assessment wheel.**

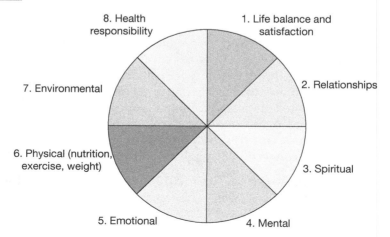

Source: Reprinted from Dossey, Luck, and Schaub (2015). Permission granted by the International Nurse Coach Association.

The IHWA is a questionnaire that explores each of the above life areas in depth, assists the user in acknowledging their readiness for and priorities related to change, and provides the opportunity to create an action plan based on current lifestyle. If we are going to be "global" in our work, we must commit to be "global" in our assessments of self and other, addressing all social and environmental determinants of health, as well as the mental, emotional, and spiritual aspects of well-being. The IHWA (short form) is located at the end of this chapter for reader use, and is an important assessment for global nurses to utilize in their care of self and in their holistic assessment of others.

One cannot positively impact health and well-being on a global scale until that same level of attention and care is focused inward. Beyond self-use, the IHWA can be employed in part or in whole as an assessment of clients during both the introductory phases and throughout the trajectory of ongoing partnerships. It is intended to be a tool for self-development as the global nurse continues to promote improved health behaviors and health awareness for both self and others. Dossey and Luck (2016) remind us that, "When one strives to develop in one or several areas, a sense of wholeness emerges, one's self-worth increases, and action plans for healthier lifestyle behaviors and goals are actualized" (pp. 714–715).

In the transnational context, it is important that the global nurse takes the time to understand what "health" means to the client and what treatment plan is most appropriate for the client and his or her family/population/nation. Well-being is determined not only by individual factors of health and the clients' sense of purpose in life, but also by the quality of relationships, power of community, and the environment in which they work and live (Kreitzer & Koithan, 2014). Nurses are in the privileged position to translate the caring–healing ethic of the profession to those working to implement SDG 3 so that all human beings may live healthy lives and experience an improved sense of vitality and well-being.

In closing, commit to completing the IHWA (short form) shown in Figure 14.2. Familiarize yourself with the areas of assessment, and look for opportunities to integrate them into client assessments, interactions, and provisions of care.

REFLECTION AND DISCUSSION

- How can I procure health and well-being for myself, first and foremost, and then for others?
- Am I intentional about demonstrating a caring ethic in the practice of global nursing?
- What are the challenges in assessing the unique needs of populations, including the double burden of disease?
- How do I cocreate meaningful and useful solutions for the community at hand?
- In what ways might I promote a more integrative definition of well-being, beyond the individual mental–emotional–physical–spiritual factors, to include relationships and the environment?

| Figure 14.2 | Integrative Health and Wellness Assessment (short form). |

INTEGRATIVE HEALTH AND WELLNESS ASSESSMENT™

This **INTEGRATIVE HEALTH and WELLNESS ASSESSMENT** (short form) is intended for informational purposes only. It is not a substitute for professional medical advice, diagnosis or treatment.

DIRECTIONS: This questionnaire contains statements about your present way of life, feelings, and personal habits. Please respond to each item as accurately as possible, and try not to skip any item. Indicate the frequency with which you engage in each item by shading (●) one of the following:

1 = Never   2 = Rarely   3 = Occasionally   4 = Frequently   5 = Always

Life Balance/Satisfaction   / 20   ❶ ❷ ❸ ❹ ❺

1. I have balance between my work, family, friends, and self.   ◯ ◯ ◯ ◯ ◯

2. I can release anxiety, worry, and fear in a healthy way.   ◯ ◯ ◯ ◯ ◯

3. I use strategies (breathing, stretching, relaxation, meditation and imagery) to manage stress daily.   ◯ ◯ ◯ ◯ ◯

4. I recognize negative thoughts and reframe them.   ◯ ◯ ◯ ◯ ◯

Relationships   / 15

5. I create and participate in satisfying relationships.   ◯ ◯ ◯ ◯ ◯

6. I feel comfortable sharing my feelings/opinion without feeling guilty.   ◯ ◯ ◯ ◯ ◯

7. I easily express love and concern to those I care about.   ◯ ◯ ◯ ◯ ◯

Spiritual   / 15

8. I feel that my life has meaning, value, and purpose.   ◯ ◯ ◯ ◯ ◯

9. I feel connected to a force greater than myself.   ◯ ◯ ◯ ◯ ◯

10. I make time for reflective practice (affirmation, prayer, meditation).   ◯ ◯ ◯ ◯ ◯

Mental   / 15

11. I prioritize my work and set realistic goals.   ◯ ◯ ◯ ◯ ◯

12. I ask for help/assistance when needed.   ◯ ◯ ◯ ◯ ◯

13. I can accept circumstances and events that are beyond my control.   ◯ ◯ ◯ ◯ ◯

①

(continued)

Figure 14.2 *(continued)*

	1	2	3	4	5
Emotional / 20					
14. I recognize my own feelings and emotions.	○	○	○	○	○
15. I express my feelings in appropriate ways.	○	○	○	○	○
16. I practice forgiveness.	○	○	○	○	○
17. I listen to and respect the feelings of others.	○	○	○	○	○
Physical/Nutrition / 20					
18. I eat at least 5 servings of fruits and vegetables, and recommended whole foods (beans, nuts, etc.) daily.	○	○	○	○	○
19. I drink 6-8 glasses of water daily.	○	○	○	○	○
20. I eat real food.	○	○	○	○	○
21. I eat mindfully (concentrate on eating and not multi-tasking or eating in front of the TV).	○	○	○	○	○
Physical/Exercise / 15					
22. I do stretching or flexibility exercises (head, neck, shoulders, back, legs) for at least 5 minutes, 3 days a week.	○	○	○	○	○
23. I do strength exercises (use strength-training equipment, sit-ups, push-ups) regularly.	○	○	○	○	○
24. I do aerobic exercise (jogging, swimming, fitness walking using arms, aerobic dance, active sports) regularly, using at least moderate intensity, 3 or more days a week for at least 30 minutes.	○	○	○	○	○
Physical/Weight / 10					
25. I maintain an ideal weight.	○	○	○	○	○
26. I have gained no more than 11 pounds in adulthood.	○	○	○	○	○
Environmental / 15					
27. I have a healthy non-toxic home environment.	○	○	○	○	○
28. I have a healthy non-toxic work environment.	○	○	○	○	○
29. I am aware of how my external environment affects my health and wellbeing.	○	○	○	○	○

2

(continued)

Figure 14.2 (*continued*)

Health Responsibility / 35   ① ② ③ ④ ⑤

30. I believe I am key to my wellbeing and overall health. ◯ ◯ ◯ ◯ ◯

31. I know my blood pressure, triglycerides, cholesterol and glucose levels. ◯ ◯ ◯ ◯ ◯

32. I am aware of my risk factors for disease. ◯ ◯ ◯ ◯ ◯

33. I pay attention to my physical wellbeing and address symptoms as they arise. ◯ ◯ ◯ ◯ ◯

34. I can work and do regular activities of daily life. ◯ ◯ ◯ ◯ ◯

35. I avoid smoking or using smokeless tobacco. ◯ ◯ ◯ ◯ ◯

36. I discuss/formulate a wellness plan with my primary healthcare provider and take (if needed) and know prescribed medications and possible side effects. ◯ ◯ ◯ ◯ ◯

Total Score / 180

3

(*continued*)

Figure 14.2 (*continued*)

AREAS TO ADDRESS	SCORE	MY READINESS TO CHANGE 1= In one year 2= Within 6 months 3= Next month 4= In two weeks 5= Now	PRIORITY FOR MAKING CHANGE (1-5) 1= Never a priority 2= Very low priority 3= Medium priority 4= Priority 5= Highest priority	CONFIDENCE IN MY ABILITY TO DO IT (1-5) 1= Not at all confident 2= Not very confident 3= Somewhat confident 4= Confident 5= Very confident
Life Balance/Satisfaction	/ 20			
Relationship	/ 15			
Spiritual	/ 15			
Mental	/ 15			
Emotional	/ 20			
Physical/Nutrition	/ 20			
Physical/Exercise	/ 15			
Physical/Weight	/ 10			
Environment	/ 15			
Health Responsibility	/ 35			

©2014. International Nurse Coach Association. www.inursecoach.com

④

(continued)

Figure 14.2 (*continued*)

ACTION PLAN

Please list 3 changes that you can implement into your current lifestyle over the next 3 months:

1.

2.

3.

Additional changes, comments, thoughts:

REFERENCES

Acumen Fund. (2016). About Acumen: Who we are, what we do, how we do it, and why. Retrieved from http://acumen.org/content/uploads/2013/02/Acumen-Leadership -model.png

Ahmad, N. (2015). *Translating Sustainable Development Goals (SDGs) at the country level*. Islamabad: Leadership for Environment And Development Pakistan. Retrieved from http://www .lead.org.pk/lead/Uploaded_images/Events/Policy%20Note%20-%20Translating%20 Sustainable%20Development%20Goals%20(SDGs)%20at%20the%20National%20Level.pdf

American Association of Nurse Practitioners. (2012-2017). Core purpose and values. Retrieved from https://www.aanp.org/press-room/press-releases/163-about-aanp/strategic -focus-tabs/1860-core-purpose-and-values

Bhattacharya, D. (2015). The agenda of Sustainable Development Goals: Implementation challenges for Bangladesh. Retrieved from http://cpd.org.bd/wp-content/uploads/ 2015/10/The-Agenda-of-Sustainable-Development-Goals-Implementation-Challenges -for-Bangladesh-CPD-Debapriya-Bhattacharya.pdf

Brassard, A., & Smolenski, M. (2011). Removing barriers to advanced practice registered nurse care. *Insight on the Issue, 55*. Washington, DC: AARP Public Policy Institute. Retrieved from http://campaignforaction.org/sites/default/files/RemovingBarriers -HospitalPrivileges.pdf

Brennan, F., Gwyther, L., Lohman, D., Kiyange, F., Ezer, T., & Mwangi-Powell, F. N. (2015). Palliative care as a human right. In B. R. Ferrell, N. Coyle, & J. A. Paice (Eds.), *Oxford textbook of palliative nursing* (4th ed., pp. 1174–1178). New York, NY: Oxford University Press.

Bygbjerg, I. C. (2012). Double burden of noncommunicable and infectious diseases in developing countries. *Science, 337*(6101), 1499–1501.

Cappuccio, F. P., & Miller, M. A. (2016). Cardiovascular disease and hypertension in sub-Saharan Africa: Burden, risk and interventions. *Internal and Emergency Medicine, 11*(3), 299–305.

Cherny, N. I. (2015). Palliative care in situations of conflict. In B. R. Ferrell, N. Coyle, & J. A. Paice (Eds.), *Oxford textbook of palliative nursing* (4th ed., pp. 1168–1173). New York, NY: Oxford University Press.

Connor, S. R. (2015). International palliative care initiatives. In B. R. Ferrell, N. Coyle, & J. A. Paice (Eds.), *Oxford textbook of palliative nursing* (4th ed., pp. 1056–1057). New York, NY: Oxford University Press.

Dossey, B. M., & Luck, S. (2016). Self-assessments. In B. M. Dossey & L. Keegan (Eds.), *Holistic nursing: A handbook for practice* (7th ed., pp. 703–715). Burlington, MA: Jones & Bartlett.

Dossey, B. M., Luck, S., & Schaub, B. G. (2015). *Nurse coaching: Integrative approaches for heath and well-being*. North Miami, FL: International Nurse Coach Association.

Farmer, P., Basilico, M., Kerry, V., Ballard, M., Becker, A., Bukhman, G., . . . Yamamoto, A. (2013). Global health priorities for the early twenty-first century. In P. Farmer, J. Y. Kim, A. Kleinman, & M. Basilico (Eds.), *Reimagining global health: An introduction* (pp. 302–339). Berkeley and Los Angeles: University of California Press.

Frenk, J., Bobadilla, J. L., Sepuúlveda, J., & Cervantes, M. L. (1989). Health transition in middle-income countries: New challenges for health care. *Health Policy & Planning, 4*(1), 29–39.

International Council of Nursing. (n.d.). Definition and characteristics of the role. Retrieved from http://international.aanp.org/Practice/APNRoles

Iwelunmor, J., Blackstone, S., Veira, D., Nwaozuru, U., Airhihenbuwa, C., Munodawafa, D., . . . Ogedegbe, G. (2016). Toward the sustainability of health interventions implemented in sub-Saharan Africa: A systematic review and conceptual framework. *Implementation Science, 11*, 1–27.

Keegan, L., & Drick, C. A. (2011). *End of life: Nursing solutions for death with dignity*. New York, NY: Springer Publishing.

Keegan, L., & Drick, C. A. (2013). *The golden room: A practical guide for death with dignity*. Charleston, SC: CreateSpace.

Keegan, L., & Drick, C. A. (2016). *Dying in peace*. In B. M. Dossey & L. Keegan (Eds.), *Holistic nursing: A handbook for practice* (7th ed., pp. 415–435). Burlington, MA: Jones & Bartlett.

Kleinpell, R., Scanlon, A., Hibbert, D., Ganz, F., East, L., Fraser, D., . . . Beauchesne, M. (2014). Addressing issues impacting advanced nursing practice worldwide. *Online Journal of Issues in Nursing, 19*(2), manuscript 5. doi:10.3912/OJIN.Vol19No02Man05

Koithan, M. (2014). Concepts and principles of integrative nursing. In M. J. Kreitzer & M. Koithan (Eds.), *Integrative nursing* (pp. 3–16). New York, NY: Oxford University Press.

Kreitzer, M. J., & Koithan, M. (Eds.). (2014). *Integrative nursing.* New York, NY: Oxford University Press.

Manjrekar, P. (2016). Resourceful and unified: Partnering across cultures and worldviews. In W. Rosa (Ed.), *Nurses as leaders: Evolutionary visions of leadership* (pp. 345–358). New York, NY: Springer Publishing.

Misganaw, A., Mariam, D. H., & Araya, T. (2012). The double mortality burden among adults in Addis Ababa, Ethiopia, 2006–2009. *Preventing Chronic Diseases, 9.* doi:10.5888/pcd9.110142

Murray, C. J. L., & Lopez, A. D. (Eds.). (1996). *The global burden of disease: A comprehensive assessment of mortality and disability from diseases, injuries, and risk factors in 1990 and projected to 2020.* Cambridge, MA: Harvard University Press.

Newhouse, R. P., Stanik-Hutt, J., White, K. M., Johantgen, M., Bass, E. B., Zangaro, G., . . . Weiner, J. P. (2011). Advanced practice nurse outcomes 1998–2008: A systematic review. *Nursing Economic$, 29*(5), 1–21.

Ngalesoni, F., Ruhago, G., Norheim, O. F., & Robberstad, B. (2015). Economic cost of primary prevention of cardiovascular diseases in Tanzania. *Health Policy & Planning, 30*(8), 875–884.

Pesut, D. J. (2016). Tranformed and in service: Creating the future through renewal. In W. Rosa (Ed.), *Nurses as leaders: Evolutionary visions of leadership* (pp. 165–178). New York, NY: Springer Publishing.

Plough, A. & Chandra, A. (2015). *From vision to action: A framework and measures to mobilize a Culture of Health.* Princeton, NJ: Robert Wood Johnson Foundation. Retrieved from http://www.rwjf.org/content/dam/COH/RWJ000_COH-Update_CoH_Report_1b.pdf

Pulcini, J., Jelic, M., Gul, R., & Loke, A. Y. (2010). An international survey on advanced practice nursing education, practice, and regulation. *Journal of Nursing Scholarship, 42*(1), 31–39.

Robert Wood Johnson Foundation. (n.d.). What is a culture of health? Retrieved from http://www.evidenceforaction.org/what-culture-health

Robert Wood Johnson Foundation. (2013). Improving patient access to high quality care: How to fully utilize the skills, knowledge, and experience of advanced practice registered nurses. Retrieved from http://www.rwjf.org/content/dam/farm/reports/issue_briefs/2013/rwjf405378

Rosa, W. (2014). Conscious dying and cultural emergence: Reflective systems inventory for the collective processes of global healing. *Beginnings, 34*(5), 20–22.

Rosa, W. (2016). Dying and caring in a Rwandan intensive care unit. *Journal of Art and Aesthetics in Nursing and Health Sciences, 3*(2), 10–13.

Rosa, W., & Estes, T. (2016). What end-of-life care needs now: An emerging praxis of the sacred and subtle. *Advances in Nursing Science, 39*(4), 333–345.

Rosa, W., Estes, T., & Watson, J. (2017). Caring science conscious dying: An emerging meta-paradigm. *Nursing Science Quarterly, 30*(1). doi:10.1177/0894318416680538

Rosa, W., & Lubansky, S. (2016). The advanced practice holistic nurse: A leader in the implementation of core values. *Beginnings, 36*(3), 10–13.

Shields, D. A., & Stout-Shaffer, S. (2016). Self-development: The foundation of holistic self-care. In B. M. Dossey & L. Keegan (Eds.), *Holistic nursing: A handbook for practice* (7th ed., pp. 683–702). Burlington, MA: Jones & Bartlett.

Sliney, A. (2015). Global health partnerships. In S. Breakey, I. B. Corless, N. L. Meedzan, & P. K. Nicholas (Eds.), *Global health nursing in the 21st century* (pp. 103–111). New York, NY: Springer Publishing.

United Nations. (2015). Transforming our world: The 2030 Agenda for Sustainable Development. Retrieved from https://docs.google.com/gview?url=http://sustainabledevelopment.un.org/content/documents/21252030%20Agenda%20for%20Sustainable%20Development%20web.pdf&embedded=true

United Nations Development Programme. (2016). Goal 3: Good health and well-being. Retrieved from http://www.undp.org/content/undp/en/home/sdgoverview/post-2015-development-agenda/goal-3.html

Wilkinson, A., & Matzo, M. (2015). Palliative care in mass casualty events with scarce resources. In B. R. Ferrell, N. Coyle, & J. A. Paice (Eds.), *Oxford textbook of palliative nursing* (4th ed., pp. 823–833). New York, NY: Oxford University Press.

World Health Organization. (1998). *The world health report 1998: Life in the 21st century: A vision for all.* Geneva, Switzerland: Author. Retrieved from http://www.who.int/whr/1998/en/whr98_en.pdf

World Health Organization. (1999). *The world health report 1999: Making a difference.* Geneva, Switzerland: Author. Retrieved from http://www.who.int/whr/1999/en/whr99_en.pdf?ua=1

World Health Organization. (2017). WHO definition of palliative care. Retrieved from http://www.who.int/cancer/palliative/definition/en

Worldwide Palliative Care Alliance. (2014). Global atlas of palliative care at the end of life. Retrieved from http://www.who.int/nmh/Global_Atlas_of_Palliative_Care.pdf

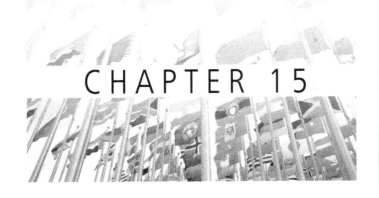

CHAPTER 15

Goal 4. Ensure Inclusive and Equitable Quality Education and Promote Lifelong Learning Opportunities for All

William Rosa

The right to a quality education is, I believe, the perfect path to bridge the gap between different cultures and to reconcile various civilizations. Without such a right, the values of liberty, justice, and equality will have no meaning. Ignorance is by far the biggest danger and threat to humankind. (Al Missned, 2009, p. 2)

Nursing's role in educating the public has forever been a cornerstone of the profession. It is an ethical prerogative to procure quality education for those we serve, and deliver it in a contextually relevant manner for clients across cultures. But how do we know our education is effective? How do we assure that education is given in a way clients, be they individuals or populations, can receive it? What is nursing's duty in promoting equitable educational access on a transnational scale? Quality education as a human right is one of the pressing changes needed to transform the world as we know it; and global nurses are at the forefront of its delivery.

Box 15.1 provides a list of the associated targets for Sustainable Development Goal (SDG) 4 (see the Appendix to view the Sustainable Development Agenda in its entirety). Quality education is vital in order to change people's lives from the root level and aid human beings to rise beyond the economic opportunity limitations inherent in poverty-stricken countries. Of the 103 million youth lacking basic literacy skills, 60% of them are women, 57 million children remain unable to attend school in developing nations, and roughly 50% of primary school–aged children currently not enrolled in school live in conflict-affected areas (UNSD, 2016).

Box 15.1   Sustainable Development Goal 4 and Its Associated Targets

Goal 4. Ensure inclusive and equitable quality education and promote lifelong learning opportunities for all

4.1 By 2030, ensure that all girls and boys complete free, equitable, and quality primary and secondary education leading to relevant and effective learning outcomes.

4.2 By 2030, ensure that all girls and boys have access to quality early childhood development, care, and preprimary education so that they are ready for primary education.

4.3 By 2030, ensure equal access for all women and men to affordable and quality technical, vocational, and tertiary education, including university.

4.4 By 2030, substantially increase the number of youth and adults who have relevant skills, including technical and vocational skills, for employment, decent jobs, and entrepreneurship.

4.5 By 2030, eliminate gender disparities in education and ensure equal access to all levels of education and vocational training for the vulnerable, including persons with disabilities, indigenous peoples, and children in vulnerable situations.

4.6 By 2030, ensure that all youth and a substantial proportion of adults, both men and women, achieve literacy and numeracy.

4.7 By 2030, ensure that all learners acquire the knowledge and skills needed to promote sustainable development, including, among others, through education for sustainable development and sustainable lifestyles, human rights, gender equality, promotion of a culture of peace and nonviolence, global citizenship, and appreciation of cultural diversity and of culture's contribution to sustainable development.

4.a Build and upgrade education facilities that are child sensitive, disability sensitive, and gender sensitive and provide safe, nonviolent, inclusive, and effective learning environments for all.

4.b By 2020, substantially expand globally the number of scholarships available to developing countries, in particular least developed countries, small island–developing states and African countries, for enrolment in higher education, including vocational training and information and communications technology, technical, engineering, and scientific programs, in developed countries and other developing countries.

4.c By 2030, substantially increase the supply of qualified teachers, including through international cooperation for teacher training in developing countries, especially least developed countries and small island–developing states.

Source: Reprinted with permission from the United Nations (2015).

Without appropriate educational training, young people in low- and middle-income countries (LMICs) are limited in their abilities to create a healthier and safer life for themselves and their families.

Fiscella and Kitzman (2009) noted that, "Academic achievement and education seem to be critical determinants of health across the life span and disparities in one contribute to disparities in the other" (p. 1073). This powerful and fundamental point is instrumental in guiding our partnerships with populations that may not have access to equitable educational resources. Health experts continue to validate the lifelong sequelae of insufficient education: shorter lives, higher incidence of chronic diseases, increased risk factors, such as smoking and obesity, and greater disabilities (Virginia Commonwealth University Center on Society and Health, 2014). Global nurses advocate for educational parity among all individuals in a given context, across genders, ages, and socioeconomic strata, and provide influential parties with the evidence that substantiates a converse relationship between health and education. We are the change agents charged with informing policy makers and community leaders about the deeper connections between educational resource equity and health indicators related to life quality. With nursing's commitment to prevention and professional focus on holistic individual/community assessments, education becomes an inextricable aspect of the human right to a healthy life.

Global nurses contribute to improved health-specific educational quality by partnering with various in-country affiliates throughout the world, and fostering standards of excellence in health care professional training and preparation. We play an integral role in developing the global health workforce from the ground up. The Global Health Workforce Alliance (GHWA) and World Health Organization (WHO; 2013) addressed that human resources for health (HRH) are in need of substantial growth, in terms of both quality and quantity. As the title of their report suggests, we are left to confront *A Universal Truth: No Health Without a Workforce* (GHWA & WHO, 2013). They described the current worldwide HRH scenario:

- 83 countries with less than 22.8 skilled health professionals per 10,000 population
- 100 countries with less than 34.5 skilled health professionals per 10,000 population
- 118 countries with less than 59.4 skilled health professionals per 10,000 population
- 68 countries with more than 59.4 skilled health professionals per 10,000 population

True, there is no health without a workforce, but there is certainly no workforce without nurses (Shamian, 2015). Nurses and midwives account for over 19 million HRH worldwide (Sarna, Wolf, & Bialous, 2012), and are called to fulfill their roles as educators in countries that fall below the more dire thresholds mentioned earlier. As collaborating educators, we aid in preparing an upcoming cadre of adequately trained clinicians, researchers, educators, and future nurse leaders. Ultimately, there is no global health without HRH (Shamian, Murphy, Rose, & Jeffs, 2015).

Shamian et al. (2015, p. 2) urge us to reflect on what is needed to support this emerging transnational and interdependent health system:

- What are the educational systems required to educate health professionals to work in a new health system?
- What are the legislative and regulatory frameworks and policies that need to be in place?
- What data need to be collected and analyzed to monitor progress on an iterative and ongoing basis?

Many cross-cultural initiatives are already underway in this endeavor. For example, organizations such as Seed Global Health (2016) "strive to strengthen health education . . . in places facing a dire shortage of health professionals by working with partner countries to meet their long-term health care human resource needs." Seed is currently working in Malawi, Tanzania, and Uganda and will be launching new programs in Liberia and Swaziland later in 2016. The provision of high-quality education for nurses brings with it the hope of safer health care services and improved systemwide mechanisms for populations at large. Additionally, Seed and other HRH programs strive to decrease health care–worker shortages, improve quality care at point of delivery, and promote host country workforce autonomy (Binagwaho et al., 2013; Cancedda et al., 2015; Kerry, Cunningham, Daoust, & Sayeed, 2015). These organizations are addressing the four main areas impacting HRH highlighted by the GHWA and WHO (2013):

- Availability: refers to a quantity of health workers that is appropriate for the setting, possessing the required competencies and skills to deliver the necessary health care for the population at hand;
- Accessibility: addresses the distribution of health workers toward a more equitable equation in terms of travel time and transport, facility hours and workforce presence, physical attributes of the facility's infrastructure, referral mechanisms, and both formal and informal cost of services;
- Acceptability: calls for a workforce that is able to provide dignified, human care to all, create trusting relationships, and provide culturally sensitive services that respect cultural norms, values, and considerations;
- Quality: promotes guiding standards to measure and evaluate competencies, skills, knowledge, and behavior of health workers.

There are substantial challenges to increasing the quality of nursing education in LMICs, and therefore, the health education of the public in those countries. For instance, in Egypt, although master's and doctoral degrees in nursing are possible, secondary school training and associate degrees are the norm, with bachelor's degrees requiring more money and time for students who may not have the means (Elcokany & Hussein, 2014). Obstacles such as the unequal distribution of nurses throughout Egypt, improper role delineation, long working hours, poor working conditions, and low wages significantly hinder nursing advancement. Global health advocacy and the ability of nurses to build partnerships at the policy and regulatory levels are integral to overcoming these barriers and achieving appropriate educational standards.

GLOBAL PARTNERSHIPS TO ADVANCE EDUCATION

As global nurses, we must not hesitate to use out-of-the-box and big-picture thinking to fill educational gaps for nurses worldwide. During my time working in Rwanda, I spearheaded an effort to create a miniconsortium of national and international nursing organizations that would provide otherwise unavailable resources to graduate students at the University of Rwanda (UR) in Kigali. With the cocreative partnerships and willingness of organizations such as the Academy of Medical–Surgical Nurses (AMSN), American Association of Critical-Care Nurses (AACN), American Nephrology Nurses Association (ANNA), Association of periOperative Registered Nurses (AORN), and Oncology Nursing Society (ONS), well over half of the UR graduate students in the first Masters of Science in Nursing cohort received access to gratis association memberships, books and e-books, journal databases and evidence-based practices, core curriculums for different specialties, continuing education offerings, and global networking opportunities via social media platforms. This miniconsortium of invested organizations initiated a commitment to the global community of nurses that promoted educational advancement and professional development for the discipline worldwide.

The articles that follow, by Mukamana, Niyomugabo, and Rosa (2016) and Mukamana, Dushimiyimana, et al. (2016), give prominence to the voices of those involved in these efforts, and of the students themselves. These exemplars demonstrate the impact of professional solidarity and quality education procurement for all.

GLOBAL PARTNERSHIP ADVANCES MEDICAL–SURGICAL NURSING IN RWANDA[1]

Background and Context

Rwanda is one of the fastest economically developing nations in sub-Saharan Africa and a hub for global health partnerships.

In 1994, the genocide against the Tutsi claimed the lives of roughly 1 million Tutsi and moderate Hutu leaving behind destruction, poverty, a fractured economic system, and devastating consequences for the health care scenario.

In the past 22 years, the Rwandan government, under the auspices of the Ministry of Health (MOH) and in collaboration with countless international nongovernmental organizations (NGOs), has dramatically bettered health access and delivery in keeping with the United Nations (UN) Millennium Development Goals (MDGs; UN Development Programme [UNDP], 2013).

Incredible progress has been made in halting and reversing HIV, tuberculosis, and malaria. There is increased access to improved sanitation and a significant reduction in maternal mortality and mortality rates in children under 5 years (WHO, 2015).

Rwanda is now primed to readily achieve the UN's Sustainable Development Goals (SDGs) by 2030, a global development agenda that strives to address the root causes of poverty and ensure all citizens' rights to peace, well-being, and environmental/planetary health (UNDP, 2016).

---

[1] *Source:* Reprinted from Mukamana, Niyomugabo, and Rosa (2016).

Nursing in Rwanda

Rwanda's current population is approximately 11.5 million (National Institute of Statistics of Rwanda, 2016). Throughout the health care system, there continue to be major barriers to sufficient staffing, resources, and necessary educational preparation.

In 2012, the MOH collaborated with global partners to create the Human Resources for Health (HRH) Program, a 7-year initiative between Rwandan health care affiliates and a U.S.-based consortium of medical centers and nursing, public health, and dentistry schools.

The goals: increase the quality of health care services; increase the total number of adequately trained professionals in nursing, medicine, health management, and oral health throughout the country; and increase the autonomy of Rwandan health care professionals (Binagwaho et al., 2013; Republic of Rwanda, Ministry of Health [MOH], n.d.).

Of specific consideration to nursing education is to increase the total number of nurses and midwives prepared at the A0 level (baccalaureate equivalent) and the number of nurses with A1 level (associate degree equivalent) qualifications upgraded from A2 (secondary school training program).

Nursing is advancing quickly in Rwanda. In the past, students have been mandated to nursing as a vocation based on secondary school marks. Now, however, it is becoming a desirable and sought-after career path. Young people are now choosing to become nurses to help their families and communities, improve health care access and delivery, alleviate the suffering of the vulnerable, and to make a reliable decision toward economic autonomy (Figures 15.1 and 15.2).

Rwandan nurses are now held to standards of practice and licensure by the National Council of Nurses and Midwives, formed in 2008, and represented by the Rwanda Nurses and Midwives Union.

Due to many of these efforts, nursing is becoming respected by both the MOH and society at large as a responsible and powerful profession. Nurses are now leading or being targeted to lead health initiatives, organizations, accreditation programs, monitoring and evaluation services, performance-based financing, and community health offices. Nurses are being recognized as unique contributors to health care capable of influencing the necessary changes for improved quality services.

Rwanda's First MScN Program and the Medical–Surgical Specialty

As a result of the HRH Program, U.S. faculty and Rwandan colleagues partnered to create the country's first Masters of Science in Nursing (MScN) program. This 2-year degree program grants students specialty certification in one of eight tracks: critical care, oncology, nephrology, pediatrics, leadership and management, neonatology, perioperative, and medical–surgical nursing. Previously, nurses desiring advanced education were required to travel out of the country. Currently over 100 students are preparing to end their first year of education and, as of this writing, are taking part in their first focused clinical rotations.

The MScN program brings new hope for the autonomy and expertise of nursing practice in Rwanda. Nurses have always been viewed as subservient to physicians and caught in the confines of a hierarchical society. This makes true interdisciplinary communication and collaboration challenging, if not impossible.

As students are trained to be graduate-level medical–surgical nurses, there is an opportunity to advance critical thinking, leadership, and research skills. These

Figure 15.1	Med-surg MScN students gather at the University Teaching Hospital of Kigali (CHUK) for clinical rotations. Back row, from left: Eugenie Nyirabazungu, Vestine Mukayoboka, Fulgence Maniriho, Priscille Yamuragiye, Aloys Niyomugabo, Deborah Mukamuhirwa, Diane Muhimpundu. Front row from left: Sylvestre Ntirenganya and Leontine Ingabire.

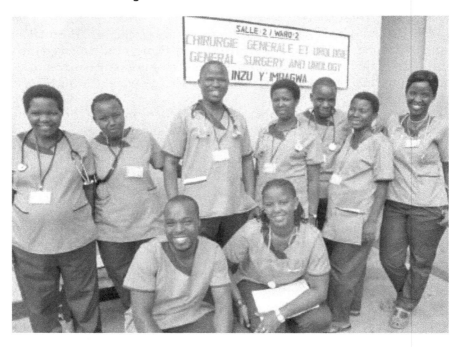

Figure 15.2	Authors Aloys Niyomugabo (left) and William Rosa.

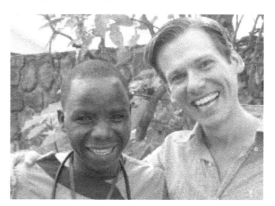

graduates will be accountable for improving medical–surgical protocols and empowering nursing with evidence-based practices to change irrelevant habits and systems.

Nurses did not previously feel they possessed the skills to perform research, but now these advanced clinicians will be able to lead research initiatives, create new knowledge, and improve patient safety. There is a renewed pride in nursing, nursing ethics, and nursing language.

For example, students in the MScN program now take pride in nursing care plans to promote the role of nursing among interdisciplinary colleagues, demonstrate the depth of nursing knowledge, and provide evidence to improve overall care delivery.

Many of the medical–surgical nursing students are determined to become change agents and role models to transform patient care. They are committed to becoming global nurse citizens, creating new possibilities of contributing to health care throughout the East African Region and worldwide. Graduate education in medical–surgical nursing gives clinicians the knowledge in scientific concepts, patient care applications, and the systems leadership needed to advance nursing as both a discipline and a profession.

AMSN AND RWANDA

In April 2016, AMSN graciously donated 16 2-year virtual memberships for the current Rwandan MScN medical–surgical track students. In addition, AMSN has donated a copy of their *Core Curriculum for Medical-Surgical Nursing, 5th Edition*, to the University of Rwanda library. These memberships fill a dire professional development gap in the careers of these future graduates.

With access to continuing education, updates and practice standards for medical–surgical practitioners, *MEDSURG Nursing Journal* and other AMSN publications, students will have unprecedented resources in realizing their potential as change agents, role models, and global nurse citizens. Through AMSN's provision of information on policymaking, evidence-based knowledge, scope of practice, and the laws affecting American nursing, Rwandan medical–surgical nurses can gain the valuable information needed to guide and build an advanced level of practice for themselves and their patients, an opportunity to which they simply would not have access otherwise.

In addition to AMSN, many other international organizations have joined this collaborative to support the first cohort of MScN students in Rwanda. The ANNA, the ONS, the AACN, and the AORN have all made generous donations to advancing the practice and education of their respective specialty track students.

Because of these associations' willingness to make a positive impact on the global well-being of the nursing profession, the Rwandan students will receive opportunities and resources that were previously unavailable due to financial restrictions.

AMSN, in conjunction with this miniconsortium of American associations, has redefined what it means to advocate for nurses and nursing worldwide. These organizations have proven that we are so much stronger together than apart and that we are so much more alike than different. Because of these efforts, it is safe to say that the future of nursing in Rwanda is bright, to say the least.

ONWARD

The only way forward is to ensure that Rwandan faculty are equipped to become autonomous leaders of the University of Rwanda MScN program. Clear goals and measures need to be established to ensure sustainability.

This program is the product of cross-cultural contributions and major financial investments, and without planning for sustainability, it will make all of these efforts useless. Sustainability will become the reward.

Rwandan autonomy is a way to perpetuate the legacy of global partnerships, a way of saying "thank you" to all of those individuals and organizations who have contributed their time and energy for the betterment of Rwandan health care and the nursing profession.

The journey is still long but the first steps are being taken. PhD preparation needs to be promoted to advance nursing science and sustain a thriving MScN program run by adequately prepared Rwandan faculty.

As the collaboration with international partners continues, the long-term plan needs to focus on the continued development of educational opportunities. Rwandans need to become their own role models to maintain sustainability for the benefit of the nation.

When they graduate, the MScN medical–surgical students will have the ability and opportunity to provide a more holistic and comprehensive education for a tremendous portion of the Rwandan population. They will be the ones advancing skills and awareness for patients, empowering families to care for their loved ones with accurate knowledge, and addressing how to prevent both communicable and noncommunicable diseases in rural and urban areas throughout Rwanda.

They are the change agents and the leaders of nursing. AMSN's role in their professional development makes this possible. It is a contribution that will be long remembered and celebrated not only by the MScN program students and faculty at the University of Rwanda, but by every patient who receives the informed, expert, and compassionate care of an MScN-prepared medical–surgical nurse

NEPHROLOGY NURSING IN RWANDA: CREATING THE FUTURE THROUGH EDUCATION AND ORGANIZATIONAL PARTNERSHIP[2]

The Human Resources for Health Program was launched in Rwanda to improve health care services and decrease overall dependence on foreign aid. In partnership between U.S. academic institutions and Rwandan educational affiliates, nursing resources have become centered primarily on the design and implementation of Rwanda's first MScN Program at the School of Nursing and Midwifery, College of Medicine and Health Sciences, University of Rwanda, Kigali. The nephrology track consists of seven students with a wealth of clinical and educational experience who will receive the training needed to become advanced, ethical, and capable leaders in the nephrology nursing field. Faculty member, William Rosa, collaborated with ANNA to provide these students with the

---

[2] *Source:* Reprinted from Mukamana, Dushimiyimana, et al. (2016).

online community, continuing education, practice standards, and journal access required to be proficient as graduate nurses through the donations of virtual memberships and copies of necessary texts. This is the University of Rwanda's MScN Nephrology Track story.

William Rosa, MS, RN, LMT, AHN-BC, AGPCNP-BC, CCRN-CMC

I arrived in Rwanda as a U.S. faculty member of the Human Resources for Health (HRH) Program on August 1, 2015. There was no way of foreseeing the relationships I would create and the joy I would have working in this incredible country. Rwanda was a mystery to me at the time. I mistakenly thought I would be the one making the contributions. Rather, my colleagues, the patients, and the sheer resilience of the Rwandan people have contributed to my life in countless ways. It has been an honor to partner with faculty from around the globe to improve the health and well-being of the population.

The innovations in nursing education began with partnerships between HRH and eight institutional affiliates throughout the country focused on improved undergraduate preparation and curriculum/content development. Over the past year, nursing educational resources have become centered primarily on the design and implementation of Rwanda's first MScN Program at the School of Nursing and Midwifery, College of Medicine and Health Sciences at the University of Rwanda in Kigali. This first of its kind program in Rwanda gives more than 100 A0 nurses, who possess at least 2 years of practice experience and exceptional academic credentials, the chance to receive graduate-level preparation in one of eight specialty tracks: critical care, leadership and management, medical–surgical, neonatology, nephrology, oncology, pediatrics, and perioperative nursing. As of this writing, the students have finished their first year of didactic preparation and are now completing their first semester of focused clinical.

The nephrology track consists of seven students with a wealth of clinical and educational experience who are receiving the training needed to become advanced, ethical, and capable leaders in the nephrology nursing field (see Figure 15.3). As the U.S. faculty lead for the nephrology track, I have been responsible for creating content and planning the clinical experience for these students in collaboration with Rwandan colleagues. In assessing the learning needs and understanding the future expectations of these MScN students at the national, policy, and administrative levels, there was additional support required to ensure their success. Socioeconomic constraints in Rwanda do not allow many nurses to pay for association memberships or purchase additional education to fill the gaps.

The ANNA was the first organization to which I reached out in order to provide these students with the online community, continuing education, practice standards, and journal access required to be proficient as graduate nurses, and assist them to carry out individual research studies in their second year. ANNA generously donated 2-year virtual memberships for each of the seven students and mailed several copies of their *Core Curriculum for Nephrology Nursing* (6th ed.) for the university library. This gift will not only see them through to graduation but will continue to guide them into their first year of practice as advanced nephrology nurses, and will be a cherished reference for future MScN cohorts. As

Figure 15.3	MScN Nephrology Track Nurses With Their Instructor, William Rosa, After a Pediatric Nephrology Presentation at Africa Health Care Network, Kimihurura, Rwanda

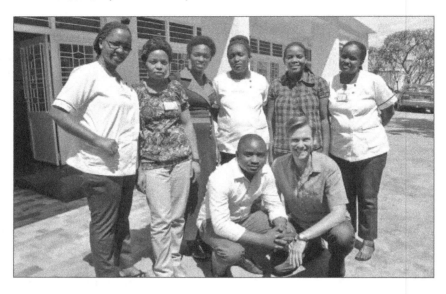

Notes: Front row: Flavien Ngendahayo, William Rosa. Back row: Gisele Mudasumbwa, Violette Dushimiyimana, Marie Jeanne Tuyisenge, Josiane Nibagwire, Olive Gashumba Uwambajimana, Jacqueline Kayitesi.

a nurse colleague, educator, and leader, I am honored to partner with ANNA to procure the highest quality resources for these students and am humbled by the willingness and enthusiasm ANNA has demonstrated in celebrating the education advances being made in Rwanda and in global nephrology nursing. Since ANNA signed on to partner with us, several other organizations have enlisted as a part of this association consortium with resources for their respective specialties, including the AACN, the AMSN, the AORN, and the ONS.

Flavien Ngendahayo, BScN, RN

For the past 5 years, I have worked as a tutorial assistant at the University of Rwanda, School of Nursing and Midwifery at Byumba campus. I teach A1 level students nursing ethics, pharmacology, and the nursing care process, and I guide them in their clinical experiences throughout various health facilities in Rwanda. Previously, I had background in HIV research and provided mentorship to district hospital and health center nurses through partners in health (PIH) programs.

The progress of nursing in Rwanda has moved slowly in its educational and practice standard development, but I believe it has started to advance with great power. There is now organizational representation at a national level. In 2008, the National Council of Nurses and Midwives was formed to promote increased safety and quality of nursing practice through attention to educational improvements, scope of practice delineation, and licensure requirements. In 2013, the Nurses and Midwives Association became the Rwanda Nurses and Midwives Union to provide professional advocacy and labor organization. The MOH is mandating A2 nurses receive the education required to become proficient at the A1 level and assisting them to achieve this goal. Today, we as nurses finally have a chance to attain specialty training at the master's level. The social and governmental recognition of nursing as a unique career has dramatically increased. For example, people used to believe that nurses simply assisted physicians, and now they understand that nursing and medicine are collaborative but distinct professions.

Olive Gashumba Uwambajimana, BScN, RN

Over my past 8 years as a nurse, I have worked in the Ngoma District Health Center and as a pediatric bedside nurse at Kibagabaga Hospital and the University Teaching Hospital in Kigali. Prior to the creation of the MScN program, there were very few nurses in Rwanda who held a graduate degree, and they had to travel out of country to attain it. Those master's-prepared nurses very often hold the position of director of nursing at a referral hospital or are relegated to an educational setting. The opportunity to attend University of Rwanda for my MScN creates a host of new leadership and educational possibilities. This program gives master's-prepared nurses the chance to take advanced practice into the clinical setting for the first time!

Nephrology is a growing field in Rwanda. I chose this specialty track because I will be able to take the skills learned at the graduate level and improve delivery of services to renal patients throughout the country. This education provides me with the resources I will need to improve the systems in which nurses work and the way nurses think about their practice. With the research skills I gain in the program, I hope to identify the risk factors for chronic kidney disease and design prevention mechanisms for nurses to improve patient outcomes.

Gisele Mudasumbwa, BScN, RN

Over the past 16 years, I have worked at the Rwanda Military Hospital in internal medicine and surgical wards, and most recently, in the adult intensive care unit. My favorite part of being a nurse is when I am able to help patients in the midst of their health challenges, in those times when they cannot help themselves. This is when I feel like I have contributed something important. Throughout my years as a direct care nurse, I've seen many patients suffering from kidney complications who could not afford the proper treatments. My hope is that through this advanced education, I will help patients prevent kidney disease, but also help them gain access to the necessary resources in the event my patients require them.

Currently, the MScN students are in second semester and have completed studies in global health, research design and biostatistics, leadership and management, nursing theory, pathophysiology and clinical management, and advanced health assessment. We are now in our first focused clinical for 200 hours. The goal for nephrology students in Focused Clinical I is to apply the education received thus far in the program to medical–surgical, intensive care, and outpatient dialysis clients. In the fall of 2016, Semester 3 will dive deeper into education regarding change agency in the Rwandan health care system, complex studies of renal conditions and emergencies, renal replacement therapies, and clinical management, and an additional focused clinical that will emphasize dialysis treatment.

While still in the beginning stages of our MScN education, I am already seeing the benefits of advanced training. I have been able to see peritoneal dialysis being performed in medical–surgical units at a referral hospital and the positive impacts on the patient condition. I am currently rotating in an outpatient dialysis clinic where I am learning the broad implications of chronic kidney disease on clients and how they live their lives. The MScN program will empower me to make a difference in patient outcomes, the future of nursing, and the state of nephrology practice in Rwanda.

Violette Dushimiyimana, BScN, RN

Since I was a young girl, I observed that people in the villages would initially go to the local health centers when they were ill. The health centers are run completely by nurses. The health center in my village of Kivumu was managed by nuns who were nurses and were organized, kind, and always kept the center and patients clean. As a little girl, I wanted to be like those nurses.

I had a background in biology and chemistry, which I studied in secondary school, and then completed my A0 preparation in 2011. Since graduation, I have worked in outpatient consultations and in-patient settings at a health center in Western Province, and worked as an internal medicine and then neonatology nurse in a district hospital. I am currently working at University of Rwanda, Byumba Campus, as a tutorial assistant.

The MScN program is training us to conduct and lead research in nephrology. Right now, we are using evidence from other countries, using equipment based on that evidence, and educating nurses based on external or international standards and practices. We need to create our own knowledge and evidence so our practices are relevant to patients in Rwanda. Our nurse-led research can improve the quality of care to which people have access and guide the development of the profession.

Because Rwanda is experiencing a double burden of disease from communicable and noncommunicable pathologies, we must research ways to mitigate implications of these illnesses on patients at risk for renal disorders. For example, diabetes and hypertension lead to renal failure, but so does malaria. I don't believe nurses in Rwanda fully understand the breadth of risk factors for patients regarding renal complications. As MScN-prepared nurses, we will be able to improve care delivery, prepare nurses throughout the country with the necessary knowledge, and be sure nurses in the health centers who care for the majority of village populations know how to assess and when to escalate care for renal disease.

Josiane Nibagwire, BScN, RN

Because of the history of nursing education in Rwanda, until recently people who wanted to become nurses had to start their nursing education in secondary school. In 1999, I started my 3-year certificate A2 program; in 2004, I was able to begin an additional 3-year A1 training; and then from 2009–2011, I was able to achieve my A0. When I complete the MScN program, I will have been studying nursing in school for 10 years! Prospective nursing students today have the option of choosing direct entry into A1 or A0 programs that will significantly decrease their schooling time. For the past 9 years, I have worked as an accident and emergency nurse at King Faisal Hospital.

After I finished my A0 education, I had time to continue my independent studies and became extremely interested in the functions of the kidney. In practice, I would see countless patients suffering from renal conditions who had no understanding of how the kidney worked, impacted their health, or what they could do to prevent complications. I also noticed that nurses in Rwanda needed more education regarding kidney injury prevention and the unique needs of these patients.

I am passionate about kidney injury prevention. The nephrology program will prepare me with the skills needed to save lives. If I can teach clients and nurses prevention education, it will help in the early identification of renal complications and acute kidney injury, and preserve resources in the long run. This work will have a direct impact on the well-being of the nation. Expert nephrology nursing education impacts all patients at all stages of life, and determines outcomes related to a host of diseases. The MScN program is offering us the unique, once-in-a-lifetime opportunity to leave our mark on the health of those we serve.

Jacqueline Kayitesi, BScN, RN

I have been a nurse for the past 10 years and received both my A1 and A0 training at University of Rwanda, Nyarugenge Campus. Since graduation, I have worked at the University Teaching Hospital in Butare as a bedside nurse in ear, nose, and throat, and as a tutorial assistant at the Kibungo School of Nursing teaching pediatrics. I have worked in the surgical ward at King Faisal Hospital in Kigali for the past 5 years. My favorite part of being a nurse is being able to witness patients who are very ill, and after receiving nursing care, are able to return to the quality of life they knew before.

My ANNA membership is and will continue to be invaluable to me as a clinician and teacher. Their practice updates can be adapted to my practice in Rwanda so that my patients are receiving evidence-based care. Access to ANNA's *Nephrology Nursing Journal* is an incredible adjunct to my MScN training, providing me with cutting-edge research in topics that interest me, such as prevention of acute and chronic kidney disease. The continuing education offered by ANNA will help me to better understand the therapies utilized by renal patients and how to prevent complications.

Nephrology nursing in Rwanda is an emerging specialty, so we don't yet have role models to follow or learn from. ANNA's generous donation of their Core Curriculum fills this gap and will aid in guiding us as we create and implement nephrology nursing in our country. Being connected to them through online platforms and having access to their expertise will continue to inform and influence my practice and positively impact patient care outcomes in nephrology.

Marie Jeanne Tuyisenge, BScN, RN

I became an RN in 2006 and have worked as a nurse in maternity wards, operating theatres, medical–surgical units, in family planning and immunization programs, and outpatient consultations throughout all provinces in Rwanda. My practice experience ranges from village health centers to district and referral hospitals. I am currently a tutorial assistant at the University of Rwanda, College of Medicine and Health Science at Nyarugenge Campus. In this role, I teach students hands-on skills in the simulation center, evaluate their practice-based competencies, and supervise them during their clinical rotations at various sites.

I believe the future of nursing is bright. In the past, nursing education was insufficient to provide holistic patient-centered care. We have now shifted from informal to formal nursing education in Rwanda. The shift has taken place from A2-level–prepared nurses to professionals who now have the opportunity to complete a master's degree. I believe when nurses are trained with the appropriate level of education, leadership, and research skills, we will be capable of providing the quality health care services to which our patients are entitled. Nurses will become forces for change. They will lead evidence-based initiatives that improve care delivery. Existing curricula and practices will be assessed and revised for relevance and accuracy.

With the advent of this nephrology specialty, nephrology nursing will see the preparation of its first seven MScN-prepared nurses. As the program continues, I hope the number of MScN-prepared nephrology nurses will increase to adequately care for renal patients throughout the East African Region. When we reach a sufficient number, we will be able to form our own nephrology nursing association in Rwanda and develop specialty scope and standards, organize conferences, and create certification requirements. These efforts will increase the awareness of our contribution to nursing and educate the public regarding the services we can provide to renal patients. We will use our means to contribute to the reduction in the morbidity and mortality of noncommunicable diseases, particularly renal pathologies. We will positively impact the information delivery, education, and communication provided to the public at large regarding lifestyle changes needed for those suffering from renal conditions. We are only seven now, but we are just the beginning. We may be a small number, but we have the potential to impact significant change in the field of nephrology nursing throughout Rwanda, the East African Region, and beyond.

Donatilla Mukamana, PhD, RN

As the dean of the School of Nursing and Midwifery, College of Medicine and Health Sciences, University of Rwanda, I have witnessed tremendous progress in the development of the nursing profession. I started my basic education in the health care professions in Rwanda before 1990. After the genocide against the Tutsi in 1994, Rwanda needed mental health nurses to care for and attend to the nation. At that time, I was finishing my studies in psychiatric nursing school in Geneva, Switzerland. In 1996, I returned to aid those patients with psychological posttraumatic stress related to the genocide at the National Center of Trauma in Kigali. Shortly after my arrival, Kigali Health Institute, now a part of the University of Rwanda, required my reassignment to a new mental health nursing program. And there, I began my work as an educator.

In 2004, I completed my master's degree in South Africa, and in 2014, PhD studies that explored the long-term psychological effects of rape among women survivors of the 1994 genocide against the Tutsi. In August 2014, I was appointed dean. My personal mission was to implement innovative and creative approaches using the resources available to improve education for nursing. I wanted my nursing students to be able to make a difference within their countries and the East African Region, and to train them to think globally through cross-cultural collaboration.

The MScN program represents a transformation in nursing practice and health care. It will increase the ability of Rwandans to stay in-country for necessary treatment, whereas in the past, they needed to travel abroad for expert services. With advanced practice nurses, there will be skilled clinicians available to care for these patients at the bedside, facilitating follow-up, decreasing costs, and helping families and friends to remain together during times of vulnerability and suffering. As a collectivist society, our families and friends are our reason for living; they are our happiness. The MScN program will produce nurses who will bring healing to the nation as they promote family-centered care for all Rwandans.

My hope for the nephrology nursing MScN students is that they will raise awareness throughout the country regarding renal disease and complications. The public needs this education desperately. They will improve the quality of preventative services and mitigate the complications associated with end-stage renal diseases. As the science of nephrology advances in Rwanda, these graduates will be the ones to lead nursing through to the future: transplantation, widespread dialysis access, and community knowledge that will save lives.

We are educating global nurses. ANNA's donation makes this standard of excellence possible. These emerging leaders will be the advocates to translate international nephrology standards to the context of Rwanda and throughout Africa. This collaboration is the innovation and creativity I continue to dream of: global partnerships that share our vision for quality health care in Rwanda. The generosity of ANNA will continue to impact the education and professional development of future MScN nephrology nursing cohorts. I look forward to continued partnership and celebrating the achievements of these students for years to come.

FINAL THOUGHTS

As we mobilize efforts to ensure that SDG 4 is achieved by 2030, we must begin to develop a new understanding of what education means to those living in LMICs and cultures different from our own. By cocreating and implementing improved educational opportunities for nurse colleagues in brother and sister countries, we indirectly contribute to those countries' improved health education status. The health knowledge left behind by global nurses nurtures a new future informed by a better-prepared workforce, and subsequently, a more well-informed citizenship. The systems they hope to build may not look like those in higher income nations. Their educational aspirations will undoubtedly include alignment with the broader sociopolitical goals of the nation and take significant resource constraints into consideration. The programs and initiatives that will be implemented to carry out the goal of quality education for all and an environment of lifelong learning will require a commitment to true and culturally humble collaboration in order to create sustainable change for those we serve.

REFLECTION AND DISCUSSION

- Do I believe quality education is a human right?
- How does nursing educational standards in LMICs increase overall global health literacy?
- In what ways must education be tailored to the broader sociopolitical landscape of a country?
- Is "human resources for health" a professional and global health priority? How so?
- How does health education play into the broader spectrum of targets proposed by SDG 4?

REFERENCES

Al Missned, S. M. b. N. (2009, March 18). Speech of Her Highness Sheikha Mozah bint Nasser Al Missned of Qatar. Opening session of the thematic and interactive debate on education in emergencies. United Nations General Assembly, New York, NY. Retrieved from http://www.un.org/ga/president/63/interactive/education/unesco_special_envoy.pdf

Binagwaho, A., Kyamanywa, P., Farmer, P. E., Nuthulaganti, T., Umubyeyi, B., Nyemazi, J. P.,. . . Goosby, E. (2013). Human Resources for Health Program in Rwanda: A new partnership. *New England Journal of Medicine, 369*(21), 2054–2059.

Cancedda, C., Farmer, P. E., Kerry, V., Nuthulaganti, T., Scott, K. W., Goosby, E., & Binagwaho, A. (2015). Maximizing the impact of training initiatives for health professionals in low-income countries: Frameworks, challenges, and best practice. *PLOS Medicine, 12*(6). doi:10.1371/journal.pmed.1001840

Elcokany, N., & Hussein, A. (2014). Seeking higher education: From Egypt to the United States. In M. J. Upvall & J. M. Leffers (Eds.), *Global health nursing: Building and sustaining partnerships* (pp. 34–44). New York, NY: Springer Publishing.

Fiscella, K., & Kitzman, H. (2009). Disparities in academic achievement and health: The intersection of child education and health policy. *Pediatrics, 123*(3), 1073–1080.

Global Health Workforce Alliance & World Health Organization. (2013). A universal truth: No health without a workforce. Retrieved from http://www.who.int/workforcealliance/knowledge/resources/hrhreport_summary_En_web.pdf

Kerry, V., Cunningham, L., Daoust, P., & Sayeed, S. (2015). Addressing medical and nursing clinical education gaps in East Africa: The first year experience of the Global Health Service Partnership. *World Population and Health, 1*(16), 24–35.

Mukamana, D., Dushimiyimana, V., Kayitesi, J., Mudasumbwa, G., Nibagwire, J., . . . Rosa, W. (2016). Nephrology nursing in Rwanda: Creating the future through education and organizational partnership. *Nephrology Nursing Journal, 43*(4), 311–315.

Mukamana, D., Niyomugabo, A., & Rosa, W. (2016, June). Global partnership advances medical-surgical nursing in Rwanda. *Med-Surg Nursing Connection*, 1–5.

National Institute of Statistics of Rwanda. (2016). Size of the resident population. Retrieved from http://www.statistics.gov.rw/publication/size-resident-population

Republic of Rwanda, Ministry of Health. (n.d.). Human Resources for Health Program, Republic of Rwanda: Program overview. Retrieved from http://www.hrhconsortium.moh.gov.rw/about-hrh/program-overview

Sarna, L., Wolf, L., & Bialous, S. A. (2012). Enhancing nursing and midwifery capacity to contribute to the prevention, treatment and management of noncommunicable diseases. *Human Resources for Health Observer*, (12). Retrieved from http://www.who.int/hrh/resources/observer12.pdf

Seed Global Health. (2016). About Seed Global Health. Retrieved from http://seedglobalhealth .org/about/#.VzWOl2M0G8U

Shamian, J. (2015). No health without a workforce, no workforce without nurses. *British Journal of Nursing, 25*(1), 54–55.

Shamian, J., Murphy, G. T., Rose, A. E., & Jeffs, L. (2015, June). No global health without human resources for health (HRH): The nursing lens. *Nursing Leadership.* doi:10.12927/ cjnl.2015.24204

United Nations. (2015). Transforming our world: The 2030 Agenda for Sustainable Development. Retrieved from https://docs.google.com/gview?url=http://sustainabledevelopment .un.org/content/documents/21252030%20Agenda%20for%20Sustainable%20 Development%20web.pdf&embedded=true

United Nations Development Programme. (2013). Millennium Development Goals: Rwanda: Final Progress Report. Retrieved from http://www.rw.undp.org/content/dam/rwanda/ docs/Rwanda_MDGR_2013.pdf

United Nations Development Programme. (2016). A new sustainable development agenda. Retrieved from http://www.rw.undp.org/content/rwanda/en/home/post-2015

United Nations Sustainable Development. (2016). Goal 4: Ensure inclusive and quality education for all and promote lifelong learning. Retrieved from http://www.un.org/ sustainabledevelopment/education

Virginia Commonwealth University Center on Society and Health. (2014). *Education: It matters more to health than ever before.* Retrieved from http://www.rwjf.org/content/dam/farm/ reports/issue_briefs/2014/rwjf409883

World Health Organization. (2015). *World health statistics: 2015.* Geneva, Switzerland: Author. Retrieved from http://apps.who.int/iris/bitstream/10665/170250/1/9789240694439_ eng.pdf

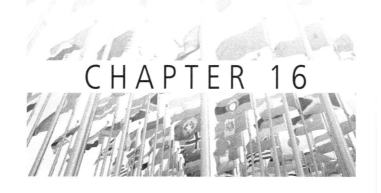

CHAPTER 16

Goal 5. Achieve Gender Equality and Empower All Women and Girls

William Rosa

The extremists are afraid . . . of women . . . afraid of the equality that we will bring into our society. . . . [T]oday I am focusing on women's rights . . . because they are suffering the most. . . . I am focusing on women to be independent. . . . To ensure freedom and equality for women so that they can flourish. We cannot all succeed when half of us are held back. We call upon our sisters around the world to be brave—to embrace the strength within themselves and realize their full potential. (Yousafzai, 2013)

Equality between men and women is a major focus of the Sustainable Development Agenda, seeking to ensure equity in health care, education, economic security, governance, and the right of all women to be compensated fairly for their work. In order to implement systems that are based on and continually promote gender equality, many systems related to socioeconomic and political decision making need to be examined at both local and global levels. Box 16.1 provides the associated targets of Sustainable Development Goal (SDG) 5 (see the Appendix to view the Sustainable Development Agenda in its entirety).

There are countless systems and traditions that continue to demoralize and dehumanize women. Female genital mutilation/cutting (FGM/C) is just one of these offenses. "FGM/C" refers to any and "all procedures involving partial or total removal of the external female genitalia or other injury to the female genital organs for non-medical reasons" (United Nations International Children's Fund [UNICEF], n.d.). It is documented that at least 200 million girls and women have experienced FGM/C in over 30 countries on three continents. A World Health Organization (WHO) study group showed that obstetrical outcomes for women with FGM/C include increased risks of caesarean section, postpartum hemorrhage, extended maternal hospital stay, infant resuscitation, stillbirth or early neonatal death, and low birthweight, as well as an estimated extra 1 to 2 perinatal deaths per 100 deliveries (WHO Study Group on Female Genital Mutilation and

---

Box 16.1 **Sustainable Development Goal 5 and Its Associated Targets**

Goal 5. Achieve gender equality and empower all women and girls

5.1 End all forms of discrimination against all women and girls everywhere.

5.2 Eliminate all forms of violence against all women and girls in the public and private spheres, including trafficking and sexual and other types of exploitation.

5.3 Eliminate all harmful practices, such as child, early and forced marriage, and female genital mutilation.

5.4 Recognize and value unpaid care and domestic work through the provision of public services, infrastructure and social protection policies, and the promotion of shared responsibility within the household and the family as nationally appropriate.

5.5 Ensure women's full and effective participation and equal opportunities for leadership at all levels of decision making in political, economic, and public life.

5.6 Ensure universal access to sexual and reproductive health and reproductive rights as agreed in accordance with the Programme of Action of the International Conference on Population and Development and the Beijing Platform for Action and the outcome documents of their review conferences.

5.a Undertake reforms to give women equal rights to economic resources, as well as access to ownership and control over land and other forms of property, financial services, inheritance and natural resources, in accordance with national laws.

5.b Enhance the use of enabling technology, in particular information and communications technology, to promote the empowerment of women.

5.c Adopt and strengthen sound policies and enforceable legislation for the promotion of gender equality and the empowerment of all women and girls at all levels.

Source: Reprinted with permission from the United Nations (2016).

Obstetric Outcome, 2006). SDG 5.3 directly calls for an end to harmful practices on women, including FGM/C, reminding the world that it is a human rights violation that remains a global concern. UNICEF (2016) reports that the current progress being made is not sufficient to keep up with current rates of increasing population growth, and that if the trends continue, the number of females experiencing FGM/C will rise substantially over the next 15 years.

Another mechanism that keeps women disempowered is gender-based violence (GBV). According to the United Nations Population Fund (n.d.), "Violence against women and girls is one of the most prevalent human rights violations in the world . . . [it] undermines the health, dignity, security and autonomy of its victims, yet it remains shrouded in a culture of silence." The health implications of GBV victims include sexual and reproductive health complications, unwanted pregnancies and unsafe abortions, sexually transmitted infections, psychosocial trauma, and, in the worst of cases, death. Intimate partner violence (IPV), the mental, emotional, or physical violence experienced by those individuals participating in an intimate relationship, plagues women worldwide. The WHO (2013) showed that 35% of women worldwide have been victims of physical or sexual violence, up to 30% of women in a relationship have experienced violence at the hands of an intimate partner, and that up to 38% of the murders of women are perpetrated by intimate partners. This violence has a host of effects on women's health, including adverse mental–emotional effects, reproductive health difficulties, and increased exposure to HIV (O'Connor, Conley, & Breakey, 2015).

As women's health services continue to be severely resource constrained in low-income countries worldwide, nurses play an integral role in the screening and identification of GBV and IPV, and in mitigating the associated long-term psychological and physical traumas (O'Connor et al., 2015). This requires that all victims are treated with the same health delivery standards as other members of the community and that nurses are prepared to care for victims of GBV and IPV without shame or judgment. Support services should include sexual violence protocols and staff training, a secure, clean, and private treatment area, female forensic examiners, a full range of options (including abortion where relevant), a medical/legal report free of charge, and strict confidentiality (Council of Europe, 2008).

Malaysia was the first country to create and implement a "one-stop center" so that all of the services needed for women survivors of domestic or sexual violence were centralized in one location. These centers provide women with immediate physician examination and treatment, consultation with a counselor within 24 hours, and reference to an emergency shelter or admission into the accident and emergency ward for an additional 24 hours if going home is not safe (United Nations Women, 2012). Global nurses can partner with hospital management, staff, and providers across the spectrum of care to create and sustain welcoming, private, caring, and effective one-stop centers for the safety and protection of GBV and IPV victims.

Women and girls are continuously objectified by an overly medicalized system that views and treats them as objects rather than fully functioning, thinking, feeling human beings (da Cruz Leitão, 2015). This unconscious dehumanization reinforces discriminatory practices in communities and inadvertently substantiates norms and values that sanction the subservience and inferiority of females. While the dehumanization of human beings in health care extends across gender lines (Watson, 2008, 2012), women may be more vulnerable than men in communities where inequality is inflamed and female rights are considered more the exception than the rule.

Global nurses are the frontline workers who can discourage social inequality by *rehumanizing* health care, promoting practical, authentic, and human-centered care, unhindered by gender labels and biases. Human-centered care may very well be one of the primary interventions of global nurses in the journey toward gender equality. Rosa and Estes (2016) define *evolving human-centered care* as

> compassionate and empathic care that responds, attends, and conforms to the human as a living, breathing, evolving experience; human as a fluctuating phenomenological being of engagement; human as history, as

story, and as narrative; human as presence, emergence, and possibility; human as fellow sojourner; human as caring-healing . . . human as LOVE.

Human-centered care returns us to our moral/ethical starting point as nurses in service to a dignified and caring society where healing is honored and celebrated. By breaking the cycles of discrimination through rehumanizing care, we simultaneously partner with communities to identify the social impetuses that promote unquestioned biases, and cocreate new worldviews rooted in social justice that are culturally appropriate and sensitive.

EXPANDING THE GENDER CONVERSATION

We must not overlook what it means to be truly gender equitable in a globally conscious world, beyond the targets identified by the United Nations (UN) in regards to females. This means we must include in the conversation all individuals who identify as gender nonconforming and transgender. This population is potentially subject to harsh discrimination across political, religious, social, and economic settings. However, in nursing and health care, exclusionary opinions and judgments simply have no place in a caring–healing relationship (Boykin & Schoenhofer, 2015). There is pervasive stigma and discrimination against gender nonconforming and transgender clients that negatively impacts, and even obstructs, their access to quality, safe, and respectful care (Bockting et al., 2016). For example, if an anatomically male patient identifies as a female, she is considered transgender. If, then, she lives in a country where "transgender" is considered categorically equivalent to "homosexuality" due to lack of knowledge, and homosexuality is a crime in said country, the client will be restricted from openly discussing health concerns, accessing resources for safe sex practices, or self-advocating for psychosocial well-being openly. She is then subject to a host of inequalities based on her gender identity that is not recognized nor accepted. Gender inequalities transcend the more parochial notions of "male–female" and exist along a broader spectrum of human expression. Permissive discrimination in health care toward any population, as mentioned above, promotes the social stigma that binds and oppresses.

By rehumanizing engagement with these clients, we have another opportunity to become role models for compassionate care delivery. However, the global nurse must integrate cultural humility and discretion in openly advocating for these individuals based on the context, as those marginalized due to sexual identity may not be capable of accessing their human health rights in certain countries and may, furthermore, face criminalization or other discriminatory responses as a result of their identity being made public (Ash & Mackereth, 2013; Campbell, 2013). The shame politically enforced upon this community in countries around the world has sparked fears of client secrecy leading to mental and physical health barriers, honest client–provider relationship becoming discouraged, and epidemics, such as HIV/AIDS, continuing to spread due to stifled health care systems and oppressive bureaucracies (Clark, 2014). Table 16.1 provides definitions of basic terms that may be useful in caring for clients across the gender spectrum. It is important that all nurses use appropriate language in referring to clients and understand how they feel about their gender identity and experience.

Table 16.1 Terms in Caring for Clients Across the Gender Spectrum

Term	Definition
Cisgender	A term used to describe a person whose gender identity aligns with those typically associated with the sex assigned to them at birth
Closeted	Describes a lesbian, gay, bisexual, transgender, queer or questioning (LGBTQ) person who has not disclosed their sexual orientation or gender identity
Coming out	The process in which a person first acknowledges, accepts, and appreciates his or her sexual orientation or gender identity and begins to share that with others
Gay	A person who is emotionally, romantically, or sexually attracted to members of the same gender
Gender dysphoria	Clinically significant distress caused when a person's assigned birth gender is not the same as the one with which they identify. According to the American Psychiatric Association's *Diagnostic and Statistical Manual of Mental Disorders (DSM)*, the term—which replaces gender identity disorder—"is intended to better characterize the experiences of affected children, adolescents, and adults"
Gender-expansive	Conveys a wider, more flexible range of gender identity and/or expression than typically associated with the binary gender system
Gender expression	External appearance of one's gender identity, usually expressed through behavior, clothing, haircut or voice, and which may or may not conform to socially defined behaviors and characteristics typically associated with being either masculine or feminine
Gender-fluid	According to the Oxford English Dictionary, a person who does not identify with a single fixed gender; of or relating to a person having or expressing a fluid or unfixed gender identity
Gender identity	One's innermost concept of self as male, female, a blend of both or neither—how individuals perceive themselves and what they call themselves. One's gender identity can be the same or different from their sex assigned at birth
Gender nonconforming	A broad term referring to people who do not behave in a way that conforms to the traditional expectations of their gender, or whose gender expression does not fit neatly into a category
Homophobia	The fear and hatred of or discomfort with people who are attracted to members of the same sex
LGBTQ	An acronym for "lesbian, gay, bisexual, transgender, and queer."
Living openly	A state in which LGBTQ people are comfortably out about their sexual orientation or gender identity—where and when it feels appropriate to them
Outing	Exposing someone's lesbian, gay, bisexual, or transgender identity to others without their permission. Outing someone can have serious repercussions on employment, economic stability, personal safety, or religious or family situations
Sexual orientation	An inherent or immutable enduring emotional, romantic, or sexual attraction to other people
Transgender	An umbrella term for people whose gender identity and/or expression is different from cultural expectations based on the sex they were assigned at birth. Being transgender does not imply any specific sexual orientation. Therefore, transgender people may identify as straight, gay, lesbian, bisexual, and so forth
Transphobia	The fear and hatred of, or discomfort with, transgender people

Source: Human Rights Campaign (2016). Reprinted with permission.

CONCLUSION

Gender inequality worsens the health care disparities already impacting women and other minorities on a global scale. It places these groups in high-risk situations that compromise their autonomy and mental, emotional, and physical well-being. Global nurses must identify opportunities to effectively prevent GBV and IPV, and also assess the readiness to educate communities about the link between gender and sexual identity equity, and access to quality health care. In this way, nurses become advocates for both the equality and empowerment of all gender minorities in all nations where gender-based discrimination continues to corrode the vision of a shared and inclusive humanity.

REFLECTION AND DISCUSSION

- What actions can I take to raise awareness of gender inequalities?
- How can I promote gender equity in professional and community settings?
- Is GBV and IPV prevalent in my current personal–professional setting? What is needed to decrease and stop it?
- How can a more inclusive health system aid transgender and nonconforming people in the journey toward equality?
- In what ways can I empower gender minorities to take their places as equal global citizens?

REFERENCES

Ash, M., & Mackereth, C. J. (2013). Assessing the mental health and wellbeing of the lesbian, gay, bisexual and transgender population. *Community Practitioner, 86*(3), 24–27.

Bockting, W., Coleman, E., Deutsch, M. B., Guillamon, A., Meyer, I., Meyer, W., . . . Ettner, R. (2016). Adult development and quality of life of transgender and gender nonconforming people. *Current Opinion in Endocrinology, Diabetes and Obesity, 23*(2), 188–197. doi:10.1097/MED.0000000000000232

Boykin, A., & Schoenhofer, S. O. (2015). Theory of nursing as caring. In M. C. Smith & M. E. Parker (Eds.), *Nursing theories & nursing practice* (4th ed., pp. 341–356). Philadelphia, PA: F. A. Davis.

Campbell, S. (2013). Sexual health needs and the LGBT community. *Nursing Standard, 27*(32), 35–38.

Clark, F. (2014). Discrimination against LGBT people triggers health concerns. *The Lancet, 383*(9916), 500–502.

Council of Europe. (2008). Combating violence against women: Minimum standards for support services. Retrieved from http://www.coe.int/t/dg2/equality/domesticviolence campaign/Source/EG-VAW-CONF(2007)Study%20rev.en.pdf

da Cruz Leitão, M. N. (2015). Health, sex, and gender: The inequalities as challenges. *Revista Da Escola De Enfermagem Da USP, 49*(1), 10–11.

Human Rights Campaign. (2016). Glossary of terms. Retrieved from http://www.hrc.org/resources/glossary-of-terms

O'Connor, A. L., Conley, K. A., & Breakey, S. (2015). Violence against women. In S. Breakey, I. B. Corless, N. L. Meedzan, & P. K. Nicholas (Eds.), *Global health nursing in the 21st century* (pp. 193–210). New York, NY: Springer Publishing.

Rosa, W., & Estes, T. (2016). What end-of-life care needs now: An emerging praxis of the sacred and subtle. *Advances in Nursing Science, 39*(4), 333–345.

United Nations. (2015). *Transforming our world: The 2030 agenda for sustainable development.* Retrieved from https://docs.google.com/gview?url=http://sustainabledevelopment. un.org/content/documents/21252030%20Agenda%20for%20Sustainable%20 Development%20web.pdf&embedded=true

United Nations International Children's Fund. (n.d.). Female genital mutilation/cutting. Retrieved from http://www.unicef.org/protection/57929_58002.html

United Nations International Children's Fund. (2016). UNICEF's data work on FGM/C. Retrieved from http://www.unicef.org/media/files/FGMC_2016_brochure_final_ UNICEF_SPREAD(2).pdf

United Nations Population Fund. (n.d.). Gender-based violence. Retrieved from http://www .unfpa.org/gender-based-violence

United Nations Sustainable Development. (2016). Goal 5: Achieve gender equality and empower all women and girls. Retrieved from http://www.un.org/sustainabledevelopment/ gender-equality

United Nations Women. (2012). Intimate partner violence and/or sexual assault (one-stop) centres. Retrieved from http://www.endvawnow.org/en/articles/683-intimate-partner -violence-and-or-sexual-assault-one-stop-centres.html

Watson, J. (2008). *Nursing: The philosophy and science of caring* (Rev. ed.). Boulder: University Press of Colorado.

Watson, J. (2012). *Human caring science: A theory of nursing* (2nd ed.). Sudbury, MA: Jones & Bartlett.

World Health Organization. (2013). *Global and regional estimates of violence against women: Prevelance and health effects of intimate partner violence and non-partner sexual violence.* Geneva, Switzerland: Author.

World Health Organization Study Group on Female Genital Mutilation and Obstetric Outcome. (2006). Female genital mutilation and obstetric outcome: WHO collaborative prospective study in six African countries. *The Lancet, 367*(9525), 1835–1841.

Yousafzai, M. (2013, July 12). Malala Yousafzai's speech at the Youth Takeover of the United Nations. Retrieved from https://secure.aworldatschool.org/page/content/the-text-of- malala-yousafzais-speech-at-the-united-nations

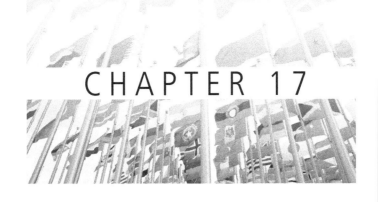

CHAPTER 17

Goal 6. Ensure Availability and Sustainable Management of Water and Sanitation for All

William Rosa

Facilitating health by preventing contact with hazardous waste, human and otherwise, was the cornerstone of Nightingale's action plan at Scutari. . . . Sanitation and hygiene were Nightingale's essential pillars of public health. . . . A competent nursing staff was equally essential to a sanitary environment; the former was responsible to ensure the latter. (Ward, 2016, p. 31)

The legacy of nursing is deeply rooted in environmental activism. Nightingale (1860) discussed the link between environmental determinants of health and individual wellness and well-being. As global nurses, we look for ways to elevate the awareness of populations to understand the connection between their external environment and their health. Water and sanitation pollution can worsen and prolong noncommunicable diseases (NCDs), increasing the double burden of disease experienced by people living in low- and middle-income countries (LMICs). We must continue to form innovative models of knowledge exchange between the disciplines, mitigate harmful environmental exposures that protract NCDs, and elevate the global community's consciousness regarding the interplay between pollution and health outcomes (Suk & Mishamandani, 2016). From education to policy changes, to advocating for infrastructure improvements that will address water and sanitation deficits, global nurses are integral to the realization of Sustainable Development Goal (SDG) 6, the associated targets of which are listed in Box 17.1 (see the Appendix to view the Sustainable Development Agenda in its entirety).

The World Health Organizaiton (WHO; 2016) reported that 2.3 billion people gained access to better quality drinking water between 1990 and 2012. However,

| Box 17.1 | **Sustainable Development Goal 6 and Its Associated Targets** |

Goal 6. Ensure availability and sustainable management of water and sanitation for all

6.1 By 2030, achieve universal and equitable access to safe and affordable drinking water for all.

6.2 By 2030, achieve access to adequate and equitable sanitation and hygiene for all and end open defecation, paying special attention to the needs of women and girls and those in vulnerable situations.

6.3 By 2030, improve water quality by reducing pollution, eliminating dumping, and minimizing release of hazardous chemicals and materials, halving the proportion of untreated wastewater, and substantially increasing recycling and safe reuse globally.

6.4 By 2030, substantially increase water-use efficiency across all sectors and ensure sustainable withdrawals and supply of freshwater to address water scarcity and substantially reduce the number of people suffering from water scarcity.

6.5 By 2030, implement integrated water resources management at all levels, including through transboundary cooperation as appropriate.

6.6 By 2020, protect and restore water-related ecosystems, including mountains, forests, wetlands, rivers, aquifers, and lakes.

6.a By 2030, expand international cooperation and capacity-building support to developing countries in water- and sanitation-related activities and programs, including water harvesting, desalination, water efficiency, wastewater treatment, recycling and reuse technologies.

6.b Support and strengthen the participation of local communities in improving water and sanitation management.

Source: Reprinted with permission from the United Nations (2015).

continued access is becoming a worldwide dilemma, impacting every continent on the planet. It is projected that by 2050, one in four people is likely to be impacted by recurring water shortages (United Nations Sustainable Development [UNSD], 2016). So how does inadequate clean water and sanitation currently impact the world's population? According to UNSD (2016):

- At least 1.8 billion use a drinking water source with fecal contamination;
- Water scarcity affects more than 40% of the global population;
- 2.4 billion lack basic sanitation services, such as toilets or latrines;
- Roughly 1,000 children die daily due to preventable water and sanitation-related diarrheal diseases.

Without safe water and sanitation mechanisms, health promotion becomes largely irrelevant and health care delivery spirals toward futility (Prevost & Dye, 2015).

Several countries' populations suffer due to water and sanitation challenges. In Kenya, water-, sanitation-, and hygiene-related diseases are the number one cause of hospitalization in children under 5 years of age (Water.org, 1990–2016a). Of Peru's 31 million people, 4 million lack access to safe drinking water and nearly 8 million lack adequate sanitation (Water.org, 1990–2016b). It is vital that global nurses understand the economic implications of providing clean water and sanitation for all. The WHO (2017) states that "worldwide capital financing would need to triple to US $114 billion per annum, and operating and maintenance costs need to be considered in addition," and that there are significant variations between countries and regions requiring nuanced strategies and approaches to achieving SDG 6 (p. iv).

Nursing's ethical commitment to procure the human dignity of all peoples in all settings (Watson, 2008, 2012) is directly related to the statistics and goals mentioned earlier. By rediscovering the environmental advocacy inherent to the profession, nurses can work to improve educational services regarding water and sanitation and lead initiatives in partnership with initiatives being implemented to accomplish SDG 6. Global nurses are in direct alignment with organizations like Water.org. Water.org strives to deliver clean and safe water to the world's poor by delivering them the financial capital they need so they can be self-reliant in developing water and sanitation solutions (Meedzan, Nicholas, Nreakey, & Corless, 2015). With capital in hand, women and girls are freed from water scavenging and gathering, and able to focus on education or attaining other work opportunities for increased economic gain. Gary White, chief executive officer (CEO) of Water.org identifies nursing's role in the clean water and sanitation effort and suggests that we look at water "as the most basic *medicine*," and, he believes,

> The more that nurses, particularly in developing countries, view water as a medical intervention and sanitation as a medical intervention the more proactive nurses will be in addressing some of these waterborne diseases. . . . I turn to the . . . nursing profession in particular to lobby and educate so that the facts and the connection between the water that people are drinking and the health impact on them and their children are being circulated and understood. (Meedzan et al., 2015, p. 131)

Frankly, health education regarding dietary guidelines of water consumption mean little if the quality of water is not adequately managed and procured (Van Graan, Bopape, Phooko, Bourne, & Wright, 2013).

There are other hopeful initiatives underway that are integral to SDG 6 progress. The Sulabh Sanitation Movement in India has constructed 1.3 million household toilets, 54 million government toilets, and over 8,500 community block toilets since 1970 (Sulabh International Social Service Organisation, 2015). The Right to Sanitation Challenge is improving access, elevating awareness, and taking action to ensure sanitation as a human right throughout India (Right to Sanitation, n.d.). We can also partake in and support the efforts of nurse-led organizations, such as the Alliance of Nurses for Health Environments (ANHE; n.d.), whose mission is to "promot[e] healthy people and healthy environments by educating and leading the nursing profession, advancing research, incorporating

Table 17.1 American Nurses Association's Principles (ANA's) of Environmental Health for Nursing Practice

1. Knowledge of environmental health concepts is essential to nursing practice.
2. The precautionary principle guides nurses to use products and practices that do not harm human health or the environment and to take preventative action in the face of uncertainty.
3. Nurses have a right to work in an environment that is safe and healthy.
4. Health environments are sustained through multidisciplinary collaboration.
5. Choices of materials, products, technology, and practices in the environment that impact nursing practice are based on the best evidence available.
6. Approaches to promoting a healthy environment respect the diverse values, beliefs, cultures, and circumstances of patients and their families.
7. Nurses participate in assessing the quality of the environment in which they practice and live.
8. Nurses, other health care workers, patients, and communities have the right to know relevant and timely information about the potentially harmful products, chemicals, pollutants, and hazards to which they are exposed.
9. Nurses participate in research of best practices that promote a safe and healthy environment.
10. Nurses must be supported in advocating and implementing environmental health principles in nursing practice.

Source: Adapted from ANA (2007).

evidence-based practice, and influencing policy." As nurses learn about the various programs being implemented worldwide, they can partner with organizations that align with their personal and professional vision for a healthy and equitable world. Supporting water supply and sanitation projects that believe in community-driven leadership and community ownership of sustainability corresponds with global nursing ethics of respect for autonomy and beneficence (Montgomery, 2016).

SDG 6 invites all nurses to become more environmentally conscious in practice, education, and research. It is one of many SDGs that relate to environmental health and maintain direct implications for global nursing practice (other environmentally relevant SDGs include 7, 9, and 11–15). The American Nurses Association's (ANA's) Principles of Environmental Health for Nursing Practice specify environmental health as foundational to nursing practice, key to optimal health and well-being, and promote nursing's full participation in the procurement of environmental safety for all. ANA's Principles of Environmental Health for Nursing Practice are listed in Table 17.1. Specifically, ANA Principle 6 highlights that respect and inclusion of diversity in environmental education and promotion is a keystone of global nursing.

Lack of access to clean water and adequate sanitation services directly impacts the health of the families and communities we serve as global nurses. Luck (2015) articulates the connection between global nursing and our collective Nightingalean heritage:

> At the heart of Florence Nightingale's (1820–1910) legacy is a knowing that our external environment is inextricably interconnected to the health and well-being of all species and ecosystems. There is both the urgency and opportunity to address environmental factors that affect the lives of our clients/patients, families, and communities. (p. 166)

We need to understand our roles in communicating environmental awareness and leading health policy changes to clients and communities at large. Nurses must elevate the understanding of how individual and global health are interrelated and challenge the status quo in order to create healing environments for all (Luck, 2016). Clean water and sanitation services are just one step in realizing global well-being for all human beings on the planet.

REFLECTION AND DISCUSSION

- How do I begin to educate the public about the dilemma of clean, safe, and reliable water?

- In what ways can I partner with environmental agencies to improve sanitation practices?

- Do I actively promote the Nightingalean legacy of environmental activism?

- Are ANA's Principles of Environmental Health applicable across cultures and in LMICs? Why or why not?

- What is the relationship between clean water and sanitation, individual health, and global well-being?

REFERENCES

Alliance of Nurses for Health Environments. (n.d.). About. Retrieved from http://envirn.org/pg/groups/4104/alliance-of-nurses-for-healthy-environments

American Nurses Association. (2007). Principles of environmental health for nursing practice with implementation strategies. Retrieved from http://www.nursingworld.org/MainMenuCategories/WorkplaceSafety/Healthy-Nurse/ANAsPrinciplesofEnvironmentalHealthforNursingPractice.pdf

Luck, S. (2015). Environmental health. In B. M. Dossey, S. Luck, & B. G. Schaub (Eds.), *Nurse coaching: Integrative approaches for health and wellbeing* (pp.165–177). North Miami, FL: International Nurse Coach Association.

Luck, S. (2016). Informed and impactful: Stewarding the environmental determinants of health and well-being. In W. Rosa (Ed.), *Nurses as leaders: Evolutionary visions of leadership* (pp. 333–343). New York, NY: Springer Publishing.

Meedzan, N. L., Nicholas, P. K., Breakey, S., & Corless, I. B. (2015). Access to clean water and the impact on global health: An interview with Gary White, CEO and Cofounder, Water.org. In S. Breakey, I. B. Corless, N. L. Meedzan, & P. K. Nicholas (Eds.), *Global health nursing in the 21st century* (pp. 123–136). New York, NY: Springer Publishing.

Montgomery, M. J. (2016). What works in water supply and sanitation projects in developing countries with EWB-USA. *Review on Environmental Health, 31*(1), 85–87.

Nightingale, F. (1860). *Notes on nursing: What it is and what it is not.* London, UK: Harrison.

Prevost, S. S., & Dye, T. (2015). The importance of water for global nursing. In S. Breakey, I. B. Corless, N. L. Meedzan, & P. K. Nicholas (Eds.), *Global health nursing in the 21st century* (pp. 115–122). New York, NY: Springer Publishing.

Right to Sanitation. (n.d.). Why RTS? Retrieved from http://www.cafindia.org/pages/why-rts.htm

Suk, W. A., & Mishamandani, S. (2016). Changing exposures in a changing world: Models for reducing the burden of disease. *Reviews on Environmental Health, 31*(1), 93–96.

Sulabh International Social Service Organisation. (2015). Home. Retrieved from http://www.sulabhinternational.org

United Nations. (2015). Transforming our world: The 2030 agenda for sustainable development. Retrieved from https://docs.google.com/gview?url=http://sustainabledevelopment.un.org/content/documents/21252030%20Agenda%20for%20Sustainable%20Development%20web.pdf&embedded=true

United Nations Sustainable Development. (2016). Goal 6: Ensure access to water and sanitation for all. Retrieved from http://www.un.org/sustainabledevelopment/water-and-sanitation

Van Graan, A., Bopape, M., Phooko, D., Bourne, L., & Wright, H. (2013). "Drink lots of clean, safe water": A food-based dietary guideline for South Africa. *South African Journal of Clinical Nutrition, 26*(3), S77–S86.

Ward, F. (2016). Florence Nightingale: Where most work is wanted. In D. A. Forrester (Ed.), *Nursing's greatest leaders: A history of activism* (pp. 21–54). New York, NY: Springer Publishing.

Water.org. (1990–2016a). Kenya. Retrieved from http://water.org/country/kenya

Water.org. (1990–2016b). Peru. Retrieved from http://water.org/country/peru

Watson, J. (2008). *Nursing: The philosophy and science of caring* (Rev. ed.). Boulder: University Press of Colorado.

Watson, J. (2012). *Human caring science* (2nd ed.). Sudbury, MA: Jones & Bartlett.

World Health Organization. (2016). Drinking water. Retreived from http://www.who.int/mediacentre/factsheets/fs391/en

World Health Organization. (2017). *Financing universal water, sanitation and hygiene under the Sustainable Development Goals: UN-Water global analysis and assessment of sanitation and drinking water: GLAAS 2017 report*. Geneva, Switzerland: Author. Retrieved from http://apps.who.int/iris/handle/10665/254999

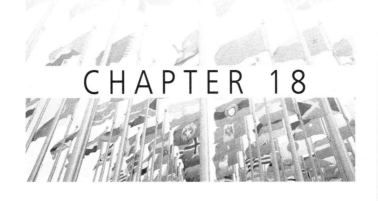

CHAPTER 18

Goal 7. Ensure Access to Affordable, Reliable, Sustainable, and Modern Energy for All

William Rosa

[Many are] without the . . . power to insulate themselves from the negative consequences of the world's energy production and consumption. . . . While the immediate . . . consequences are felt by the poor, there are long-term implications for future generations of [all] species, and the earth systems on which . . . life depends—a moral challenge if there ever was one . . . . (Sharpe, 2008, p. 16)

Energy is the heartbeat of the modern industrialized world. Access or lack of access to energy determines how well we live, work, eat, deliver health care services, and communicate. When one in five people lack access to electricity, 3 billion people still rely on wood, coal, charcoal, or animal waste as an energy source, and unethical energy practices are contributing toward 60% of the global greenhouse gas emissions that are causing climate change, something must be done (UNSD, 2016). Sustainable Development Goal (SDG) 7 and its associated targets are provided in Box 18.1 (see the Appendix to view the Sustainable Development Agenda in its entirety).

In 2007, Wilkinson and colleagues acknowledged the tremendous advancements energy has provided to the world over the past 250 years, but also clearly indicted fossil fuels as a major determinant of the global health burden and the primary contributor to climate change (Wilkinson, Smith, Joffe, & Haines, 2007). For instance, household air pollution (HAP), secondary to the energy sources aforementioned, negatively impacts chronic illnesses, such as cardiovascular disease; increased research on the relation between HAP and health complications may be key to driving policy changes that improve patient education and access to energy alternatives in low- and middle-income countries (LMICs) (Noubiap, Essouma, & Bigna, 2015). And as with many other worldwide health challenges, the initiatives

| Box 18.1 | Sustainable Development Goal 7 and Associated Targets |

Goal 7. Ensure access to affordable, reliable, sustainable and modern energy for all

7.1 By 2030, ensure universal access to affordable, reliable and modern energy services

7.2 By 2030, increase substantially the share of renewable energy in the global energy mix

7.3 By 2030, double the global rate of improvement in energy efficiency

7.a By 2030, enhance international cooperation to facilitate access to clean energy research and technology, including renewable energy, energy efficiency and advanced and cleaner fossil-fuel technology, and promote investment in energy infrastructure and clean energy technology

7.b By 2030, expand infrastructure and upgrade technology for supplying modern and sustainable energy services for all in developing countries, in particular least developed countries, small island developing States and landlocked developing countries, in accordance with their respective programmes of support

Source: Reprinted with permission from the United Nations (2015).

we support and lead as global nurses that further the goals of SDG 7 must be rooted in collaborative and culturally sensitive partnerships.

When it comes to environmental education, including the impact of energy sources on individual and population health, there is a critical knowledge gap in the preparation of health care professionals (Sattler, 2003). Global nurses must learn to gather reliable information on sources of energy, identify how energy fits into political agendas, and work with communities to ensure reliable, consistent access (Nicholas, Breakey, Winter, Pusey-Reid, & Viamonte-Ros, 2015). Energy use and sourcing must be a part of health promotion, education, assessment, and evaluation in order to become a meaningful consideration to clients.

Data suggests that up to 3.3 million deaths per year are a secondary cause of outdoor air pollution and as many as 3.5 million deaths per year are due to indoor smoke (World Health Organization [WHO], 2012). Much of this air pollution is the result of ineffective and outdated energy technologies and sources. There are several health indicators that can help global nurses assess progress toward SDG 7: percentage of households with affordable and clean energy access, amount of electricity produced with minimal pollutants, health facilities supplied with 24-hour water and electricity, the health burden attributable to pollution, and health equity and its relation to energy policy (WHO, 2012).

While the impacts of energy access at resource-constrained health facilities and in LMICs on patient outcomes are not well known, lack of access to reliable electricity may negatively affect health worker recruitment and retention and delay emergency response time (WHO, 2014). The correlation between energy access and effective health care delivery is clear. Energy impacts cold-chain storage of blood, vaccines, and medicines, lighting, ability to sterilize equipment, insufficient communication options, inadequate water and hygiene resources, and also the number of health care workers attracted to living and working in more rural areas, where staff shortages are dire (WHO, 2014). In the future, more research needs to be completed to accurately illustrate the link between energy access and patient outcomes in order to drive policy improvements and influence large scale change.

There is a myth that clean, otherwise known as "green," sources of energy are economically inaccessible for most and require an advanced level of scientific development for implementation. However, all countries, including LMICs, are encouraged to start transitioning toward these sources in ways that are in alignment with their technological capabilities and economic status (Matatiele & Gulumian, 2016). Ultimately, global nurses can promote populations to start where they are in relation to clean sources of energy and assist in community assessments to suggest possible financial rerouting and identify methods of affordability. For example, the role of nurses in educating the public about opportunities for improved cook stoves and clean fuels that reduce HAP can help clients in understanding the positive impacts not only on family health, but also on improving environmental well-being and lessening negative climate implications (Lewis & Pattanayak, 2012).

At first glance, the everyday clinical nurse may not understand his or her role in reaching the targets of SDG 7. But make no mistake, nurses play a critical role in all of the SDGs, including the creation of new knowledge through research design, navigating the implementation of systems improvements, and sharing global health implications at the tables where policy decisions are made (WHO, n.d.). By closing our own knowledge gap in regards to energy access and delivery, we can more adequately embrace the meaningful leadership roles before us.

REFLECTION AND DISCUSSION

- How can I educate health care professionals regarding energy sources and their impact on individual/global health?

- How can I evaluate my information about energy sources and how they fit into various political agendas?

- What are the health indicators related to energy usage?

- In what ways can I link patient outcomes and energy access to drive policy changes?

- Am I prepared to create new knowledge and lead research related to the impact of energy delivery on population health?

REFERENCES

Lewis, J. J., & Pattanayak, S. K. (2012). Who adopts improved fuels and cookstoves? A systematic review. *Environmental Health Perspectives, 120*(5), 637–645.

Matatiele, P., & Gulumian, M. (2016). A cautionary approach in transitioning to "green" energy technologies and practices is required. *Reviews on Environmental Health, 31*(2), 211–223.

Nicholas, P. K., Breakey, S., Winter, S., Pusey-Reid, E., & Viamonte-Ros, A. M. (2015). Climate change, climate justice, and environmental health issues. In S. Breakey, I. B. Corless, N. L. Meedzan, & P. K. Nicholas (Eds.), *Global health nursing in the 21st century* (pp. 25–40). New York, NY: Springer Publishing.

Noubiap, J. N., Essouma, M., & Bigna, J. (2015). Targeting household air pollution for curbing the cardiovascular disease burden: A health priority in sub-Saharan Africa. *Journal of Clinical Hypertension, 17*(10), 825–829.

Sattler, B. (2003). Environmental health education. In B. Sattler & J. Lipscomb (Eds.), *Environmental health and nursing practice* (pp. 311–320). New York, NY: Springer Publishing.

Sharpe, V. A. (2008). "Clean" nuclear energy? Global warming, public health, and justice. *Hastings Center Report, 38*(4), 16–18.

United Nations. (2015). Transforming our world: The 2030 agenda for sustainable development. Retrieved from https://docs.google.com/gview?url=http://sustainabledevelopment.un.org/content/documents/21252030%20Agenda%20for%20Sustainable%20Development%20web.pdf&embedded=true

United Nations Sustainable Development. (2016). Goal 7: Ensure access to affordable, reliable, sustainable, and modern energy for all. Retrieved from http://www.un.org/sustainabledevelopment/energy

Wilkinson, P., Smith, K. R., Joffe, M., & Haines, A. (2007). A global perspective on energy: Health effects and injustices. *The Lancet, 370*(9591), 965–978.

World Health Organization. (n.d.). Health workforce. Retrieved from http://www.who.int/hrh/news/2015/global_nurse_conf-kor/en

World Health Organization. (2012, May 17–18). Health indicators of sustainable energy in the context of the Rio+20 UN Conference on Sustainable Development. Retrieved from http://www.who.int/hia/green_economy/indicators_energy2.pdf

World Health Organization. (2014). *Access to modern energy services for health facilities in resource-constrained settings: A review of status, significance, challenges and measurement*. Geneva, Switzerland: Author. Retrieved from http://apps.who.int/iris/bitstream/10665/156847/1/9789241507646_eng.pdf

CHAPTER 19

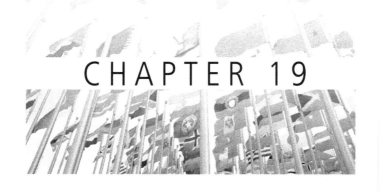

Goal 8. Promote Sustained, Inclusive, and Sustainable Economic Growth, Full and Productive Employment, and Decent Work for All

William Rosa

[Human dignity] starts by standing with the poor, listening to voices unheard, and recognizing potential where others see despair. It demands investing as a means, not an end, daring to go where markets have failed and aid has fallen short. It makes capital work for us, not control us. (Acumen, 2016a)

The world has become all too familiar with economic disparities, depression, and stagnation. In 2007 to 2008, the world experienced a financial crisis that left millions of people grappling to get by, pay mortgages, sustain their livelihoods, and find reliable sources of income to meet their needs. On a global scale, across governments and private investors, there has been a noted "economic terrorism," which deprives the poor of food, water, electricity, health care, education, and creates institutionalized imbalances in economic welfare (Roy, 2008). This incapacitation of the majority public further divides humanity, creating gaps in interpersonal and cross-cultural understanding, and keeping the ideals of peace and unity far at bay. Sustainable Development Goal (SDG) 8 and its associated targets are provided below in Box 19.1 (see the Appendix to view the Sustainable Development Agenda in its entirety).

In a global economy where about half of the world's population lives on the equivalent of roughly $1 to $2 per day, this struggle is not a hypothetical or a temporary hardship—it is reality. It impacts children, men, and women of all ages and challenges them in every way possible. It prevents them from getting the nutrition

Box 19.1   Sustainable Development Goal 8 and Its Associated Targets

Goal 8. Promote sustained, inclusive, and sustainable economic growth, full and productive employment, and decent work for all

8.1   Sustain per capita economic growth in accordance with national circumstances and, in particular, at least 7 percent gross domestic product growth per annum in the least developed countries.

8.2   Achieve higher levels of economic productivity through diversification, technological upgrading, and innovation, including through a focus on high–value added and labor-intensive sectors.

8.3   Promote development-oriented policies that support productive activities, decent job creation, entrepreneurship, creativity and innovation, and encourage the formalization and growth of micro-, small-, and medium-sized enterprises, including through access to financial services.

8.4   Improve progressively, through 2030, global resource efficiency in consumption and production and endeavor to decouple economic growth from environmental degradation, in accordance with the 10-Year Framework of Programmes on Sustainable Consumption and Production, with developed countries taking the lead.

8.5   By 2030, achieve full and productive employment and decent work for all women and men, including for young people and persons with disabilities, and equal pay for work of equal value.

8.6   By 2020, substantially reduce the proportion of youth not in employment, education, or training.

8.7   Take immediate and effective measures to eradicate forced labor, end modern slavery and human trafficking, and secure the prohibition and elimination of the worst forms of child labor, including recruitment and use of child soldiers, and by 2025 end child labor in all its forms.

8.8   Protect labor rights and promote safe and secure working environments for all workers, including migrant workers, in particular women migrants, and those in precarious employment.

8.9   By 2030, devise and implement policies to promote sustainable tourism that creates jobs and promotes local culture and products.

8.10   Strengthen the capacity of domestic financial institutions to encourage and expand access to banking, insurance, and financial services for all.

8.a   Increase Aid for Trade support for developing countries, in particular least developed countries, including through the Enhanced Integrated Framework for Trade-Related Technical Assistance to Least Developed Countries.

8.b   By 2020, develop and operationalize a global strategy for youth employment and implement the Global Jobs Pact of the International Labour Organization.

Source: Reprinted with permission from the United Nations (2015).

they need, the safe living quarters they deserve, and the health care that is a human right (United Nations Sustainable Development, 2016). It is an unending cycle of poverty, where finding work does not necessarily mean security and the number of quality jobs available require educational preparation simply too expensive for many people to afford. The setbacks can be insurmountable and may carry with them damaging and lifelong health implications.

Along with social considerations, the impact of the environment, and an individual's own characteristics and actions, one's economic reality is a prime determinant of health. The World Health Organization (WHO; 2016a) acknowledges that higher income and social status are related to greater levels of health, and that the more substantial the divide between the rich and poor, the more substantial the discrepancies in health quality. Those individuals and communities who are unable to access reliable employment opportunities and maintain even base notions of economic security are, indeed, a vulnerable population. People considered to have a low socioeconomic status (SES) experience higher levels of physical and mental health challenges and may have difficulty in meeting basic psychological needs, potentially leading to emotional exhaustion and elevated stress levels (González, Swanson, Lynch, & Williams, 2016).

Global nurses must focus not only on the amelioration of health consequences that occur secondary to economic instability, but also on prevention mechanisms, early identification of barriers to optimal health, and community assessments that explore individual well-being in relation to family and community factors. It is never too early to start both assessment and intervention related to the economic contributors of client health. In fact, there is strong evidence that links low income and SES in the first 5 years of life with adverse physical health outcomes later on (Spencer, Thanh, & Louise, 2013). In addition to the health outcomes of decreased access to education, financial security, and decent work, the subjective perception of lower social rank has been linked to diminished psychological well-being, depression, and other physical symptoms (Quon & McGrath, 2014). A more integrative, whole-person/whole-system approach to care (Kreitzer & Koithan, 2014) will assist the global nurse in identifying not only the objective markers of SES classification, but also the mental, emotional, spiritual, and social implications of economic poverty, and their overall impact on health and well-being.

Global nurses are vital to the procurement of the aforementioned targets while maintaining human dignity and ensuring the health of all involved. By partnering with and educating about organizations that seek to accomplish these goals, global nurses become integral to clients' economic well-being: a prime indicator of their overall health. In the health sector alone, the WHO (2016b) suggests there will be an estimated 40 million new health sector jobs and a shortage of about 18 million health workers in LMICs by 2030.

The newly appointed High-Level Commission on Health Employment and Economic Growth (HLCHEEG), a transnational collaborative venture of the WHO (2016b), will focus on developing the infrastructures and relationships needed for widespread economic well-being, and will promote the global economic development called for by the SDGs. The HLCHEEG will guide the creation of health and social sector jobs as a means to advance inclusive economic growth, paying specific attention to LMICs (WHO, 2016b). Global nurses play a role in the HLCHEEG's efforts to recommend institutional reforms, determine sources of financing, assess and analyze the effects of global health worker imbalances and uneven distributions, and generate political support for sustainability. As a recently instated advisory body, the HLCHEEG (2016) is currently consulting on questions regarding:

- Health workforce investments that will achieve universal health coverage and the SDGs;
- Gender-sensitive policies that are respectful and inclusive of women and girls in the health and social sectors;
- Risks and benefits related to international migration of health workers and increased retention of health workers in home country;
- Multisector collaboration to enhance work being done in relation to decent work and related health and workforce considerations;
- Strengthened governance in the health and social sectors.

Skills in advocacy and leadership, as well as boardroom involvement with the sectors, investors, and policy makers mentioned earlier, put global nurses in a pivotal role for change related to SDG 8. We must be sitting at the tables where decisions are made and be involved in the policy deliberations that impact health care, health care workers, global nurses, global health, and economic development; it is an inherent component of our role and an ethical obligation for exacting long-term change and health quality improvement (Nickitas, 2016; Patton, Zalon, & Ludwick, 2014).

Outside of health care, not-for-profit ventures are doing their part in cocreating a global community of economic inclusivity and autonomy. Acumen (2016b) is one such organization that seeks to invest in people as entrepreneurs in their own right, providing them with the resources needed to start their businesses, the training required to successfully manage new ventures, and the skills to become valuable leaders in their communities. Founder and chief executive officer (CEO), Jacqueline Novogratz (2009), had witnessed the trappings and insufficiency of traditional philanthropic investments: ventures that focused on short-term financial fixes to poverty and did little to nurture human dignity or autonomy. Acumen provides investees with a long-term repayment plan at an extremely low interest rate called "patient capital." The funds gained from the repayment are then reinvested into the same communities to foster sustainability and spread opportunities for others. They offer investees the economic and interpersonal tools required to become self-reliant role models for their families and communities. It is not just about helping people create jobs; it is about supporting them to find their unique voice as a person, professional, and member of society. In this way, the economic morale of a population is not only elevated, but the human spirit becomes both empowered and fully expressed.

Acumen is rooted in an ethical foundation of moral imagination and is about emboldening investees to affect meaningful change with dignity. "Moral imagination" is the

> . . . the humility to see the world as it is, and the audacity to imagine the world as it could be. It's having the ambition to learn at the edge, the wisdom to admit failure, and the courage to start again . . .

(Acumen, 2016a; see Chapter 4 for more information on moral imagination). Acumen's manifesto (Acumen, 2016b), which was the introductory quote for this chapter, ends by saying:

> It requires patience and kindness, resilience and grit: a hard-edged hope. It's leadership that rejects complacency, breaks through bureaucracy, and challenges corruption. Doing what's right, not what's easy . . . the radical idea of creating hope in a cynical world. Changing [how] the world tackles poverty and building a world based on dignity.

As global nurses seek opportunities to impact change through SDG 8, organizations such as Acumen become viable partners. Moral imagination and deeply listening to the needs of those we serve, combined with financial skills and a heightened socioeconomic awareness, will not only promote economic well-being for global communities, but it will also continue to shift health delivery toward a more humanistic model of holism, respect, and humility. Being a part of these initiatives is an opportunity for nursing to educate the public and policy makers about the relationship between economic well-being, access to dependable employment, and overall health. By engaging with those most affected by poverty through a lens of moral imagination, we contribute to SDG 8 with integrity, dignity, and the skill set necessary to invite global health advancement.

REFLECTION AND DISCUSSION

- How can I, as a global nurse, improve my assessment skills regarding the health indicators related to economic status?
- How can I ensure community treatment plans are considerate of the whole system and the individual considerations within that system?
- What are my responsibilities in leading initiatives that break the cycle of poverty and economic destitution?
- What are my opportunities to integrate moral imagination for improved relationships, opportunities, and outcomes?
- How can I create hope in a cynical world?

REFERENCES

Acumen. (2016a). What we do. Retrieved from http://acumen.org
Acumen. (2016b). Manifesto. Retrieved from http://acumen.org/manifesto
González, M. G., Swanson, D. P., Lynch, M., & Williams, G. C. (2016). Testing satisfaction of basic psychological needs as a mediator of the relationship between socioeconomic status and physical and mental health. *Journal of Health Psychology, 21*(6), 972–982.
High-Level Commission on Health Employment and Economic Growth. (2016, May 27). High-Level Commission on Health Employment and Economic Growth: Open consultation. Retrieved from http://globalhealth.org/wp-content/uploads/High-Level-Commission-on-Health-Employment-and-Economic-Growth-Open-Cons-.pdf
Kreitzer, M. J., & Koithan, M. (Eds.). (2014). *Integrative nursing.* New York, NY: Oxford University Press.

Nickitas, D. M. (2016). Ethical and economical: Calling the profession to social justice. In W. Rosa (Ed.), *Nurses as leaders: Evolutionary visions of leadership* (pp. 149–163). New York, NY: Springer Publishing.

Novogratz, J. (2009). *The blue sweater: Bridging the gap between rich and poor in an interconnected world.* New York, NY: Rodale.

Patton, R. M., Zalon, M. L., & Ludwick, R. (Eds.). (2014). *Nurses making policy: From bedside to boardroom.* New York, NY: Springer Publishing.

Quon, E. C., McGrath, J. J. (2014). Subjective socioeconomic status and adolescent health: A meta-analysis. *Health Psychology, 33*(5), 433–447.

Roy, A. (2008). *The shape of the beast: Conversations with Arundhati Roy.* New Delhi, India: Viking Press.

Spencer, N., Thanh, T. M., & Louise, S. (2013). Low income/socio-economic status in early childhood and physical health in later childhood/adolescence: A systematic review. *Maternal & Child Health Journal, 17*(3), 424–431.

United Nations. (2015). Transforming our world: The 2030 agenda for sustainable development. Retrieved from https://docs.google.com/gview?url=http://sustainabledevelopment.un.org/content/documents/21252030%20Agenda%20for%20Sustainable%20Development%20web.pdf&embedded=true

United Nations Sustainable Development. (2016). Goal 8: Promote inclusive and sustainable economic growth, employment and decent work for all. Retrieved from http://www.un.org/sustainabledevelopment/economic-growth

World Health Organization. (2016a). The determinants of health. Retrieved from http://www.who.int/hia/evidence/doh/en

World Health Organization. (2016b). High-level commission on health employment and economic growth. Retrieved from http://www.who.int/hrh/com-heeg/en

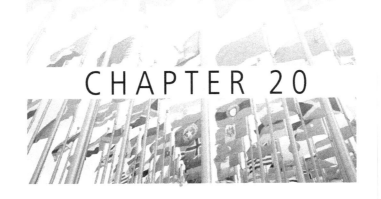

CHAPTER 20

Goal 9. Build Resilient Infrastructure, Promote Inclusive and Sustainable Industrialization, and Foster Innovation

William Rosa

Rural communities in [low- and middle-income] countries often face severe health problems. . . . Lack of access to health care in rural areas contributes to high mortality rates among children, who often die from treatable illnesses such as dehydration, pneumonia, and malaria . . . developing innovative strategies for health care delivery to rural communities [is key].
(Fund for Global Health, 2015)

The 2014 Ebola outbreak in west Africa showed the world the devastating and frightening implications of geographic and economic isolation where infrastructure is obsolete, industry remains absent, and innovation is an afterthought to crisis and is rarely, if ever, preventative. The epidemic quickly spread throughout Guinea, Sierra Leone, and Liberia, and, as of April 13, 2016, resulted in 11,310 deaths (Centers for Disease Control and Prevention, 2016). By February 9, 2014, Liberia alone had reported 8,864 cases of Ebola, just over 3,000 of which were laboratory confirmed, and many outbreaks in remote areas that lacked phone or communication services, basic road infrastructure, and adequately prepared community health teams (Kateh et al., 2015). Provinces throughout the affected countries experienced delays in treatment and continued to spread the virus due to lack of community knowledge and resources, and health education access. In short, the health systems in west Africa were unprepared to control the outbreak due to a lack of material and human resources, but also infrastructure access that made containment possible. As the Ebola crisis has quieted, Guinea, Sierra Leone, and Liberia have all experienced a degradation in the social fabric of their communities and observed an increase in poverty and population vulnerability (United Nations Development Group, 2015). What would a more substantially developed infrastructure have made possible? Would countries that were thriving from a firmly rooted industrial presence and related innovations been able to provide help more quickly, prevent deaths, and contain the spread more effectively? Box 20.1 provides more about Sustainable Development Goal (SDG) 9 and its associated targets (see the Appendix to view the Sustainable Development Agenda in its entirety).

An evolving question: what is the global nursing role in promoting safe and responsible industry, innovation, and infrastructure? As suggested earlier, poor infrastructure may restrict access to health care delivery and a host of other services needed for survival. It may limit those nurses in low- and middle-income countries (LMICs) willing or able to educate rural communities or provide in-person support when needed (Manjrekar, 2016). If there is a nurse available, he or she may be the only primary care provider for miles, and the determining factor of a client's survival (Jones, 2010). Where infrastructure is insufficient, industry is lacking and innovation is not likely to be encouraged. This leaves impoverished residents in those areas without opportunities for social and economic development and without the resources needed to become an empowered and healthy population, omitting them from the development of their nation that occurs in urban and more centralized locations. This is a problem not only in LMICs, but also in substantially more industrialized nations. The National Rural Health Association (NRHA; 2016) of the United States notes that due to the access limitations of more rural and geographically isolated residents, there are higher rates of smoking, obesity, physical inactivity, higher death rates, and an overall higher prevalence of heart disease, cancer, suicide, injury, and stroke. Global nurses carry the solution for inclusive health care delivery to even the most remote areas through partnership and innovation. All of the initiatives that are evolving from the changes called for by SDG 9 will improve the quality of communication between and within nations and foster a sense of unity throughout provinces and rural areas that might otherwise be excluded.

There are many companies applying innovative strategies worldwide to overcome the barriers to health care delivery posed by poor infrastructure. One such company is Zipline (n.d.), an organization seeking to improve medication, vaccine, and blood access through drone delivery. Zipline is surpassing the obstacles of long travel times, substandard roads, hazardous weather, and challenging topography, altogether. The organization recently embarked on an exciting collaboration with the government of Rwanda, becoming the first to provide drone blood delivery to transfusion centers throughout the country. Zipline's initiative significantly decreases the time of blood product delivery from up to 4 hours by car to somewhere between 15 to 35 minutes anywhere in Rwanda. The company is currently working on several ventures in other countries, looking to transform the way health care is practiced, and decrease the mortality rates associated with delayed wait times for blood and other emergent medications.

Global nurses should invite partnership with these organizations to assess how health care systems will need to adapt in order to accommodate and safely

| Box 20.1 | Sustainable Development Goal 9 and Its Associated Targets |

Goal 9. Build resilient infrastructure, promote inclusive and sustainable industrialization, and foster innovation

9.1 Develop quality, reliable, sustainable, and resilient infrastructure, including regional and transborder infrastructure, to support economic development and human well-being, with a focus on affordable and equitable access for all.

9.2 Promote inclusive and sustainable industrialization and, by 2030, significantly raise industry's share of employment and gross domestic product, in line with national circumstances, and double its share in least developed countries.

9.3 Increase the access of small-scale industrial and other enterprises, in particular in developing countries, to financial services, including affordable credit, and their integration into value chains and markets.

9.4 By 2030, upgrade infrastructure and retrofit industries to make them sustainable, with increased resource-use efficiency and greater adoption of clean and environmentally sound technologies and industrial processes, with all countries taking action in accordance with their respective capabilities.

9.5 Enhance scientific research, upgrade the technological capabilities of industrial sectors in all countries, in particular developing countries, including, by 2030, encouraging innovation and substantially increasing the number of research and development workers per 1 million people, and public and private research and development spending.

9.a Facilitate sustainable and resilient infrastructure development in developing countries through enhanced financial, technological, and technical support to African countries, least-developed countries, landlocked developing countries, and small island–developing states.

9.b Support domestic technology development, research and innovation in developing countries, including by ensuring a conducive policy environment for, inter alia, industrial diversification and value addition to commodities.

9.c Significantly increase access to information and communications technology and strive to provide universal and affordable access to the Internet in least developed countries by 2020.

Source: Reprinted with permission from the United Nations (2015).

implement these innovations. For example, in Rwanda, as blood delivery wait time is substantially decreased, global nurses can work with companies such as Zipline to develop and employ the quality improvement protocols required to ensure responsible handling and transfer of blood, ethical and transparent practices in the ordering and distribution of blood products, and safe patient monitoring pretransfusion, intratransfusion, and posttransfusion. Due to decreased wait times, many centers not previously able to retrieve blood will be receiving these products with increased frequency. This means that local nursing staff and interprofessional partners may not be initially prepared to safely handle and deliver blood: a procedure that may have been rare in the past. Global nurses have a role in assessing the systems that partake in such initiatives, identifying gaps in patient safety, providing education to professional health colleagues as well as key stakeholders, and evaluating the ability of transfusion centers to realize the vision of Zipline and like-minded organizations. Through such partnerships, global nurses can help steer businesses and investors to understand the role of nursing worldwide, create new approaches to quality health care innovations, promote whole-systems thinking, and identify barriers and solutions to real-time implementation. In turn, businesses like Zipline have the opportunity to tap into the holistic knowledge and wealth of clinical understanding that nurses possess to advance sustainability and continue ongoing collaborations with international health ministries.

The contributions of global nursing can become the translational determinant between businesses like Zipline and the unfolding healthcare scenario in LMICs. They are the link between the theory of improved delivery that innovators strive for and the creation of measurable and positive outcomes in practice. We are the leaders who take a singular idea and integrate it systemwide in a way that creates meaningful and lasting change for all involved. The notion of decreasing blood delivery times and increasing access to blood transfusion as a treatment is an honorable and celebrated endeavor. But without a nursing sensibility, without the background understanding of how hospitals work or the knowledge of how nurses in diverse cultures function, the idea falls short. Global nursing is the missing link.

Bleich (2016, p. 46) shares his vision for the future of nursing and health care that is particularly relevant in this context:

> . . . health systems will be designed to be seamless and continuous rather than needlessly complex and disjointed. Nurses will play a strong role in the design of these systems through education, training, and presence in the settings where care is needed. . . . Our role in care design at the institutional level will not be trumped at the policy level, as we bridge institutional policies and practices with state and national policies and practices. Our contribution will be to bring coalitions together to afford needed change in the health system.

It is the unique contribution of nursing in these interdisciplinary collaborations that makes the realization of SDG 9 possible. It is the global nurse as partner, leader, and advocate that imbeds industry and infrastructure innovations into systems in order to improve health and well-being for individuals, populations, and nations worldwide.

REFLECTION AND DISCUSSION

- How does global nursing assure the safe and appropriate implementation of health advances in infrastructure and industry?

- What global nurse partnerships with cutting-edge industries looking to improve health care are needed?

- In what ways can I steer businesses to understand the role of nursing and promote sustainability with a nursing lens?

- How can I help organizations translate innovative theories and visions into practical outcomes?

- What is my role in designing health systems to be seamless and continuous?

REFERENCES

Bleich, M. (2016). Translational and indispensible: Using the gift of foresight to re-envision nursing. In W. Rosa (Ed.), *Nurses as leaders: Evolutionary visions of leadership* (pp. 33–47). New York, NY: Springer Publishing.

Centers for Disease Control and Prevention. (2016). 2014 Ebola outbreak in West Africa: Case counts. Retrieved from https://www.cdc.gov/vhf/ebola/outbreaks/2014-west-africa/case-counts.html

Fund for Global Health. (2015). Rural health care. Retrieved from http://www.fundforglobalhealth.org/what-we-do#rural

Jones, P. (2010). Health workers on the frontline. *British Journal of Healthcare Assistants*, 4(9), 460.

Kateh, F., Nagbe, T., Kieta, A., Barksey, A., Gasasira, A. N., Driscoll, A., . . . Nyenswah, T. (2015). Rapid response to Ebola outbreaks in remote areas—Liberia, July–November 2014. *Morbidity and Mortality Weekly Report, 64*(7), 188–192.

Manjrekar, P. (2016). Resourceful and unified: Partnering across cultures and worldviews. In W. Rosa (Ed.), *Nurses as leaders: Evolutionary visions of leadership* (pp. 345–358). New York, NY: Springer Publishing.

National Rural Health Association. (2016). *National Rural Health Association policy brief: Rural public health.* Retrieved from https://www.ruralhealthweb.org/getattachment/Advocate/Policy-Documents/NRHARuralPublicHealthPolicyPaperFeb2016.pdf.aspx?lang=en-US

United Nations. (2015). *Transforming our world: The 2030 Agenda for Sustainable Development.* Retrieved from https://docs.google.com/gview?url=http://sustainabledevelopment.un.org/content/documents/21252030%20Agenda%20for%20Sustainable%20Development%20web.pdf&embedded=true

United Nations Development Group. (2015). Socio-economic impact of Ebola virus disease in West African countries: A call for national and regional containment, recovery and prevention. Retrieved from http://www.africa.undp.org/content/dam/rba/docs/Reports/ebola-west-africa.pdf

Zipline. (n.d.). The future of healthcare is out for delivery. Retrieved from http://flyzipline.com/product

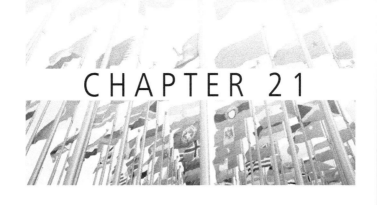

CHAPTER 21

Goal 10. Reduce Inequality Within and Among Countries

William Rosa

The stage is set for more of the same, even though we are reassured by the powerful that the age of barbarism is behind us. . . . Rights violations are, rather, symptoms of deeper pathologies of power and [reflect] the social conditions that . . . determine who will suffer . . . and who will be shielded. (Farmer, 2005, p. 7)

Inequality negatively and powerfully impacts the quality of life for people worldwide. It becomes relentlessly treacherous when it has been adopted as a norm or value of a particular society through the inaction, silence, and apathy of its citizens. Box 21.1 provides more information on Sustainable Development Goal (SDG) 10, which addresses inequalities and its associated targets (see the Appendix A to view the Sustainable Development Agenda in its entirety).

Inhumane laws and enforced discriminatory norms bound African Americans as slaves in the United States for more than 300 years, officially reduced them to subhuman status until the advent of civil rights in the 1960s, and continue to be an impetus for racially motivated bias and violence throughout the country. As slaves, African Americans were officially the "property" of their masters and could be bought or sold and passed on as inheritance as their owners saw fit. Slave trades around the world have been the ultimate affront to civil society; the radical dehumanization of a thinking, seeing, hearing, feeling person to object; to thing; to "it."

Legalized inequality in the United States kept same-sex couples from lawful marriage for generations, keeping human rights and social justice out of reach for thousands and debilitating the overall social and economic well-being of life partners across the nation. This institutionalized phobia of individuals across the sexual orientation and gender identity spectrum has resulted in politically condoned aggression against homosexuals in Uganda and the Middle East, the stripping

Box 21.1   Sustainable Development Goal 10 and Its Associated Targets

Goal 10. Reduce inequality within and among countries

10.1   By 2030, progressively achieve and sustain income growth of the bottom 40% of the population at a rate higher than the national average.

10.2   By 2030, empower and promote the social, economic and political inclusion of all, irrespective of age, sex, disability, race, ethnicity, origin, religion or economic or other status.

10.3   Ensure equal opportunity and reduce inequalities of outcome, including by eliminating discriminatory laws, policies and practices and promoting appropriate legislation, policies and action in this regard.

10.4   Adopt policies, especially fiscal, wage and social protection policies, and progressively achieve greater equality.

10.5   Improve the regulation and monitoring of global financial markets and institutions and strengthen the implementation of such regulations.

10.6   Ensure enhanced representation and voice for developing countries in decision-making in global international economic and financial institutions in order to deliver more effective, credible, accountable and legitimate institutions.

10.7   Facilitate orderly, safe, regular and responsible migration and mobility of people, including through the implementation of planned and well-managed migration policies.

10.a   Implement the principle of special and differential treatment for developing countries, in particular least developed countries, in accordance with World Trade Organization agreements.

10.b   Encourage official development assistance and financial flows, including foreign direct investment, to States where the need is greatest, in particular least developed countries, African countries, small island developing States and landlocked developing countries, in accordance with their national plans and programmes.

10.c   By 2030, reduce to less than 3% the transaction costs of migrant remittances and eliminate remittance corridors with costs higher than 5%.

Source: Reprinted with permission from the United Nations (2015).

of marriage rights in India, the June 2016 murder of at least 49 (with another 53 injured) in a gay nightclub in Orlando, Florida, and the public humiliation and social abandonment of openly known lesbian, gay, bisexual, transgender, and gender nonconforming people across countries and civilizations.

On a global scale, inequality and its counterpart, hatred, have become unfortunate and predominant threads throughout cross-cultural settings. Whether it is the political endorsement of female subservience in nations around the globe or the hostile schism between Sunni and Shia Islamic sects in countries such as

Syria and Pakistan, inequality leads to the devastation of both humanity and the human spirit. The divisiveness of hatred has devolved fragments of the world into a modern-day and brutalized city of Babel; a kaleidoscope of confusion and misunderstanding that continues to foment violence in the global village. Violence is the ultimate voice of inequality. An estimated 475,000 people per year around the world are murdered, and millions of other victims receive health care services related to countless types of assault and abuse: physical, sexual, child, elder, intimate partner, the list goes on (World Health Organization [WHO], 2014). The most graphic examples of violence the world has known come from the accounts we know of wars and genocides.

Genocide is the ultimate consequence of inequality and hatred; whether it be the attempted eradication of the Cambodian intellectuals and artists, the Armenians under the Ottoman empire, or the Jews throughout Europe in the early half of the 20th century, inequality leads to the categorization of human beings as "other," "less than," and "inhuman." And once this happens, destruction in all its forms becomes possible and acceptable.

The cultural and tribal fabric of Rwanda was deeply wounded when, over the course of generations and under the influence of colonization, Tutsis and Hutus were segregated, murder between civilians became politically sanctioned and economically motivated, and the 1994 Genocide Against the Tutsi resulted in the murder of over 1 million human beings.

Countless genocides and so-called ethnic cleansings have strained world history throughout the past century, claiming the lives of over 15 million targeted people all over the world (United to End Genocide, 2015). Currently, there are statistically evident genocides unfolding in Syria, Ethiopia, Sudan, Democratic Republic of Congo, and Burma, with imminent and early warning signs of potential genocide activity progressing in over a dozen other nations worldwide (Genocide Watch, n.d.). The effects extend far past the survivors themselves, who may be continuing to confront posttraumatic stress disorder (PTSD) among other mental–emotional–spiritual challenges. The literature is now showing that the descendants of these survivors may be at an increased risk for anxiety disorders and psychosocial dysfunction due to the transmission of trauma at a cellular level (J. Atkinson, Nelson, Brooks, C. Atkinson, & Ryan, 2014; Rodriguez, 2015).

In this way, genocide impacts not only direct survivors, but also refugees unable to return home, rehabilitating communities and nations, neighboring countries, and generations yet to be born. It leaves few untouched. This information infers that a significant portion of the world's population is experiencing the aftermath of genocide or widespread persecution in some way, whether socially, politically, personally, or economically. There is no statistic that provides information regarding just how many people have been affected by the devastating consequences of the genocide continuum.

THE REFUGEE CRISIS: ASSESSING A POPULATION

One of the most glaring consequences of inequality within and among countries is the worldwide refugee crisis. In addition to the death tolls and budding crises listed earlier, 65.3 million people are now forcibly displaced due to "persecution, conflict, generalized violence, or human rights violations" (United Nations High

Commissioner for Refugees [UNHCR], 2016). Roughly 21 million refugees are currently seeking protection in asylum countries due to inequality or active or looming conflict (UNHCR, n.d.), and many are experiencing the debilitating and broad-spectrum health deficits resultant of collective violence (Krug, Dahlberg, Mercy, Zwi, & Lozano, 2002). Global nursing is required not only to introduce the science and advances needed to meet the unique needs of such a population, but also to rehumanize settings where the threads of shared humanity have been shredded and torn.

We must use culturally inclusive tools that equip us to cohesively assess and understand those we serve, particularly if they have experienced the hardship of refugee displacement. Boyle and Baird (2016) provide a Transcultural Nursing Assessment Guide for Refugees to aid in the process. By using such a cultural assessment tool, global nurses can better promote healing inclusive of cross-cultural beliefs, experiences, and values for refugees and for any population receiving health care in a transcultural context. This level of human-centered care is essential to ending inequalities and promoting ethical systems invested in delivering individualized and contextually relevant health care. The components of the Boyle/Baird Transcultural Nursing Assessment Guide with brief descriptions include:

- **Migration Experience:** Acknowledge that many refugees have often emigrated from LMICs, escaped settings of conflict, and lack sufficient economic means. Inquiring about these background domains helps to more thoroughly assess needs related to health, trauma, and difficulties with resettlement. Common questions to ask should be directed to the migration experience itself, challenges faced in the current health care system, and the appropriate languages/dialects and traditions most important to the person and family.

- **Traditional Beliefs and Practices of Healing:** Assess the patient's understanding of the disease—causes, meaning, implications, and how the illness impacts self-identity and role in family/societal structure. What the patient believes and practices, and the barriers to maintaining those beliefs and practices in the current context, fills in vital information relevant to developing safe and effective treatment options.

- **Family/Kinship Assessment:** What is the story of this family? This person likely serves a particular function within and is an integral part of the broader family dynamic. Strive to clearly understand if family was left behind or killed, how the family is recovering as a whole, and whether the family makes decisions as a unit or if individual autonomy is promoted within the culture.

- **Social Life and Networks:** For many collectivist cultures, engagement with society is the premise of identity and determines how life unfolds. Ask about roles of individuals and families within the societal structure, who the community leaders are and their involvement in family welfare, educational aspirations for children and adults, and if there are culture-specific concerns related to substance abuse, violence, safety, or health and well-being.

- **Religious Beliefs and Practices:** Note that religion and society around the world are often inextricably interconnected. Inquire about the ways religion impacts daily life, cultural occasions and rites of passage related to religious faith, and what major life events, such as births or deaths, will require heightened attention to intensive religious and/or spiritual care.

- **Trauma/Torture:** Mental and emotional health secondary to trauma or torture can often be overlooked and/or underreported aspects of providing care for refugees and other vulnerable populations. Attend to mental and emotional needs; provide a safe space for the patient/family to share difficult experiences; refer to appropriate medical specialties for additional support; follow-up routinely. Boyle and Baird (2016) recommend using a validated tool such as "The Harvard Trauma Questionnaire" (HTQ) or "The Hopkins Symptom Checklist- 25" (HSCL-25).

CONCLUSION

Global nursing must commit to its part in realizing SDG 10 by continually assessing, articulating, and identifying solutions that mitigate the effects of inequality on health and well-being. In order to do this, we must realize "that health and human rights are inextricably linked; and that social exclusion exacerbates the relationship between human rights violations and negative health impacts" (Tripathi, Hoodbhoy, & Rosenthal, 2011, p. 253).

As vanguards of human caring (Watson, 2008, 2012) and peacemakers in service to the dignity of the global village (Lane, 2016; Lane, Samuels, & Watson, 2012), nurses have an ethical responsibility to address inequalities wherever they may exist and advocate for those who are vulnerable to the consequences. The very act of nursing—that art of healing—is peacemaking in the process. The ideals we promote reflect humanistic ideals of wholeness, inclusivity, generosity, gentleness, kindness, compassion, and respect. These characteristics must be paired with an equally skillful determination and political savvy if we are to effectively promote the safety and equality deserved by the world's people. Nursing must make a moral commitment to procure human rights and social justice (Nicholas, 2015), foster effective partnerships and collaborations through trust building and the identification of sustainability mechanisms (Sliney, 2015), and understand cultural contexts in order to promote community engagement (Dieckmann, 2012). By having honest conversations about the ways inequality deteriorates health and well-being on a global scale, we can lead and copartner initiatives that seek to heal individuals, populations, and nations.

A nursing sensibility goes a long way toward achieving the targets of SDG 10. However, we must start by clarifying the harmful misnomers regarding nursing as a profession, which keep nurses servile and "less than" throughout global health infrastructures. Global nurses have an obligation to address their own experienced inequality among the health professions that prevent us from "equal opportunity" participation in policy, practice, and research arenas. We must learn self-advocacy; speak clearly and proudly about our practice; clarify our role to the public; empower colleagues across nations to become autonomous as knowledgeable and capable nurses they are; mend the fences of interprofessional disagreement; and celebrate the unique contribution of nursing to global health. By tending to the inequalities that enfeeble nursing, we take personal–professional accountability toward realizing the goals of SDG 10 as they relate our current status as a discipline and our abilities to influence global health standards and outcomes in the future.

REFLECTION AND DISCUSSION

- What are my strengths and abilities in advocating for the marginalized?
- In what ways does the public need clarification regarding nursing's global role?
- How can I support my cross-cultural colleagues in their autonomy as practitioners, researchers, and educators?
- As a health care system, how do we go about mending the fences of interprofessional disagreement?
- What can I do to raise the visibility of nursing's part in reducing inequalities?

REFERENCES

American Psychiatric Association. (2000). *Diagnostic and statistical manual of mental disorders* (4th ed., text rev.). Washington, DC: Author

Atkinson, J., Nelson, J., Brooks, R., Atkinson, C., & Ryan, K. (2014). Addressing individual and community transgenerational trauma. In N. Purdie, P. Dudgeon, & R. Walker (Eds.), *Working together: Aboriginal and Torres Strait Islander mental health and wellbeing principles and practice* (2nd ed., pp. 135–144). Bruce, Australia: Australian Institute of Health and Welfare.

Boyle, J. S., & Baird, M. B. (2016). Boyle/Baird transcultural nursing assessment guide for refugees. In M. M. Andrews & J. S. Boyle (Eds.), *Transcultural concepts in nursing care* (7th ed., pp. E1–E4). Philadelphia, PA: Wolters Kluwer Health/Lippincott Williams & Wilkins.

Dieckmann, J. L. (2012). Challenges in program implementation. In A. L. Cupp Curley & P. A. Vitale (Eds.), *Population-based nursing: Concepts and competencies for advanced practice* (pp. 239–265). New York, NY: Springer Publishing.

Farmer, P. (2005). *Pathologies of power: Health, human rights, and the new war on the poor.* Berkeley and Los Angeles: University of California Press.

Genocide Watch. (n.d.). Alerts. Retrieved from http://www.genocidewatch.org/alerts/newsalerts.html

Kleinman, A. (1980). *Patients and healers in the context of culture: An exploration of the borderland between anthropology, medicine and psychiatry.* Berkeley: University of California Press.

Krug, E. G., Dahlberg, L. L., Mercy, J. A., Zwi, A. B., & Lozano, R. (Eds.). (2002). *World report on violence and health.* Geneva, Switzerland: World Health Organization. Retrieved from http://apps.who.int/iris/bitstream/10665/42495/1/9241545615_eng.pdf

Lane, M. R. (2016). Authentic and creative: Walking the Caritas path to peace. In W. Rosa, *Nurses as leaders: Evolutionary visions of leadership* (pp. 323–332). New York, NY: Springer Publishing.

Lane, M. R., Samuels, M., & Watson, J. (2012). *The Caritas path to peace: A guidebook to creating world peace with caring, love, and compassion.* North Charleston, SC: CreateSpace.

Nicholas, P. K. (2015). Health, human rights, and social justice: An interview with Paul Farmer and Sheila Davis. In S. Breakey, I. B. Corless, N. L. Meedzan, & P. K. Nicholas (Eds.), *Global health nursing in the 21st century* (pp. 73–83). New York, NY: Springer Publishing.

Rodriguez, T. (2015). Descendants of Holocaust survivors have altered stress hormones. *Scientific American, 26*(2). Retrieved from http://www.scientificamerican.com/article/descendants-of-holocaust-survivors-have-altered-stress-hormones

Sliney, A. (2015). Global health partnerships. In S. Breakey, I. B. Corless, N. L. Meedzan, & P. K. Nicholas (Eds.), *Global health nursing in the 21st century* (pp. 103–111). New York, NY: Springer Publishing.

Tripathi, V., Hoodbhoy, M. O., & Rosenthal, M. (2011). Promoting human rights in public health programs: Lessons learned from HealthRight International. In E. Beracochea, C. Weinstein, & D. P. Evans (Eds.), *Rights-based approaches to public health* (pp. 253–269). New York, NY: Springer Publishing.

United Nations. (2015). Transforming our world: The 2030 agenda for sustainable development. Retrieved from https://docs.google.com/gview?url=http://sustainabledevelopment.un.org/content/documents/21252030%20Agenda%20for%20Sustainable%20Development%20web.pdf&embedded=true

United Nations High Commissioner for Refugees. (n.d.). Figures at a glance. Retrieved from http://www.unhcr.org/figures-at-a-glance.html

United Nations High Commissioner for Refugees. (2016). *Global trends: Forced displacement in 2015*. Geneva, Switzerland: Author. Retrieved from http://www.unhcr.org/statistics/country/576408cd7/unhcr-global-trends-2015.html

United to End Genocide. (2015). Past genocides and mass atrocities. Retrieved from http://endgenocide.org/learn/past-genocides

Watson, J. (2008). *Nursing: The philosophy and science of caring* (Rev. ed.). Boulder: University Press of Colorado.

Watson, J. (2012). *Human caring science: A theory of nursing* (2nd ed.). Sudbury, MA: Jones & Bartlett.

World Health Organization. (2014). *Global status report on violence prevention 2014*. Geneva, Switzerland: Author.

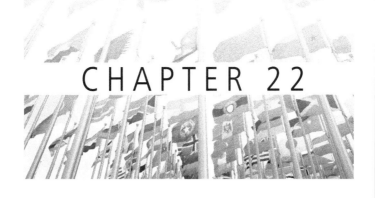

CHAPTER 22

Goal 11. Make Cities and Human Settlements Inclusive, Safe, Resilient, and Sustainable

William Rosa

[E]fforts to tackle urban environmental health problems in the . . . world . . . must involve the formulation of realistic policies that integrate the relevant issues such as sanitation, poverty, education . . . housing and health. [This] can be . . . ensured by [placing] people at [the] community level at the centre of every stage of the process. (Konteh, 2009, pp. 76–77)

With roughly half of the world's population—3.5 billion people—living in cities and over 828 million people living in slums, cities across the world comprise about 3% of the Earth, but account for up to 80% of all energy consumption and 75% of carbon emissions (United Nations Sustainable Development, 2016). As low- and middle-income countries (LMICs) focus their industry and innovation efforts on the modernization of their cities, their respective communities must continue to have access to safe housing, clean water, effective sanitation mechanisms, and adequate health care delivery. As urbanization continues to be the priority for many countries seeking economic advancement, quality of life for all metropolis inhabitants should be enhanced along with the city's progress. Box 22.1 lists Sustainable Development Goal (SDG) 11's associated targets (see the Appendix to view the Sustainable Development Agenda in its entirety).

The urbanization movement carries with it varied and complex health and climate implications for many nations, and it requires early identification measures and preventative health promotion strategies on the part of global nurses (Patrick, Noy, & Henderson-Wilson, 2015). China's rapid urbanization and subsequent environmental changes have led to an epidemiological shift from infectious to chronic diseases, and increases in both air and water pollution that are

| Box 22.1 | **Sustainable Development Goal 11 and Its Associated Targets** |

Goal 11. Make cities and human settlements inclusive, safe, resilient, and sustainable

11.1 By 2030, ensure access for all to adequate, safe and affordable housing and basic services, and upgrade slums.

11.2 By 2030, provide access to safe, affordable, accessible and sustainable transport systems for all, improving road safety, notably by expanding public transport, with special attention to the needs of those in vulnerable situations, women, children, persons with disabilities and older persons.

11.3 By 2030, enhance inclusive and sustainable urbanization and capacity for participatory, integrated and sustainable human settlement planning and management in all countries.

11.4 Strengthen efforts to protect and safeguard the world's cultural and natural heritage.

11.5 By 2030, significantly reduce the number of deaths and the number of people affected and substantially decrease the direct economic losses relative to global gross domestic product caused by disasters, including water-related disasters, with a focus on protecting the poor and people in vulnerable situations.

11.6 By 2030, reduce the adverse per capita environmental impact of cities, including by paying special attention to air quality and municipal and other waste management.

11.7 By 2030, provide universal access to safe, inclusive and accessible, green and public spaces, in particular for women and children, older persons and persons with disabilities.

11.a Support positive economic, social and environmental links between urban, peri-urban and rural areas by strengthening national and regional development planning.

11.b By 2020, substantially increase the number of cities and human settlements adopting and implementing integrated policies and plans toward inclusion, resource efficiency, mitigation and adaptation to climate change, resilience to disasters, and develop and implement, in line with the Sendai Framework for Disaster Risk Reduction 2015–2030, holistic disaster risk management at all levels.

11.c Support least developed countries, including through financial and technical assistance, in building sustainable and resilient buildings utilizing local materials.

Source: Reprinted with permission from the United Nations (2015).

contributing to both morbidity and mortality (Li et al., 2016). There has been a strong and positive correlation found between overweight/obesity and urban dwelling throughout geographic regions in India (Siddiqui, Kandala, & Stranges, 2015). And, in Italy, it has been found that living in a rapidly developing urban setting leads to a perceived sense of uncertainty, feelings of distress, poor social functioning, and harmful implications related to mood, anxiety, and psychological well-being (Luciano et al., 2016).

Through deliberate planning and the creation of efficient cross-cultural partnerships, cities have the potential to push the global development envelope while remaining cognizant and responsive to the diverse needs of their people. It is essential that throughout the urbanization process and the economic–environmental changes that accompany it, global nurses advocate for strategies, policies, and activities considerate of local and culturally relevant realities over, and possibly in contrast to, larger global, transnational priorities and goals, particularly in LMICs (Konteh, 2009).

Using a holistic wellness model, global nurses can help to identify community strengths and nurture resilience throughout the change process of urbanization. Clark (2002a) calls for nurses to assess for and further develop physiological, psychological, social, and spiritual community strengths, such as education, coping skills, support systems, and problem-solving abilities. In this way, we become advocates who strengthen positive community characteristics and foster a sense of resilience within cities and populations.

Global nurses may use a community development approach in helping implement SDG 11. This approach "views health and wellness within the broader context of social and economic improvement, and it views resident empowerment as a vital element in achieving health and wellness" (Clark, 2002b, p. 35). In continuing to assess the health and wellness of urbanized cities and communities, several in-depth considerations need to be given. However, Clark (2002b) suggests starting with these reflections:

- With whom do I work to collect needed information?
- How can I work most effectively with the identified community representatives?
- How can I understand the processes that affect health and wellness in this community?

A fundamental understanding of available resources is needed to successfully proceed with a community assessment and respond with contextually appropriate solutions.

The global nurse will need to consider key aspects of the community, from geographical composition and vital statistics regarding births and deaths, to morbidity and mortality and communicable disease rates, to available education, employment opportunities, marriages, divorces, accessible health services, and police reports (Benjamin, 2012). It is vital to understand the community's history and the progress they have made toward their goals to date in order to acknowledge accomplishments and strategically plan for the future. Furthermore, it is essential to assess the readiness of individuals and larger cities for the radical transformation indicative of urban development. By doing so, we will be better able to support them as they move through the fluctuations inherent to any change process.

Jeffreys and Antoine (2016) urge us to consider the "cultural revolution" in health care by availing ourselves to the concerns and challenges experienced by clients worldwide, from their perspective and context. At the heart of this process, we are required to become attuned to our own cultural arrogance, surrender ways of being that are fixed and culturally insensitive, and embrace strategies that are both inclusive and humble (Soulé, 2016). The World Health Organization (WHO, 2010) suggests the following as action steps to procure more sustainable cities and communities:

- Aid health ministries in: addressing social determinants of health and which policy changes impact health; identifying multisector partners for effective strategy building; and considering environmental impact in urban planning.
- Work with local governments to champion physically active community-based activities; involve volunteer, professional, and local government organizations that will provide a forum for health education and transparency; share data freely; and encourage community participation in the planning and implementation of programs.
- Engage civil society to be inclusive of residents across socioeconomic differences to find practical solutions to community well-being; collaborate with governments to be a part of policy development and budgetary design.
- Lead and facilitate research that fills the many knowledge gaps regarding urbanization, health disparities across rural and urban areas, prevention mechanisms, and the contribution of citizens in decision-making processes.
- Collaborate with urban planners to ensure proper respect of zoning and land-use regulations; adopt building practices that protect urban health; and create compact and easily accessible cities.
- Form relationships with international agencies to invite support regarding healthy environment policies, relate experiences and learn from one another, support equality across the board, and encourage policy makers to use accurate and more diverse sociodemographic data in urban planning and future development.

By maintaining this sensibility and remaining open and available, we can come to understand our role in procuring safe and inclusive cities that promote health and well-being for all by 2030.

REFLECTION AND DISCUSSION

- Do I believe I have a part in the establishment of safe cities and communities around the world?
- How can urbanization occur with respect to the diverse needs of people and populations in my local community?
- In what ways can I ensure that social and economic improvement is inclusive of health and wellness?

- Why is knowledge of a community's history and present challenges essential in determining relevant health goals?

- What does the "cultural revolution" mean to me? What challenges might it pose in adopting new practices and innovative approaches to relationship building and global health promotion?

REFERENCES

Benjamin, B. B. (2012). Building relationships and engaging communities through collaboration. In A. L. Cupp Curley & P. A. Vitale (Eds.), *Population-based nursing: Concepts and competencies for advanced practice* (pp. 211–237). New York, NY: Springer Publishing.

Clark, C. C. (2002a). A model for health and wellness promotion in communities. In C. C. Clark (Ed.), *Health promotion in communities: Holistic and wellness approaches* (pp. 3–14). New York, NY: Springer Publishing.

Clark, C. C. (2002b). Community self-assessment. In C. C. Clark (Ed.), *Health promotion in communities: Holistic and wellness approaches* (pp. 35–45). New York, NY: Springer Publishing.

Jeffreys, M. R., & Antoine, K. (2016). Overview of key issues and concerns. In M. R. Jeffreys (Ed.), *Teaching cultural competence in nursing and health care: Inquiry, action, and innovation* (3rd ed., pp. 3–39). New York, NY: Springer Publishing.

Konteh, F. H. (2009). Urban sanitation and health in the developing world: Reminiscing the nineteenth century industrial nations. *Health & Place, 15,* 69–78.

Li, X., Song, J., Lin, T., Dixon, J., Zhang, G., & Ye, H. (2016). Urbanization and health in China: Thinking at the national, local and individual levels. *Environmental Health, 15,* 113–123.

Luciano, M., De Rosa, C., Del Vecchio, V., Sampogna, G., Sbordone, D., Atti, A. R., . . . Fiorillo, A. (2016). Perceived insecurity, mental health and urbanization: Results from a multicentric study. *International Journal of Social Psychiatry, 62*(3), 252–261.

Patrick, R., Noy, S., & Henderson-Wilson, C. (2015). Urbanisation, climate change and health equity: How can health promotion contribute? *International Journal of Health Promotion and Education, 54*(1), 34–49.

Siddiqui, S. T., Kandala, N.-B., & Stranges, S. (2015). Urbanisation and geographic variation of overweight and obesity in India: A cross-sectional analysis of the Indian Demographic Health Survey 2005–2006. *International Journal of Public Health, 60*(6), 717–726.

Soulé, I. (2016). Flexible and responsive: Applying the wisdom of "It depends." In W. Rosa (Ed.), *Nurses as leaders: Evolutionary visions of leadership* (pp. 417–430). New York, NY: Springer Publishing.

United Nations. (2015). *Transforming our world: The 2030 agenda for sustainable development.* Retrieved from https://docs.google.com/gview?url=http://sustainabledevelopment.un.org/content/documents/21252030%20Agenda%20for%20Sustainable%20Development%20web.pdf&embedded=true

United Nations Sustainable Development. (2016). Goal 11: Make cities inclusive, safe, resilient, and sustainable. Retrieved from http://www.un.org/sustainabledevelopment/cities

World Health Organization. (2010). *Why urban health matters.* Geneva, Switzerland: Author. Retrieved from http://www.who.int/world-health-day/2010/media/whd2010background.pdf

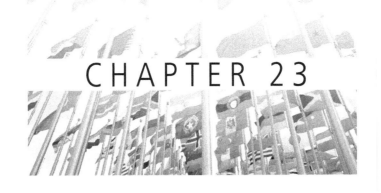

CHAPTER 23

Goal 12. Ensure Sustainable Consumption and Production Patterns

William Rosa

*We are in a new dawn regarding environmental health and activism . . .
[there is] a demand for nurses to understand and become more involved in
the relationship between human health and the environments in which we
live, learn, work, and play. We have moved beyond questioning the science
of whether we are in an environmental health peril to almost unanimous
consensus that we must act and act now on many of the risks we are all
experiencing in our present and for future generations. (Luck, 2016, p. 338)*

The statement quoted in the following paragraph should concern you. Hopefully,
it will throw you into action. You might find yourself reflecting on what you can do
or how you can procure future global well-being while mitigating the potential risk
of human suffering ahead. You might wonder if you have the skills and resources
necessary to impact positive change for individuals and populations at large. If you
are like me, you may lose your breath for a moment only to soon realize that we are
capable, as impossible as it may seem, of both reversing this trend and preventing
the complications and human-made disasters implied by such a projection.

Here it is: "Should the global population reach 9.6 billion by 2050, the equivalent
of almost three planets could be required to provide the natural resources needed
to sustain current lifestyles" (United Nations Sustainable Development, 2016).
Personally, I will be 67 years old in 2050. My spouse will be 81. What about you?
What about your partner? How old will your children and your children's children
be? What will be left for them to eat and breathe and drink? What will be the quality of their lives as they struggle to maintain optimal health and well-being? While
these questions might be intimidating to reflect upon, they could not be more essential to ask at this pivotal time in human development and globalization. Sustainable
Development Goal (SDG) 12 and its associated targets are listed in Box 23.1 (see the
Appendix to view the Sustainable Development Agenda in its entirety).

Box 23.1 **Sustainable Development Goal 12 and Its Associated Targets**

Goal 12. Ensure sustainable consumption and production patterns

12.1   Implement the 10-Year Framework of Programmes on Sustainable Consumption and Production Patterns, all countries taking action, with developed countries taking the lead, taking into account the development and capabilities of developing countries.

12.2   By 2030, achieve the sustainable management and efficient use of natural resources.

12.3   By 2030, halve per capita global food waste at the retail and consumer levels and reduce food losses along production and supply chains, including postharvest losses.

12.4   By 2020, achieve the environmentally sound management of chemicals and all wastes throughout their life cycle, in accordance with agreed international frameworks, and significantly reduce their release to air, water and soil in order to minimize their adverse impacts on human health and the environment.

12.5   By 2030, substantially reduce waste generation through prevention, reduction, recycling and reuse.

12.6   Encourage companies, especially large and transnational companies, to adopt sustainable practices and to integrate sustainability information into their reporting cycle.

12.7   Promote public procurement practices that are sustainable, in accordance with national policies and priorities.

12.8   By 2030, ensure that people everywhere have the relevant information and awareness for sustainable development and lifestyles in harmony with nature.

12.a   Support developing countries to strengthen their scientific and technological capacity to move toward more sustainable patterns of consumption and production.

12.b   Develop and implement tools to monitor sustainable development impacts for sustainable tourism that creates jobs and promotes local culture and products.

12.c   Rationalize inefficient fossil-fuel subsidies that encourage wasteful consumption by removing market distortions, in accordance with national circumstances, including by restructuring taxation and phasing out those harmful subsidies, where they exist, to reflect their environmental impacts, taking fully into account the specific needs and conditions of developing countries and minimizing the possible adverse impacts on their development in a manner that protects the poor and the affected communities.

Source: Reprinted with permission from the United Nations (2015).

Imagine, if you will, a world where water scarcity becomes a daily reality for even the most affluent of nations: bare store shelves and empty refrigerators. Think about the food deprivation that may occur as farmland is further degraded as a result of unsustainable practices, overfishing continues to pillage lakes and oceans, and food is wasted at exponential, almost unthinkable, rates. Consider breathing air so polluted by the irresponsibility of industrial waste emissions that respiratory diseases become the norm and not the exception.

Waste and wasteful practices are endemic in the health care sector. Kwakye, Brat, and Makary (2011) noted that health care is the second largest contributor to waste production. Incineration of medical waste products leads to the release of dioxin, a well-studied carcinogen. Though there has been much study regarding the health consequences of dioxin exposure and guidance on safer, more environmentally friendly methods of waste disposal for health facilities (United States Environmental Protection Agency, 2016; World Health Organization, 2015), unsafe incineration practices and subsequent dioxin release continue to be a health issue in low- and middle-income countries (LMICs) (Njagi, Oloo, J. Kithinji, & M. J. Kithinji, 2012). Global nurses have a role in promoting environmentally responsible health care consciousness. Table 23.1 provides a list of sustainability measures environmentally responsible nurses can promote and the undesirable practices they can discourage in regard to energy consumption, water use, and consumption/disposal of products and materials, as identified by Kangasniemi, Kallio, and Pietilä (2014). Through an ongoing commitment to focused educational initiatives, interprofessional and organizational collaboration, continuous research, leading planning strategies, and updating protocols and guidelines, global nurses can make formidable contributions to ensuring sustainable consumption and production (Kangasniemi et al., 2014).

Table 23.1 Environmentally Responsible Nursing Actions

Category	Environmentally Responsible Actions
Energy consumption	• Share knowledge regarding amount of electricity used due to increased use of technologies • Turn off unused lights and devices (i.e., monitors, pumps, computers) • Promote the purchase of "green" resources and equipment • Educate investors regarding clean energy options and eco-friendly hospitals
Water use	• Avoid unnecessary linen laundering and running water • Reduce costs and energy consumption related to water heating by identifying clean energy sources for delivery and heating purposes
Consumption of products and materials	• Audit purchasing lists and reduce excessive inventory to minimize waste and promote conservation • Buy easily recyclable materials and shift toward the purchase of recycled materials • Opt for reusable products when safe and possible (no current evidence that reused devices pose health risks) • Reduce the number of products used and included in prepackaged "sets" of products or instruments • Sort waste disposal and recycle when possible

Source: Kangasniemi et al. (2014).

Worldwide initiatives are under way that environmentally responsible nurses need to be coleading and supporting. For example, the Healthier Hospitals Initiative (HHI; Healthier Hospitals, n.d.) is a collaboration between the organizations Practice Greenhealth and Health Care Without Harm, and 11 major U.S. health care systems that strives to increase sustainability and promote responsible consumption and production through attention to engaged leadership, healthier food, leaner energy, less waste, safer chemicals, and smarter purchasing. Practice Greenhealth provides ongoing education and resources to help hospitals improve consumption practices through initiatives like Greening the OR® (operating room; Practice Greenhealth, 2016a) and Greening the Supply Chain™ (Practice Greenhealth, 2016b). Health Care Without Harm (2016) is committed to reducing the environmental footprint of health care around the world by raising awareness regarding environmentally responsible practices in building, chemical use, energy consumption, food production and waste, pharmaceutical management and disposal, patient and staff transportation, waste policies and sustainable disposal options, and water conservation.

Previous chapters have addressed the partnerships and initiatives in which global nurses can engage to achieve and address many of these targets. One additional and crucial role includes promoting self-reflection for individuals and communities to better understand their responsibilities in sustainable consumption. This includes the dissemination of accurate information for all people to understand the implications of their lifestyle choices on the health and well-being of the global village.

Self-reflection in this regard means that we are able to gauge our individual and communal contributions to the greater environmental status of the world at large. Luck and Keegan (2016, p. 559) provide these questions for consideration:

- What does it mean to be human?
- What does it mean to be an Earth citizen?
- How can we face the great ecological crises of our time?
- How do each of our stories contribute to the larger story?
- How does changing our own story lead to planetary change?

As we identify the places and spaces where our lives intersect with the priorities of global well-being, we gain the opportunities to improve the choices we make and affect meaningful, positive changes for both self and others.

The considerations of SDG 12 are not the problems of some far off and unlikely future of which we will not be a part. On the contrary, many of us will be alive and well to reap the consequences of the choices we are making and the industrial practices we are supporting right now. We have a duty, as global citizens, to take a hard and uncomfortable look at how we live, eat, drink, work, play, and sustain ourselves in respect to the natural resources of the planet. This self-reflection is a part of responsible living: a vital component of the desire we have to see our families and communities thrive in health and happiness.

REFLECTION AND DISCUSSION

- How am I called to promote environmental consciousness?
- What strategies can I employ to aid my facility in adopting more responsible consumption and production practices?

- What can I do right now to create new knowledge regarding the relationship between environmental practices and health?
- In what ways can I facilitate client and community self-reflection?
- How can I change the planetary narrative?

REFERENCES

Health Care Without Harm. (2016). Mission and goals. Retrieved from https://noharm-uscanada.org/content/us-canada/mission-and-goals

Healthier Hospitals. (n.d.). HH challenges. Retrieved from http://www.healthierhospitals.org/hhi-challenges

Kangasniemi, M., Kallio, H., & Pietilä, A.-M. (2014). Towards environmentally responsible nursing: A critical imperative synthesis. *Journal of Advanced Nursing, 70*(7), 1465–1478.

Kwakye, G., Brat, G. A., & Makary, M. A. (2011). Green surgical practices for health care. *Archives of Surgery, 146*(2), 131–136.

Luck, S. (2016). Informed and impactful: Stewarding the environmental determinants of health and well-being. In W. Rosa (Ed.), *Nurses as leaders: Evolutionary visions of leadership* (pp. 333–343). New York, NY: Springer Publishing.

Luck, S., & Keegan, L. (2016). Environmental health. In B. M. Dossey & L. Keegan (Eds.), *Holistic nursing: A handbook for practice* (7th ed., pp. 557–587). Burlington, MA: Jones & Bartlett.

Njagi, N. A., Oloo, M. A., Kithinji, J., & Kithinji, M. J. (2012). Health-care waste incineration and related dangers to public health: Case study of the two teaching and referral hospitals in Kenya. *Journal of Community Health, 37,* 1168–1171.

Practice Greenhealth. (2016a). Greening the operating room. Retrieved from https://practicegreenhealth.org/initiatives/greening-operating-room

Practice Greenhealth. (2016b). Greening the supply chain initiative. Retrieved from https://practicegreenhealth.org/initiatives/greening-supply-chain

United Nations. (2015). Transforming our world: The 2030 agenda for sustainable development. Retrieved from https://docs.google.com/gview?url=http://sustainabledevelopment.un.org/content/documents/21252030%20Agenda%20for%20Sustainable%20Development%20web.pdf&embedded=true

United Nations Sustainable Development. (2016). Goal 12: Ensure sustainable consumption and production patterns. Retrieved from http://www.un.org/sustainabledevelopment/sustainable-consumption-production

United States Environmental Protection Agency. (2016). Learn about dioxin. Retrieved from https://www.epa.gov/dioxin/learn-about-dioxin

World Health Organization. (2015). Health-care waste. Retrieved from http://www.who.int/mediacentre/factsheets/fs253/en

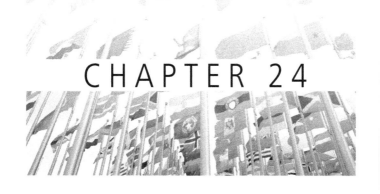

CHAPTER 24

Goal 13. Take Urgent Action to Combat Climate Change and Its Impacts

William Rosa

For [the Maldives] it is so difficult to imagine that we might not exist. We have been living in the middle of the Indian Ocean for the last 2000 years. We have a written history of 2000 years. We have a culture, we have a civilisation and it is just simply impossible for us to comprehend and digest that we will not be around during the next century. . . . In our minds, climate change is not just an environmental issue. It is a human rights issue. It is the right to live. It is a fundamental right. Therefore, it is non-negotiable. We cannot negotiate with our lives. . . . [I]f you cannot save the Maldives today, you will not be able to save yourselves tomorrow.
(Nasheed, 2010)

In 2012, a film was released that showed the tip of the future devastation possible if the global community does not awaken to the evolving threats resulting from climate change. Jon Shenk's *The Island President* documents former President Mohamed Nasheed's quest to protect his country, the Maldives, from annihilation. As the lowest lying country on the planet, the Maldives is dangerously impacted by the rise in sea level, which is occurring at rapid rates secondary to global warming. The Maldives is an endangered civilization that is now advocating for the world to adopt more sustainable industry options and reduce greenhouse gas emissions for their survival. *The Island President* offered a glimpse into humanity's future if climate change is not urgently addressed on a global scale. It is safe to say: We are not responding quickly enough. Box 24.1 lists Sustainable Development Goal (SDG) 13 along with its associated targets (see the Appendix to view the Sustainable Development Agenda in its entirety).

| Box 24.1 | **Sustainable Development Goal 13 and Its Associated Targets** |

Goal 13. Take urgent action to combat climate change and its impacts*

13.1 Strengthen resilience and adaptive capacity to climate-related hazards and natural disasters in all countries.

13.2 Integrate climate change measures into national policies, strategies and planning.

13.3 Improve education, awareness-raising and human and institutional capacity on climate change mitigation, adaptation, impact reduction and early warning.

13.a Implement the commitment undertaken by developed-country parties to the United Nations Framework Convention on Climate Change to a goal of mobilizing jointly $100 billion annually by 2020 from all sources to address the needs of developing countries in the context of meaningful mitigation actions and transparency on implementation and fully operationalize the Green Climate Fund through its capitalization as soon as possible.

13.b Promote mechanisms for raising capacity for effective climate-change-related planning and management in least developed countries and small island developing States, including focusing on women, youth and local and marginalized Communities.

*Acknowledging that the United Nations Framework Convention on Climate Change is the primary international, intergovernmental forum for negotiating the global response to climate change.

Source: Reprinted with permission from the United Nations (2015).

Table 24.1 lists the key elements of climate change, their updated scientific records, predictions of their trajectories, the global regions most affected, and the health impacts that will be felt in urban settings around the world, compiled by Patrick, Noy, and Henderson-Wilson (2016, pp. 39–41). It illustrates the connection between urbanization, as discussed in Chapter 22, and climate change. Though Table 24.1 is specifically related to an urban context, the data is truly reflective of human interference with ecosystems and subsequent stress placed upon the environment across settings and considerations; it is a future glimpse of what is in store if timely and adequate global change is not prioritized.

The U.S. Environmental Protection Agency (EPA; 2016) has been clear that global warming is occurring at an alarming rate due to human activities that emit greenhouse gases, such as carbon dioxide, into the atmosphere. Burning fossil fuels for energy, deforestation, poor industrial processes, and agricultural practices that emit high amounts of such gases lead to the signs and symptoms of climate change worldwide: more intense heat waves, dangerous floods and droughts, melting of glaciers, increased warming and acidity of the oceans, rising sea level, and an elevation in the average global temperature. Health and climate changes are inextricable. The World Health Organization (WHO, 2016) has acknowledged that climate change:

Table 24.1 Key Elements of Climate Change Information and Modeling, and Predicted or Actual Health-Related Impacts Relevant to Urban Settlements

Phenomenon	Scientific Record	Predictions/Modeling	Region	Health Impacts in an Urban Context
Global warming *Example:* climate changes over the past 30 years have led to the loss of over 154,000 lives and approximately 5.5 million DALYs per year throughout the world	Global mean warming 0.8% above preindustrial levels	Global surface temperature rise of between 1.1 and 6.4 degrees by 2100; higher temperature increases rates of spread and multiplication of pathogens and changes to the ranges and survival of nonhuman host species (e.g., malaria, cholera, and dengue fever); increased air pollution and particulate matters; ozone-related deaths increase by 4.5%	All regions	Uncontrolled urbanization (deforestation drives up GHG levels); increase range (prevalence of communicable/infectious diseases associated with urban crowding (poor sanitation); warmer temperatures increase air pollution from vehicle (industrial sources in cities); increased particulate matters in cities exacerbate chronic diseases (i.e., asthma)
More heat waves *Example:* Europe 2003 death toll exceeding 70,000; Russia 2010 death toll estimated at 55,000, 11,000 of which were in Moscow	Changes in some extreme events particularly daily temperature and heat waves; past decade an exceptional number of extreme heat waves have been observed around the world	Increases in frequency of warm daily temperatures; decreases in cold extremes throughout the 21st century; heat waves will increase in length, frequency and/or intensity; in a double CO_2 climate, extreme hot days 20 times more frequent	Global scale, over most land areas, particularly North and South America and Eurasia	Aggravated by "heat-island" effect of cities 5 °C–11°C warmer than surrounding areas; heat amplified effects of urban–industrial air pollutants cause respiratory disease and exacerbate CVD; urban population (i.e., older adults, children, women, and low SES) at greater risk of suffering because of higher inner-city temperatures, population density, and inadequate sanitation and freshwater services
Increased extreme wind events *Example:* Hurricane Katrina 2005 winds caused storm surges and 80% of New Orleans was inundated with contaminated floodwater; 1,833 deaths, 711,698 acute impacts and long-term morbidity issues; millions displaced	Uncertainties in tropical cyclone records, incomplete understanding of mechanisms linking cyclone metrics to climate change and degree of cyclone variability mean *low confidence* for attribution of detectable changes in cyclone activity, or occurrence of single event, to anthropogenic influences	Increases in maximum wind speed of tropical cyclones (typhoons or hurricanes); increased intensity of tropical cyclones; but possible decrease in number of cyclones or same number is predicted	Possibly not every ocean basin; high-intensity tropical cyclone concentrated in North America, East Asia, the Caribbean and the Central American region	Social inequities and poor disaster response worsen health impacts especially for vulnerable populations (i.e., poor and African Americans, children and older adults); economic losses from cyclone damage

(continued)

Table 24.1 Key Elements of Climate Change Information and Modeling, and Predicted or Actual Health-Related Impacts Relevant to Urban Settlements (*continued*)

Phenomenon	Scientific Record	Predictions/Modeling	Region	Health Impacts in an Urban Context
Increased droughts and aridity *Example:* Mediterranean experienced 10 of the 12 driest winters since 1902 in the past two decades	Warming-induced drying has increased areas under drought by 8% since the 1970s	Droughts will intensify in the 21st century; total drought affected area to increase from current 15.4% of global cropland to 44% (+/−6%) by 2100	Africa and Oceania, Southern Europe and Mediterranean region, central Europe, central North America, Central America and Mexico, northeast Brazil, Southern Africa; Australia	Food and water security impacts; severe losses to agricultural yields (i.e., maize and wheat production); decreasing food availability to cities; repeated drought contributes to the migration of families from rural/agricultural areas to urban areas, which may result in a loss of rural livelihoods
Rising sea levels *Example:* small island developing states	Acceleration of sea-level rise over the past two decades; sea-level rise of 20+ cm since preindustrial times to 2009	Forced abandonment of small island states, e.g., Tuvalu; average sea-level rise will contribute to extreme coastal high water levels; predicted 1 m sea-level rise in the Caribbean by 2080 will cause total GDP loss of U.S. $68.2 billion	Low latitudes, i.e., Indian Ocean, Western Pacific; northeastern North America, eastern Asian coasts; coastal cities in developing regions (e.g., Mozambique, Mexico, India, Bangladesh)	Loss of livelihood in coastal towns and cities; e.g., fisheries, tourism and agriculture; increased health care costs; salinization of freshwater supply and arable land that cities depend on
Increased extreme precipitation events (leading to floods, storms, and heavy rains). *Example:* Pakistan 2010 rainfall records, worst flooding in its history, approximately 3,000 deaths, affected 20 million people	Increased number of major flood events globally from 2000 to 2010	Increased frequency of heavy precipitation during the 21st century; projected precipitation and temperature changes imply changes in floods; uncertainty about magnitude or frequency of river-related flooding (limited evidence and complex regional dynamics); 20%–30% increases in precipitation during wet months in affected regions (e.g., tropics)		Urban development that promotes deforestation and destruction of protective coastal wetlands/estuarine environments will exacerbate human impacts; floods, storms, heavy rain disproportionately impact on those living in poor-quality housing and/or urban areas with poor flood protection infrastructure and drainage; flash flooding in built-up areas may lead to risk of severe ill-health and disrupted livelihoods

CVD, cardiovascular disease; DALY, disability-adjusted life year; GDP, gross domestic product; GHG, greenhouse gas; SES, socioeconomic status.

Source: Patrick et al. (2016). Reprinted with permission from Taylor & Francis Ltd.

- Impacts all social and environmental determinants of health and creates barriers to attaining the basics of a dignified life: safe and adequate air, water, food, and shelter;
- Is projected to cause 250,000 deaths between 2030 and 2050 related to diseases such as malaria and malnutrition, as well as factors such as heat stress;
- Will cost the health sector roughly $2 to $4 billion by 2030;
- Poses tremendous risk to areas lacking adequate health infrastructure and challenges their ability to cope, prepare, and respond.

Global nurses and health worker colleagues are responsible for communicating the health risks associated with climate change through education, leading research efforts, and partnering directly with the communities in which they work and live to design relevant health promotion plans (Chadwick, 2016). Influential communication regarding climate change extends beyond the mere imparting of knowledge and statistics; it involves deeply listening to clients while assessing their understanding of and perceived risk related to climate change.

The Intergovernmental Panel on Climate Change (IPCC, 2015) warns that "[c]limate change will amplify existing risks and create new risks for natural and human systems," and acknowledges that the economically disadvantaged are the most vulnerable (p. 13). Climate change poses a formidable barrier to ending poverty, one of the cornerstones of the Post-2015 Agenda (Hallegatte et al., 2016). Its immediate attention requires cooperative action at local, national, and international levels, and must address the extreme outcomes projected for all people, particularly those living in low- and middle-income countries (LMICs; IPCC, 2012).

Preventing further complications associated with climate change requires the interprofessional collaboration of health, law, policy, financial, and educational sectors to address its widespread effects, and a shared global vision across governments and countries (Krueger, Biedrzycki, & Hoverter, 2015; The World Bank, 2016). Global collaboration is mandatory since the atmospheric and environmental fallouts of the harmful practices mentioned earlier affect all human beings everywhere. Environmentalism and prevention are two keystones of the nursing profession that directly relate to the planetary efforts being taken to secure a future of health and well-being for all.

Efforts are, indeed, underway. Organizations such as the IPCC, The World Bank, and international partnerships, such as the Asian Cities Climate Change Resilience Network (ACCCRN), seek innovative ways to mitigate the consequences of climate change across demographics and cultures. The ACCCRN (n.d.) looks "to build inclusive urban climate change resilience" and currently has networks in Bangladesh, India, Indonesia, Thailand, and Vietnam. Despite these multifaceted and transnational initiatives there is a tremendous gap in leadership. Health professionals—global nurses—must be willing to answer this call to leadership and coordinate the strategies that will link education, the facilitation of research, and the inclusion of policy makers to deepen partnerships among the international community and continue to raise awareness regarding climate change (Mayhew, Van Belle, & Hammer, 2014).

Florence Nightingale was a staunch environmentalist who developed a tenet known as "the precautionary principle" (Luck, 2016; Luck & Keegan, 2016). This principle implies that "if there is a suspicion about a harmful environment or exposure, even though all of the evidence is not in, remove the person from the situation or stop the use of suspected harmful exposures" (Luck & Keegan, 2016, p. 561). In regard to climate change, since it is impossible to remove people from the global environmental situation, the answer is simple: We must stop the use of these detrimental contributors to our health.

Nightingale was what Forrester (2016) calls an "exemplary leader": a future-oriented and active change agent who sought improved future outcomes for nursing, health care, and society. She was not content with merely discussing mechanisms for improved health; she took intentional action to impact change. Global nurses must constantly assess their abilities to demonstrate the traits associated with exemplary leadership, such as being trustworthy, credible, fearless, shrewd, and politically aware (Forrester, 2016). Exemplary leadership is the beanstalk we need to climb to effectively face the giant that is climate change. By continuing to role-model excellence and ethical values, enrolling communities in the creation of a shared vision, challenging the current norms and processes, empowering others to act wisely and deliberately, and demonstrating courage and hope (Kouzes & Posner, 2012), global nurses can create powerful advocacy initiatives to improve climate change.

When it comes to the consequences mentioned previously, we must look beyond our country's borders to what is happening worldwide, employing a global awareness that we are all in this together (R. L. Goldsteen, K. Goldsteen, & Dwelle, 2015). The world can no longer afford to think of itself as a landscape of individual nations and governments living side by side. We are, indeed, interconnected. The future sequelae of climate change will be as devastating to high-income and LMICs alike. If the planetary population is to not merely survive—but thrive—in the years to come, we must accept responsibility for how we contribute to these problems and what solutions we can implement in realistic ways. A first small step is to calculate your household carbon footprint (www3.epa.gov/carbon-footprint-calculator) and learn which of your daily activities can be adjusted to lower greenhouse gas emissions.

It starts and ends with each one of us.

REFLECTION AND DISCUSSION

- In what ways is the work of global nursing related to environmental health?
- How can global nurses fill the leadership gap in climate change?
- How do I demonstrate exemplary leadership?
- How can climate change education be integrated into health promotion activities and client/community educational programs?
- How do individual actions contribute to planetary health and well-being?

REFERENCES

Asian Cities Climate Change Resilience Network. (n.d.). About the ACCCRN Network. Retrieved from http://acccrn.net/about-acccrn

Chadwick, A. E. (2016). Climate change, health, and communication: A primer. *Health Communication, 31*(6), 782–785.

Forrester, D. A. (2016). Exemplary nursing leadership. In D. A. Forrester (Ed.), *Nursing's greatest leaders: A history of activism* (pp. 3–17). New York, NY: Springer Publishing.

Goldsteen, R. L., Goldsteen, K., & Dwelle, T. L. (2015). Public health: Promise and prospects. In R. L. Goldsteen, K. Goldsteen, & T. L. Dwelle (Eds.), *Introduction to public health: Promises and practices* (2nd ed., pp. 235–260). New York, NY: Springer Publishing.

Hallegatte, S., Bangalore, M., Bonzanigo, L., Fay, M., Kane, T., Narloch, U., . . . Vogt-Schlib, A. (2016). *Shock waves: Managing the impacts of climate change on poverty. Climate change and development.* Washington, DC: World Bank.

Intergovernmental Panel on Climate Change. (2012). *Managing the risks of extreme events and disasters to advance climate change adaptation: Special report of the Intergovernmental Panel on Climate Change.* New York, NY: Cambridge University Press. Retrieved from http://www.ipcc.ch/pdf/special-reports/srex/SREX_Full_Report.pdf

Intergovernmental Panel on Climate Change. (2015). *Climate change 2014: Synthesis report.* Geneva, Switzerland: Author. Retrieved from http://www.ipcc.ch/pdf/assessment-report/ar5/syr/SYR_AR5_FINAL_full_wcover.pdf

Kouzes, J. M., & Posner, B. Z. (2012). *The leadership challenge* (5th ed.). San Francisco, CA: Jossey-Bass.

Krueger, J., Biedrzycki, P., & Hoverter, S. P. (2015). Human health impacts of climate change: Implications for practice and law of public health. *Journal of Law, Medicine & Ethics, 43,* 79–82.

Luck, S. (2016). Informed and impactful: Stewarding the environmental determinants of health and well-being. In W. Rosa (Ed.), *Nurses as leaders: Evolutionary visions of leadership* (pp. 333–343). New York, NY: Springer Publishing.

Luck, S., & Keegan, L. (2016). Environmental health. In B. M. Dossey & L. Keegan (Eds.), *Holistic nursing: A handbook for practice* (7th ed., pp. 557–587). Burlington, MA: Jones & Bartlett.

Mayhew, S., Van Belle, S., & Hammer, M. (2014). Are we ready to build health systems that consider the climate? *Journal of Health Services Research & Policy, 19*(2), 124–127.

Nasheed, M. (2010, July). Speech by his excellency President Mohamed Nasheed, at the Commonwealth Parliamentary Association's conference on climate change. Copenhagen, Denmark. Retrieved from https://thimaaveshi.files.wordpress.com/2009/10/speech-by-his-excellency-president-mohamed-nasheed-at-the-commonwealth-parliamentary-association_s-conference-on-climate-change.pdf

Patrick, R., Noy, S., & Henderson-Wilson, C. (2016). Urbanisation, climate change and health equity: How can health promotion contribute? *International Journal of Health Promotion and Education, 54*(1), 34–49.

United Nations. (2015). *Transforming our world: The 2030 agenda for sustainable development.* Retrieved from https://docs.google.com/gview?url=http://sustainabledevelopment.un.org/content/documents/21252030%20Agenda%20for%20Sustainable%20Development%20web.pdf&embedded=true

United States Environmental Protection Agency. (2016). Climate change: Basic information. Retrieved from https://www3.epa.gov/climatechange/basics

The World Bank. (2016). Catalyzing climate action. Retrieved from http://www.worldbank.org/en/topic/climatechange/overview#2

World Health Organization. (2016). Climate change and health. Retrieved from http://www.who.int/mediacentre/factsheets/fs266/en

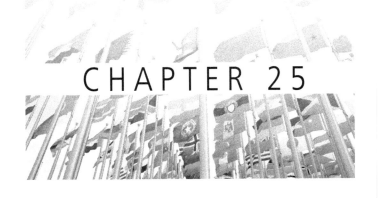

CHAPTER 25

Goal 14. Conserve and Sustainably Use the Oceans, Seas, and Marine Resources for Sustainable Development

William Rosa

But as the unthinkable keeps happening—as water disappears from rivers and lakes and the aquifers beneath our feet—I believe we will begin to awaken to our kinship with water, which springs from knowing at a cellular level that water's gift is life. No water, no life. (Postel, n.d.)

Biodiversity refers to the diversity indicated by the numbers of plant and animal species in a particular environment. Both Sustainable Development Goals (SDGs) 14 and 15 pertain to biodiversity preservation and recognize its essential role in planetary health. More specifically, SDG 14 addresses the well-being of the biodiversity and life below water, and the vitality of international marine ecosystems. Box 25.1 lists SDG 14 with its associated targets (see the Appendix to view the Sustainable Development Agenda in its entirety). As global nurses, we must be clear about how we can use our roles as leaders, educators, and advocates to protect the biodiversity of the oceans and marine systems and elevate consciousness regarding prevention and conservation.

The global community is a little more than halfway through the United Nations Decade on Biodiversity and the Strategic Plan for Biodiversity 2011–2020, an initiative created before the Post-2015 Agenda in order to halt and reverse the loss of biodiversity worldwide (Convention on Biological Diversity [CBD], 2010). The vision of this decade-long work is that, "By 2050, biodiversity is valued, conserved, restored and wisely used, maintaining ecosystem services, sustaining a health planet and delivering benefits essential for all people" (CBD, 2010). The five

Box 25.1 Sustainable Development Goal 14 and Its Associated Targets

Goal 14. Conserve and sustainably use the oceans, seas, and marine resources for sustainable development

14.1 By 2025, prevent and significantly reduce marine pollution of all kinds, in particular from land-based activities, including marine debris and nutrient pollution.

14.2 By 2020, sustainably manage and protect marine and coastal ecosystems to avoid significant adverse impacts, including by strengthening their resilience, and take action for their restoration in order to achieve healthy and productive oceans.

14.3 Minimize and address the impacts of ocean acidification, including through enhanced scientific cooperation at all levels.

14.4 By 2020, effectively regulate harvesting and end overfishing, illegal, unreported and unregulated fishing and destructive fishing practices, and implement science-based management plans, in order to restore fish stocks in the shortest time feasible, at least to levels that can produce maximum sustainable yield as determined by their biological characteristics.

14.5 By 2020, conserve at least 10% of coastal and marine areas, consistent with national and international law and based on the best available scientific information.

14.6 By 2020, prohibit certain forms of fisheries subsidies which contribute to overcapacity and overfishing, eliminate subsidies that contribute to illegal, unreported and unregulated fishing and refrain from introducing new such subsidies, recognizing that appropriate and effective special and differential treatment for developing and least developed countries should be an integral part of the World Trade Organization fisheries subsidies negotiation.

14.7 By 2030, increase the economic benefits to small island developing States and least developed countries from the sustainable use of marine resources, including through sustainable management of fisheries, aquaculture and tourism.

14.a Increase scientific knowledge, develop research capacity and transfer marine technology, taking into account the Intergovernmental Oceanographic Commission Criteria and Guidelines on the Transfer of Marine Technology, in order to improve ocean health and to enhance the contribution of marine biodiversity to the development of developing countries, in particular small island developing States and least developed countries.

14.b Provide access for small-scale artisanal fishers to marine resources and markets.

14.c Enhance the conservation and sustainable use of oceans and their resources by implementing international law as reflected in the United Nations Convention on the Law of the Sea, which provides the legal framework for the conservation and sustainable use of oceans and their resources, as recalled in paragraph 158 of "The future we want."

Source: Reprinted with permission from the United Nations (2015).

Table 25.1 Goals of the Strategic Plan for Biodiversity 2011–2020

Strategic Goal	Purpose
Strategic Goal A	Address the underlying causes of biodiversity loss by mainstreaming biodiversity across government and society
Strategic Goal B	Reduce the direct pressures on biodiversity and promote sustainable use
Strategic Goal C	Improve the status of biodiversity by safeguarding ecosystems, species and genetic diversity
Strategic Goal D	Enhance the benefits to all from biodiversity and ecosystem services
Strategic Goal E	Enhance implementation through participatory planning, knowledge management, and capacity building

Source: Convention on Biological Diversity (2010).

strategic goals of the plan (Table 25.1) were designed in order to assist humanity in living more harmoniously with nature, and guiding individuals and governments to protect the ecosystems and the variety of life on the planet.

In order to contribute toward SDG 14 and foster environmental efforts toward conserving sustainable use of the oceans, global nurses must first gain an understanding of the current marine preservation mechanisms in place and the challenges posed by existing infrastructures. According to Ban et al. (2013), the United Nations Convention on the Law of the Sea (UNCLOS) is the overarching governing body for all human activities on oceans. A foundational barrier to global collaboration is that the research guiding the leadership of UNCLOS is based on a 1970s worldview focused on pollution, unaware of deep-water ecosystems, and not yet focused on the threats of climate change (Gjerde, 2012). The number of organizations leading various and independent initiatives on the high seas—the areas beyond national jurisdiction—has led to an overly fragmented system, "a limited, regional, sector-by-sector approach, with multiple authorities managing parts of the same regions, extensive areas without governance arrangements, and few attempts to coordinate activities, mitigate conflicts, address cumulative impacts or facilitate communication" (Ban et al., 2013, p. 42). Table 25.2 provides a list and description of the global agreements and United Nations bodies that are relevant to marine biodiversity and sustainable use of the high seas.

By knowing the key players and stakeholders in marine preservation, global nurses will be better able to advocate effectively and drive policy changes that seek collaborative efforts and strengthen fragmented partnerships.

We are equipped to educate the public and create evidence-based interventions that contribute toward biodiversity preservation while raising worldwide awareness of the interconnections between optimal health, quality of life, and environmental well-being; they are, in fact, one and the same and not mutually exclusive endeavors. The Population–Health–Environment (PHE) method is a holistic and interdisciplinary model of care that addresses the interconnectedness between ecosystems and dependent communities (Mohan et al., 2014).

Table 25.2 Key Global Agreements and UN Bodies Relevant to Marine Biodiversity and Sustainable Use in the High Seas

Key Global Agreement	Description
United Nations Convention on the Law of the Sea (UNCLOS), 1982, in force 1994	Provides the legal order for the oceans to promote peaceful uses, equitable and efficient utilization of resources, conservation of living resources, and study, protection, and preservation of the marine environment. Includes high seas freedoms (Article 87), such as the freedom to fish and navigate, and environmental duties (Articles 192–196 and 204–206), including duty to protect and preserve the marine environment.
Convention on International Trade in Endangered Species of Wild Fauna and Flora (CITES), 1973, in force 1975	Objective is to promote international cooperation to protect threatened and endangered wildlife species against overexploitation from international trade.
International Whaling Convention (IWC), 1946, in force 1948	Ensures conservation of whale species.
International Convention for the Prevention of Pollution from Ships (MARPOL), 1973, and modified by Protocol of 1978	Seeks the elimination of intentional pollution of the marine environment by oil and other substances, and minimization of accidental discharge.
International Convention for the Control and Management of Ships' Ballast Water and Sediments (Ballast Water Convention), 2004, not yet in force	Seeks to prevent, minimize, and eliminate transfer of harmful aquatic organisms and pathogens through the control and management of ships' ballast water and sediments.
Convention on the Prevention of Marine Pollution by Dumping Wastes and Other Matter (London Convention), 1972, in force 1975, and its Protocol to the London Convention, 1996, in force 2006	Promotes all practical steps to prevent pollution of the sea by dumping of wastes and other matter. The London Protocol modernized the convention by calling for a precautionary approach.
Convention on the Conservation of Migratory Species (CMS), 1979, in force 1983	Objective is to protect migratory listed species, conserve, or restore habitat and mitigate impacts that may impinge on their migration or survival.
Convention on Biological Diversity (CBD), 1992	Objectives are conservation of biodiversity, sustainable use of its components, and fair and equitable sharing of benefits. In the high seas, applies only to processes and activities carried out under the control of parties, which may have an adverse impact on biodiversity.
UN Fish Stock Agreement (UNFSA, an implementing agreement under UNCLOS), 1995, in force 2001	Ensure long-term conservation and sustainable use of straddling and highly migratory fish stocks through improving the implementation of relevant provisions of UNCLOS.
Agreement to Promote Compliance with International Conservation and Management Measures by Fishing Vessels on the High Seas (FAO Compliance Agreement), 1993, in force 2003	Objective is to deter the practice of flagging and reflagging as a means to avoid compliance with national conservation and management measures. Does not apply to vessels fishing in areas where there are no RFMOs or agreed international conservation and management measures.

(continued)

Table 25.2 Key Global Agreements and UN Bodies Relevant to Marine Biodiversity and Sustainable Use in the High Seas (*continued*)

Key UN Bodies	Description
United Nations General Assembly (UNGA)	The key political forum for member states to raise issues relevant to oceans and Law of the Sea.
UN Division on Oceans and Law of the Sea (DOALOS or the Division)	Serves as the secretariat of UNCLOS.
UN Informal Consultative Process on Oceans and Law of the Sea (UNICPOLOS)	Was established in 2000 for informal discussions on pressing issues regarding ocean affairs.
UN-Oceans	Interagency coordinating mechanisms within the UN system, established in 2003.
International Seabed Authority (ISA)	Established under UNCLOS as the organization through which states organize and control activities for exploration for and exploitation of nonliving resources.
UN Food and Agriculture Organization (FAO), Committee on Fisheries (COFI)	Global intergovernmental forum where major international fisheries and aquaculture problems and issues are examined and recommendations developed.
International Maritime Organization (IMO)	The UN specialized agency with responsibility for the safety and security of shipping and the prevention of marine pollution by ships.
Intergovernmental Oceanographic Commission (IOC)	Focuses on international oceanographic research programs; part of the UN Educational, Scientific and Cultural Organization (UNESCO).
United Nations Environment Programme (UNEP)	Supports and coordinates activities and major international programs for conservation and sustainable use of oceans, including the Regional Seas Conventions and Action Plan.

RFMO, regional fisheries management organization; UN, United Nations.
Source: Reprinted with permission from Ban et al. (2013).

PHE makes clear the undeniable interplay between the causes of poverty, poor health, inequalities, food insecurity, population growth concerns, irresponsible resource utilization, and biodiversity degradation. It is a whole system approach that merges social, economic, and environmental factors into an integrated community-based care plan for sustainability and inclusivity (Mohan et al., 2014). Many themes are consistently being addressed through PHE methods but two stand out: family planning and environmental conservation.

Sinaga, Mohammed, Teklu, Stelljes, and Belachew (2015) explain the relationship: Family planning is all about balancing population growth with sustainable economic development and responsible resource utilization; the greater the population growth, the more demand there are for natural resources and the quicker said resources are exploited; population growth that is disproportionate to economic development leads to food insecurity and its potential sequelae such as increased malnutrition and poor health; and finally, "[f]ood insecurity. . . obliges people to [further] encroach into the natural environment leading to a spiraling progress to destitution" (Sinaga et al., 2005, p. 1). Through access to reproductive health and family planning education, as well as involving populations in conservation efforts, PHE has been shown to be effective in several countries:

- Ethiopia: In the rural communities in Gurage Zone, women now demonstrate increased knowledge of family planning methods with strong spousal support, and there is now a more effective integration of health, family planning, and environmental issues at the grassroots level (Sinaga et al., 2015).
- Kenya: Environmental volunteers have reported a greater understanding of family planning, the need for committed conservation efforts, an expanded range of contraceptive options, and improved dialogue between spousal partners regarding family planning (Hoke et al., 2015).

And, more specifically to marine environments:

- Madagascar: Family planning services have been well adopted in an isolated and biodiverse coastal region in the southwestern part of the country due to the work of Blue Ventures. The services provided, integrated into a preexisting community-based conservation program, have led to autonomy in family planning choices, long-term support for conservation efforts, and increased awareness regarding the correlations between reproductive health, family size, and food security (Mohan & Shellard, 2014).
- Malawi: The Lake Chilwa Basin Climate Change Adaptation Programme (LCBCCAP), implemented by Leadership for Environment and Development (LEAD), was able to identify reasons for local women's low environmental project participation rates and the factors that contribute to their increased vulnerability. In this fragile ecosystem, important for both biodiversity and the population's livelihoods, LEAD has been able to improve women's involvement and address the health needs of the community (Mohan et al., 2014).
- Philippines: The Integrated Population and Coastal Resource Management (IPOPCORM) initiative, led by PATH Foundation Philippines Inc. (PFPI), has focused efforts in areas of primary marine conservation concerns with exorbitant population growth levels. The IPOPCORM focused on coastal resource management actions that took a stand regarding overfishing, destructive fishing practices, and the consistently declining productivity of fisheries, coral reefs, sea grasses, and so on, and raised policy maker and community awareness of the interconnection with sexual reproductive health and rights. IPOPCORM has demonstrated the increased involvement of women in conservation efforts and improved participation of men and adolescent boys regarding reproductive health education (Mohan et al., 2014).

Global nurses have the opportunity to participate and colead in the design, planning, implementation, and evaluation of PHE models to ensure not only reproductive and family health, but also increased environmental awareness and community involvement in conservation efforts. Being a part of these initiatives simultaneously contributes toward the achievement of SDGs 1 (poverty eradication), 2 (hunger alleviation through food security), 3 (good health and well-being), 5 (gender equality), and 12 (sustainable consumption and production patterns).

REFLECTION AND DISCUSSION

- How does biodiversity impact my local community? How do those considerations extend to the national and international levels?

- Why have the connections between biodiversity health and human health remained widely unaddressed for so long?

- What communities do I know of that could benefit from a PHE model?

- How can I integrate biodiversity knowledge and preservation consciousness into existing client and community educational programs?

- How will I communicate the impact of environmental policy on the health of all species to decision makers and those in power?

REFERENCES

Ban, N. C., Bax, N. J., Gjerde, K. M., Devillers, R., Dunn, D. C., Dunstan, P. K., . . . Halpin, P. N. (2013). Systematic conservation planning: A better recipe for managing the high seas for biodiversity conservation and sustainable use. *Conservation Letters, 7*(1), 41–54.

Convention on Biological Diversity. (2010). X/2. Strategic plan for biodiversity 2011–2020. Retrieved from https://www.cbd.int/decision/cop/?id=12268

Gjerde, K. M. (2012). The environmental provisions of the LOSC for the high seas and seabed area beyond national jurisdiction. *International Journal of Marine Coastal Law, 27*, 839–847.

Hoke, T. H., Mackenzie, C., Vance, G., Boyer, B., Canoutas, E., Bratt, J., . . . Waceke, N. (2015). Integrating family planning promotion into the work of environmental volunteers: A population, health and environment initiative in Kenya. *International Perspectives on Sexual and Reproductive Health, 41*(1), 43–50.

Mohan, V., Castro, J., Pullanikkatil, D., Savitzky, C., Teklu, N., De Souza, R.-M., & Fisher, S. (2014, September 17–18). *Population Health Environment Programmes: An integrated approach to development post-2015*. A Population and Sustainable Development Alliance (PSDA) Panel Presentation and Paper for the 2nd International Conference on Sustainable Development Practice, New York, NY. Retrieved from http://psda.org.uk/wp-content/uploads/2014/09/PSDA-SDSN-paper-FINAL.pdf

Mohan, V., & Shellard, T. (2014). Providing family planning services to remote communities in areas of high biodiversity through a Population-Health-Environment programme in Madagascar. *Reproductive Health Matters, 22*(43), 93–103.

Postel, S. (n.d.). Honest hope. Retrieved from http://environment.nationalgeographic.com/environment/freshwater/honest-hope/#page=1

Sinaga, M., Mohammed, A., Teklu, N., Stelljes, K., & Belachew, T. (2015). Effectiveness of the population health and environment approach in improving family planning outcomes in the Gurage Zone South Ethiopia. *BMC Public Health, 15*(1). doi:10.1186/s12889-015-2484-9

United Nations. (2015). Transforming our world: The 2030 Agenda for Sustainable Development. Retrieved from https://docs.google.com/gview?url=http://sustainabledevelopment.un.org/content/documents/21252030%20Agenda%20for%20Sustainable%20Development%20web.pdf&embedded=true

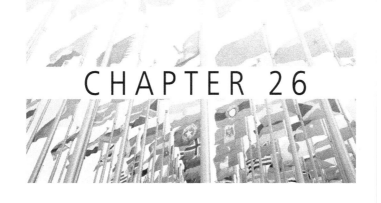

CHAPTER 26

Goal 15. Protect, Restore, and Promote Sustainable Use of Terrestrial Ecosystems, Sustainably Manage Forests, Combat Desertification, and Halt and Reverse Land Degradation and Halt Biodiversity Loss

William Rosa

Environmental justice was a term coined in the early 1990s to denote the application of fair strategies and processes in the resolution of inequality related to environmental contamination. The fact that such a term exists suggests several things: (a) that we as a [global society] have done things to our environment that place people at risk; (b) that remedies have been enacted to rectify environmental contamination and the associated threats to health and well-being; and (c) that all people have not been treated the same when it comes to enacting these remedies. . . . Well-informed [global] nurses using the vast array of environmental resources and networks can assist vulnerable communities to address real and potential environmental threats. (Powell & Slade, 2003, pp. 321, 333)

Sustainable Development Goal (SDG) 15 attends to life on land: life beyond the human race and inclusive of both animal species and ecosystems. Box 26.1 provides the associated targets of SDG 15 (see the Appendix to view the Sustainable Development Agenda in its entirety).

Box 26.1 **Sustainable Development Goal 15 and Its Associated Targets**

Goal 15. Protect, restore and promote sustainable use of terrestrial ecosystems, sustainably manage forests, combat desertification, and halt and reverse land degradation and halt biodiversity loss

15.1   By 2020, ensure the conservation, restoration and sustainable use of terrestrial and inland freshwater ecosystems and their services, in particular forests, wetlands, mountains and drylands, in line with obligations under international agreements.

15.2   By 2020, promote the implementation of sustainable management of all types of forests, halt deforestation, restore degraded forests and substantially increase afforestation and reforestation globally.

15.3   By 2030, combat desertification, restore degraded land and soil, including land affected by desertification, drought and floods, and strive to achieve a land-degradation-neutral world.

15.4   By 2030, ensure the conservation of mountain ecosystems, including their biodiversity, in order to enhance their capacity to provide benefits that are essential for sustainable development.

15.5   Take urgent and significant action to reduce the degradation of natural habitats, halt the loss of biodiversity and, by 2020, protect and prevent the extinction of threatened species.

15.6   Promote fair and equitable sharing of the benefits arising from the utilization of genetic resources and promote appropriate access to such resources, as internationally agreed.

15.7   Take urgent action to end poaching and trafficking of protected species of flora and fauna and address both demand and supply of illegal wildlife products.

15.8   By 2020, introduce measures to prevent the introduction and significantly reduce the impact of invasive alien species on land and water ecosystems and control or eradicate the priority species.

15.9   By 2020, integrate ecosystem and biodiversity values into national and local planning, development processes, poverty reduction strategies and accounts.

15.a   Mobilize and significantly increase financial resources from all sources to conserve and sustainably use biodiversity and ecosystems.

15.b   Mobilize significant resources from all sources and at all levels to finance sustainable forest management and provide adequate incentives to developing countries to advance such management, including for conservation and reforestation.

15.c   Enhance global support for efforts to combat poaching and trafficking of protected species, including by increasing the capacity of local communities to pursue sustainable livelihood opportunities.

Source: Reprinted with permission from the United Nations (2015).

There are several examples (Keesing et al., 2010; Rountree, 2015) of how biodiversity loss is already impacting and will continue to affect human health:

- When deforestation occurs and bird biodiversity is lost, the remaining birds become an increased reservoir for mosquito-borne West Nile Virus: more birds become infected, increasing contact with human beings, and the human infection rate rises.

- Some scientists hypothesize that HIV made the leap from chimpanzees to human beings because usual food sources were not available, forcing people to consume increased quantities of bush meat, and exposing themselves to the virus they otherwise would not have encountered.

- Ebola is a virus carried by fruit bats in Africa, but as their forests are decimated, they are more likely to come in contact with humans and pass along the virus.

There are other countless health implications related to biodiversity loss and secondary to the extinction of plant species, pollution, and other harmful environmental and agricultural practices (Rountree, 2015).

SDG 15, along with 14 (as discussed in Chapter 25), highlights the links between health, human rights, and the need for global cooperation in order that all people across the planet are considered and cared for. Kent (2011) wrote,

> Health is not only a series of separate national issues; it is also a global issue. The process has accelerated the intensity and diversity of ways in which actions in one part of the globe can affect health conditions in other parts. Even if there were no such linkages, health everywhere should be a matter of global concern in moral terms. The fact that life is nasty, brutish, and short in many places should trouble all of us. (p. 103)

As global nurses, we need to consider the health and well-being of the 35 million people who depend on Lake Victoria in Uganda for survival as it is continually debilitated by overfishing, pollution, and sewage (Ryan, 2015). We need to think about Indonesia, a country that lost 15 million acres of forest between 2000 and 2012, and now has the highest deforestation rate in the world due to the greed and lumber needs of developers (Landen, 2014). Most importantly, we must remember that this is not Uganda or Indonesia's problem; it is ours.

Global nurses need to include the initiatives and targets of SDGs 14 and 15 in their community health education. The World Health Organization (WHO, 2015) suggested that we identify areas where biodiversity targets intersect with other SDGs and health outcomes. For example, more sustainable agricultural practices will positively impact the environment but may also improve nutrition (SDG 2) and reduce noncommunicable disease burdens (SDG 3; WHO, 2015). The populations we serve have the right to understand how irresponsible businesses and practices—and the silence that is kept to protect their investments—impact billions of people worldwide.

Our obligation to advocate is foundational to global nursing and a required component of environmental justice. We must use our observational skills to accurately articulate inequities and harmful practices, question environmentally deleterious policies and continually re-assess community awareness, become politically astute regarding the system in place and the legislative processes, remain culturally sensitive and appropriate, and use every possible advocacy outlet available, from lobbying, media, and mediation, to providing expert testimony, organizing community coalitions and clinically relevant programs (Powell & Slade, 2003). We are not just advocating for the health of the human species but also for the innumerable other species that depend on us and on whom we depend for sustainable outcomes and long-term well-being. The quality of life both under water and on land does not just influence our survival—it determines it.

REFLECTION AND DISCUSSION

- What does environmental justice mean to me? How does it relate to my current role?

- In what ways does biodiversity awareness intersect with the education I provide as a global nurse?

- How do I help to transform the notion of health from a series of separate national issues to a cohesive global one?

- What new methods of advocacy can be designed and implemented to engage nurses in biodiversity conversation?

- How can I translate the global issues happening in ecosystems such as Uganda and Indonesia to local communities and stakeholders to promote environmental health?

REFERENCES

Keesing, F., Belden, L. K., Daszak, P., Dobson, A., Harvell, C. D., Holt, R. D., . . . Ostfeld, R. S. (2010). Impacts of biodiversity on the emergence and transmission of infectious diseases. *Nature, 468*(7324), 647–652.

Kent, G. (2011). Global plans of action for health. In E. Beracochea, C. Weinstein, & D. P. Evans (Eds.), *Rights-based approaches to public health* (pp. 103–115). New York, NY: Springer Publishing.

Landen, X. (2014). Indonesia reaches highest deforestation rate in the world. Retrieved from http://www.pbs.org/newshour/rundown/indonesia-reaches-highest-deforestation-rate-worldwide

Powell, D., & Slade, D. (2003). Advocating for environmental justice: Protecting vulnerable communities from pollution. In B. Sattler & J. Lipscomb (Eds.), *Environmental health and nursing practice* (pp. 321–338). New York, NY: Springer Publishing.

Rountree, R. (2015). Monoculture and loss of biodiversity: Effects on human health. *Alternative and Complementary Therapies, 21*(1), 6–12.

Ryan, R. (2015, April 2). Africa's biggest lake is on the verge of dying. Retrieved from http://www.news.com.au/travel/world-travel/africas-biggest-lake-is-on-the-verge-of-dying/news-story/364bdb4e810ab33aa6434f3b71a473dc

United Nations. (2015). Transforming our world: The 2030 Agenda for Sustainable Development. Retrieved from https://docs.google.com/gview?url=http://sustainabledevelopment.un.org/content/documents/21252030%20Agenda%20for%20Sustainable%20Development%20web.pdf&embedded=true

World Health Organization. (2015). Connecting global priorities: Biodiversity and human health: A state of knowledge review. Retrieved from http://apps.who.int/iris/bitstream/10665/174012/1/9789241508537_eng.pdf

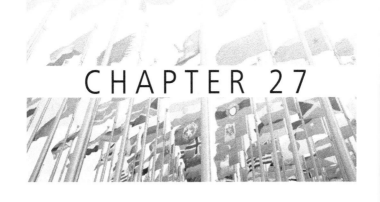

CHAPTER 27

Goal 16. Promote Peaceful and Inclusive Societies for Sustainable Development, Provide Access to Justice for All and Build Effective, Accountable, and Inclusive Institutions at All Levels

William Rosa

Look into your own heart, discover what it is that gives you pain, and then refuse under any circumstance whatsoever to inflict that pain on anybody else. . . . If we don't manage to implement The Golden Rule, globally, so that we treat all peoples . . . whoever they may be, as though they were as important as ourselves, I doubt that we'll have a viable world to hand on to the next generation. . . . One of the great tasks of our time is to build a global society. . . where people can live together in peace. . . . Educate and stimulate compassionate thinking. . . . We don't have to fall in love with each other but we can become friends. (Armstrong, 2009)

The right to peace and the right to health are deeply interwoven: peace and peaceful circumstances being central determinants of health and well-being (Perry, Fernández, & Puyana, 2015). The United Nations Office of the High Commissioner for Human Rights (OHCHR; 2013, 2014, 2015) has been drafting an intergovernmental declaration on the global right to peace since 2008, and has described peace not only as the absence of conflict but as an ongoing and participatory process involving mutual engagement and a shared vision for cooperation and understanding. The third principle articulated by the World Health Organization (WHO) constitution states: "The health of all peoples is fundamental to the attainment of peace and security and is dependent upon the fullest co-operation of individuals and states" (WHO, 2006, p. 1). Justice may be one mechanism for instituting peace and, conversely, peace may be the way justice is restored. They are reciprocal and complementary forces. For in an unjust world there can be no real peace; and the lack of peace is often symptomatic of unjust treatment, policies, laws, or inflictions of aggression.

This Sustainable Development Goal (SDG) recognizes that peace and justice are just as necessary to the well-being of the global village as improving utilization of sustainable resources, the eradication of poverty, and the responsible modernization of industry and infrastructure. Peace and justice are the indicators that reflect quality of life, feelings of safety, and ensure that disparities of all kinds are addressed in the quest for equality. Box 27.1 provides SDG 16 along with its

---

Box 27.1 Sustainable Development Goal 16 and Its Associated Targets

Goal 16. Promote peaceful and inclusive societies for sustainable development, provide access to justice for all and build effective, accountable, and inclusive institutions at all levels

16.1 Significantly reduce all forms of violence and related death rates everywhere.

16.2 End abuse, exploitation, trafficking and all forms of violence against and torture of children.

16.3 Promote the rule of law at the national and international levels and ensure equal access to justice for all.

16.4 By 2030, significantly reduce illicit financial and arms flows, strengthen the recovery and return of stolen assets and combat all forms of organized crime.

16.5 Substantially reduce corruption and bribery in all their forms.

16.6 Develop effective, accountable and transparent institutions at all levels.

16.7 Ensure responsive, inclusive, participatory and representative decision making at all levels.

16.8 Broaden and strengthen the participation of developing countries in the institutions of global governance.

16.9 By 2030, provide legal identity for all, including birth registration.

16.10 Ensure public access to information and protect fundamental freedoms, in accordance with national legislation and international agreements.

16.a Strengthen relevant national institutions, including through international cooperation, for building capacity at all levels, in particular in developing countries, to prevent violence and combat terrorism and crime.

16.b Promote and enforce nondiscriminatory laws and policies for sustainable development, including for conservation and reforestation.

Source: Reprinted with permission from the United Nations (2015).

associated targets (see the Appendix to view the Sustainable Development Agenda in its entirety). Each global nurse has the fundamental capacity and responsibility to become a representative of peace and contribute to the goals listed in Box 27.1 through his or her practice and ethic of caring.

Peace and peacemaking are inherent to the foundations of caring, dignity, health, well-being, and advocacy for human betterment that give meaning to the profession of nursing. Global nurses may not often think of ourselves as peacemakers, but maybe it is time to expand our self-definition to include the concept. We contribute to the healing of clients, be they individuals or communities, regardless of age, religious affiliation, gender, sexual orientation, race, ethnicity, socioeconomic status, education level, or disability. We do this work for those whose political views differ from ours and maybe even for those with criminal histories. If we were called to care for those involved in a violent altercation, we would be ethically bound to deliver equitable and quality care to both the aggressor and the victim. It is the very act of nursing—that of caring for others out of a commitment to service and covenant with society—that makes peace in the world. And with 20.7 million nurses and midwives working in countries across the planet (Sarna, Wolf, & Bialous, 2012), what a formidable statement of peace we have the opportunity to proclaim!

Anselmo (2016) tells the story of caring for two patients affected by cancer: one, an elderly survivor of the Holocaust and, the other, the child of a Nazi soldier. She writes,

> . . . together they opened my heart to a deeper calling and understanding of nursing: the gifts of compassion, going beyond all concepts of discrimination, views of right and wrong, touching our shared humanity, and cultivating true openhearted inclusiveness within ourselves. (p. 21)

Through her nursing and the demonstration of equanimity in her provision of care, she became a representative of peace for her patients, their families, and the community in which she worked. She did not espouse a mere theory or philosophy of peace, but became a living, breathing example of its healing power: peace in action.

A commitment to peace and justice can become a moral and ethical foundation for practice. It can be what drives nurses to create new knowledge, deliver exemplary care, and educate the next generation of peacemakers. Peace and justice are the rationales for client advocacy and the goals for policy changes. They are the most respectable of personal and professional aspirations.

Chinn (2013) defines the acronym PEACE as both the underlying intention of any group working together and also the hoped for outcome. The letters of PEACE stand for **P**raxis, **E**mpowerment, **A**wareness, **C**ooperation, and **E**volvement. Chinn (2013) uses these terms to define "PEACE":

- *Praxis*: the merging of knowing and doing; living life in a way that actions are consistent with personal values and ideals
- *Empowerment*: supporting each person in a given community with regard to his or her individual abilities and strengths through a lens of respect
- *Awareness*: guiding consciousness to search for meaning beneath the surface; engaging with self and others while remaining committed to the values of peace and mutual empowerment

- *Cooperation*: honoring the diversity of those contributing to the context at hand while remaining committed to group solidarity
- *Evolvement*: honoring and celebrating the growth and change needed for all individuals and communities as a part of their continued development

Nurses maintain an ethical obligation to openly address the behaviors and circumstances that promote disrespect and incivility across contexts (Chinn, 2016). The concepts of *peace* and *power* may be socially construed as in conflict with each other. *Power* can be described as "the energy from which human action and interaction arises" and is further expressed by individuals in response to learned social and cultural norms over time (Chinn & Falk-Rafael, 2015, p. 64). Specifically in regard to conflict resolution, a "power-over" worldview suggests that one party is viewed as a "winner" and the other as a "loser"; but from a "peace power" perspective, conflict is an opportunity to grow and develop, and an invitation to achieve outcomes representative of shared values (Chinn & Falk-Rafael, 2015). In this framework, power-over practices tend to be practiced in public spheres and are often symptomatic of rules, laws, and hierarchical structures, whereas peace powers are often witnessed in private domains of human interaction and act as a guide in recreating one's definition of "power" through a peaceful lens. Table 27.1 compares the contrasting powers derived from public (power-over powers) and private (peace powers) spheres of human interaction (Chinn & Falk-Rafael, 2015, p. 66).

While all powers listed in Table 27.1 can be seen in both public and private spheres of interaction, both types should be acknowledged as a part of the human experience in order to resolve conflict, respectfully acknowledge another's experience and context, and develop collaborative and peaceful solutions for a shared humanity. By gaining an understanding of these power demonstrations, and how they interact with each other, one can develop a more compassionate paradigm through which to know and see the world.

The role of compassion in delivering ethically sound and equitable health care has been previously discussed in the literature, including compassionate engagement as a central theme of artful and humane nursing and compassion as intention, action, rationale, and outcome (Rosa, 2016a; Sinclair et al., 2016). Compassion has been cited as the very element capable of halting and potentially reversing the global cycles of egoism, violence, division, and hatred, and elevating the world toward an experience of peace and justice (Armstrong, 2010). Lane (2016, p. 329) describes the connection between nursing, compassion, and peace when she writes:

> Compassion is a kind of love; it joins your light with another's. If you are ill, it joins you to a healer; if you are a healer, it joins you to the person you are healing; if you are making peace, it joins you to your enemy. . . . The . . . [n]urse for peace who sees with compassion sees the enemy in a different way. . . . Compassion breaks the cycle of violence that leads to more violence. There is nothing more ethical than practicing and embracing this way of being and becoming in the world.

Compassion is not something to be merely theorized or written about; it exists in practice and thrives in its exchange between and among human beings. Tippett (2010) said that the healing force of compassion can be felt, known, and seen through its component parts: lived demonstrations of tenderness, kindness,

Table 27.1 Contrasting Powers Derived From Public and Private Spheres of Human Interaction

Power-over Powers	Peace Powers
Power of results—the means justify the ends	Power of process—how we work together is equally important to what we accomplish
Power of prescription—actions and goals defined by rules or authority figures	Power of letting go—actions and goals are negotiated for the best interest of the group as well as each individual
Power of division—a few are privileged while others lack knowledge, skills, and resources	Power of the whole—knowledge, skills, and resources flow among all for the benefit of all
Power of force—penalties and negative consequences are used to ensure conformity	Power of collectivity—each person's participation is valued for reaching strong decisions that everyone values
Power of hierarchy—linear chain of command with layers of privilege and responsibility	Power of solidarity—responsibility is distributed in a lateral network of interaction
Power of command—leaders set the agenda and followers comply without question	Power of sharing—leadership shifts according to talent, skills, and interest
Power of opposites—decisions are polarized into "for" or "against" choices	Power of integration—decisions are examined in context to consider both/and possibilities
Power of use—accepts exploitation of resources and people	Power of nurturing—values respect and protection for all people and for the environment
Power of accumulation—material goods and resources are hoarded and used for personal gain	Power of distribution—goods and resources are shared to benefit all according to need
Power of causality—relies on technology as a solution for problems regardless of the consequences	Power of intuition—attuned to the long-term potential well-being of all when considering solutions
Power of expediency—makes choices based on what is easy and readily available	Power of consciousness—choices are derived from values that protect life, growth, and peace
Power of xenophobia—restricts participation to those who willingly conform to group norms	Power of diversity—values equal participation of those with alternative and dissenting views
Power of secrets—relies on mystification of processes in the interest of gaining conformity	Power of responsibility—values demystification so that all can make informed choices to promote the well-being of each individual and the group
Power of rules—policies, norms, and laws govern what is done without consideration of the situation or context	Power of creativity—values actions that arise from ingenuity to form solutions best fitting the situation
Power of fear—focuses on imaginary future disaster and harm to control the behavior of others	Power of trust—focuses on building and maintaining relationships that nurture understanding of one another

Source: Adapted from Chinn (2013).

Figure 27.1	The component parts of compassion as identified by Tippett (2010).

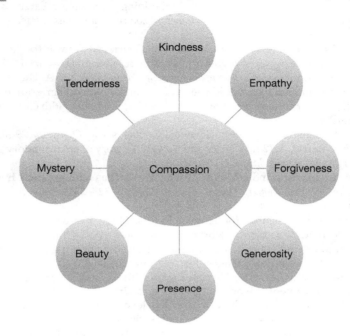

Source: Reprinted from Rosa (2016b).

empathy, forgiveness, generosity, and by being present to the beautiful and myste-rious. The component parts of compassion are illustrated in Figure 27.1.

Global initiatives, such as the Charter for Compassion (n.d.), promote compassion-ate thinking and doing throughout the global village as a premise for shared humanity "to honour the inviolable sanctity of every single human being, treating everybody, without exception, with absolute justice, equity and respect" (all nurses and global citizens can affirm a commitment to a more compassionate way of life by signing and sharing the charter at www.charterforcompassion.org/index.php/charter).

Peace and justice. And so it is.

REFLECTION AND DISCUSSION

- What are the inequities related to peace and justice that I observe in the global village?
- How are peace and peacemaking foundational to my roles as a global nurse and as a healer?
- How does quality of health influence peace and justice? How do peace and justice determine health, health access, and health outcomes?
- How can I integrate the concepts of the acronym PEACE into both my personal and professional settings?
- Why does compassion matter in the journey toward peace and justice?

REFERENCES

Anselmo, J. (2016). Mindful and intentional: Embodying interbeing awareness in grassroots leadership. In W. Rosa (Ed.), *Nurses as leaders: Evolutionary visions of leadership* (pp. 17–31). New York, NY: Springer Publishing.

Armstrong, K. (2009). Let's revive the Golden Rule. Retrieved from https://www.ted.com/talks/karen_armstrong_let_s_revive_the_golden_rule?language=en#t-179544

Armstrong, K. (2010). *Twelve steps to a compassionate life.* New York, NY: Anchor Books.

Charter for Compassion. (n.d.). Home. Retrieved from http://www.charterforcompassion.org

Chinn, P. L. (2013). *Peace & power: New directions for building community* (8th ed.). Burlington, MA: Jones & Bartlett.

Chinn, P. L. (2016). Dialogue on peace and power. *Nursing Science Quarterly, 29*(3), 208–210.

Chinn, P. L., & Falk-Rafael, A. (2015). Peace and power: A theory of emancipatory group process. *Journal of Nursing Scholarship, 47*(1), 62–69.

Lane, M. R. (2016). Authentic and creative: Walking the Caritas path to peace. In W. Rosa (Ed.), *Nurses as leaders: Evolutionary visions of leadership* (pp. 323–332). New York, NY: Springer Publishing.

Office of the High Commissioner for Human Rights. (2013, February). First session of the open-ended intergovernmental working group on a draft United Nations declaration on the right to peace, Geneva, Switzerland. Retrieved from http://www.ohchr.org/EN/HRBodies/HRC/RightPeace/Pages/FirstSession.aspx

Office of the High Commissioner for Human Rights. (2014, June). Second session of the open-ended intergovernmental working group on a draft United Nations declaration on the right to peace, Geneva, Switzerland. Retrieved from http://www.ohchr.org/EN/HRBodies/HRC/RightPeace/Pages/SecondSession.aspx

Office of the High Commissioner for Human Rights. (2015, April). Third session of the open-ended intergovernmental working group on a draft United Nations declaration on the right to peace, Geneva, Switzerland. Retrieved from http://www.ohchr.org/EN/HRBodies/HRC/RightPeace/Pages/thirdsession.aspx

Perry, D. J., Fernández, C. G., & Puyana, D. F. (2015). The right to life in peace: An essential condition for realizing the right to health. *Health & Human Rights: An International Journal, 17*(1), 148–158.

Rosa, W. (2016a). Awakened and conscious: Reclaiming lost power and intraprofessional identity. In W. Rosa (Ed.), *Nurses as leaders: Evolutionary visions of leadership* (pp. 359–376). New York, NY: Springer Publishing.

Rosa, W. (2016b). Public health nursing series: Sustainable Development Goal #16—Peace and justice. Retrieved from http://www.springerpub.com/w/nursing/blog-public-health-nursing-series-sustainable-development-goal-16-peace-justice-part-18

Sarna, L., Wolf, L., & Bialous, S. A. (2012). Enhancing nursing and midwifery capacity to contribute to the prevention, treatment and management of noncommunicable diseases. *Human Resources for Health Observer,* (12). Retrieved from http://www.who.int/hrh/resources/observer12.pdf

Sinclair, S., McClement, S., Raffin-Bouchal, S., Hack, T. F., Hagen, N. A., McConnell, S., & Chochinov, H. M. (2016). Compassion in health care: An empirical model. *Journal of Pain and Symptom Management, 51*(2), 193–203. doi:10.1016/j.jpainsymman.2015.10.009

Tippett, K. (2010). Reconnecting with compassion. Retrieved from https://www.ted.com/talks/krista_tippett_reconnecting_with_compassion?language=en

United Nations. (2015). *Transforming our world: The 2030 Agenda for Sustainable Development.* Retrieved from https://docs.google.com/gview?url=http://sustainabledevelopment.un.org/content/documents/21252030%20Agenda%20for%20Sustainable%20Development%20web.pdf&embedded=true

World Health Organization. (2006). *Constitution of the World Health Organization* (45th ed.). Geneva, Switzerland: Author. Retrieved from http://www.who.int/governance/eb/who_constitution_en.pdf

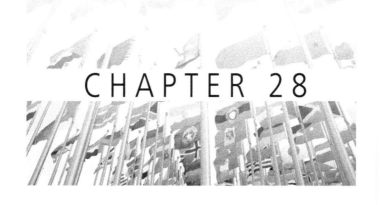

CHAPTER 28

Goal 17. Strengthen the Means of Implementation and Revitalize the Global Partnership for Sustainable Development

William Rosa

Partnership is the central element of global nursing practice. Nurses must collaborate closely as an integrated team with . . . partners to achieve optimum cross-cultural care reaching beyond disease management to build the capacity of partners and to avoid leaving holes in health care services upon departure. That partnerships occur both within a country's borders and across borders emphasizes the transnational component of global health. Through partnership we address health problems and their underlying social determinants, which affect all of us in varying degrees. Dichotomistic terminology such as "third world" and "first world" as well as "developing" versus "developed" nations distances partners and promotes an attitude of "us" and "them.". . . [P]ower imbalances persist among those receiving assistance and those providing it. [Some] strongly, and correctly, [condemn] using the term partner in cases in which no partnership truly exists. (Upvall & Leffers, 2014, p. xviii)

Partnerships in global nursing are discussed in great detail in the literature (Upvall & Leffers, 2014; see Chapter 32 for more information from Upvall and Leffers on raising consciousness through global collaboration). Partnerships can be a bit of a tricky business. Under the guise of very good intentions and altruistic motives, I have observed time and time again health professionals who often state,

"Let's partner together," while subconsciously (or consciously) meaning, "Let's work together, I'll take the lead and show you how it's done, and please ask if there are any questions along the way." There may at times be an inherent presumption of the nurse's superior knowledge and the client's need for education: reflections of the cultural arrogance discussed earlier in this book. We see these paternalistic remnants throughout medicine and in environments where expertise is sought after to improve systems and practices, particularly in global health care settings. But a true partnership implies mutual participation, shared accountability, equal contributions, and a joint commitment toward achieving the subjectively identified goals of the recipient party (Sliney, 2015).

Box 28.1 lists Sustainable Development Goal (SDG) 17 and its associated targets (see the Appendix to view the Sustainable Development Agenda in its entirety). Since the SDGs are, indeed, Global Goals to transform the world, partnerships across socioeconomic status, gender, age, culture, religion, and between nations are vital to their successful realization by 2030. According to United Nations Sustainable Development (UNSD; 2016), the SDG 17 partnership targets include radical and progressive outcomes in finance, technology, capacity building, trade, and global systems.

Box 28.1 Sustainable Development Goal 17 and Its Associated Targets

Goal 17. Strengthen the means of implementation and revitalize the global partnership for sustainable development

Finance

17.1 Strengthen domestic resource mobilization, including through international support to developing countries, to improve domestic capacity for tax and other revenue collection.

17.2 Developed countries to implement fully their official development assistance commitments, including the commitment by many developed countries to achieve the target of 0.7% of gross national income for official development assistance (ODA/GNI) to developing countries and 0.15%–0.20% of ODA/GNI to least developed countries; ODA providers are encouraged to consider setting a target to provide at least 0.20% of ODA/GNI to least developed countries.

17.3 Mobilize additional financial resources for developing countries from multiple sources.

17.4 Assist developing countries in attaining long-term debt sustainability through coordinated policies aimed at fostering debt financing, debt relief and debt restructuring, as appropriate, and address the external debt of highly indebted poor countries to reduce debt distress.

17.5 Adopt and implement investment promotion regimes for least developed countries.

(continued)

Box 28.1 **Sustainable Development Goal 17 and Associated Targets (*continued*)**

Technology

17.6   Enhance North–South, South–South and triangular regional and international cooperation on and access to science, technology and innovation and enhance knowledge sharing on mutually agreed terms, including through improved coordination among existing mechanisms, in particular at the United Nations level, and through a global technology facilitation mechanism.

17.7   Promote the development, transfer, dissemination and diffusion of environmentally sound technologies to developing countries on favorable terms, including on concessional and preferential terms, as mutually agreed.

17.8   Fully operationalize the technology bank and science, technology and innovation capacity-building mechanism for least developed countries by 2017 and enhance the use of enabling technology, in particular information and communications technology.

Capacity building

17.9   Enhance international support for implementing effective and targeted capacity building in developing countries to support national plans to implement all the Sustainable Development Goals, including through North–South, South–South and triangular cooperation.

Trade

17.10   Promote a universal, rules-based, open, nondiscriminatory and equitable multilateral trading system under the World Trade Organization, including through the conclusion of negotiations under its Doha Development Agenda.

17.11   Significantly increase the exports of developing countries, in particular with a view to doubling the least developed countries' share of global exports by 2020.

17.12   Realize timely implementation of duty-free and quota-free market access on a lasting basis for all least developed countries, consistent with World Trade Organization decisions, including by ensuring that preferential rules of origin applicable to imports from least developed countries are transparent and simple, and contribute to facilitating market access.

Systemic issues

Policy and institutional coherence

17.13   Enhance global macroeconomic stability, including through policy coordination and policy coherence.

17.14   Enhance policy coherence for sustainable development.

17.15   Respect each country's policy space and leadership to establish and implement policies for poverty eradication and sustainable development.

(*continued*)

| Box 28.2 | Sustainable Development Goal 17 and Associated Targets (*continued*) |

Multi-stakeholder partnerships

17.16   Enhance the Global Partnership for Sustainable Development, complemented by multi-stakeholder partnerships that mobilize and share knowledge, expertise, technology and financial resources, to support the achievement of the Sustainable Development Goals in all countries, in particular developing countries.

17.17   Encourage and promote effective public, public–private and civil society partnerships, building on the experience and resourcing strategies of partnerships.

Data, monitoring and accountability

17.18   By 2020, enhance capacity-building support to developing countries, including for least developed countries and small island developing States, to increase significantly the availability of high-quality, timely and reliable data disaggregated by income, gender, age, race, ethnicity, migratory status, disability, geographic location and other characteristics relevant in national contexts.

17.19   By 2030, build on existing initiatives to develop measurements of progress on sustainable development that complement gross domestic product, and support statistical capacity building in developing countries.

Source: Reprinted with permission from the United Nations (2015).

Global nurses are vital to capacity building throughout international health care systems. We have the "intellectual and numeric power" to partner with global colleagues and create viable and successful health outcomes worldwide (Fulmer, 2016, p. 97). Partnerships are needed every step of the way: with global health workers, governments, policy makers, and interprofessional contributors in finance and education.

However, we must be clear about how to build equitable and relevant partnerships to achieve the outcomes required. First, global nurses need to know the resources available to them, be they human, financial, or material (Leffers, 2014). Nurses leverage each of these resources in their professional partnerships to maintain standards of excellence, and a shortage of any one may result in thwarted or unrealized target achievements. Identifying the resources available and the mechanisms needed to retrieve them, along with understanding the relationships necessary for and barriers related to their implementation, give global nurse partners an opportunity to successfully and efficiently plan.

Second, the elements that constitute an effective partnership should be clearly delineated, practiced, and supported. Table 28.1 lists the characteristics of effective and ineffective partnerships as identified by Sliney (2015).

Table 28.1 Effective and Ineffective Partnerships

Elements of Effective Partnerships	Common Pitfalls of Ineffective Partnerships
• Clearly defined reasons for the partnership • Trust • Shared vision • Shared goals • Clearly articulated roles and responsibilities • In-country leadership • Equity • Accountability • Shared evaluation process • Recognition of the particular strengths and weaknesses of each partner • Sustainability as a key value for all parties	• Priorities driven by the donor agency • Imbalance in commitment to the project • Partners not fulfilling their commitments • Lack of transparency related to finances • Cultural misunderstandings or insensitivity • Poor planning for sustainability

Source: Sliney (2015).

In continually reassessing the pattern developments occurring within partnerships and responding with appropriate solutions, global nurses will be able to consciously sway unhealthy partnerships in the right direction.

Third, global nurses should be aware that not all cultures view partnerships the same. Scholars Upvall and Leffers (2016) are currently working with professional nurses in Cambodia, Haiti, India, Kenya, Lesotho, Pakistan, Thailand, Uganda, and Vietnam to better understand how the concept of partnership is perceived and understood through diverse cultural contexts. Through this qualitative and descriptive work, they hope to create an integrative and inclusive perspective on partnership that is respectful of the voices of nursing colleagues in low- and middle-income countries (LMICs). The professional nurse study participants acknowledge several differences from how partnership has been defined in the literature, which is often contributed using a Western-based construct. Some of the emerging findings include the resource inequities that lead to power differentials in cross-cultural partnerships; geopolitical influences (e.g., an unstable national climate) that may result in some encountering difficulty attracting international partners to work in person; the idea that many in different cultures may liken "partnership" to the idea of "friendship"; and how colleagues in LMICs have felt marginalized both within the profession of nursing and by country leadership that does not acknowledge the full scope of nursing's capabilities and potential (Upvall & Leffers, 2016).

It may be helpful to adopt a holistic orientation toward communication in our approach to relationship building and partnership development. A holistic communication process builds on therapeutic communication skills of empathy, unconditional regard, and caring with two additional concepts: being centered in one's self and creating intention before engaging with another (Thornton & Mariano, 2016). *Centering* refers to any practice that brings us back to the moment at hand and allows us to be authentic and present. This might include deep breathing, meditation, reflective journaling, or just mindful attention to what is

Table 28.2 Be CLEAR: A Guide to Holistic Communication

Processes	Explanation
Center yourself	Take a moment to pause and connect with your breath. Consider your intention and ask yourself how you can best be of service.
Listen wholeheartedly	Release personal agendas, judgments, and distractions. Open your mind and heart to what is being said. Connect to the other person's views and perspectives.
Empathize	Strive to see the situation and world from the others' point of view. Create safety for them and feel the meaning of their words as they express their thoughts.
Attention: be fully present	Return to the moment at hand again and again. Stay aware of the fluctuations of your thoughts, feelings, reactions, and judgments. Be here now.
Respect	Invite diversity and all it implies. Respect all that evolves from this interaction and partnership. Respect yourself and your needs, being clear about boundaries if needed. Respect the other person and the cultural differences that present themselves. Respect the process of partnership and growth.

CLEAR, Choosing Life: Empowerment! Action! Results!

Source: Adapted from Thornton (2013, pp. 190–191) and Thornton and Mariano (2016, p. 474).

happening "right now." *Creating intention* allows us to clarify our purpose, evaluate our motives, and identify new ways we may be of value and service. CLEAR communication guides us in the processes of holistic communication and stands for: **Center yourself, Listen wholeheartedly, Empathize, Attention: be fully present, and Respect** (Thornton, 2013; Thornton & Mariano, 2016). Table 28.2 spells out the CLEAR acronym with explanations of each.

Additionally, employing a nurse coach sensibility is particularly useful in nurturing the ongoing, interpersonal, and sensitive needs of any developing partnership. *Professional nurse coaching* can be defined as, "A skilled, purposeful, results-oriented, and structured relationship-centered interaction with clients provided by. . . nurses for the purpose of promoting achievement of client goals" (Dossey & Luck, 2016). Nurse coaches have an integral part in ensuring health and well-being on a global scale and in assisting all clients/communities across cultures in achieving their self-identified goals (Dossey & Hess, 2013). Nurse coaching is guided by a thoroughly delineated practice scope and competencies (Hess et al., 2013), and allows partnerships to be client-centered and client-guided. The art and science of nurse coaching relies on healthy partnerships with clients in order to remain fully present to the work unfolding, create actionable and realistic goals appropriate to the context at hand, remain in authentic communication, and maintain positive change long term.

While the holistic communication process suggested above aids in consistently present and respectful interactions on a moment-to-moment basis, the nurse coaching process provides a "big picture" approach to client-centered partnerships that can aid global nurses in building deeper and more meaningful relationships (Dossey, Luck, & Schaub, 2015). Table 28.3 lists the traditional and linear steps of the nursing process in the left-hand column; the more circular and continuous processes of the nurse coaching process in the middle column (Dossey et al., 2015);

Table 28.3 Nursing Process, Nurse Coaching Process, and Methods to Engage the Nurse Coaching Process

Traditional Nursing Process	Nurse Coaching Process	Methods to Engage the Nurse Coaching Process to Build Partnerships
Assessment	Establishing the relationship and identifying readiness for change	• Be fully present to self and other • Acknowledge assessment as premise for ongoing partnership • Understand assessment as a continuous and dynamic process • Identify change readiness and resistance
Diagnosis	Identifying opportunities, issues, and concerns	• Share results of assessment data with client and identify change priorities • Refrain from assigning labels or passing judgments • Guide the client in considering how he or she can grow in relation to overall health and well-being • Acknowledge what is currently working for the client to promote future success and encourage continued growth
Outcomes identification	Establishing client-centered goals	• Help the client in identifying the goals that will lead to the desired change • Nurture the relationship through supportive interactions, allowing client change and barriers to change to evolve as they will • Design coaching interactions to facilitate realization of the goals
Plan	Creating the structure of the coaching interaction	• Cocreate responsibilities of both coach and client • Clearly articulate and agree upon the shared vision and shared accountability • Allow client to identify goals with your assistance • Support the client in creating realistic and resource-considerate strategies
Implementation	Empowering clients to reach goals	• Be open to new goals and priorities as they emerge • Continue to provide the client with opportunities for reflection and personal assessment • Listen deeply • Respectfully and continuously share feedback related to progress and accountability • Remain curious and client-centered
Evaluation	Assisting clients to determine the extent to which goals were achieved	• Support the client in leading the evaluation process regarding progress and achievement • Explore the client's perceptions of success • Continue to cocreate new goals, plans, and outcomes based on evaluation • Remain available as new client-centered goals emerge

Source: Adapted from Dossey et al. (2015).

and methods the global nurse can use to engage the client each step of the way. Notice how the language shifts between the nursing process and the nurse coaching process, suggesting a more human and personal interaction.

Partnerships that are guided by the nurse coach process are individualized, personal, and invite true collaboration to take root and flourish.

Reconfiguring our understanding of what it means to "collaborate" may be one pertinent, yet missing, component to successful partnership development. It is not in any way similar to the verbs commonly ascribed to many global health donor–recipient dyads: "instruct," "guide," "mentor," and "inform." It requires a commitment beyond mundane collegiality. True collaboration requires our determination to transform what could be an ordinary professional relationship into something meaningful for ourselves, our coworkers, the communities we serve, and the health systems we maintain. Hills provides an inspiring definition of "collaboration" for us to consider:

> Collaboration is the creation of a synergistic alliance that honors and utilizes each person's contribution in order to create collective wisdom and collective action. Collaboration is not synonymous with co-operation, partnership, participation or compromise. Those words do not convey the fundamental importance of being in relationship nor the depth of caring that is collaboration. Collaborators are committed to, care about and trust in each other. They recognize that despite their differences, each has unique and valuable knowledge, perspectives and experiences to contribute to the collaboration. (Hills, 1992, p. 14, 2016, p. 298; Hills & Watson, 2011, p. 71)

Partnership—true partnership—is beyond "working together." It is collaboration in its highest form.

REFLECTION AND DISCUSSION

- How do I honor and utilize the uniqueness of others?
- Am I interested in creating a collective wisdom?
- Does collaboration require a caring ethic and ethos?
- Do I invite and embrace the knowledge, perspectives, and experiences of others?
- Am I willing to do it differently?

REFERENCES

Dossey, B. M., & Hess, D. (2013). Professional nurse coaching: Advances in national and global healthcare transformation. *Global Advances in Health and Medicine, 2*(4), 10–16.

Dossey, B. M., & Luck, S. (2016). Nurse coaching. In B. M. Dossey & L. Keegan (Eds.), *Holistic nursing: A handbook for practice* (7th ed., pp. 501–511). Burlington, MA: Jones & Bartlett.

Dossey, B. M., Luck, S., & Schaub, B. G. (2015). *Nurse coaching for health and wellbeing.* North Miami, FL: International Nurse Coach Association.

Fulmer, T. (2016). Influential and determined: Assuring integrity in the care of older adults and beyond. In W. Rosa (Ed.), *Nurses as leaders: Evolutionary visions of leadership* (pp. 87–99). New York, NY: Springer Publishing.

Hess, D. R., Dossey, B. M., Southard, M. E., Luck, S., Schaub, B. G., & Bark, L. (2013). *The art and science of nurse coaching: A provider's guide to scope and competencies.* Silver Spring, MD: Nursesbooks.org.

Hills, M. (1992). Collaborative nursing project. Development of generic integrated nursing curriculum in collaboration with four partner colleges. Report to Ministry of Advanced Education, Centre for Curriculum and Professional Development.

Hills, M. (2016). Emancipatory and collaborative: Learning to lead from beside. In W. Rosa (Ed.), *Nurses as leaders: Evolutionary visions of leadership* (pp. 293–309). New York, NY: Springer Publishing.

Hills, M., & Watson, J. (2011). *Creating a caring science curriculum: An emancipatory pedagogy for nursing.* New York, NY: Springer Publishing.

Leffers, M. J. (2014). Resources for global health partnerships. In M. J. Upvall & J. M. Leffers (Eds.), *Global health nursing: Building and sustaining partnerships* (pp. 123–132). New York, NY: Springer Publishing.

Sliney, A. (2015). Global health partnerships. In S. E. Breakey, I. B. Corless, N. L. Meedzan, & P. K. Nicholas (Eds.), *Global health nursing in the 21st century* (pp. 103–111). New York, NY: Springer Publishing.

Thornton, L. (2013). *Whole person caring: An interprofessional model for healing and wellness.* Indianapolis, IN: Sigma Theta Tau International.

Thornton, L., & Mariano, C. (2016). Evolving from therapeutic to holistic communication. In B. M. Dossey & L. Keegan (Eds.), *Holistic nursing: A handbook for practice* (7th ed., pp. 465–478). Burlington, MA: Jones & Bartlett.

United Nations. (2015). Transforming our world: The 2030 Agenda for Sustainable Development. Retrieved from https://docs.google.com/gview?url=http://sustainabledevelopment.un.org/content/documents/21252030%20Agenda%20for%20Sustainable%20Development%20web.pdf&embedded=true

United Nations Sustainable Development. (2016). Goal 17: Revitalize the global partnership for sustainable development. Retrieved from http://www.un.org/sustainabledevelopment/globalpartnerships

Upvall, M. J., & Leffers, J. M. (2014). Preface. In M. J. Upvall & J. M. Leffers (Eds.), *Global health nursing: Building and sustaining partnerships* (pp. xvii–xviii). New York, NY: Springer Publishing.

Upvall, M. J. & Leffers, J. M. (2016, October). *Perspectives of partnership from nurses in low and middle resource countries.* Paper presented at the Seed Global Health Conference, Boston, Massachusetts.

A Global Health Vision for 2030 and Beyond

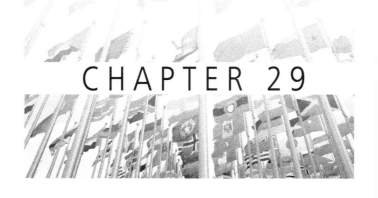

CHAPTER 29

Global Nursing Wisdom: Notes From the Field

Julie K. Anathan, Busisiwe Rosemary Bhengu,
Olivia Bahemuka, Kelly Burke, Maureen E. Connell,
Carole Ann Drick, Helen Ewing, Lynn Keegan,
Susan Luck, Phalakshi Manjrekar, Patricia Moreland,
Jasintha T. Mtengezo, William Rosa, and Deborah Wilson

*[C]hange takes time and change begets change. It takes one nurse, one unit,
one system, one nursing organization to create the spark; to fire up the
conversation; to share caring wisdom and to bring that wisdom to practice;
and to stand up, speak out to other nurses, health care professionals, and
the public through dialogue, publications, and action to say, I have had
enough of being defined by others. I am a healer whose expertise is nursing
. . . [my work] . . . sustains human dignity. I am a nurse who makes a
difference in people's lives like no other profession. (Wagner, 2016; p. 448)*

We *must* tell our stories.

In many ways, sharing our experiential knowledge with health care colleagues, students, and the public is a moral requisite of nursing; a responsibility to elevate the profession, inform the collective about the global concerns confronting each of us, and unify the broader community of nurses and midwives through the narratives of our nurse–client, nurse–nurse, nurse–self relationships. These relationships are central to the ethical foundations of nursing (Helming, 2016), and openly sharing the stories we have in regard to them allows us, and our listeners, to come "face-to-face with quandaries, insights, struggles, joy, suffering, pain, and healing moments" (Burkhardt & Nagai-Jacobson, 2016, p. 148). The acts of both telling our stories and being present to receive the story of another is just one way of practicing courage, compassion, and connection: the elements needed to reflect, learn, and become whole persons (Brown, 2010, 2012). Our stories reflect the *courage* it takes to be a global nurse, demonstrate the *compassion* needed for self and other amid the complex nature of global nursing work, and strengthen our *connection* with the world around us.

Storytelling is just one method of reflective practice. *Reflective practice* is a form of self-care and self-renewal that has been shown to promote self-efficacy, improve patient outcomes and the quality of care delivery, and transform nursing education and work environments at the organizational and systems level (Freshwater, Taylor, & Sherwood, 2008; Sherwood & Horton-Deutsch, 2012, 2015). Reflective practice guides us to continue our personal and professional development toward becoming conscientious, ethically grounded leaders (Horton-Deutsch, 2016); see Chapter 30 for more on reflective practice.

Every single day, at bedsides, in classrooms and boardrooms, in villages, cities, and countries all around the world, nurses are contributing to the healing of patients, families, groups, and communities. It is not necessary to work in Uganda to increase our understanding of the health barriers faced by children there, or to become a rural nurse in India to make the connections between the lack of economic opportunity and the poor health outcomes faced by the population majority. Being a competent global nurse requires us to share our stories and to be authentically present to the stories of others: to reflect and learn so that the initiatives we create, support, and implement are culturally inclusive of our colleagues and their efforts and worldviews. It gives us the opportunity to grow in our awareness of global and planetary considerations that face other nations, health systems, and people from all walks of life.

WISDOM FROM THE FIELD: OPPORTUNITIES TO CONTRIBUTE TO SUSTAINABLE DEVELOPMENT

This chapter brings together global nurses who have lived and worked in many parts of the world, from the United States, Canada, and the United Kingdom, to various countries in Africa, and in South Asia. All contributors tell their stories of global nursing, sharing their observations and the lessons learned from their work, through the lens of each of the 17 Sustainable Development Goals (SDGs). Each testament has merit because each is based on lived experiences that cannot be refuted. Each gives us a glimpse of global health challenges as they relate to each of the 17 SDGs, the real-world barriers facing the achievement of sustainable development, and imparts skills each of us can cultivate to work intelligently and collaboratively in striving to realize a safe and inclusive existence for all human beings on the planet.

In and of itself, this chapter is an exercise in peace and inclusiveness as we respect and provide space for different voices, styles, and experiences while understanding the importance and validity of all. Some authors employ a more scholarly tone, supporting ideas with critical application of data while others speak more candidly and succinctly about how we can make small changes today, right here, and right now. This chapter makes one thing evident about the global profession of nursing: We are made of many but we are stronger together than apart. In celebrating our diversity in how each articulates self and service, we come to recognize the myriad opportunities we each have to participate in SDG attainment around the world in both simple/personal and large-scale/collective endeavors.

The following sections are based on the critical areas of importance identified by the United Nations (UN) 2030 Agenda for Sustainable Development (2015): People, Planet, Prosperity, Peace, and Partnership. Within each of these areas can be found the relevant SDGs and each author's contributions (see the Appendix to read the complete UN 2030 Sustainable Development Agenda). These writings do not attempt to address all 169 targets of the 2030 Agenda, but rather to enlighten us with intimate and firsthand experiential wisdom that addresses different aspects of each of the SDGs. Though the SDGs are categorized under specific critical areas for organizational purposes within this chapter, it is important to remember that many SDGs have targets that cross over and impact People, Planet, Prosperity, Peace, and Partnership simultaneously.

To help guide you through this chapter, the following is a list of the critical areas, relevant SDGs, and the contributing authors addressing them:

- **People**
  - No Poverty, End Hunger (SDGs 1 and 2)—Maureen E. Connell
  - Good health and well-being (SDG 3)—William Rosa
  - Equitable and Inclusive Quality Education (SDG 4)—Julie K. Anathan and Jasintha T. Mtengezo
  - Achieve Gender Equality and Reduce Inequalities of All Kinds for All Peoples and Countries (SDGs 5 and 10)—Busisiwe Rosemary Bhengu
  - Clean Water and Sanitation (SDG 6)—Olivia Bahemuka
  - Cities and Communities (SDG 11)—Patricia Moreland
- **Planet**
  - Clean Energy (SDG 7)—Lynn Keegan
  - Responsible Consumption and Production (SDG 12)—Lynn Keegan
  - Climate Change (SDG 13)—Carole Ann Drick
  - Life Below Water (SDG 14)—Susan Luck
  - Life on Land (SDG 15)—Susan Luck
- **Prosperity**
  - Decent Work and Economic Growth (SDG 8)—Phalakshi Manjrekar
  - Infrastructure, Industry, and Innovation (SDG 9)—Deborah Wilson
- **Peace**
  - Peace and Justice for All (SDG 16)—Kelly Burke
- **Partnership**
  - Revitalize the Global Partnership (SDG 17)—Helen Ewing

It is true, we must *tell* our stories. But we must also *listen* deeply to another's.

PEOPLE

No Poverty, End Hunger (SDGs 1 and 2)

Maureen E. Connell

Mother Theresa once said, "The greatest poverty was to be unloved and uncared for." "Poverty" is officially defined in economic terms based on income levels and access to basic necessities such as food, water, and sanitation. People living on less than $2.25 a day are said to be experiencing "extreme poverty." However, each of us has our own perception of what it is to be poor.

I once lived in a remote part of Scotland. My neighbor was a 90-year-old man who had worked as a shepherd all his life; he told me that he began his married life in a small two-room cottage. His employer provided him with oatmeal, flour, sugar, and tea, and he had a cow for milk. He worked for 6 months before he received his salary. So, for the first 6 months of his married life he had no money whatsoever. I asked if he considered himself poor; he looked at me with surprise and replied, "Not at all, we had a house, food, firewood, and each other. They were the happiest days of my life."

Poverty is a relative concept, although "absolute poverty" is absolute! I grew up in deprived circumstances and, as a family, we were poor. However, I was always aware that there were other families who were much poorer, so in relative terms we counted ourselves "lucky" with the little we had.

In a globalized world, we are constantly reminded that there are people living in extreme poverty, both in high- and LMICs. However, as Sir Michael Marmot (2006), states, poverty in a rich country and poverty in a poor country are different and we need to address them in different ways. We all know instinctively that poverty is not just a lack of money or resources, but a combination of factors that affect our ability to flourish as human beings and reach our full potential. SDG 1 states that we should try to end poverty in *all* its forms because poverty certainly has myriad expressions and a multitude of features. Poverty and hunger go hand in hand.

One aspect of poverty is clear, however: It is inherently unhealthy. The poor, in whatever setting, experience more ill health, have less access to health care, and invariably die earlier than their more economically sound neighbors. This is profoundly unfair and preventable. As nurses working in a global setting, we need to be aware of and ready to tackle the wider issues of poverty, such as loss of dignity and self-esteem, lack of opportunity, disempowerment, and insecurity.

I cannot claim to possess the solutions to these issues, but my work as a nurse in various humanitarian situations in severely resource-constrained settings has given me the firsthand knowledge to address them and offer suggestions of how we, as a global nursing community, can aid in the efforts of SDGs 1 and 2. Overall, my experience taught me that it is not enough to simply provide *relief* to the poor and hungry (e.g., money, food, resources). We need to seek new ways of creating an equal world where the poor no longer experience the greater burden of disease and death.

I began my career as a nurse midwife in Sudan during the famine of 1984–1985. I worked in one of the many refugee camps along the border with Ethiopia. We provided relief to the refugees through food, medicine, and material goods. As in all emergency situations, we focused on basic needs; we did nothing to address the root causes of poverty and distress. However, we were always aware of the wider issues around poverty and hunger, and worked to provide care with dignity and respect. For example, each camp had a refugee council made up of men and women who helped make the decisions around services for the population. The council participated in meetings between government and UN officials and was seen as a participatory approach to the day-to-day functioning of the camp. Similarly, before we began any new health or social initiative, we would consult with local elders to determine if it was both acceptable and appropriate. Nothing was done without prior discussion, consultation, and consensus.

I witnessed a good example of this while working in the tuberculosis (TB) "hospital." The 6-week trek from Ethiopia to Sudan, coupled with severe malnutrition and overcrowding, resulted in a very high prevalence of TB in the camp. The TB "hospital" consisted of one long room filled with straw beds. Family members cared for the sick and often slept on the floor beside the patient. TB treatment at that time consisted of daily streptomycin injections together with oral medication. Due to malnutrition and muscle wasting, the injections were very painful and the medication often made patients nauseous and lethargic. To this day, I will never forget the suffering endured in that hospital ward.

The refugees were convinced that the hot dry climate of Sudan had caused TB; they said they had never experienced a disease such as TB in the mountains of Tigray. Consequently, some people refused treatment and did not believe that the disease was contagious. So we began a program of education to raise community awareness. We identified a number of community elders who were well respected. We trained them as teachers and taught them about TB: how it was transmitted and why people became infected. When one teacher-training course was complete we would begin again with another group of elders. Each participant received a certificate of training. Armed with their new knowledge and skills, they passed on health education and promotion messages in culturally acceptable ways. One elder told us, "I will never forget the people from the West who came to tell us about the disease called TB and how to stop it spreading. Now I am teaching my own people about this disease."

The refugees lived in simple canvas tents with two openings at each side. In the day the heat was unbearable; at night it was very cold. Some families had 10 to 12 members living in each tent. Yet the refugees told us that after sleeping in the open for 6 weeks, they were simply grateful to have some form of shelter.

Each day I visited patients in the community. Ethiopian hospitality is legendary; a guest is always offered food and drink, no matter how poor or destitute a family may be. This was my experience in the camps. Each family would provide me with something out of the little they had, (literally, their camp food ration), usually a crude form of *tella* (a drink made from grain), which tasted like charcoal, and a plate of *injura* (bread). To refuse would be a direct insult to their code of hospitality. By accepting to share and eat with them, we were upholding their dignity and self-esteem. I realized that I was never taught this in nursing school. My training was mainly about what I could do to help heal and treat patients. But our nursing code and considerations must extend further; they must enable us to engage those who are searching for acceptance, kindness, and a sense of meaning amid their illnesses and contexts. Our duty of care must be to uphold human dignity and respect.

After about 2 years, a program of repatriation began in the camp. All of the refugees wanted to return home. They yearned to see the green meadows and mountains of Tigray. The UN provided trucks to transport them to the border; however, due to lack of space in the trucks, each adult refugee was allowed to take only one small bag. This did not deter them, they were so happy to return home, and simply let go of anything they could not take. Again, I reflected: It is indeed possible for someone to possess, literally, no material thing, and yet to be content. This experience illustrates that poverty is not only about a lack of money or resources, it is also about a sense of belonging, community, and integration, as well as the ability to embody a purpose or pursue a goal in life.

The repatriation program created an ethical dilemma in regard to the TB patients. The UN High Commissioner for Refugees (UNHCR) stipulated that anyone undergoing TB treatment, an 18-month treatment at the time, should be actively discouraged from returning to Ethiopia. If they did decide to return, their TB treatment would be terminated. The explanation was that refugees undergoing treatment would have to take their TB medication with them and take it unsupervised. The UN decided that this was unacceptable and, therefore, made a policy that if a refugee with TB decided to return home, his or her treatment would stop. The nongovernmental organization (NGO) I worked for made an official complaint against the policy, and provided arguments around the morality of the decision, including the fundamental human rights issue based on Article 25 of the United Nations Declaration of Human Rights (UN, 1948), which states that,

> Everyone has the right to a standard of living adequate for the health and well-being of himself and of his family, including food, clothing, housing and medical care and necessary social services, and the right to security in the event of . . . lack of livelihood in circumstances beyond his control.

However, the UN insisted that it was unsafe for TB medication to be so freely available among the population returning home. We insisted that the educational program had equipped people with the knowledge and skills necessary for safe TB medication self-administration. The UN disagreed and the policy prevailed. Despite encouraging the TB patients to stay in the camps and finish their course of treatment, many refugees decided to return home and, consequently, did not complete their treatment. Likewise, newly diagnosed patients who were planning to return home were not offered treatment. I remember, especially, one young girl who was sputum positive. Her family was due to return to Ethiopia the following day and because of this she was refused treatment. She had no part in any decision regarding her future life, to return home, or to be treated. That young girl was totally disempowered and had no voice. That is true poverty.

My time in the camps taught me a great deal about how poverty and hunger affect those who are caught in the aftermath of war, disaster, and famine. It taught me how to view particular rules and regulations with skepticism and to question authority that conflicts with my ethical values. It also taught me that we, as nurses, have the potential to help foster resilience within those we serve, despite the terrible consequences of poverty and hunger—not simply by providing food and medication, but through our attitude to others, openness to difference, defiance in the face of injustice, and our love of humankind.

Over the years, I have worked in many different situations, mainly emergencies of one kind or another. In 1993 I went to Nepal to help with the little known and unreported refugee crisis in Nepal when thousands of ethnic Nepalese were expelled from Bhutan. The situation was so well managed that we had few issues with malnutrition. However, one incident remains with me, and again taught me a great deal about poverty and loss, and how it affects individuals in different ways.

One day, the feeding center staff reported that a young girl aged 9 years had been admitted and was refusing to eat. It is very unusual for a child above 5 years to be admitted to a feeding center. Usually children below 5 years are the most vulnerable to malnutrition and concomitant disease. So we tried to determine why this child was malnourished and, of course, why she was refusing to eat, but she would not tell us. We examined her background to see if she had experienced a particular trauma. Her mother had died and her father had abandoned the family; she had been brought to the camp by her two older brothers, both of whom had disappeared. She was totally alone. I could only imagine the sense of abandonment and loneliness she must have felt. It was hardly surprising that she refused to eat. But I had to try to help her regain some purpose in life.

Eventually, I asked her with the help of a translator what it was she wanted. I said, "I cannot bring your parents back, but I will try to get whatever it is you want." She looked up and said something to the translator, who turned to me and said, "She wants clothes. She wants a dress, pants, socks, and shoes." I remember thinking how stupid I had been to overlook a basic need. She did have some clothes, but they were old and worn; she clearly wanted clothes that were new and clean. We bought her the clothes. As soon as she put them on she said, "Now, you can give me the food."

In times of war and disaster people do need basic materials such as food, water, and shelter. However, they also need to have their dignity and self-esteem recognized and respected. I thought I was doing everything possible for that young girl. But her individual need at that time was to be recognized for who she was: a young girl who simply wanted a clean dress and some new shoes.

SDG 2 urges the need to end hunger and improve nutrition. But we must also address the terrible consequences of poverty: lack of dignity, and abandonment. It is not enough for us to "feed" people. We must nourish their innermost need for a sense of belonging, recognition, and love.

A great deal of my time working in LMICs was spent as a relief nurse working in feeding centers. These could be places of great sadness when lots of babies were dying, and great joy when children improved and went home fit and well. In 1993, I worked in a feeding center in a remote part of South Sudan. Most of the population had traveled to the small town to seek security as the army commander was stationed in the same town. It was one of the most desolate places on earth. There was no road in or out, no vegetation, nor resources of any kind. Everything had to be transported by plane from the now famous Lokichogio airbase in neighboring Kenya. Even the water was flown in each day. There were many children dying of malnutrition and something had to be done. I was asked to set up a therapeutic and supplementary feeding center. There were no facilities to open an intensive feeding center where children would ideally stay overnight. So children would come to the feeding center in the morning and go home in the evening. I went to the feeding center every day and there were always problems: no buckets, no water, and no charcoal. It was a daily struggle to keep the feeding center functioning.

Many of the children were orphans, and one particular orphan captured my heart. He was about 7 years old and desperately ill. Someone used to bring him to the feeding center every morning and take him back to the orphanage each evening. Sometimes I would carry him back myself and make sure he was comfortable for the night. One morning I arrived at the feeding center early and found him dead. The image of that boy lying on the floor has remained with me over the past 23 years. The day before I had asked someone to take him back to the orphanage, but this clearly had not happened. He had stayed in the feeding center all night, and died alone, without anyone to comfort him. That young boy was buried in an unmarked grave, somewhere in South Sudan, mourned by one person, myself, who often thinks of him and his great unachieved potential. This death was just one among the approximately 10 million child deaths that occurred that year, of which 70% were preventable.

The situation in South Sudan at that time was catastrophic; each day more people arrived and more children needed feeding. It was necessary to maintain good relations with the army commander, but at times this was difficult. For example, the NGO sent blankets, which were then distributed to the mothers and children. I asked that they bring their blankets to the feeding center each day so they could lie down and rest. However, the next day there were no blankets to be seen and, instead, the soldiers and local men all carried the blankets around their shoulders. When I asked the army commander, he said this was a much better use of the blankets. He also complained that the well children in the camp were not being fed, only the sick children. He questioned me: "Why was this? Why not feed the well children and keep them strong since the sick ones are going to die anyway?" I explained that we could not let the malnourished children die; there was an admission criterion for the feeding center, and we were required to follow that criterion. The commander responded that he was in charge of the town and, therefore, I should obey him. I again explained that I worked for the NGO and was answerable to them. It was difficult but I stood my ground. Later I received more blankets from the NGO, but this time I cut them in half so that they were too small to be used by any adult. This time I told the mothers, these are for your children only. The next day the commander came to the feeding center demanding to know why I had cut up the blankets. The UN representative (who usually stayed in Lokichogio) was with him. I explained that the blankets were for the children, so I cut them to the children's size. The commander was furious and threatened to close the feeding center. Later, I was warned by the UN representative that I should be "careful"—people had been killed in the past for disobeying orders.

I am sometimes asked if I was ever afraid while working in these settings. When I look back I cannot remember feeling afraid. I think the needs of the moment take over and one often loses a sense of oneself in the fight for justice. I know that was my feeling as I squared up to the commander.

Again, we are not really taught how to deal with these kinds of situations in nursing school, but what we are taught is the importance of defending the weak, safeguarding the vulnerable, and speaking for the voiceless. I hope that is what I was doing that day in a small village in South Sudan.

Another experience of intensive feeding was with Somali refugees in Eastern Ethiopia (1991–1992). The camps were situated along the Ethiopian border with Somalia, and were very remote and difficult to access. There were huge logistical problems around the provision of food and water. Roads were nonexistent and in the rainy season were often impassable. There were also problems with security, frequent hijacking, and shootings with people being killed. The feeding program had over 1,000 registered children and each day more were admitted. Many children died. The needs were overwhelming. Often the water trucks could not get to the camps, or food supply was delayed. At times the security situation meant that we could not travel or stay in the camps. This led to a feeling of powerlessness and impotence. It made me question my purpose. One particular incident made me reflect on my role as a nurse and the long-term effects of my efforts.

It happened just after the Ethiopian People's Revolutionary Democratic Front (EPRDF) had taken power and their soldiers had come to the camp in which I was working. They provided much needed security in the camp. One day a soldier came to speak with me. He said, "I remember your face; you worked in the TB hospital when I was in the refugee camp in Sudan in 1985; I was a patient there." I was astonished, and remember being overwhelmed by the understanding of how our actions impact others in ways we cannot imagine, and how our lives go full circle. As Elliot (1995) says in the poem *Little Gidding*, "We shall not cease from exploration, and the end of all our exploring will be to arrive where we started and know the place for the first time" (p. 43). This is both our gift and privilege as global nurses: to realize this interconnectedness in real, tangible, and sacred ways.

Of all my experiences, the one that epitomizes the inequities and injustices of poverty has to be my work in Haiti. I first worked in Haiti in 1999. I went to evaluate a program and to try to write a project proposal for further funding. I carried out the evaluation in the bidonvilles in Port au Prince and rural villages in Port Salut. The bidonvilles are shanty towns surrounding the city of Port au Prince. At that time, they were overcrowded and unsafe with minimal water and sanitation services. I had worked in many refugee camps that had basic water and sanitation resources, but I had never seen anything like the bidonvilles before. Whole families lived in one-room shacks with no running water or toilet facilities. I asked one family where they went to use the bathroom. They took me to a hill with some cardboard boxes and a group of teenagers there told me that they would defecate into an empty plastic bag, tie it up, and then throw it into Petionville, an affluent part of Port au Prince. The teenagers picked up plastic bags and demonstrated the action. I remember laughing with them—I could see their point of view. There were plastic bags everywhere, pinned down by rubbish and excrement, noisily flapping in the wind; the smell was nauseating. In the distance, I could see great expanse of blue sea. Haiti is so beautiful. Yet, this squalid place was where thousands of people lived, worked, went to school, and worshipped their God, trying to make something of their lives.

The project I evaluated was a small development program designed to help women make healthy meals on a budget. Initially, I thought it was an insult to presume to teach women how to cook; after all they were the experts in their culture. However, as I got to know more about the project, I realized there was a great deal more to the program. It was managed entirely by Haitian women, and as it developed, it broadened in scope and purpose. Many of the women learned how to read and write; they were then taught how to teach and inspire others. With this newfound confidence, they began to develop women's groups, which met regularly to talk about other issues in the community. One of these was the problem of gender-based violence (GBV). In Port Salut the women told me they had found the courage to say *Non!* to their partners. I was concerned that this might engender more abuse; however, the women were adamant and they told me, "We have each other now. We are stronger." In a small way the program helped to facilitate the process of empowerment among the women—a huge weapon against poverty. Nevertheless, despite my efforts, I was told by the donor organization that the program would not receive further funding. In the end, it had to close. I often think of those women I was privileged to meet and wonder: Are they still together, saying *Non* to domestic abuse?

I found the situation in Haiti shocking because I witnessed great poverty directly beside great wealth. In my earlier experiences, I had worked in situations where almost all the people were poor. But in Haiti, the disparities were glaringly obvious.

Final Thoughts

People often ask me how I cope seeing so much death and suffering caused by poverty and hunger? This is difficult to answer. Like all nurses, I have a particular job to do. It would be impossible to do that job if I became overwhelmed by the suffering and pain around me. However, it would also be impossible to do the job if I was somehow detached from the pain and suffering. I was always disturbed by the death of each child; I was distressed by the immense suffering I witnessed. But it did not affect my ability to go on working. All I can say is that these experiences have "marked" me in some way, and have colored how I look at the world and my own life. There are certain things I cannot enjoy without a tinge of guilt. When I think about buying something, I often compare the price with the basic salary or a school fee of someone living in Africa.

My experiences have marked the person I am and the decisions I make. So much so that years after "retiring" from humanitarian work I decided to return to Africa. I now teach nurses in Rwanda, and love my job and feel so privileged. Every day I witness a new generation of nurses striving to become effective global citizens, upholding the virtues and principles of our nursing profession. Each of us has the responsibility to fill the gaps for which nursing school has not been able to prepare us: to immerse ourselves in cultures and open our minds to new ways of seeing the world, more deeply understand the implications of poverty and hunger and their bearing on individual and global health and well-being, and to humanize each provision of care with dignity and compassion. Without such efforts, the targets of SDGs 1 and 2, along with the remainder of the 2030 Agenda, will fail to be achieved.

Good Health and Well-Being (SDG 3)

William Rosa

The third goal of the Sustainable Development Agenda—good health and well-being—is the one most often familiar to nurses and midwives. It is discussed thoroughly and in great detail throughout this book, as it very often becomes nurses' fundamental lens for evaluating clients, systems, outcomes, resources, and the world around us. For the purpose of this section, I would like to discuss my experiences working for the Human Resources for Health (HRH) Program in Rwanda as it relates to creating a culture of safety and the questions we must continue to ask ourselves as global nurses to ensure optimal health and well-being.

A Culture of Safety

The American Nurses Association (ANA, 2016) declared 2016 as the Culture of Safety Year, and defines a *culture of safety* as "core values and behaviors resulting from a collective and sustained commitment by organizational leadership, managers, and health care workers to emphasize safety over competing goals." There has been much talk about creating a culture of safety since the Institute of Medicine's (IOM, 2000) report, *To Err Is Human: Building a Safer Health System*, citing that anywhere between 44,000 and 98,000 people die each year in American hospitals as a result of medical errors. The IOM (2000) made it clear that not only do medical errors debilitate patients' trust in the system, they also decrease satisfaction for patients and staff alike. In many low- and middle-income countries (LMICs), the focus tends to be on timely access and delivery of quality care, with specific targets related to the prevalent diseases at hand. Maintaining patient safety is always a concern in resource-constrained environments due to any or all of the following: staff shortages, patients' and families' inadequate financial means to pay for necessary diagnostics and interventions, mixed educational preparation of staff, and/ or lack of access to equipment or technology that would promote seamless and optimal patient care (World Health Organization [WHO], 2016).

The ANA (2016) identifies the attributes of a positive safety culture as (a) openness and mutual trust when discussing safety concerns and solutions without individual blame; (b) marshaling of appropriate resources, such as safe staffing- and skill-mix levels; (c) a learning environment in which health care professionals learn from errors and proactively detect systemic weaknesses; and (d) transparency and accountability. Each of these attributes is discussed in what follows, with regard to my experiences in Kigali, Rwanda.

Openness, Mutual Trust, and a Blame-Free Culture

In 1994, the Genocide Against the Tutsi resulted in the murder of over 1 million Tutsi citizens and moderate Hutus in just 100 days. The Hutu extremist government sought to exterminate the Tutsi population, inciting mass civilian violence to carry out their plan. The 1994 genocide came on the heels of decades of discriminatory and oppressive policies, and ethnic pogroms that started as early as 1959 (Kinzer, 2008). By the end of the genocide, virtually all sectors of the country had collapsed and Rwanda faced the challenges of assembling a new government, fostering peace, pursuing justice, and rebuilding reliable and sustainable mechanisms for economic growth, education, finance, agriculture, and health care. Rwanda has made tremendous strides in all of these areas and continues to develop itself in solidarity and with the support of countless NGOs and foreign diplomatic relationships.

The history of the Rwandan people has created difficulty for some to remain open and be able to trust again. This is evident in the health system. Many patients, particularly those who experienced trauma during 1994, can become retraumatized by complications of an illness or the sequelae of a motor vehicle accident. The fear caused by a lack of control or the vulnerability inherent to the experience of being a patient can induce isolation, refusal to comply, or the willingness to seek medical attention altogether.

After the genocide, the local community courts, known as the *gacaca*, were responsible for assigning prison sentences based on crimes committed. The culture is one of efficiency, hard work, and collectivist ideals. Everyone is responsible for very specific duties and held accountable for expectations not met. This can result in the tendency to assign blame, particularly in a health care setting where errors can result in patient harm. Very often the focus is on individuals rather than system breakdowns.

This is not a "Rwandan" problem but an experience had by nurses and systems worldwide. We must learn to support colleagues and identify potential improvement areas for organizations that promote team building and a sense of openness and trust.

As global nurses, we must continue to ask ourselves:

- How do we role-model openness to colleagues and clients?
- What approaches to trust building can we employ that transcend cultures and contexts?
- What is needed to support a given culture in moving toward a blame-free work environment?

Appropriate Resources

What working environment is not constrained in some way? In the complex world of health care, there will always be some need for better technology, more equipment, additional staff, accessible leaders, more effective communication mechanisms, and/or universal health coverage. The goal as global nurses is to become experts in assessing the needs of the environment, celebrating accomplishments and strengths, and ushering in innovative approaches to help fill the gaps specific to the context and meet the self-identified needs of the organization at hand.

We must never underestimate the power of promoting innovation in the face of resource constraints (Brysiewicz, Hughes, & McCreary, 2015). In Rwanda, for example, innovative strategies have been employed to implement a blended learning model of classroom and online approaches (Mulaudzi & Chyun, 2015), and in acquiring much needed resources for graduate students in the Master's of Science in Nursing program at the University of Rwanda through partnerships with major inter/national professional organizations (Mukamana, Dushimiyimana, et al., 2016; Mukamana, Karonkano, & Rosa, 2016; Mukamana, Niyomugabo, & Rosa, 2016).

As global nurses, we must continue to ask ourselves:

- What resources are needed to improve care based on the self-identified goals of the organization at hand?
- How can I think outside the box to obtain the resources needed?
- In what ways can I remain solutions-focused to find resources that will serve the greatest good for all involved?

A Learning and Proactive Environment

My clinical and academic experiences in Rwanda frequently led to the "not enough" experience: not enough staff, not enough space, not enough rooms, not enough beds, not enough medications, and so on. Creating a proactive and exciting environment in which to learn and practice nursing in a "not enough" headspace is challenging. Throughout the year, I learned I had to somehow translate the "not enough" rant into the acceptance that all was "as it should be." No matter what setting I was in, what assistance I had (or did not have), what tools I found (or did not find), or how discouraged I felt, I reminded myself—day in and day out—that all was exactly "as it should be." This shift in mentality allowed me to create new possibilities in education, partnership, and nursing practice under any circumstances and allowed my colleagues and me to accomplish more than we had anticipated. "As it should be" is a mantra I have used in professional settings to surrender to "what is" so that I can focus on finding realistic and contextually appropriate solutions to help move health care forward to "where we need to be."

As global nurses, we must continue to ask ourselves:

- What is the "not enough" rant I see in my professional setting? How does it prevent me from contributing my best?
- What do I need to accept so that I can continue to be of service to the goals at hand?
- What are the challenges I face in accepting resource constraints and working within the framework being presented to me right now?

Transparency and Accountability

Medical errors scare health care workers. Aside from dealing with the fear of administrative sanction, they must confront their feelings of guilt that accompany patient harm. But how do you promote an environment of transparency and accountability when the consequences may reap substantial and long-term difficulties for you and your family?

I worked with a nurse in Rwanda who was simply brilliant—let us call him Jean Paul. One day, I stood at a bedside with Jean Paul after a patient had cardiac arrested and been resuscitated for the third time in 48 hours. I had assessed the patient on my own and noticed that her pupils were dilated and fixed, suggesting anoxic brain injury. Alone in the room with Jean Paul, the patient unresponsive to even noxious stimuli, this is the conversation that ensued:

Billy: Jean Paul, have you assessed her pupils?

Jean Paul: No, I'm not interested in her pupils because we still don't know why she was admitted to the hospital. We must find out this information and treat the underlying cause.

Billy: I understand, but what her pupils are suggesting may make the underlying cause irrelevant.

Jean Paul: I don't want to look at her pupils because I am focused on finding how we can treat her if she has a pneumonia or infection.

Billy: Jean Paul, I really think we should address what's going on with her pupils sooner rather than later.

Jean Paul: Billy, if I look at her pupils and acknowledge what it is you're saying, myself and every other nurse on duty right now will go right to jail. So I'm glad you assessed her pupils and are aware of the implications, but right now, I need to find and treat an underlying cause.

And there it was. There was never going to be real transparency or full accountability because the system was set up to assign disproportionate blame accordingly. Again—this is not a "Rwandan" problem. All around the world, nurses face life-changing consequences for errors and patient outcomes that are not their fault; we must partner with colleagues to shift the consciousness from "Who failed?" to "What system broke down?"

As global nurses, we must continue to ask ourselves:

- How can I demonstrate compassion and understanding to colleagues who face disproportionate consequences for medical errors and negative patient outcomes?
- How can I support professional relationships to become transparent and accountable by focusing on system strengths and weaknesses?
- In what ways do I contribute to a blame culture? How can I rectify those behaviors today?

Final Thoughts

A culture of safety is the right of every patient and every global nurse. We must search for opportunities to create partnerships based on openness and trust. We must be creative and think outside the box when it comes to obtaining necessary resources and inviting new possibilities within the context. We must continue to be innovative in how we promote learning environments that are proactive and make the best of the resources at hand. And, finally, we must continue to promote environments that are transparent and accountable to patients and their families, always promoting a unified front for nursing while striving for a culture of safety.

Equitable and Inclusive Quality Education (SDG 4)

Julie K. Anathan

The aim of SDG 4 is to "Ensure inclusive and equitable quality education and promote lifelong learning opportunities for all." As it currently stands, a student enrolled in a baccalaureate nursing program in the United States has access and opportunities for learning that may not be available to the same student in a limited resource setting. One important reason for this is a significant shortage of HRH in LMICs. The HRH constraints lead to a dearth of nurses, midwives, and faculty, crippling both the health care systems and the nursing educational systems. In Malawi, for example, there is less than one nurse for every 1,000 people (in the United States, there are 10 nurses per 1,000 people), and faculty shortages are also acute. Faculty do not have enough time and the resources required to design and teach a well-integrated and student-centered curriculum, conduct research, and continue their clinical practice simultaneously. Students often struggle to receive the attention and support from faculty that is essential to developing the competencies and skills required for patient care.

The United States is not immune to challenges within nursing education. There is a serious faculty shortage related to cuts in funding, an aging nursing workforce, poor compensation, and limited mentorship for new faculty. We have a growing student demographic that is culturally, ethnically, linguistically, and racially more diverse. A greater number of faculty—and one that is more diverse—is needed to ensure an educational system that is responsive and inclusive, ensuring that every student has an equal chance to achieve academically.

In recognition of the shortage of nurses and midwives, ministries of health and education in Malawi (and other limited-resource countries facing HRH shortages) are encouraging nursing schools to absorb more students. In one government university in Malawi, there are now over 200 nursing students in class. While student enrollment increases, faculty numbers have not increased to meet the demand. The student class with over 200 students may have just one faculty member responsible for both classroom and clinical teaching. As student numbers rise, clinical sites are overwhelmed and crowded. Additional clinical sites are identified, and students are spread across several distant sites, some up to 5 or more hours away. The ability to provide clinical instruction becomes financially and logistically impossible for faculty. Students are at times left alone in the clinical setting unsupervised, learning "by trial and error" (Msiska, Smith, & Fawcett, 2014). New graduates are known for strong theoretical knowledge but struggle with critical thinking and clinical competencies.

One way we can advance SDG 4 is to recognize the impact the faculty shortage has on both the quality of student learning and the ability of faculty to fully engage in their role, and respond by partnering with nursing academic institutions to build their capacity to provide excellence in nursing education that is responsive to national and local priorities and impacts individual and population health.

My work with Seed Global Health (Seed) hopes to support that need. Our mission is to strengthen health education and delivery of health care in countries facing such HRH shortages by working with partner countries to meet their long-term health care human resource needs. Our flagship program, the Global Health Service Partnership (GHSP), is a joint initiative with the Peace Corps, the U.S. President's Emergency Plan for AIDS Relief (PEPFAR), and our country sites. We work with partner countries to place U.S. nurses and doctors to work alongside local faculty to educate and mentor the next generation of medical and nursing professionals in Liberia, Malawi, Swaziland, Tanzania, and Uganda.

I have been humbled by the success stories that illustrate the power of this partnership to fortify local faculty efforts, giving local faculty the support they need to teach to their full role and provide students the attention they need to achieve academically. One of my favorite stories recently comes from Malawi. This is a case report of a third-year bachelor's of nursing student to her class and clinical faculty, a GHSP nurse educator who has focused the majority of her time with students in the skills lab and on the wards:

> I noticed my patient was very lethargic, had pale palms and conjunctiva, so I asked the nurse in charge if it would be OK to check his hemoglobin. It was 4.6, so we got a type and cross match and an order for a blood transfusion. I went to the lab to pick up the blood and they said it wouldn't be ready until tomorrow. I told them this child was very sick and needed it now and I wasn't leaving until they had it ready. The blood was hung right before the end of my shift. When I came back today, the child is awake, alert and had stable vital signs . . . he was ready for discharge.

Taken out of context, it may be hard to imagine why I tell this story again and again, celebrating the success of a nursing student who successfully made a critical assessment, advocated for timely interventions, safely administered a transfusion, and saved a little boy's life. Her story demonstrates the critical thinking skills and competencies that are the result of an educational system that has prioritized closing the gap in these areas, and we hope our partnership has helped, even just a small amount, toward that end.

Within our partner countries, I have had the privilege to work with nurse policy makers, deans, and faculty, such as Ms. Jasintha Mtengezo in Malawi: committed and passionate leaders in advancing equitable, quality nursing education. They educate us about the unique landscape of the state of nursing and nursing education in regard to the policies, education, and health care systems that inform our work. We listen and learn so that we can be responsive to the need—to the task. As Ms. Mtengezo comments: "Sustainability is living on the interest, not the principal." There will be no interest—no sustainability—if our fundamental approach is not responsive to the needs of our partners.

Ms. Mtengezo provides her perspective on SDG 4 and its application to nursing.

Quality Education and Nursing

Jasintha T. Mtengezo

Quality education is a tool to achieve sustainability in the health of individuals, communities, societies, and globally. In LMICs such as Malawi, there is a critical shortage of faculty to provide quality education to student nurses. If quality education is a tool to achieve sustainability, will LMICs with a significant shortage of HRH, like Malawi, achieve SDG 4? Education provides people the opportunity for lifelong learning, to help them find new solutions to the economic, societal, and environmental problems affecting their health. Sustainable development should be able to meet the needs of the society to improve the quality of life. Nurses operate through a lens of quality and safe care for the betterment of all they serve. Quality education both in the classroom and clinical area requires adequate faculty and clinical nurses to promote critical thinking skills in students. Critical thinking development is essential for the application of theory into practice. There is often a gap, particularly in countries with severe HRH shortages including Malawi. Critical thinking helps nurses solve problems they encounter in the field so that they can improve the delivery of nursing care for individual patients and families, and elevate the overall health care system and society's quality of life.

People should have a healthy and productive life. Eradicating poverty and reducing disparities in living standards is essential to achieve sustainable development and to meet the needs of the people. Global health organizations, such as Seed, support sustainable development by deploying nurses and other financial resources to these resource-constrained countries to ensure equity in human resources. Seed has been working in Malawi to address the critical shortage of health care human resources in the country to ensure equitable quality education and promote lifelong learning opportunities for all. To achieve sustainable development, LMICs including Malawi should think of ways of sustaining themselves with adequate local faculty to teach nurses rather than depending on donors or developmental partners to deploy nurses. The donor partners should think of investing in scholarships to train local faculty. About economics, sustainability is living on the *interest* rather than the *principal*. Sustainability means to be able to continue the work beyond the initial funding or support after the donor or partner has phased out. There is a need to have expatriate nurses at the same time train our local faculty for skills transfer so that we have enough human capital to provide sustained quality education to student nurses. Sustainable development requires societies' improved scientific understanding of their problem and requires them to be involved in self-directed mechanisms for ensuring sustainability. All people have natural rights to quality education and life supported by fairness and equality. Quality education has an impact on the individuals, communities, and society quality of life.

Education and Quality of Life

Quality education is the key to a nation's ability to develop and achieve sustainability. If basic education is low, the country's development remains low and hinders plans for sustainability. Quality education can enhance society's health status, reduce population growth rates, and raise the standards of living. Education facilitates the socialization process and participation in society, which in turn is associated with better health. Education reduces poverty by preparing individuals to contribute productively in work environments, increases opportunities for sustainable income and other opportunities, and lowers the risk of diseases and health problems. Education also improves decision making, which has a bearing on the quality of life. Good decision making depends on an educated society. Educational attainment strongly influences disease mortality and morbidity rates, health-related behaviors, economic status, and health knowledge in the following ways.

Education, Morbidity, and Mortality

Social determinants of health, such as level of education, directly correlate to health outcomes (Heiman & Artiga, 2015). Those with lower levels of education in all countries are more likely to have poorer general health and functional limitations. They will die at a younger age than those with higher education. In Malawi, in my clinical experience, I have observed that people with low education have been associated with communicable diseases like TB, HIV/AIDS, and other diseases such as diabetes and malnutrition due to lack of resources and poverty at different stages of the life cycle.

Education and Health Behaviors

With my experience in studying in the United States, I have also learned that in high-income countries, those with lower levels of education are less likely to engage in healthy behaviors and more likely to adopt unhealthy habits like physical inactivity, unhealthy diet, smoking, and risky sexual activity. In fact, research has confirmed my observation (Zimmerman, Woolf, & Haley, 2015). Physical activity maintains and improves health. It contributes to personal, social, and physical development. Knowledge of healthy dietary requirements is beneficial for maintaining and improving health, and avoiding obesity. Those with greater levels of education are more likely to eat more fruits, vegetables, and fiber and less fat than those with lower education levels. Those with lower levels of education are poor and more likely to be engaged in sex at a younger age, less likely to use contraceptives, and more likely to contract sexually transmitted diseases. Teaching people how to avoid dangers of contracting diseases is important in preventing the spread of diseases. While the provision of health care services is an important determinant of health, research has found that it is relatively weak when compared to the choices individuals make regarding behavior such as exercise, diet, and smoking in predicting health outcomes (Heiman & Artiga, 2015).

Education and Health Knowledge

Those with higher levels of education are likely to have greater knowledge of health conditions, adherence to treatments, better self-management skills, and are more likely to participate in prevention programs than those with lower levels of education. Even knowing what to do during emergency situations contributes to health. From experience as a nurse, those with lower levels of education have higher rates of hospital visits, hospitalization, and increased direct and indirect health care costs.

Education and Socioeconomic Status

Appropriate educational attainment strongly influences employment chances and income. Low family income can be a barrier to educational attainment. As is the case in Malawi, the population is socioeconomically disadvantaged leading to challenges for families to raise finances to send their children to school and colleges, which creates a critical shortage of health personnel. This fact greatly emphasizes the need for global nurses to partner with local nurses in improving human resources. In LMICs, students are less likely to benefit from quality education than their peers in high-income countries.

How Can Global Nurses Improve the Educational System?

The shortage of HRH worldwide adds to the challenges of providing safe and quality care to the public, especially in LMICs. The demand for higher education in the nursing profession has increased globally due to the increasing labor markets for highly skilled nurses. There is an expansion of educational qualifications for nurses both within and across countries, and transnational nursing organizations like the International Council of Nurses (ICN), which promotes standards for nursing and nursing education worldwide.

The nursing colleges in Malawi are engaged in various partnerships to raise the standards of nursing education in the country. The partnerships involve exchange programs for faculty and students. Global nurses are contracted as instructors in both classroom and clinical areas working in pairs with local faculty and staff. The skills are transmitted to local staff and ensure sustainability of the skills once the contracts expire. The higher income countries like the United States, Britain, and Australia accelerate the mobility of HRH, like global nurses, in resource-constrained settings where there is a great need. There is circulation of information, resources, and people, which improves on the numbers that teach and supervise student nurses in the clinical area.

As other people and nurses see how expatriate nurses discharge their duties, people start encouraging their children to seek quality education overseas from where those nurses come. Student nurses often travel overseas to attain their education or can be educated through distance learning. Some universities in Malawi have established branches overseas to provide quality education that contributes to the skills of an individual and improves individual income. Income is related to the level of education that people have. Higher education means higher lifetime income. Some educational partnership is provided through financial support through scholarships to nursing students with the aim of meeting the critical shortage of HRH. There is also a need for nurses to have international tools to improve the quality of education on a global scale.

Tools Needed to Improve the Quality of Education Worldwide

The tools needed to improve the status of quality of education include global standards for education, accreditation and regulatory bodies, resources, and strong leadership support. Global standards for nursing education ensure that practitioners are competent and provide quality care, and promote positive health outcomes among the populations they serve. Strong regulatory and accreditation bodies, both internationally and locally, are important to make sure that quality systems are in place, and that monitoring of the educational standards and quality of nurses is implemented. Resources include adequate financial, material and human resources, books, and computers. In LMICs, the material resources in colleges are inadequate. Global nursing and strong global partnerships within the profession will help in improving these resources and quality of education where the nurses are deployed. Strong leadership support is necessary for implementing policies. The leadership and subordinates need to share a unified commitment to the way duties are discharged, and how resources are allocated.

Education gives people lifelong learning to help them find new solutions to their economic, environmental, and societal problems that affect their health. Sustainable development should be able to meet the needs of the society to improve the quality of life. Quality education can lead to higher chances of finding better paying employment and more opportunities for sustainable development with health benefits for individuals, communities, and society.

Final Thoughts

It has been demonstrated that the more highly educated the nurse is at the bedside, the better the patient outcomes (American Association of Colleges of Nursing, 2015). The pediatric patient discussed earlier, cared for by a nursing student in a bachelor's of nursing program and supported by a master's-prepared clinical instructor, was discharged healthy and able to return to school, learn, grow, and contribute to his society. I will never forget the quiet words of a little Ugandan girl with cancer sitting on her hospital bed. "I just want to go back to school," she said. Having a compassionate and well-educated nurse at her bedside will increase the likelihood of her wish coming true and ensuring she becomes a future productive contributor to her community.

Through authentic, meaningful partnerships that honor reciprocity and bidirectional benefits, low-, middle-, and high-income countries can work together toward the common goal of ensuring inclusive and equitable education (including nursing education) and promote lifelong learning opportunities for all. To that end, Seed, GHSP, Malawi, and other partner country nursing institutions are committed to promoting excellence in nursing education that is responsive/ responsible to local priorities and impacts individual and population health, and will, ultimately, yield a positive influence on the education of communities across Africa and the world.

Achieve Gender Equality and Reduce Inequalities of All Kinds for All Peoples and Countries (SDGs 5 and 10)

Busisiwe Rosemary Bhengu

My point of departure is two SDGs as developed by the UN (2015), namely, SDG 5: Achieve gender equality and empower all women and girls, and SDG 10: Reduce inequality within and among countries. Literature maintains that poverty, gender, and place of birth are grave barriers to getting schooled. To be exact, poor, rural girls are the least likely to be in school (60 Million Girls, n.d.). Furthermore, this organization maintains that 56% of girls will never enter a classroom, compared to 41% out-of-school boys (60 Million Girls, n.d.). Besides being a girl, brought up in a rural area under very poor conditions, I lived in the peak of the apartheid regime in South Africa. There are things I never dreamt of but my quest for education made it possible, thanks to my father who seems to have been convinced by the saying that: "If you educate a man you educate an individual, but if you educate a woman you educate a family (nation)" (Kwegyir-Aggrey [1895–1927] as cited by Nyamidie, 1999). Dr. James Emmanuel Kwegyir-Aggrey was a scholar from Ghana most likely trying to convince parents to send their daughters to school and bring gender equality to the school system.

My History

I was born in Boksburg near Johannesburg in a family of 11 children though we grew up as eight children after three did not make it through infancy. My father was a migrant laborer who worked for a Catholic boarding school as a driver and handyman. He had a small house of two rooms built for our family within the premises of this boarding school. I was the sixth child in the family but grew up as number four after two of my siblings died before I was born.

When I turned 5 years old, my father decided we should relocate to the province from which he originally came because I was about to start school and he would not trust that I would like schooling in the city where "children do not behave well," according to him. *He* believed his girl must go to school in violation of the *cultural* belief that girls must not go to school. Indeed, we moved but he himself could not move with us because he was a laborer; he was not able to get a job on the farm to which we moved.

Schooling

I started school the following year in KwaZulu-Natal, then Natal. The place to which we moved had no school within a closer distance. We had to walk more than 10 kilometers every day to and from school, even when a school was eventually erected across the road; as Catholics we had to attend a Catholic school according to our church. Thunderstorms would find us walking and I am grateful today that we were never struck by lightning. Despite his minimal salary, my father managed to take us to a prestigious boarding school for high school. At the time, one did not even realize that this was a prestigious school, but it produced excellent results. I was lucky to excel and achieve for myself bursaries from the second year of high school on. I remember at one time having to choose between two offers of bursaries, but one required me to move to another school. I later learned in my adult age that this movement would have required me to become a spy for the apartheid government. Luckily my father would not allow me to change from a Catholic school. He would rather struggle with the fees not covered by my bursary.

Even as an adult, I cannot believe it myself when I saw the house I grew up in. How a family of six children (at the time) and two parents fit in that house is a wonder. But we had no choice; apartheid was at its peak with the Group Areas Act of 1950 and amended allocating residences according to racial groups. How the nuns kept us in that small house with this act . . . I still wonder.

A time most painful came when I realized how apartheid was really affecting me. It was a norm to have no identity document until 16 years. I could not complete high school final examinations without some identity document. This was not an identity document that my White counterparts carried. It was called a reference book, but locally it became known as a *dompas*. I am not sure which language this was because it is a mixture of Afrikaans and English. *Dom* means "stupid" in Afrikaans and *pas* as in "pass law." To get my reference book I had to produce a birth certificate. It became difficult to get this certificate and I could not understand why. I knew my birth date and gave it. They just had to trace my name.

I later found out that the names I have were not the names recorded when I was born. My mother explained that when we were born in hospital, she had to wait for the nuns who employed my father to name us from the names of the saints. The midwives who assisted my mother could not wait for the names, so they just gave us any name. Many as we were, my mother could not remember these names because they were hurriedly given and no record was given to her. She could remember only our firstborn brother who was named after the doctor who delivered him. Hence our names could not be traced to issue the reference books. This was difficult for me, but thanks to God, I could secure a birth certificate with current names and wrong place of birth. Otherwise I would not be able to secure a reference book to be able to write the final high school examination. I would have dropped out of school at that stage. I was later able to secure my real identity document when I was married in 1978, at the peak of the struggle for liberation from apartheid.

While apartheid hit me so much with schooling, staying in a rural area had its impact in my life. As indicated earlier, I landed in a prestigious boarding school with students coming from well-known cities like Johannesburg, Durban, and so on. They wore fashion, they spoke rich, and had exposure to some amenities we had never seen. They would call us names such as *plaas japitjies,* meaning "farm girls." But here we are, survived.

Choosing a Career

My other sore point in my life was choosing a career. My choice was not dependent on my own cognitive ability but my family circumstances, which was emphasized in our career guidance at school. My second brother had been to a university for medicine but could not complete because he had become engaged with apartheid struggle movements and failed. My father could not take another family member to a university to "waste his money." I had to divert to something else. I opted for laboratory science, then called "medical technology" and offered in technical colleges. These colleges had residences for male students and I was informed that I had to rent a room outside the school as a girl. But I would get a minimal salary. My father could not accept a young girl renting a room outside school. I then had to divert to nursing, which was also paying minimal salary. I could not enjoy my salary, though, because I had to support my family. I think this has to do with being a woman. However, this was a blessing in disguise because I have made such progress in my nursing career that I still doubt it would have been possible to make in medicine.

Nursing Practice and Education

As fate would have it, as a nurse, I had to work with the White male–dominated medical counterparts in a city where I trained. We would be called "nursie" (small nurse) to minimize us. At some stage in my training career, a White male doctor gave me a clap, frustrated from a failed resuscitation. I will not detail the circumstances under which he clapped me. This was 2 weeks after a Black RN was clapped in the operating room. On reporting, a Black matron was requested to give me a talk on how in nursing we must expect such. To this matron it was normal. What brainwashing!

I worked with an RN at some stage who was afraid of any authority in the hospital. She would even run away from a phone call. One day a young doctor who had realized that this RN was running away refused to be assisted by me for ward rounds as I was still a student nurse. He waited until the RN had to show. When the RN came, he yelled nonsensical orders at her, one after the other. He shouted at her and kept saying to her "trolley" and she would jump to the trolley without instruction on what to do at the trolley. He then would say "patient" and she would jump to the patient without having established what his exact request pertaining to this patient included. In the end the doctor repeated: "trolley," "patient," "trolley," "patient," and so on. The RN kept jumping between the trolley and the patient just touching these. Mind you, this was not a young RN and the doctor was very young, and this happened in front of the patients. This was one of the motivations to study and advance professionally. I was thinking of a different career because at the time university education did not exist for Black nurses. As fate would have it, when I completed training, I approached a distance education university (University of South Africa) for a bachelor of science degree because I was interested in mathematics and physiology and zoology. In response, I was given a prospectus for what I requested, including information on a graduate nursing degree. By then I was married and I agreed with my husband that I continue with what I had started, that is, nursing. I have never regretted the decision.

Work Career

My work career, though progressive, was not smooth either. I worked for 5 years as an RN in an intensive care hospital for neurosurgery, cardiothoracic surgery, and coronary care. This hospital had separate sections for Whites and Blacks. I obviously worked in a Black section but soon neurosurgery units were merged with much publicity, mixing even male and female patients. I remember this story in an old newspaper reporting interviews with the hospital management. This was all due to a very forceful professor of neurosurgery who would shout at us and throw things all over. I was moved when I met him years later after 1994, the year of liberation in South Africa. I was also a university lecturer then and he was dean of the medical school. We met at a workshop in the hospital in which we both worked. And he said we needed our own Truth and Reconciliation Committee (TRC), probably remembering what he did to us. It was heartwarming, in the spirit of Mandela, to know that he realized the wrong he did to us as a doctor and a White.

I grew and developed in this college including going back to my previous workplace to study for an intensive care diploma, which I passed with distinction. Another interesting experience of inequality at this time was when we asked the matron in charge of the hospital to present an in-service lecture. In her introductory paragraph, she said that we should understand her because she had never worked with Blacks as colleagues but as general assistants. This she was repeating from her inaugural speech.

I eventually landed at the university from which I finally retired. The nursing department was very progressive and encouraged research and scholarship. I started academic life late for research grants, which seemed to favor the younger nurse scientists. There were age restrictions in most of the applications for grants. I am proud to have resisted these rough times and I am now well published and continuing to do so.

I am afraid I have hit another form of inequality related to my age. During my teaching time I used to engage students in debates on distributive justice in which we supported a utilitarian approach to distribution of resources in hospital. With chronic illnesses one may find patients needing longer hospital stays or management; yet the hospitals are overcrowded with no beds or technology, such as dialysis machines, which are sometimes unavailable. Young patients with no comorbidities who may be discharged earlier and with fewer complications are prioritized. Money talks sometimes if you can afford a private hospital, but if you cannot, medical insurance in South Africa does not cover it.

As fate would have it, one day immediately after my retirement, I met with my cardiac surgeon colleague at the airport lounge and he shared with me how cardiac surgery had decreased because funds had been diverted to HIV and AIDS. In response, I expressed concern on how chronic diseases among the old would warrant such surgery. My colleague loudly howled at me saying, "At your age you would need aggressive treatment." For God's sake, I was 60 years old and active both physically and cognitively, and was economically sound. I was disturbed but then I have gone through that debate. It is my turn now.

Can We, as Global Nurses, Stop Inequality?

Nurses have guiding principles and ethics captured in the ICN's pledge of service that just need to be upheld. This pledge emphasizes, among others:

> I promise to take care of the sick with all the skill and understanding I possess, without regard to race, creed, color, politics, or social status, sparing no effort to conserve life, to alleviate suffering, and promote health.

The advocacy role of the nurses at different levels must be emphasized, realized, monitored, and evaluated. Nelson (1988) maintains that advocacy has moved from a posture of mediating for clients to acting as guardian of the clients' rights to autonomy and free choice both as individuals and as groups.

Person-centered care (PCC) according to the IOM (2001) emphasizes respect for a person's preferences, needs, and values, ensuring that all these guide the clinical decisions and interventions to promote self-determination and freedom of choice. PCC must go hand-in-hand with customer satisfaction surveys that are analyzed and used for improvement.

Academic institutions work in three pillars, namely practice, education, and training, including community engagement. Nurse academics could take advantage of these pillars to empower the disadvantaged, especially women, bearing in mind the benefit of teaching a girl or woman is teaching a nation.

Globalization should be encouraged to open borders and promote interconnectedness and interdependence among countries allowing free transfer of wealth, goods, and services across national borders. Sustainability should, however, be one of the objectives to be addressed from the very beginning. Higher income countries could partner with lower income countries for special projects to distribute wealth and curb inequality.

Final Thoughts

Reflection on my life journey, especially imposed by apartheid and inequality, makes me walk tall having gone through rough patches and resisted obstacles. I continue to live my life goal of reaching for the sky. This is particularly important because I fulfilled my father's wish of an educated girl irrespective of the norm at the time that girls need not be educated. That I have gone through almost all types of inequality, namely gender, racial, age, geographic, and occupational (nurse versus doctor) is a miracle well lived. I appreciate my parents, my father who actively assisted me to win this battle and my mother who was always emotionally engaged in support of my life journey. I have indeed extended my education to my siblings through financial support from my meager nursing salary. I have adopted some students at the university, assisting them financially. I have also been privileged to participate in a multimillion dollar project on primary health care for empowerment of rural women in collaboration with McMaster University in Canada. My article emanating from this project bears testimony of my contribution: Bhengu (2010). The SDGs may not directly benefit me in my lifetime, but continue to challenge me to contribute to the fight for other girls and oppressed people everywhere.

Clean Water and Sanitation (SDG 6)

Olivia Bahemuka

In its document, *The Future of Nursing: Leading Change, Advancing Health*, the IOM (2011) calls upon nurses to embrace the transformative role of leadership as full partners along with other health professions in order to achieve the vision of improved health systems in the United States. The need and significance of nursing's collaborative transformative leader role in health care for achieving improved health for all populations is further emphasized at the global level. Thus, it is worth reflecting on what nursing's role is as we move from the Millennium Development Goals (MDGs) to SDGs around the globe. To accomplish the latter, I contemplated how nursing has dealt with the practice challenges brought about due to lack of access to clean water and adequate sanitation. I considered the nursing experiences and contributions to addressing the issues of access to safe drinking water, general hygiene, and sanitation, seeking to draw some light on how nurses today can proceed to engage effectively in this matter. So, focusing on what some may call a "non-nursing issue"—clean water and sanitation—SDG 6, previously categorized under "environmental sustainability" (MDG 7), I will attempt to suggest how nurses as transformative leaders can contribute to this goal attainment.

Nurses Taking on the Challenge of Access to Clean Water and Sanitation in LMICs

The world rejoiced at the resolve by world leaders in 2000 to fight poverty and to improve the well-being for all, which resulted in the eight MDGs. Specifically, a focus was put on LMICs where these challenges are most pronounced. Not only is water and sanitation recognized as a basic human right, but also as essential for services rendered for any given population's health and well-being (Cumming, Elliot, Overbo, & Bartram, 2014). Despite the major strides made, it is known worldwide that access to improved water sources and quality sanitation remains a challenge facing many LMICs (Bain et al., 2012). The contribution to the burden of disease due to lack of access to good drinking water and adequate sanitation is well documented (Bliss, 2009). Reflecting on my personal experience in global health involvement, I recalled witnessing nurses at the forefront grappling with challenges of access to clean water and sanitation (ACWS), both in practice and in their patients' communities.

The problem of clean water, hygiene, and sanitation as faced by nurses in the care of their patients, is due largely to ill-equipped health facilities. From 2000 to 2004, while visiting Uganda, East Africa with various health teams and providing support to health centers and sometimes rural hospitals, I observed that nurses did not have handwashing stations nor toilet facilities that were adequate for both staff and patients. On many occasions nurses had to depend on the patient's family to provide adequate water to meet the patient's needs: hydration, medication administration, bathing, and so on. Working in this type of environment made it difficult for nurses and other health professionals to provide the necessary patient teaching on hygiene, thus enabling missed opportunities for quality health service provision. In addition, nurses were unable to role-model best practice hygiene for their patients and families, which in turn also contributed to both nurse and patient/family dissatisfaction, as well as distrust in the system at large.

It was inadequate access to water and poor sanitation of health facilities that escalated the spread of the Zimbabwe cholera outbreak in 2008, leading to rioting of health workers—including nurses and the residents of affected communities. Much effort has since been rendered in both Uganda and Zimbabwe where handwashing and safe drinking water stations have been improvised on ward facilities in most of the health centers and hospitals. However, much is still needed for the sustainability of the provision of adequate, safe, and accessible drinking water and toileting facilities in the health care infrastructure in many LMICs. Hence the urgent need for nursing to be innovative and lead the necessary interventions to make sure nursing practice role-models the message of safe drinking water and adequate sanitation to all and continues to educate the public regarding its importance.

Furthermore, the issue of clean water and sanitation has challenged nurses as they worked among their communities seeking to improve the health of the populations. The latter is mostly in relation to children under age 5 and maternal health. A Cochrane systematic review on decreasing diarrhea in children by improving water quality emphasized the lack of good sources of water and sanitation as contributing to diarrhea and mortality in children under age 5 (Clasen et al., 2015). Similarly, studies have associated childhood problems like dysentery and helminths infections to lack of access to safe drinking water, sanitation, and hygiene (WASH; Hutton & Chase, 2016). Community health nurses in LMICs have been providing and continue to provide patient/family education in communities where accessing clean water or having adequate sanitary facilities is a problem.

As a nursing student with a team from the Vial Program of Nursing in North Carolina, in collaboration with two stakeholders (the First Presbyterian Church of Uganda [FPCU] and the then young Makerere University [UM] School of Nursing), I participated in such endeavors in the summers of 1998–2000. Our visiting teams supported and worked closely with one of the first baccalaureate students in Uganda (then a community health nurse—Dr. Rose Chalo Nabirye, the current acting dean of the school of health sciences at University of Makerere); we provided health education on general hygiene, teaching about boiling drinking water and its safekeeping, prevention of anthelmintics, and malaria. Additionally, joined by local village leaders, small teams went house to house discussing safe distances and ideal locations for toiletry facilities, demonstrating how and what should be done in Mpigi and Wakiso districts respectively.

Although not documented, as is the case for many nursing contributions in LMICs nurses in Uganda had been involved in such projects for years, collaborating with visiting public health personnel. In my formative and school-aged years in Kampala district in Uganda, I remember health personnel visiting my home bringing nutritious "soya" muffins and iron-enriched powdered milk from "Mwana Mugimu" (Health Child), a program that would teach parents about good nutritious foods for children, prevention of malnutrition, and safekeeping of food; and they would check our teeth as well, making referrals to the dental school when needed. These same people carried and would give us deworming medications. I have a vivid childhood memory of the small, brownish, terrible-tasting pills for worms and "Antepar" Syrup (which I grew to know as "oral piperazine citrate" by Glaxo). Recalling my primary boarding school days in Gayaza, a town of Wakiso district where regulation did not check schools to attest to the safety of drinking and bathing water sources, students received water from unsafe sources and most of us had worms. Indeed, like in most elementary schools then and a few now, toileting facilities were inadequate for the number of students; thus, schools did nothing to model the significant message of safe drinking water and sanitation to students.

In Mpigi district, nurses were involved not only in bringing awareness and in teaching communities about the significance of clean water sources to family health, but also mobilized the people to help each other in building ventilated pit latrines for improved sanitation. Similarly, working with faith-based organizations in the area, nurses spearheaded train-the-trainer sessions for young people to spread the word in the communities about sources of safe drinking water, general hygiene, and recommended safe sanitation options. In 2005, with a team from Charlotte, North Carolina, a group of nurses, nurse practitioners, and other health professions in collaboration with Kibale hospital, conducted village-to-village house visits in Kaswa, Fort Portal, and Kagadi, Bunyoro district, providing health education, talking to residents about clean water sources, adequate sanitation, and malaria prevention, in addition to performing well-check clinics.

Nurses have addressed the clean water challenge in maternity wards by buying charcoal to boil water and, at times, buying bottled water for their patients to help with hydration as well as fending off possible water infections in laboring mothers. As recent as 2015, while supporting a colleague during clinical practice supervision of her midwifery baccalaureate students at one of the district hospitals in Rwanda, we were forced not only to provide bottled water for the patients but also to purchase some passion and mango juice for the patients needing both hydration and nutrition. This midwife, while modeling for her students the need for clean water for patients in labor ward and maternity, confessed that just like safe drinking water, sanitation was still lacking in many district hospitals.

I further had the opportunity, during completion of my Afya Bora Fellowship, to work with various nurses in charge of HIV/AIDS services. I met and supported nurses working in community health clinics, caring for HIV pregnant mothers (prevention of mother-to-child transmission—PMTCT) in the central division of Kampala, Uganda. The nurses not only conducted classes for the women about the relationship of drinking clean boiled water to protect the fetuses and prevent complications of infections from poor water sources, but they collaborated with community health workers to visit these mothers at home to ensure the overall and holistic well-being of these mothers. Studies have suggested an association between poor health outcomes for pregnant women, especially HIV mothers, and the lack of water, sanitation, and hygiene (Campbell, Benova, Gon, Afsana, & Cumming, 2015).

In a rural district hospital in western Uganda, there is a sister in charge—a nurse for over 25 years—who bought and installed a drinking water station for patients and handwashing stations for staff after concluding that while waiting for the promised new building, her staff could meanwhile do their best to improve their patients' outcomes. In addition, nurses have worked in collaboration with other agencies to enlist safe water wells for the community; an example is a water well at Zana Community Center Church and School in Wakiso district. While I believe there are many nurses who have contributed to the improvement of the health of the population in LMICs, there is still much to be done.

Nursing as a Transformative Leader to Attain the Clean Water and Sanitation Goal

The IOM (2011) call mentioned earlier calls for nurses to be transformative leaders alongside other health disciplines. What does this mean to me and to us in light of achieving SDG 6 in LMICs?

Transformational leaders have been said to be visionary, with the ability to clearly communicate a vision to followers, and then motivate others to attain the vision through innovative creativity and accountability (IOM, 2011). Today's nurses, wherever they work, need to contemplate how they can engage others in health service, as well as patients and their families, and the community to achieve the overall vision of health and well-being for all. In the context of LMICs and the achieving of good water sources and adequate sanitation, though nurses have made prior contributions, we must continue to engage in this effort. So, moving forward, what actions should nurses engage in as transformative leaders to attain the vision/goal of water and sanitation in the countries with low resources? I answer the question by discussing my various global practice experiences to aid you in answering this call of transformational leading. While the measures I may describe may not be new to you, it is the approach and use of them that I request you to consider.

Global nurses must remain actively engaged with their respective initiatives, even with the trials often experienced with funding and support; this aspect in the transformational leader is that of *self-awareness*. This quality when employed by nurses as leaders can enable them to effectively work with others to accomplish not only what they are capable of but to attain more than the set goals articulated. For example, begin by urging fellow colleagues to practice within their scope and ensure best basic nursing practices within the context. While practice settings may be challenging in their provision of a safe sanitary environment, nurses have also been found to be disengaged, failing to realize that they are part of the health infrastructure that will dictate the quality necessary for change. It is possible for nurses to ensure that wards, clinics, and all equipment thereof to be used in service are kept clean, that water stations provided remain clean and are adequately supplied. Nurses should be able to actively engage cleaning services as fellow providers of the overall product of health and thus motivate them to feel as part of the team so as to take pride in their contribution to the end goal of good patient outcomes. Unfortunately, in most LMICs, the dividing lines between staff both in hospitals and outpatient services are very sharp; the cleaning crew is not regarded as part of the team, and this goes for other low-cadre members of the health staff. Nurses who are self-aware will be able to appreciate not only their role in achieving the vision of water and sanitation but will recognize the need to respectfully include others in the health sector in order to realize the common vision of SDG 6.

We must all advocate for clean water and sanitation in practice areas, as well as communities. Going forward, nursing needs to be active and persistent in advocating for the attainment of good water sources and adequate sanitation for all. Bartram and Platt (2010) point out the need for health professionals to understand their role as part of the health sector in decreasing the disease burden contributed to by lack of water and sanitation. Nurses in LMICs need to be seen at the forefront in their advocacy role for health care services and seek collaboration with NGOs: writing nursing grants, publishing to spread awareness, and offering education—efforts that, however small, bring about change in practice for the health of the people. For example, nurses today in Kenya, Rwanda, Tanzania, and Uganda can collaborate for studies through the East African Community to advocate with data relevant to issues of water and sanitation to the greater community. Sadly, the research has been left mostly to physicians in many of these countries as nursing sits aside waiting for recognition from country ministries of health, many of which still fail to accurately identify and promote nursing's significant contribution to the health of their populations. However, nursing, knowing its impact on the latter, has not documented its narrative effectively and is challenged to speak with data that supports its contributions. It is to this end that I say nursing in LMICs has to embrace the transformative role of leadership, advocating for patients and for self by making clear its contributions, and consistently documenting opportunities for improvement in water and sanitation resources. It is only through these integral steps that nursing will be able to attract other stakeholders and influence regulation and policy related to SDG 6 among others.

Nursing can lead in transformative ways by incorporating innovative measures in academic nursing education, engaging increased numbers of student nurses in thinking about their role in attaining water and sanitation for the communities in which they live and plan to work. For example, through engaging in process improvement and evidence-based practice projects between nursing schools and clinical practice areas, the nursing profession can affect much change in the current state of affairs in the health of our population. For example, in the first 6 months of my postdoc fellowship in Uganda while I worked with Dr. Peter Elyanu (at the time program officer leading the scale-up programs for Adolescent and Pediatric HIV services, AIDS Control Program [ACP], through a national supportive retrospective analysis), it was found that one of the reasons why HIV mothers were not bringing back their infants for testing as per guidelines until 18 months was their having to line up twice for their medicines at the adult clinic and then having to come also to the antenatal for the baby. A simple solution was immediately determined to keep the mothers and babies together (pairing) as part of HIV follow-up services so that both could be seen at the same time—a majority of these services were provided by nurses. If there had been engagement in process improvement on nursing's part, nurses could have easily found this on their own and contributed to the national goal of decreasing new pediatric infections! Many are such missed opportunities by nurses in LMICs that could further increase the nursing profession's advantage of being included on the health policy table.

However, to engage in such as discussed previously, nursing's image and attitude about its role as a health provider in the LMICs must be transformed. Nurses have to acknowledge the relevance and significance of their practice in bringing about positive change in the health and well-being of people. Though the wages of nurses may still be low, the saving of a human life and procuring human betterment is priceless. Nurses have to believe in their work and not measure it solely in monetary value. Thus, as they teach, mentor, and coach upcoming nurses, showing them the power and value of nursing practice in bringing about change in human lives, they would be motivating and empowering the profession to a higher call of service (IOM, 2011). The latter is one of the qualities of transformational leadership, which I argue nursing is very capable of embracing going forward to realize the vision of SDG 6. Additionally, in this role nursing can seek to work with primary, secondary, and higher institutions of learning to heighten awareness of the necessity of water and sanitation. School nurses can creatively develop ways to effectively educate younger students and help them to understand the relationship of the burden of disease and SDG 6. Borrowing from what has been done in the fight against HIV, students can be encouraged and motivated through drama and songs to participate in the fight, only this time of the necessity of water and sanitation to human life. Nursing can take the lead in ensuring that children's experiences in schools help them to become champions of hygiene, water, and sanitation in their nations.

Global nurses must continually revitalize their role in the promotion of health education at the community level. Nurses in LMICs need to spearhead network groups and task forces in the community in order to influence the change of improved water and sanitation. We must involve community health volunteers (CHVs) during health visits who can "beat the drum" for community mobilization and collaborate to achieve and maintain improved sanitation for widespread well-being. The advantage of utilizing CHVs, particularly in LMICs where culture tends to be more collectivist as opposed to individualist in nature, is that CHVs' constant presence helps patients to know they are seen and supported directly by their community, thereby leading to increased patient trust and improved patient–provider relationships. For example, in Rwanda, the position of CHV is part of the *omudugudu*, a local government cell, and is responsible to check on the health of the citizens in the cell and to communicate as per the given hierarchy any health issues to the next level. It is up to nursing to strategically use and intelligently partner with existing governing systems to realize the nursing goals; and eventually heighten the visibility of nursing's contributions as well to the uninformed public.

Last, nursing can actively seek to resurrect child health days for deworming and nutritional visits still aimed at educating, whether through demonstration or simulation, so as to empower the community for sustainability of measures employed. This can be combined with engaging the media's assistance. The media in many LMICs seeks opportunities to collaborate with the health sector in educating the community. Unfortunately, the media has been labeled as an enemy by many health professionals because of it highlighting negligence or medical error. However, as transformative leaders, nursing can leverage with one stone's throw through the media an improved image of nursing while promoting nursing's contributions as a valued team member of the health care sector and advocate for population ACWS.

Final Thoughts

In conclusion, the role of nursing as a transformational leader in achieving SDG 6 is crucial and varied. The opportunities discussed earlier are by no means the only ones, but are intended simply to introduce the conversation and promote the active involvement of more nurses serving in the countries with need. As members of the health care team, nurses today need to provide research on the impact of water and sanitation on patient care as related to nursing practice in clinical areas, educational settings, and the community. With documentation and identified measures, nursing can collaborate with interprofessional partners to influence country plans and budgets for water and sanitation as well as other related factors that affect human health and well-being. Nurses must be relentless in their pursuit of clear and consistent documentation and not allow themselves to be defined or described by medicine.

I would like to herald all those nurses laboring in LMICs who are doing great work, for though they may be unsung heroes, their patients and communities know them. My sincere argument is that even with the economic, political, and social challenges that may be posed to us in LMICs, nursing is able to collaborate and lead alongside other health professionals and interested stakeholders to achieve the improved health and optimal well-being of the populations we serve.

Cities and Communities (SDG 11)

Patricia Moreland

In 2012, I arrived in Rwanda as part of the first cohort of faculty for the HRH Program. I was assigned to Kabgayi School of Nursing and Midwifery (KASNM), located 25 miles southwest of Kigali. KASNM is the oldest school of nursing and midwifery in Rwanda, opened in 1949 by the Catholic diocese. Students at KASNM attend 3 years of training, graduating with an Advanced Diploma (A1) degree.

On arrival in Kabgayi, I was warmly greeted by highly motivated, passionate people who quickly accepted me into their homes and lives. The resilience of the Rwandan people and belief in a brighter future was moving. As part of my role, I collaborated with Rwandan colleagues on the development of courses that addressed the health needs of the Rwandan population. Through this collaboration, I learned the challenges and cultural influences that impact health outcomes and health care utilization in the rural area. Poverty, decreased access to health care, and lack of education contribute to the health disparities in the rural area.

Rwanda is largely an agrarian society with 84% of the population living in rural areas and depending on subsistence farming for their primary income. Food insecurity is a persistent problem (National Institute of Statistics of Rwanda [NISR], 2015). The rural health system includes 45,000 village-based community health workers, 478 nurse-staffed health centers, and 35 district hospitals with generalist physicians (NISR, 2015). Access to specialists (including internists and pediatricians) is largely limited to facilities in the capital, Kigali, and to the two university hospitals.

Urban–rural health disparities exist in neonatal and under-5 mortality rates, chronic malnutrition, and prevalence of malaria. Mortality in the urban areas is generally lower than in the rural areas. For example, neonatal mortality rates are 15 per 1,000 live births in the urban area compared to 24 in the rural area (NISR, 2015). The urban–rural gap is wider for under-5 mortality rates (51 deaths versus 70 deaths per 1,000 live births; National Institute of Statistics of Rwanda, 2015). Variation in children's nutrition status by residence is also quite evident. Chronic malnutrition is lower in the urban areas compared to rural areas (23.7 versus 40.6; NISR, 2015). Malaria, a major cause of morbidity and mortality in Rwanda, is lower in children aged 6 to 59 months in urban compared to rural areas (0.3 versus 2.6; NISR, 2015).

Social inequalities between urban and rural areas impact the prevention and treatment of disease. The association between poverty, disease vulnerability, and outcomes is well documented (Alsan, 2011). Unsafe water sources and inadequate sanitation and hygiene are prime contributors to infections. With respect to residence, urban households are more likely than rural households to use improved drinking water (91% vs. 69%). In addition, 31% of households in rural areas use unsafe drinking water, as compared with 9% of those in urban areas (NISR, 2015). In addition, significant gaps exist in educational attainment between urban and rural areas. In urban areas 10% of women and 7% of men have no education compared to 21% of women and 15% of men in the rural areas. Higher levels of maternal education have been positively associated with lower levels of malnutrition and increased health care utilization (NISR, 2015). As the urbanization of cities continues at the current and rapid pace, these disparities may increase and further create complications in effective care delivery.

Cultural beliefs related to traditional medicine impact access and treatment of illness. Delay in the access of care may result in worsening of health outcomes. Nurses must educate populations early in the trajectory of their illness to avoid complications and poor outcomes. Trust and confidence in nurses and other health care providers must be gained by the respectful treatment of patients. Lack of confidence in health care providers may contribute to accessing traditional healers and delay in treatment.

The disease pattern in Rwanda is changing from infectious to chronic illness (NISR, 2015). Noncommunicable diseases (NCDs) are emerging as a public health concern as urbanization and life expectancy increase. According to the Rwandan MOH *Health Management Information Systems Strategic Plan* (MOH, 2013), NCDs accounted for at least 51.86% of all district hospital outpatients' consultation and 22.3% of district hospital hospitalization during the period from January to December 2013 (NISR, 2015). Cardiovascular disease, hypertension, stroke, cancer, diabetes, chronic respiratory diseases, injuries, and disabilities are common problems (Alleyne et al., 2013).

Although the etiologies and pathologies of noncommunicable and communicable diseases may appear to be exclusively opposed, NCDs in Rwanda and other LMICs have both traditional (unhealthy diet, physical inactivity, alcohol consumption, and smoking) and nontraditional causes (rheumatic heart disease and cardiomyopathies, HIV-associated malignancies, impact of malaria on epilepsy, impact of hepatitis B and C virus on liver cirrhosis, as well as high levels of household air pollution [causing chronic respiratory disease]; NISR, 2015). This double burden of disease requires the prevention and control of risk factors related to both infectious and noncommunicable diseases.

As urbanization increases in Rwanda, the changes in the physical and social environment and lifestyle will result in an increase in NCDs and accident-related disabilities. The role of the nurse in responding to these health challenges includes the identification of joint risk factors for NCDs, including diabetes, chronic pulmonary disease, cancers, and TB, at the health center level. Vaccinating against the human papilloma virus (HPV) and hepatitis B virus (HBV) will decrease cervical cancer and prevent liver disease. Reducing infections and deficiencies in pregnancy, such as malaria and anemia, will reduce fetal and maternal mortality, prematurity, and low birth weight (Alwan, 2011). Preventing malnutrition will decrease chronic illness in adulthood.

Final Thoughts

The role of the nurse in the Post-2015 Agenda includes collaborating with governments and policy makers to recognize the relationship between disease and poverty and to drive policies that address major environmental threats and risk factors for NCDs. Improving the health system infrastructure and increasing human resources needed for the prevention and treatment of NCDs while maintaining progress in infectious diseases is a challenge faced in LMICs. Innovative programs, such as the HRH Program, currently beginning its 5th year in Rwanda as of this writing, will address capacity building in health care providers and support sustainability.

How do we educate nurses to become an active voice in the policy-making process? The ICN emphasizes the importance of nurses being politically active in health policy development to improve access to quality care and advance the profession of nursing (Benton, 2012). To participate in the political arena, nurses need leadership skills and knowledge of policy development. Nursing education must be revised to include courses and content related to political and regulatory practice. In addition to knowledge, nurses must feel empowered to speak in the public forum. Empowerment must occur at both individual and organizational levels. Individually, nurses are empowered when their voice is heard in the clinical setting and when they are recognized as an essential member of the interprofessional team. At an organizational level, nurses are empowered through participation in national organizations and associations that influence health policy development.

In the African context, empowerment of nurses is often difficult due to the traditional patriarchal system (Shariff, 2014). Recognition of the essential role that nurses play in the health care system is frequently not observed. In this environment, decisions are made from the top-down; therefore the influence of the nurse is limited. As global citizens, we must unite to support our colleagues to further advance the nursing profession. Cultural norms must be addressed with sensitivity while strengthening the role of the nurse.

PLANET

Clean Energy (SDG 7)

Lynn Keegan

We have come a long way from coal miner's black lung disease and Appalachian and northeastern cities' carbon-coated dust fallout of the past century in the United States. As a society, we have realized the need to create new industry and innovations and have invested in the necessary research and development to that end: to better clean and refine the natural resources we depend on to create the clean energy that we all use and create new products and technology.

For example, in just a few decades we have witnessed new water- and electricity-sparing appliances and devices, natural resource refining, and other technologies that have resulted in exciting new clean energy methodology. Consider in our contemporary homes and commercial industry, we now have machines that both conserve and recycle water, industrial and human waste products, as well as many new hybrid models for automobiles and other energy-driven machines that use two or more methods to deliver energy. In our family, for example, we drive a hybrid Prius car that not only uses standard gasoline fuel, but also when driving, the engine is devised to create its own battery charger thus yielding considerably less gas consumption. The hybrid models offer 40 to 50 miles per gallon of gasoline versus 18 to 22 in standard cars. Yes, its purchase price is a bit higher than a standard combustion engine, but when one keeps a vehicle in the family for many years, the cost savings by using the gas-saving hybrids save money not only for the family, but prevent tremendous negative impact on the environment. Now new all-electric cars are on the roads and, once further evolved and made available to the mass market, we will see a greater reduction in the use of fossil fuels.

As we extrapolate from our individual homes to the collective, say in our nursing day-to-day practices, how can we foster and support affordable and clean energy behaviors in the profession? First and foremost, as in most settings, we can serve as role models. For example, as our colleagues see us arrive to work in an energy-saving vehicle, we might have an opportunity to explain why we drive it. Because we are conscious and knowledgeable about the importance of clean, affordable energy, our everyday behavior will model how we use all work facilities resources. As we move through the day we can commit to simple but effective energy-saving behaviors such as adjusting window coverings to mask the heat of sunlight entering spaces during the hot summer, thus lowering the need for expensive air-conditioning to cool the room. The converse is true in the winter; adjust the environment to utilize natural sunlight to heat spaces, thereby decreasing the need to crank up the resource using energy to generate more artificial heat. In the winter we can wear sweaters and turn down the thermostat that uses fossil fuels to heat and in the summer wear lightweight, cotton fabrics so we can use less air-conditioning. All around us, every day, there are so many instances that we can apply our knowledge and learned skills to both teach and model environmentally conscious behavior.

During just this past decade, it has been a joy to observe the many new inventions moving into so many public spaces. Multiple airports are now powered by vast surrounding fields of solar panels. Throughout the United States, mountainsides, great plains, and sea coasts support legions of windmills that utilize underground pipes to transport clean energy to all regions. In Europe and Asia many communities sport solar panels on residential rooftops to heat the homes' hot water tanks.

Final Thoughts

In summary, as nurses we can call on our clean knowledge as we serve on workplace committees and contribute to our individualized settings. Let us live from a place of heightened consciousness and learned conservation skills as we live and model for a more affordable, cleaner environment for all. Let us take this knowledge about affordable, clean energy and apply it to our workplace and community-based settings. If each of us becomes an advocate at policy-making levels we can become a mighty, united force for positive change for all of us who share the planet.

Responsible Consumption and Production (SDG 12)

Lynn Keegan

One of the old adages is "you are what you eat." It is easy to add other phrases related to "you are what you: read, speak, relate, and so on" but for now, let us stick with this elemental question: What do you eat? In high-income countries, in an era of thousands of choices from hundreds of food sources, your answer would probably be complex. In lower income countries, where selection may be limited, fast foods might be being introduced into the market, and reliable meats and delicacies may be reserved for special occasions, your answer might depend more on cost and access.

The responsible and knowledgeable individual who has both access and adequate economic means would probably answer, "I eat a large selection of organic fruits and vegetables, whole grains, with occasional condiment-sized servings of fish and meats, most of which are locally grown and raised." Those who are more aware of the environmental impacts of how food is raised and prepared or who have taken particular ethical stances on food consumption may respond that they are vegetarian or vegan. But, is this really true either of you or the community at large? Unfortunately, likely neither you nor the general population follows this ideal food consumption pattern. Why is that? Probably not for lack of knowledge, for during the past few decades all of us have learned so much about where the purest, healthiest food comes from and why we should be making more socially, environmentally, and health conscious choices when it comes to dietary intake. So, why don't we *do* it?

Why we do not eat wisely can be traced to a number of factors including old habits, costly healthier choices, pallet satisfaction, and not wanting to or caring about making healthy changes. Solutions to this primary food consumption problem can be partially achieved through the delivery of intensive education from infancy to old age by showcasing good role models, increasing production of organic and unprocessed foods, teaching cooking skills right along with reading, writing, and arithmetic and behavioral modification. In other words, continue to find channels to advocate healthy eating and build new neural pathways for responsible food consumption habits.

Final Thoughts

It is not just food consumption where one does a double take in the high-income countries. Goods and services are consumed at alarming rates in many places. Many among us do not consider even the basics of conservation when it comes to using resources such as water, natural gas, electricity, automobile fuel, lawn fertilizer, pesticides, and so on. The list is huge and many individual and collective appetites gorge on these limited resources. The overuse of these precious commodities could so easily be minimized, but we must first work on changing our consumptive habits and behaviors. As a society, we must relearn the old ways to carefully choose when, where, why, and how much of any products we use. Recently there has been an introduction to minimalism with concepts such as simplicity; small houses; smart, energy-conserving appliances; carpooling or using public transportation; adding bicycle lanes for commuting; and so on. Each of us can become increasingly conscious of what resource we use and think of ways to decrease that dependence. Remember to practice and model the sustainability watchwords: "reduce, reuse, and recycle." As we grow in knowledge and use of better habits we can serve as examples to all within our sphere. As nurses, we can incorporate this knowledge into our curricula and classrooms as we model and teach these skills and behaviors.

Climate Change (SDG 13)

Carole Ann Drick

All over the planet, in every country, every city, every hospital, every clinic, every job, every person, we are experiencing to some degree a global paradigm shift (GPS). The interesting thing about change of any magnitude is that it begins in very minute ways and builds, sometimes swiftly but more often slowly until a critical mass is reached. At that point it "suddenly" becomes apparent to the majority of the people. This is also true in nursing and all of health care. For instance, the Germ Theory of Disease took a very long time to be accepted. It was not until between 1860 and 1864 that Louis Pasteur discovered the pyogenic vibrio in the blood as the cause of puerperal fever and recommended the use of boric acid to kill these microorganisms before and after confinement. That created the critical mass of information and action. The Germ Theory of Disease we now use today is the basis for medical care.

Long before the public was aware of climate change, I was already a holistic steward for this planet. My parents were first generation off the farm with college degrees and a strong environmental ethic. As the apple does not fall far from the tree, they raised three children who were awake and aware to read the signs of impending storms, early frost, preparing for winter, freshwater supply, and being one with nature. Certainly the old adage "Nature never lies . . . . Nature makes you wise" holds true within me. These leanings can be applied in nursing practice, research, and advocacy.

Starting with ourselves is the beginning of global sustainable development. The physical change is usually easier than the conscious change. Let us start with it. The question becomes: What is it that I can change in my lifestyle that will reduce my environmental impact? We start with the easy changes, say one or two, that feel comfortable with us. We do them for a couple of weeks then gradually add another and another. Our biggest hurdle is starting *now*.

Change involves taking action and responsibility. As we take action, momentum builds. We also unconsciously expand our awareness into increasingly larger spheres—our personal space, family, friends, workplace, state, national, planetary. When dropping a stone into a still lake, the ripples go out and gradually affect the entire lake. The world is our lake.

Physical Change

My northeastern U.S. home is becoming more energy efficient with such things as insulation in attic and walls, weather stripping around doors and behind electrical plates, basement pipes wrapped in insulation, adjusted hot water tank temperature, and thermal pane windows. On hot summer afternoons, the curtains and blinds on the sunny side of the home are closed and in winter the curtains are closed just before sundown and the concomitant drop in outdoor temperature. There are deciduous trees surrounding my home, which give shade in the summer and with leaves gone allow more light in the winter months. In the evening the lights are on in the room that we are in and turned off when we leave that room. All clocks are battery operated and anything with a power light is unplugged when not in use except for the refrigerator and stove.

Translating energy efficiency to nursing practice, consider at night when responding to a call bell to use the over-the-bed light rather than the ceiling light, which saves both electricity and also allows other sleeping patients to sleep rather than be abruptly awakened with the intense ceiling lights. As nurses, we need to be on planning committees for new construction or building expansion to advocate for what makes our job most efficient, gives comfort to the patient, and is overall energy efficient.

Transportation

In purchasing my homes (I have had five) one of the leading factors is location, which translates into close proximity to the resources used on a regular basis—groceries, post office, bank, and drug store. Rather than making frequent trips for one item, meals and activities are preplanned. This results in one shopping trip during the week. Anything else is placed on a list so that the errand is coordinated with at least one other activity in that area. There are very few times that a single-item trip is truly necessary. Combining trips leads to decreased fuel consumption.

When I was a staff nurse I lived fairly close to work and participated in carpooling. For the past 25 years, I have had a private practice with my office in my home and have increased my tele/Internet commute when consulting with private clients or corporations. This in itself is a tremendous savings on all levels—time, energy, and efficiency.

Consuming Less

This is probably one of the easiest ways to have less impact on the environment. This means wise purchasing considering amount of use, necessity, convenience, and practicality. It is the little things that make the difference such as reusable grocery bags stored in the trunk of the car so always available. Consuming less also translates into buying in bulk to reduce the amount of packaging—the plastic wrapping, cardboard boxes, and other unnecessary materials. Sometimes consuming less means buying more to avoid additional packaging. In addition, recycling and reusing are my first thoughts before throwing anything away. Recycling includes periodic donations of clothes, home furnishing, and small appliances.

In nursing, advocating and/or being on the committee for a successful hospital/health care facility recycling program provides an avenue to reduce operational costs, increase worker safety, enhance community relations, and sometimes even generate revenue. For me this is an easy one to be excited about since it is relatively easy and everyone can see benefits including the planet.

One of the things that my parents taught me was to *be efficient*. Rather than take things up the stairs every time you have something, place them at the bottom of the stairs. The next person going up simply takes them along. This can easily be adapted to our clinical practice as to restocking supplies for the next shift. Efficiency is also seen with putting things back where they belong immediately after use. This is certainly true in staff positions where there is shared equipment.

Eating Smart

Eating smart was a subliminal message that I received three times a day growing up. Although my parents were not vegetarians, vegetables took up two-thirds of the dinner plate plus a side salad. In the summer, we ate mainly out of the garden, which is still true today for me. Fruits and vegetables were harvested and canned or frozen for winter. I still freeze fruits and vegetables for winter. Dessert was mainly reserved for Sundays and special occasions. Today there are challenges to the environment and climate for being either vegetarian or meat eaters. Eating from the outside walls of the grocery store provides fresh fruits and vegetables. However, there is little information as to how far the apples have traveled. Processed foods are mainly in the interior aisles of the market, have Food and Drug Administration (FDA)–required nutritional information and usually synthetic ingredients and chemicals. Eating more organically is a better choice though it can be expensive. Eating organically, I consume about 25% less, which offsets the difference in cost.

Nutrition is very important for a healthy recovery from every illness or imbalance. Both staff and patients need—no, *require*—good, tasty, healthy foods that do not have the life cooked out of them. This is one area where nurses can work on self-care as a part of environmental safety for both the patient and the nurse. The watering down of school lunches to the point at which ketchup is considered a vegetable should prompt nurses to speak up and advocate for all children. Eating smart supports both our health and our planet.

Stop Cutting Down Trees!

My parents had a love for and nourished their trees, which lasted for years well beyond their own lives. For every tree that they had to cut down, they planted a new one. I also plant trees and have that delight and deep appreciation for trees and all the birds and critters that they house and protect. Plastic and synthetics are slowly replacing wood; however, they come at a price unless they are also recycled. For nurses who wear scrubs, consider ones that have the most natural fibers such as a cotton blend and a woolen blend for a sweater or jacket.

Final Thoughts

The attainment of SDG 13 requires a consciousness change—a global paradigm shift. Conservation of resources and longevity are easily understood on the physical level. Yet, there is another level of understanding that is far deeper in its effect and more elusive. Some call it "intuition," "awareness," "consciousness"—the name is not important. What is important is the result. Lasting change and sustainable global health is possible with a shift in consciousness. Einstein reminds us "we cannot solve our problems with the same level of thinking that created them." To move into sustainable development requires working from this higher level of knowing. From this larger perspective, we see the planet as a living–breathing organism that is in need of assistance to rebalance.

Coming from this expanded consciousness we can see more clearly and speak with clarity. Our words are heard and felt on two levels—within the physical mind and within the deep heart of the Universal Consciousness that is within each of us. Right now, this is the shift that we have been waiting for—and preparing for—a GPS to sustainable development to meet this universal challenge. The process is really simple as described by St. Francis, "Start by doing what is necessary, then what is possible. And suddenly you are doing the impossible." It is the "suddenly" where the shift happens and we move into a global planetary shift in consciousness.

Life Below Water (SDG 14)

Susan Luck

I have always lived near the ocean. Listening to the ebb and flow of the tides while gazing into the horizon becomes a transpersonal moment. With great reverence and respect, coastal cultures have always known the power and the fragility of this vast ecosystem that sustains life on Earth.

Living in a small island community, perched between the Atlantic Ocean and Biscayne Bay, sea-level rise along with polluted waters from a dated nuclear power plant spills acidic waste into the bay. Sewage dumped out to sea returns back with the tides. Coral reefs are disappearing at an alarming rate. Green algae slime now infects our coastline, contaminating the air above and the marine life below. As the fish disappear, so does the local economy and lifeline for so many. This is the recent story of South Florida, my home, and a microcosm to a looming global crisis.

For the 19 million nurses globally, this scenario and the urgency of "turning the tides" beg us to reflect: What is our role in this global public health crisis where clean water and air are endangered?

The world's oceans maintain temperature, chemistry, and life below the surface, driving global systems that make the Earth habitable for humankind and all living creatures. Our rainwater, drinking water, weather patterns, climate, coastlines, food supply, and the oxygen in the air we breathe, are all ultimately provided and regulated by the sea.

The UN (2016) shares these facts to consider:

- Oceans cover three-quarters of the Earth's surface, contain 97% of the Earth's water, and represent 99% of the living space on the planet by volume.
- Over 3 billion people depend on marine and coastal biodiversity for their livelihoods.
- Globally, the market value of marine and coastal resources and industries is estimated at $3 trillion per year or about 5% of global gross domestic product (GDP).
- Oceans contain nearly 200,000 identified species, but actual numbers may lie in the millions.
- Oceans absorb about 30% of carbon dioxide produced by humans, buffering the impacts of global warming.
- Oceans serve as the world's largest source of protein, with more than 3 billion people depending on the oceans as their primary source of protein.
- Marine fisheries directly or indirectly employ over 200 million people worldwide.
- Subsidies for fishing are contributing to the rapid depletion of many fish species and are preventing efforts to save and restore global fisheries and related jobs, causing an estimated loss of U.S. $50 billion per year.
- As much as 40% of the world's oceans are heavily affected by human activities, including pollution, depleted fisheries, and loss of coastal habitats.

Most of the great cities, the world over, are built along the water. So are many towns, hamlets, and villages. Sea-level rise, fueled by climate change, threatens to reclaim coastal lands and the communities that are built on them. Climate change could affect coastal areas in a variety of ways. Sensitive to sea-level rise, changes in the frequency and intensity of storms, increased precipitation, and warmer ocean temperatures along with rising atmospheric concentrations of carbon dioxide are causing the oceans to absorb more of the gas and become more acidic. This rising acidity is having significant impact on coastal and marine ecosystems.

In March 2016, the WHO published the second edition of the report, *Preventing Disease Through Healthy Environments: A Global Assessment of the Burden of Disease From Environmental Risks*, citing proven strategies for preventing disease and deaths through healthy environments (Prüss-Ustün, Wolf, Corvalán, Bos, & Neira, 2016).

Health is more than the absence of disease. Health is part of our interconnectedness to our external environment and reflects our internal world, from our microbiome to our epigenetic expression. Nurses are on the front lines: identifying, assessing, educating, and advocating for cleaner, safer, healthier environments in our communities. As nurses, we serve as health educators and coaches, empowering individuals, families, and communities to develop strategies for living healthier lives in the prevention of disease. According to the WHO, the link between our health and the environment in which we live, from the water we drink, to the air we breathe, to the food we grow and eat, are all major risk factors that contribute to the ill-health of our populations globally.

Since I live in a coastal community at the epicenter of major environmental challenges that are local issues reflecting a global crisis, I am aware each day of the potential devastation that so many communities will face if immediate action is not taken. Aware of the issues one community confronts reflects the growing health concerns we face daily as world citizens.

Here in tropical Miami, Florida, we are at ground zero for sea-level rise. I witness the flooding of our roads when the high tide full moon cycle exerts its force. During the rainy season, the flooding intensifies resulting in contamination of our surrounding bay. Our coral reefs are disappearing, an ecosystem that sustains a diversity of marine life and an important indicator of ocean health and the health of the planet overall. One might think of them as the rainforest of the sea world. Locally, sewage treatment plants cannot handle the growth and development along the coast, while old nuclear power plants sit on vulnerable coastal lands leaking their content, acidifying and polluting the ocean. From Miami to Los Angeles, from the Pacific Islands to Bangladesh, how will the changing marine ecosystem change our lives and our community's health?

Locally, we are inhaling green algae plumes surrounding our ocean coastline, giving off foul odors and increasing exposure to both skin and respiratory conditions. It is believed to be like an opportunistic infection, given the right (or wrong) conditions to thrive. Information regarding toxins from blue-green algae and risks to humans, fish, and wildlife is very limited, although it is known that the cyanotoxins produced by algae can be a threat to fish, pets, livestock, wild animals, and humans if untreated surface water is ingested. Blue-green algae can produce a number of toxins that can affect the liver, digestive system, and nervous system. Most problems happen when water containing high levels of toxin is ingested. Abdominal cramps, nausea, diarrhea, and vomiting may occur if untreated water is swallowed. Rashes can happen when skin is exposed to the algae when swimming. As nurses who live and work in every community, local to global, we are often the primary health care providers who bear witness to the devastating impact of the environment on the health and well-being of our populations throughout the life cycle. Public health measures are recommended when coming in contact with algae toxins. It is important for nurses to advise individuals, and their pets, to not ingest untreated surface water from areas experiencing blooms. Boiling water does not destroy the algae. There are currently no standards for blue-green algae toxin levels in drinking water in the United States.

The WHO's (2004) guidelines for drinking-water quality are established for potentially hazardous water constituents and provide a basis for safe water intake. Different parameters may require different priorities for management to improve and protect public health. In general, the order of priority is to: (a) ensure an adequate supply of microbially safe water, and (b) manage key chemical contaminants known to cause adverse health effects.

Priority setting should be the result of a systematic assessment based on collaborative efforts among all relevant agencies and may be applied at national and system-specific levels. It may require the formation of a broad-based interagency committee, including authorities such as health, water resources, drinking-water supply, environment, agriculture, and geological services/mining to establish a mechanism for sharing information and reaching consensus on drinking-water quality issues. Nurses should be part of this interagency approach.

Nurses, working with diverse populations, need to access current sources of information that can inform them in educating their communities in determining priorities, including industrial activities, sanitary surveys, records of previous monitoring, inspections, and access to local and community environmental concerns to address patterns for prevention and caution. The wider the range of data sources used, the more useful the results of the process will be. In many situations, authorities or consumers may have already identified a number of drinking-water quality problems, particularly where they cause obvious health effects or acceptability problems. These existing problems would normally be assigned a high priority. Nurses can interface with diverse agencies and express concerns and share information with local community organizations and become a bridge to serving public health needs.

Locally, green algae, disappearing coral, and nuclear reactor runoff into our ocean have created a growing citizen movement, which demonstrates how change can occur when community organizations join with county officials and state environmental agencies, researchers, and the public health sector to address the critical environmental issues that are responsible for the disappearance of our local marine ecosystem and contribute to the larger global seal-level rise, as we are a microcosm of the macrocosm.

Final Thoughts

We must continue to ask ourselves:

- How can we as nurses work with our local communities, public health departments, and governmental agencies and lead efforts to ensure safe water quality, safeguard our food supply, protect our waterways, and find new options for growing nutrient-dense food to support the health and well-being of our communities? How can we reduce environmental risk factors that impact human health and the economic and cultural survival of our communities?

- How can we serve as advocates to empower our citizens to safeguard their health through creating new community organizations and join existing ones to raise awareness on issues and take action for change and for healing our planet?

- How do we, as nurses, become involved in our community organizations and work with health policy analysts and researchers to cocreate innovative strategies and solutions?

From an integral perspective, nurses are essential participants in the solution-finding, interprofessional collaboration needed to address emerging environmental health crises in a timely manner.

Life on Land (SDG 15)

Susan Luck

Compounding the impact of pollution on our marine ecosystem is the multitude of chemicals on land that create havoc into our waterways. Chemicals and pesticides used on crops not only contaminate our food supply, but also "run off" spills into the local drinking-water supply for many. In Miami, nuclear regulators failed to consider a growing saltwater plume when they allowed Florida Power & Light to increase operating temperatures at the utility's Turkey Point cooling canals to prevent a reactor shutdown. The resulting plume now threatens drinking-water supplies.

As nurses, working with communities toward achieving their health goals, we can collaborate with multiple sectors including energy sources, agricultural growers, and a multitude of local industries to address root environmental causes that contribute to ill-health and lie beyond the direct auspices of the health sector. Supporting local "back to land" movements that advocate growing food and using age-old methods to avoid chemicals is critical to the health of the community and the health of our planet.

Zika Virus

As a neighbor to Central and South America, a new public/global health threat has recently emerged in our communities in South Florida with the identification of the mosquito-transmitted Zika virus. Potent, dangerous pesticides are being released intentionally into our local environment.

There are many chemicals we confront in our daily lives to kill weeds (herbicides), insects (insecticides), fungus (fungicides), rodents (rodenticides), and other creatures. Our modern world is filled with these chemicals. Research shows that they function as neurotoxins and can be found in the air we breathe, the food we eat, and the water we drink. The use of toxic pesticides to manage pest problems has become a common practice globally: in agricultural fields, homes, parks, schools, buildings, forests, and roads. It is difficult to find somewhere where pesticides are not used—from the can of bug spray under the kitchen sink to the air sprays to kill ants and mosquitoes.

In South Florida, we have become the U.S. epicenter in trying to eradicate the Zika virus through aerial spraying—sometimes daily within the same community—while local public works departments act as ground troops spraying our yards and parks and are at our door steps without warning. As fear sets into our communities, we have not had the opportunity to weigh the risks of Zika along with the risks of multiple exposures from the chemical naled, overhead. This is a potent organochlorine that is highly toxic to humans even at low concentrations and is banned in Europe while being used without warning in our communities. Naled is highly toxic to the nervous system, especially in children. It is also toxic to aquatic life, butterflies, and bees.

As nurses, we look for patterns in assessing individuals, families, and communities. Assessing for environmental exposures is an essential component in risk assessment and risk management and in understanding the myriad of often unexplained symptoms related to fatigue, memory impairment, respiratory, neurological, and digestive problems. Nurses need to have a voice and partner with public works departments in municipalities to decide on spraying along with warnings, schedules, and informing the general community as a public health response. People are being advised to bathe themselves and their children in mosquito repellent and other insecticides. Pregnant women are dousing themselves to prevent being bitten by a mosquito for fear of neurological damage from the virus to their developing fetuses. What appears to be missing from this conversation are the potentially harmful effects of pesticides, such as naled and other toxic chemicals on individuals using them on a daily basis, and on the health of our communities and on the ecosystem, already so fragile. Nursing environmental leadership to inform the public is critical.

Living on a coast, overhead daily spraying inevitably drifts to adjacent waterways. Local fish are known to have extremely high levels of the chemicals used on land. Many people still fish off piers and shoreline, especially those who have come from island communities in the Caribbean. Guidelines and precautions need to be offered to diverse populations including fisherman, young women who have not yet had children, and older adults on how to protect themselves.

In a single year in Florida, more than 6 million acres were fumigated with the chemical naled (Guarino, 2016). There is still much debate as to its effectiveness to kill larvae and there are new questions about pesticide resistance. With increasing rates of Alzheimer's disease and autism, we must ask ourselves if these chronic exposures to neurotoxic substances can contribute to our health problems, including the exponential rises of Alzheimer's and attention deficit disorders in children.

Pesticides have been linked to a wide range of human health hazards, ranging from short-term impacts, such as headaches and nausea, to chronic impacts like cancer and reproductive harm. Acute dangers include nerve, skin, and eye irritation and damage, headaches, dizziness, nausea, fatigue, and systemic poisoning, which can, occasionally, be fatal. As nurses, we can assess and monitor symptoms, but what more can we do in the advocacy and empowerment of communities to protect themselves and challenge the notion that dousing the masses is not without another set of potential health issues? Chronic health effects may occur years after even minimal exposure to pesticides in the environment, or result from the pesticide residues cumulatively that we ingest through our food and water.

A July 2007 study conducted by researchers at the Public Health Institute, the California Department of Health Services, and the UC Berkeley School of Public Health found a sixfold increase on the autism spectrum disorders (ASD) for children of women who were exposed to organochlorine pesticides in utero (Roberts et al., 2007). Highly carcinogenic pesticides can cause many types of cancer in humans. Some of the most prevalent forms include leukemia, non-Hodgkin's lymphoma, brain, bone, breast, ovarian, prostate, testicular, and liver cancers. In February 2009, the Agency for Toxic Substances and Disease Registry published a study that found that children who live in homes where their parents use pesticides are twice as likely to develop brain cancer versus those who live in residences in which no pesticides are used (Shim, Mlynarek, & van Wijngaarden, 2009). Studies by the National Cancer Institute (2011) found that American farmers, who in most respects are healthier than the population at large, had startling rates of leukemia, Hodgkin's disease, non-Hodgkin's lymphoma, and many other forms of cancer.

There is also mounting evidence that exposure to pesticides disrupts the endocrine system, wreaking havoc with the complex regulation of hormones, the reproductive system, and embryonic development. Endocrine disruption can produce infertility and a variety of birth defects and developmental defects in offspring, including incomplete sexual development, impaired brain development, behavioral disorders, and many other neurocognitive issues. Examples of known endocrine-disrupting chemicals that are present in our environment include dichlorodiphenyltrichloroethane (DDT; which still persists in abundance more than 20 years after being banned in the United States), lindane, atrazine, carbaryl, parathion, and many others.

Pesticides in Our Food Supply

Ingesting chemicals in our food chain is well-documented and the movement for local produce and natural farming practices is a growing movement globally, and an area for nurses to work with the populations with whom they partner to develop community gardens and safer methods. Growing food and using age-old methods to avoid chemicals are critical to the health of the community and the health of our planet.

A profile of the chemical in Cornell University's pesticide database shows that naled, a potent neurotoxin, is also highly toxic to bees (Extension Toxicology Network, 1993). This insect neurotoxin cannot discriminate between honey bees and mosquitoes. It was once believed that the disappearance of bees, responsible for pollinating globally to secure our food supply, was due to "colony collapse disorder," a phenomenon that occurs when the majority of worker bees in a colony disappear and leave behind a queen, plenty of food, and a few nurse bees to care for the remaining immature bees and the queen. There has been much speculation as to the disappearance of bees, our "canary in the coal mine." Naled is also a known neonicotinoid, targeting pollinators, and poisoning honeybees, bumblebees, and monarch butterflies—virtually all the species of insects. For a decade, neonics have dominated a frustrating conversation to find a cause for the loss of commercial beehives in agriculture. The issue has also moved to new scrutiny and legislation in Maryland. If the Pollinator Protection Act is signed into law by Gov. Larry Hogan, consumers will not be able to buy neonic insecticides after 2017. The pesticide industry says neonics are safe. Reported by the *Washington Post*, county aerial spraying at Flowertown Bee Farm and Supply in Summerville, South Carolina in August 2016 resulted in the instant genocide of about 2.5 million bees (Guarino, 2016). This is but one commercial bee farm where the worker bees were exposed to a single spraying of this potent neurotoxic pesticide. The danger that the decline of bees and other pollinators presents to the world's food supply was highlighted when the European Commission decided to ban a class of pesticides suspected of playing a role in bee colony collapse disorder including naled. One of every three bites of food eaten worldwide depends on pollinators, especially bees, for a successful harvest. For much of the past 10 years, beekeepers, primarily in the United States and Europe, have been reporting annual hive losses of 30% or higher, substantially more than is considered normal or sustainable. But this winter, many U.S. beekeepers experienced losses of 40% to 50% or more, just as commercial bee operations prepared to transport their hives for the country's largest pollinator event: the fertilizing of California's almond trees. This is a global health crisis.

What could be the role of educating farmers about pesticide spraying and protecting their crops, their families, and the pollinators? How do we participate in advocating for safer chemicals in our communities and workplace environments? In the United States, several national environmental advocacy organizations and commercial beekeepers filed suit in March against the U.S. Environmental Protection Agency (EPA) for its conditional registration of certain neonicotinoids, contending that the agency did not properly ensure environmental health protections, particularly with respect to pollinators.

The EPA is now reviewing its registration of neonicotinoids and has accelerated the review schedule due "to uncertainties about these pesticides and their potential effects on bees." The agency said in an e-mail that it is working with beekeepers, growers, pesticide manufacturers, and others to improve pesticide use, labeling, and management practices to protect bees and to thoroughly evaluate the effects of pesticides on honeybees and other pollinators. As part of these efforts, the EPA is working with pesticide and agricultural equipment manufacturers to reduce the release of neonicotinoid-contaminated dust during planting—a time when commercial bees are likely to encounter the insecticide.

As nurses, we can educate and advocate for community actions and join forces with farmers, community organizations, and governmental entities. We can also inform our communities of safety measures to protect ourselves when using pesticides and find safer alternatives.

Organizations such as Pesticide Action Network and Environmental Working Group lead campaigns in curbing pesticides and finding safe alternatives.

The Solution to Pesticides

The real solution to our pest and weed problems lies in nontoxic and cultural methods of agriculture, not in pulling the pesticide trigger. Organically grown foods and sustainable methods of pest control are key to our families' health and the health of the environment.

BETTER TESTING

State and federal agencies should require stricter independent testing, including testing of synergistic effects of pesticides. Pesticides known or suspected of causing human health problems should be phased out.

PROTECT OUR CHILDREN

Because our children are the most vulnerable population to pesticides, pesticide use should be prohibited in places where our children live and play, including schools, parks, and playgrounds. Strict nontoxic pest management programs are required for such places.

PESTICIDE USE REDUCTION

Provide technical assistance to farmers, local governments, businesses, and homeowners on nontoxic alternatives to pesticide use. This includes alternatives to nuisance spraying for mosquitoes and controlling West Nile virus and other pest problems.

PROHIBIT POLLUTION OF OUR WATER AND POISONING OF OUR COMMUNITIES

Ensure that aerial pesticide use does not pollute our waterways through strict rules governing spraying and buffer zones that prevent the harmful effects of drift. Prohibit the use of pesticides for purely aesthetic reasons. Prevent pesticide applications to water bodies, instead using nonchemical methods of managing aquatic invasive weeds.

RIGHT TO KNOW

Provide free and universal notification to residents about pesticide use, including who is using chemicals, where, when, how, what pesticides are being used, and why.

PROTECT WORKERS

Provide protection to workers and farmers to prevent acute and chronic pesticide poisoning.

A Global Nurse Case Study of Community Involvement

Living in a coastal community, development along the ocean and bay is unprecedented. Old buildings are being torn down, often filled with lead paint, asbestos, and arsenic-treated wood. In my town, as I saw both debris floating in the water from demolition and local fisherman seeking their catch of the day, I went to my local officials and stated that as a public health and community health nurse, and as an environmental health educator, I was deeply concerned about the lack of safeguards during this demolition of multiple buildings on our waters and on our health. I addressed that the dust overhead and being inhaled by children walking to the local school was a health hazard. I pointed out that older adults, trying to exercise as directed by their health care providers, were walking under a cloud of dust and increasing their risk of respiratory problems including asthma. I also explained that the dust being carried into our homes could be a source of lead contamination, as most buildings were built before the 1978 ban on lead in paint. With not much success in my conversations with our local elected officials, I chose to inform and mobilize my small community of 5,000 and educate them and organize a grassroots effort. I realized that having a collective voice would be more powerful and formed an Environmental Impact Committee. We showed up at public town meetings, voiced our concerns, and wrote about it in local media. Eventually, our voice was heard and led to ordinances that mandated developers to place netting around buildings at the time of demolition to contain debris and fined violators to ensure compliance. This was community-in-action led by a nurse as a concerned global citizen.

Final Thoughts

As nurses, and on the shoulders of Florence Nightingale, the voice of 20.7 million of us globally can change the course of environmental degradation, create healthier communities for our fellow citizens, and steer us toward realizing planetary health.

Through education and advocacy, whether it be for safe household water storage, better hygiene measures, safer management of toxic substances in the home and workplace, alternatives to chemicals in the food chain, or in making better choices, we hold a powerful leadership role to impact the health of present and future generations. Our time as nurses, following in Florence Nightingale's footsteps, is now!

PROSPERITY

Decent Work and Economic Growth (SDG 8)

Phalakshi Manjrekar

Health and nursing coexist to meet numerous common goals. However, availability of health resources is significantly important for the Indian nurse to practice effectively. Health availability for all is directly proportionate to the economic growth of the country, and India is a country where health may not be available equally to all—and that makes nursing the general population difficult (Sundar, Garg, & Garg, 2015). This permits people with a high socioeconomic status to afford adequate health resources as the marginalized remain unable to avail what they require (Gupta, 2016). This is the biggest hurdle for nursing. When Indian nurses compare themselves with those who are practicing in higher income countries like Europe or America, they know that those nurses have the facility to utilize the best technology, receive better education grants, pursue ongoing professional development, and practice in a safe health care setting. This is directly attributed to the better economic status these countries experience (Sundar et al., 2015). Indian nurses have a tough challenge to face when they know that they cannot cater to the health needs of all due to the economic constraints (Senior, 2010).

Based on its history, the economy of India is the seventh largest economy in the world measured by nominal GDP (Bajpai, 2016). The country is classified as a "newly industrialized country," one of the G-20 major economies, a member of an association of five major emerging national economies—Brazil, Russia, India, China, and South Africa (BRICS)—and a developing economy with an average growth rate of approximately 7% over the past two decades (DNA India, 2015). The Indian economy is growing very fast and overtaking other countries like China rapidly. This has been reflected in the growing health facilities and better nursing opportunities in the country for both the affordable population and the nonaffordable population over the past two decades. Many health care opportunities unavailable earlier are now easily accessible here; these positive shifts may be attributed to the growth in the economy.

Nursing is dependent on nursing standards developed and implemented directly by those within the profession, which in turn are related to affordable nursing education; due to the inequities throughout the economy, this education is available to a few with subsidized tuition fees and to others with a high price tag. However, the resultant outcome of practice standards has evolved and it is related to opportunities available for more nurses to pursue university education in nursing, compared to the earlier scenario when nursing education was available only at a nonuniversity diploma program called "General Nursing and Midwifery," taken after secondary school education. Opportunities to specialize and opt for higher education are better now and varied avenues for practice have also been diversified. The question that still needs to be answered is: Are opportunities to obtain affordable education available to all nurses equally throughout the country (Senior, 2010)? The economy growth is still not enough to provide equal opportunities to all.

Nurses form an integral part of the health care system in India and take the responsibility in all the sectors to achieve better patient outcomes. Job opportunities for them are definitely better than what was available two decades ago (Rao, Rao, Kumar, Chatterjee, & Sundararaman. 2011), but the opportunity still remains categorized as "fair," where "fair" is identified as a work environment with safety guidelines and measures, decent working hours, apt responsibility and authority reflective of professional expectations, minimum wage reforms respected, appropriate resting facilities, and a commitment on behalf of institutions to employ only those nurses who have a recognized official nursing education and registration.

Though these norms are widely followed, there are loopholes where needy nurses are exploited with a low salary scale and unfair working hours.

Fortunately, job opportunities are easily available for Indian nurses who are qualified. This is due to self-created improved nursing opportunities in India, but also due to the problem of international out-migration (a common barrier to a sustainable workforce faced by many LMICs). In certain cases, a nurse may be employed on a very low salary that would make meeting basic life necessities impossible, but the nurse may still accept this job as an opportunity to get one with an adequate pay scale that may not be easily available. This scenario, too, must be considered a deficiency that SDG 8 must address, as obtaining work with a humane and standard salary under the minimum wage act of each country is desirable under this goal. Nurses put in tremendous physical and mental efforts in their daily routine and being aptly paid for this is mandatory (Burns, 2014). Many nurse leaders are fighting a battle for decent wages for nurses in India, as well as in many resource-constrained settings and high-income countries alike. The fight is toward recognizing nursing professionals as equally important personnel, worthy of the respect and financial retribution of any discipline that makes life-saving decisions and contributes toward the health of human beings.

Today, nurses are the voice of nurses. We must understand this. But shouldn't the access to and delivery of quality nursing care—the systems that both promote and prevent this potential—also be the concern of society as a whole? Is it not an issue of consideration of all? It definitely calls for an appeal by all concerned and global citizens, those who believe in the cause of nurses, to voice for better recognition of nurses, and ensure them of jobs that recognize their hard work and undeniable contributions to a healthy planet. Such an appeal, when broadcasted through the appropriate channels, received a very positive response from the state of Kerala in India. Most of the Indians who decide to take up nursing belong to the state of Kerala; nursing as a profession has always been respected there and nurses receive infinite support there from all.

SDG 8.8. Protect Labor Rights and Promote Safe and Secure Working Environments for All

Reference to target 8 of SDG 8 (8.8) is directly applicable to nurses. Safety is of grave concern in LMICs. Today, all health care settings worldwide must ensure safe environments, but resource-constrained settings like in India have to do more with less and procure something with nothing on a daily basis. Many recognized large–sector hospitals, on the recommendations of accreditation committees, have implemented mandatory safety measures for all employees, including nurses. However, though a general mandate for employees exists as a part of the labor ministry, many nurse leaders take this on as a personal objective to be implemented in organizations where they have decision-making authority and the self-created responsibility to create a safe environment for nurses. This includes due consideration of the fact that the majority of the nursing workforce in India consists of women. They need: safe working hours; adequate maternity benefits, including relaxation in certain workplace demands to support the physiological demands of pregnancy; child support, such as allowing shift adjustments to promote breastfeeding; workplace support for self-health promotion and self-care, for instance, adequate patient-lifting devices to protect nurses' backs

(Gupta, 2016); sturdy and antislip shoes to prevent nurse falls; antislip floors; timely and scheduled breaks on each shift; adequate personal protective equipment; and many others.

Indian nurses belong to the low-income group who largely migrate to various international destinations in search of a better work environment, and increased remuneration and lifestyle for self and family. Most of them achieve their goals in their destination countries, and the few who do not, receive immense assistance from the respective Indian consulates.

India as a growing economy in the global scene today is seen as a country that should be making ongoing economic reforms to ensure suitable lifestyles that benefit all (Sundar et al., 2015). Unfortunately, a culture where the rich grow richer and the poor get poorer is not going to help the health care system. To the contrary, it is creating more irreparable divides and difficulties. Health care that is affordable and accessible to all seems to be a struggle.

The story of a 7-year-old child who suffered from dengue fever in India's capital city had the mother and father go from one hospital to another, as they were turned away for administrative reasons and inability to pay up front. Finally, the child succumbed to death due to lack of timely treatment, resulting in the mother and father committing suicide in frustration (Jha, 2015). This was a true tale, which brought tears of sadness to all and a backlash on the health care system of a country that has the seventh largest economy in the world, but was somehow unable to ensure health care to this child, this family, and these parents.

Nurses form the first line of the caregiver pyramid and adequacy of nurses needs to be a point of concern. A strategy to attract more young men and women to nursing is needed: one that makes nursing economically and professionally sustainable for all nurses; one that provides continual incentives to continue working in one's home country within nursing; and one that creates avenues for growth through affordable education and the establishment of various steps on the ladder for advanced designation with increased responsibility and systemic endorsement to promote the work we do. The current shortfalls may be directly related to numerous reasons. However, a movement toward a better economy, improved nursing employment opportunities, and more equitable allocations of resources may actively discourage unfair practices and inherently improve nurse–patient ratios.

The unfair distribution of nurses (Rao et al., 2011), with more of them employed in urban settings and less in the rural regions, is another cause for concern. Equality in the distribution of nurses may be addressed by encouraging incentives and safe employment assurance; the ensured opportunity to practice nursing justly and adequately will go a long way in attracting staff to geographic locations that struggle with insufficient human resources. A general objective to better nursing personnel in rural India needs to be a primary goal of nurse leaders and the health administration (Das et al., 2012). An intensive effort in all the sectors to target nurses and promote their taking up increased responsibilities in primary health care settings of villages, focused on maternal–child health, infant wellness, and noncommunicable disease management, and working with better budgets and facilities will do much to improve the overall scenario.

Will a better economy make this easier and more attainable? Once the economy and economic considerations regarding health care are addressed with the involvement and input of nursing, broad spectrum objectives need to be clarified, such as addressing the bureaucratic and hierarchical imbalances of the health system, improving transport facilities and communication modules, and directly focusing on better roads and infrastructure, particularly for villages and towns that lack these necessities altogether. A failing support system decreases the convenience of work in the rural fields. However, an economy that supports better systems in the villages, improving access to clean water, sanitation, electricity, and a stable communication network (Gupta, 2016), and convenient road and rail transport along with a good infrastructure, will gain immense respect from all, improve health outcomes, and increase access to health education and promotion. The rural population may have urgent health needs that may be different from those in cities, primarily due to the fact that most of the villages are agriculturally active and health disorders, like snake bites, waterborne diseases, and communicable diseases, are more prominent there; this calls for a brief orientation and additional educational input among nurses, physicians, and other health care workers (HCWs) who will take a position there.

In many countries, a rich investment to develop their local economies through increased rural productivity in agriculture was the way to make the economy better. Can the same work for India? This is a challenge that needs to be explored as this will pave the way for an unstoppable chain of events improving development throughout sectors. This will require a massive upgrade in the technology used in farming to increase efficiency and productivity, thus improving the economy, creating better job opportunities, and increasing the possibility of better health care systems and more professional advancement for nurses. This may also create a forum to attract nurses to practice in these settings.

Nurses may also lead various programs to meet the objectives led through the other SDG initiatives to increase employment opportunities for many. For example, a nurse-led project that addressed SDG 6 (Clean Water and Sanitation) goals looked to provide "one toilet for one house" for better sanitation in Indian villages through World Bank funding. It was able to create multiple job opportunities for a large population that was involved in making the low cost toilets (Sundar et al., 2015). We must constantly explore our opportunities that maximize our potential to reach each and every one of the SDGs.

Nurses in many higher income countries have reached a very high and respectable level of achievement and recognition. Can they assist nurses from LMICs to better their ability and professional outcomes? This would be a case of the accomplished assisting others who are on the way toward accomplishment. This may be achieved via sharing of knowledge, technology, monetary assistance, exchange programs, and mentoring toward achieving various objective sets. Sharing allows established and validated protocols being utilized in successful health systems abroad to be initiated locally without the pilot phase, thus allowing for achievement of goals more practically. Numerous initiatives by the World Bank, UN, the ICN, and the Bill and Melinda Gates Foundation have worked in this way with great success. The aims of such projects need to focus on fostering autonomy for local host participants and decrease dependence on long-term foreign aid and assistance. Any initiative that may result in a dependency culture or promote the idea that the host country "needs" others to be deemed valid as professionals can be extremely demeaning and be injurious to the dignity of all involved.

Final Thoughts

What has led to the hurdles in equal health care access in a country where some can afford the best? The issues that plague us now are low self-esteem among nurses who form a major health care workforce, inadequate baseline education and continuing education, decreased opportunities for professional development in nursing, exorbitant costs of education in the private sector that inhibit future potential nurses from enrolling, and lack of a reliable government support system for the health care recipient unable to pay upfront or overwhelming costs. The economic divides centralize the premier health care facilities and leading medical experts in the cities, leading to unfair disadvantages and the absence of necessary services at the village level.

SDG 8 is the need of the hour for so many LMICs. Its achievement has the power to impact so many and so much. In a country like India, where the economy is on the rise, it seems that with dedicated efforts, achieving the rest of the battle is possible. We must continue to bring a nursing sensibility focused on procuring human dignity, ensuring equality in care, creating healing environments, utilizing a holistic approach that includes economic considerations, and maximizing our potentials in policy and governmental forums in order to aid our respective nations and global village in realizing economic and, therefore, human equity.

Infrastructure, Industry, and Innovation (SDG 9)

Deborah Wilson

I feel fortunate to have worked all over the world over the past 20 years, from low- to middle- and high-income countries. I have been able to apply my global nursing knowledge while managing population health in incredible places, including San Francisco during the 1980s AIDS crisis and the cholera outbreak in Haiti that started in 2010. One of my most challenging missions was in Liberia, during the height of the Ebola outbreak in West Africa. I was deployed to Foya, Liberia, in September 2014 by Medecins Sans Frontieres/Doctors without Borders (MSF) and for 6 weeks worked in a 120-bed Ebola treatment unit (ETU) alongside 78 Liberian nurses. I will discuss my experiences during the Ebola outbreak here within the context of SDG 9: building resilient infrastructure, industry, and innovation. Where infrastructure is absent, so is industry and innovation. This fact poses its own unique challenges to realizing prosperity and inclusion for all people everywhere.

An HCW in a crisis such as the Ebola outbreak has little time to think of anything other than saving lives. Treating 120 sick or dying patients takes tremendous physical and mental stamina: Suiting up into full personal protective equipment (in 100 degree heat with no air-conditioning), going into the "hot" zone, cleaning patients covered in their own emesis and feces, preparing and administering oral medications, inserting intravenous lines (while double-gloved and wearing protective goggles that fog up in the heat), trying to feed patients, delivering babies, and safely removing the bodies of those patients who have expired are some examples of the day-to-day reality my colleagues and I experienced in Liberia. In such situations, no one has the time to stop and think about infrastructure. But the truth is that the lack of it can hamper humanitarian effort.

One advantage of working with an organization such as MSF is that they provide and create infrastructure when responding to an emergency. For example,

MSF provided all medications, protective equipment, and generators. They hired jeeps, sanitized water, and offered jobs for so many who had been put out of work due to the outbreak. This "imported" infrastructure protected medical teams from the extraordinary instability that exists in Liberia. Without the shipment of supplies, trained staff, and technical equipment, there would not have been an effective response to the Ebola outbreak. The weak infrastructure of the West African health care system was partly responsible for the extent of the Ebola outbreak, as illustrated in the following examples:

1. Ebola is said to have first emerged in Guinea in December 2013. The small clinics there did not have protective equipment for their staff. Sick patients came to the clinics and were treated by HCWs using their bare hands. These HCWs, in turn, became infected, unknowingly spreading the Ebola virus in their communities (Bausch & Schwarz, 2014). As Ebola began to spread, there were no facilities in Guinea, Sierra Leone, or Liberia that could test blood to determine the source of the outbreak. It was not until labs in France and Germany isolated the Ebola virus in March 2014 that the source of the outbreak was pinpointed. How many lives could have been saved if West Africa had labs that could have identified the virus months earlier?

   In Foya, we experienced the positive impact a lab can have in preventing the spread of infection. When I first arrived at the ETU, blood samples taken from patients who were displaying symptoms of Ebola (fever, headache, vomiting, aching joints) had to be transported by motorbike across the Makino River to Guinea, where our sister facility had set up a lab facility. It would take 5 days to get the test results back. During that time patients had to wait in isolation. The risk of cross-contamination was a cause of great concern. The arrival of an international team of volunteers (European Mobile Consortium) that brought and set up a laboratory at our ETU transformed the wait period from 5 days to 6 hours. The effect was dramatic: We were able to discharge patients who tested negative within hours, not days. As a result, in 2 weeks our patient census was down from 120 to 36.

2. The Liberian government was hampered at the beginning of the response with logistical challenges, including difficulties getting resources and personnel to the remote epicenters, inadequate communication networks, and significant language barriers between the three countries most affected. I was protected from these challenges by MSF's efficiency. Logisticians worked tirelessly to get us the equipment we needed. They transported it through jungles, across rivers, and along muddy roads that were often treacherous to navigate. Satellite radio was set up, even Internet, so that we could get in touch with loved ones back home. Cooks were hired to feed us—no easy task, considering that all the markets had been closed because of the concern of spreading the virus.

The infrastructure issues in a country such as Liberia can seem insurmountable, but there are things that I—and you—as a global nurse, can do to make a difference that may potentially last beyond the outbreak.

One substantial infrastructure issue I encountered in Liberia was that the local nurses working in the ETU were not being paid by the Ministry of Health. They had been promised hazard pay on top of their normal wage, but nothing was forthcoming. For 6 months they petitioned. As a result, the nurses in Sierra Leone went on strike.

As an expatriate, I had to be careful and considerate about how to deal with issues within a host country, and whether to step in and get involved. In this case, I thought it was necessary to step in. I listened to the nurses, went to the MSF management team, and set up a meeting with the Liberian nursing supervisors and the MSF administration. Pressure was brought on to the Ministry of Health, and as a result the nurses were paid part of their wages, which meant they could cover their rent and buy food. The rest of their hazard and regular pay did not come through until 5 months after the outbreak was over.

Nurses were and will always be on the front lines of medical outbreaks, risking their lives while caring for the sick. Training these nurses to protect themselves and adopt best practices is a necessary long-term strategy to fend HCWs from future infectious outbreaks. During the Ebola crisis, visits were made to the clinics where these nurses worked before the outbreak. Time was spent with the nurses designing a safe setup, so that they could triage patients who were sick while remaining safe. Putting together protective kits with gloves and masks and delivering these to the clinics were some attempts to provide these brave nurses with the kind of protection we often take for granted in the developed world—protection that should be the right of every HCW worldwide.

Final Thoughts

The Ebola outbreak further devastated a nation that already had a weak health infrastructure. Many nurses and other HCWs died, depleting an already understaffed medical community. All industry shut down during the outbreak and left Liberia with a loss of more than $106 million, and the outbreak itself was estimated to cost more than $80 million (United Nations Development Programme, 2014). To recover from this devastation, Liberia needs to rebuild its health care system. There are 10,000 orphans to be cared for, disease-surveillance systems to be developed, and HCWs to be trained. West Africa needs international support to stabilize, rebuild, and develop the infrastructure that will help prevent further devastating outbreaks.

Amid all of this devastation, one example of building resilient infrastructure that I have witnessed has arisen from the heart of global nursing. Two of my Liberian nursing colleagues who worked with me during the outbreak have been able to go on and pursue master's degrees in public health in epidemiology due to Western visiting faculty accepting positions there. Such support and international collaboration is crucial to establish and strengthen infrastructure. Without international support, the risk of another devastating outbreak remains a real concern.

It was an honor to work in Liberia among some of the finest nurses I have ever met. They continue to toil in conditions that are not for the faint of heart and demonstrate—with humor and skill—the resilience of a profession that too often goes unrecognized.

PEACE

Peace and Justice for All (SDG 16)

Kelly Burke

At the most fundamental level, it is obvious that health is impossible without peace and justice. When resources, manpower, and political will are directed toward conflict and war, many social institutions fail. In the greater sense of the word "health"—that which the WHO (1948) has defined as "a state of complete physical, mental and social well-being and not merely the absence of disease or infirmity" (p. 1)—instability and a lack of peace wreak great havoc on social well-being and cohesiveness of societies.

Nurses play a crucial role in the health systems of any country, especially in LMICs or low-resource settings. Sickness cripples families in every way imaginable, often more so in these settings, stressing their way of life. When war/conflict/instability become part of the equation, it is clear that the health of populations is compromised and threatened. Nurses play a role not only in hospital or sickness, but also in primary care, community health, and prevention.

I have seen and believe that health systems are a mirror of the society in which they work. In countries where peace, justice, and equality prevail, the health care systems often function in a manner that takes care of any and all citizens. Where conflict and injustice are more common, health care for all and the notion of health as a human right fail. People working in the health sector are the driving force and the actors who can lead to the success or failure of health systems and health care. Nurses, making up a majority of the health care workforce, therefore have a major role in peace and justice. The core nursing values that lead nurses to professionally, competently, and compassionately care for all patients and clients or community members, regardless of history, religion, ethnicity, and race are the cornerstones of dignity and humanity that contribute toward and/or maintain peaceful, just, and cohesive societies.

I received my master's of public health with a concentration in international health 4 years before I became a nurse. My interest in international public health has always been driven by my passion for improving the injustices and inequalities in the world, but it was my nursing degree and the guiding ethical principles of nursing that reinforced my steadfast beliefs in care, justice, and compassion for all people. This unwavering principle is what is often detrimentally absent or difficult to provide by local nurses in settings experiencing conflict and injustice.

I have worked in various settings and in various capacities during my career as a global health nurse: as a nurse manager, clinical trial researcher, mentor, trainer, and teacher. The underlying reason I assumed these positions was that various countries had requested donor governments or organizations to provide assistance and funding to help improve health services, rebuild health infrastructures, and/or create health systems, due to a history of conflict or instability.

One organization with which I have worked during my global nursing career stands out in my memory: MSF. The MSF extends their assistance to all individuals who are victims of armed conflicts. MSF's mission is the epitome of humanitarian action, founded on the belief that health care is a right and humanity should be served regardless of identity or affiliation. While working in Arua, Uganda, and in remote areas of Ethiopia, it was clear that although MSF may have made the independent decision to be present and provide health care and services to those in need, the health needs existed due to previous or current conflict or a lack of peace.

With MSF in 2011, I worked as a nurse manager of a 2,000+ patient HIV clinic in Arua, Uganda. Arua lies in the northwest region of Uganda, an approximate 8-hour drive from the capital of Kampala, in the West Nile region of Uganda. The West Nile region had been cut off to some extent due to political and regional issues decades before. MSF was present due to a lack of HIV prevention and treatment services and had provided the first HIV services in the region over a decade ago. In Ethiopia, where I worked as a nurse trainer on the Somali border, there was ongoing ethnic conflict in Somalia and people were fleeing across the border to Dolo Ado, Ethiopia, in order to be safe and secure. Here I spent time in transit camps along the border where MSF was assisting to provide immunizations for refugees before they would be sent to internally placed camps. In Abdurafi, in the far northwest of Ethiopia, I also trained nurses. The issue there was justice. Seasonal migrant workers coming to pick cotton and sesame, in addition to other crops, were lacking proper shelter and health services and were subjected to the bite of female sandfly that was causing the deadly neglected tropical disease known as "kala azar" or "visceral leishmaniasis." MSF was there, believing and modeling that health is a human right and that health will promote justice and peace. Most of the HCWs MSF employs and invests in are local nurses to make that happen, and I am honored to have been a part of the MSF movement.

In Rwanda as a clinical educator, working for the Rwandan Human Resources for Health Program, a 7-year U.S.-funded initiative to improve the quality of health care and education of health professionals across the country, I have seen great progress amid the past struggles. For example, in Rwanda, with a long-standing history of tribal conflict and the infamous Genocide Against the Tutsi in 1994, trust among the population was an issue. Much has been done to unite all Rwandans and this is commendable. However, trauma and stress and seeing family members killed can have negative long-term consequences for one's mental well-being, behavior, and actions. More than 20 years later, nurses are doing their best to uphold the ethics and compassion of their profession to care for all fellow Rwandans, regardless of what happened in the past, to continue to promote peace and stability. Rwanda has made major investments in health and seen successes in the years since the genocide; where, in 1994, theirs was a nonexistent or severely crippled health system due to conflict, it is now an example that health systems do, in fact, need peace and justice to succeed.

In all of the settings I have worked as a nurse there has been a degree of desensitization to death. We must not overlook the impact that the history of a nation and "nurse fatigue" plays into the care that we provide and potentially the willingness of health care professionals to deliver equitable services to all people. Serving patients and clients—regardless of the socioeconomic and cultural barriers that often cause separation—can be challenging. When death becomes a norm, either due to conflict or overwhelming amounts of untreatable disease, empathy and compassion can become tempered. I have seen this so often. Perhaps it is a protection mechanism. A global nurse must always remember this. Often we are too quick to pass it off as lack of interest or disrespect of humanity by nurses. Rather, it should be framed in a larger view of peace and justice and how conflict has shaped the people of a nation.

Final Thoughts

So how can global nurses become peacemakers through education, research, and practice? As global nurses, we can "choose" where to go and self-identify the limits of what we can handle emotionally. However, local nurses do not always have the resources or educational background to do the same. This is why, as global nurses, we must stand in solidarity with those with whom we are working. We must continue to model empathy, holistic care, and inclusiveness, in order to promote peace and justice. As global nurses, it is our duty to model and teach these behaviors and values. It is very simple to do this because as global nurses working internationally and across cultures, we are guests in a foreign country. In general, we do not have family or shared history in that country. When local nurses see the way in which we care for their own citizens, we set a shining example of care without inequality. In a small town in Rwanda, where I worked for 3 years at the district hospital, I was often told, "I saw how you took care of that patient and so I tried to give the same care," or, "It amazes me how much you can care about all of our people."

Nursing has a culture of its own. As a global nurse, working in various countries where cultures and ways of life are different, nursing values often translate. This is what we strive for. What all nurses must have in common is the characteristic of empathy. In some cultures it is not as easy, as many people carry past issues or bigger, more pressing issues we may not fully understand. But we can teach and reinforce empathy; we need not fully understand all the dynamics to model this aspect of dignity. Regardless of where a nurse works, the fundamental ethical principles are the same. If we remember that conflict and injustice can be due to ethnic, regional, or religious divisions, among other reasons, and juxtapose this with compassion and care for all people, we teach nurses to have blinders to and empathy for these divisions. Nurses can then cultivate and practice the values required for peace and justice to be realized in their communities and become leaders in creating healthy and valued citizens.

PARTNERSHIP

Revitalizing the Global Partnership (SDG 17)

Helen Ewing

Managing partnerships is a key aspect of helping others, promoting project success, and enjoying the work experience. The UN, the WHO, World Bank, NGOs, and governments from high-income countries spend millions of dollars to improve health care in LMICs. They try to deliver sustainable projects in countries that lack funding, technical expertise, and physical infrastructure. The success or failure of partnership-run projects has long-term implications at local, national, regional, and global levels.

SDG 17 recognizes that strong and revitalized partnerships are needed for projects to be successful in which many elements decide whether partnerships will work. The following analogy shows my thinking regarding the development and preservation of strong partnerships. Fabric is composed of individual pieces of thread. The strength of each thread keeps the fabric together. This section focuses on the global nurse, the thread, and his or her interaction with a project, the fabric.

When the global nurse has a successful experience, a project stays strong and resilient; when the nurse does not achieve his or her goals, projects and partnerships tear and fray, leading to unfulfilled expectations.

My intent is to go beyond standard texts and project reports and offer a personalized view of global nursing in the context of partnerships. The quality of partnerships influences a nurse's global work experience. Partners include employers, funders, governments, NGOs, educational institutions, hospitals, clinics, licensing bodies, professional associations, professionals from multiple disciplines, communities, patients, and their families.

The subsequent case studies provide a personalized way to learn about global nursing. Each case looks at project location, funding sources, partnerships, activities, notable experiences, challenges, and successes. The middle part of this section focuses on the global nurse's role in partnerships, how partnerships influenced his or her life, and the value nursing brings to partnerships. The section ends with suggestions for a successful global nursing experience.

Case Studies Related to Partnership

Case study #1: Bangladesh

Location: Urban, Dhaka, Bangladesh

Funding: Multiple sources: self, local university, international clinic

Partners: Global nurse as clinician, educator, leader, administrator, and consultant; nursing students; local university faculty and support staff; teaching hospital HCWs and support staff; teaching hospital administrators; university president and his family; local government; Ministry of Health; Ministry of Education; immigration ministry; multinational governments; nursing council, patients, and families

Activities: The goal of this international project was to support the launch of the first private nursing school in Bangladesh. My role was didactic classroom teaching, skills lab facilitation, and supervising the hospital clinical rotation. I worked on course design, curriculum, and program development. I cofacilitated and managed a 2-day workshop on cyclone disaster management delivered to midlevel government officials.

Notable experiences: On my first day of work, I met with the university president who told me I was to design and facilitate a 2-day workshop at an international conference later in the week. The attendees were midlevel East Asian government officials and the topic was cyclone disaster management from a health care standpoint, a topic of which I knew little. As a Caucasian, non-Muslim female, I would present to a group of Muslim male government officials.

I was told, and I had read, that nurses in Bangladesh were poorly regarded because their jobs involved bodily waste. The students said they were ashamed to be nurses and their family members were not proud of their career choice. Families did not want their female nurses working evening and night shifts as they would be unaccompanied females out of the home after sunset. Culturally, this behavioral pattern was seen as inappropriate and associated with being a prostitute.

The nursing students were motivated and appreciative of my help. They wondered why, as a Caucasian female, living in a high-income country, I chose a profession with low societal standing. On the last night of my stay, I organized an evening meal at a local restaurant for all the students; I saw nurses crying and others were missing. Students said they were happy but frightened because this was the first time they were served food in a restaurant while others felt overwhelmed and self-conscious because kindness was extended to them. Two invitees, with help from friends, overcame panic attacks to attend their first restaurant meal.

Challenges: There were numerous government hurdles to achieve recognition of the nursing school. There was limited money to hire faculty; therefore an allied health professional stayed in Bangladesh to run the program with help from visiting international nurses and consultants. The cultural biases against nurses were demoralizing to the students. There was a lack of physical resources; for example, the room used to teach physical health assessment was not much larger than the size of a broom closet. Only a few students could fit into the room and the examination bed was on the wrong side to show proper physical examination techniques and with temperatures above 85°F or 30°C in a very humid climate with no air-conditioning, the environment was uncomfortable. There was a lack of paper to make handouts but the university president gave special permission to allow production of the disaster management manuals. There were daily electrical brownouts, which made working on my computer difficult.

Successes: When I left, the nursing students had adopted greater pride in themselves and their profession. The students learned that nursing was perceived positively in other parts of the world and to this day thank me for my visit.

The midlevel government officials developed a country-specific disaster management manual, which they took home to their citizens. The conference participants completed feedback forms in which they articulated that they had been worried about my usefulness as an educator because I was an American, non-Muslin, Caucasian female and they were surprised I could help them. A few years later, the nursing school received accreditation. Nurses in Bangladesh and other countries volunteered countless hours to achieve this success and advance the profession of nursing. The students I taught in the first class graduated and are now working throughout Asia, many in significant administrative and academic positions.

Case Study #2: Cambodia

Location: Small city and rural, Battambang, Cambodia

Funding: Multiple sources: self and NGO

Partners: Global nurse as clinician, educator, leader; sponsoring NGO; local government; local nurses; local midwives; local doctor; local elementary schools; local government Ministry of Health; immigration services; communities; patients and their families

Activities: The intent of this international project was to partner with hospital nurses in rural areas to provide training on leadership skills. Due to monsoon rains I could not work at the assigned sites. Instead, I partnered with midwives and did outpatient wellness checks for pregnant women and well-baby clinics. Because of flooding, I was posted to local elementary schools to teach English and health and wellness for part of my stay. I developed an English health education class to teach primary health promotion and disease prevention to elementary school students.

Notable experiences: After waiting hours at the airport for a pickup, locals helped us find our transportation. My colleague and I lived in a one-room studio apartment in a two-story motel style complex for workers and their families. There was no running water or kitchen facilities and the bathroom was part of the room. Upon arrival, our itinerary was changed because of floods and we were not being granted government permission to work in certain health care centers. I was surprised and gratified at the high level of competence shown by local midwives and nurses. They welcomed me and taught me new skills; they were excellent teachers. Despite a busy clinic schedule, the nurses were dedicated, kind to their patients, and delivered necessary patient teaching.

Our *tuk-tuk* (motorized rickshaw) driver showed us the devastating effects of the civil war in Cambodia. Sadly, we were told how people were brutally killed, saw the killing fields with the skeletons and skulls still present, and heard about cannibalism. Our driver and his wife had grown up in a refugee camp in Thailand during the Cambodian civil war in the 1970s.

The main hospital did not have adequate handwashing facilities, which was a surprise and disappointment to me, yet the Internet service in Cambodia was as good as North America.

Taking pictures of a hospital's organizational chart was met with a verbal reprimand from a hospital administrator.

Challenges: I was disappointed the itinerary was changed on arrival as this eliminated the opportunity to be involved with the nursing schools or the teaching institutions. There was minimal guidance from the sponsoring organization resulting in underutilization of my skills. Until I attained a translator, language was a barrier and when asked to teach health care at the elementary schools, the local teachers left me on my own and went home. I was challenged managing third-grade boys and girls in a foreign language, with no translator, on a Friday afternoon!

Successes: I saw the local nurses efficiently carrying out WHO clinical guidelines with the skills and knowledge previously taught to them sustained, and clinic patients had confidence in the nurses who delivered excellent care. Because of Internet availability, my coworker and I were able to develop a health educational program for elementary students. Our use of the same *tuk-tuk* driver over an extended period allowed him to afford to buy a bike for his daughter and reenroll her in a private school that taught English; he knew that fluent English skills would help her succeed in life.

Case Study #3: Kenya

Location: Rural, an area close to Mombasa, Kenya

Funding: Multiple funders: participants, sponsoring NGO

Partners: Global nurse as a clinician; sponsoring NGO; elementary students; elementary teachers; local school administrators; local school systems; local nurses; local medical doctors; Kenya department of health; Kenya immigration department; community; patients and their families

Activities: This international project involved a group of volunteer multinational nurses, with different health care backgrounds, running mobile clinics in various communities in rural Kenya. The clinics were constructed and dismantled at each site and we returned to our compound nightly where we inventoried our materials, reviewed the day's events, and planned the next day's clinic. Personal risk was high and accommodations were basic. A few weeks before I arrived, volunteer workers had been kidnapped. We stayed in a compound with guards carrying weapons with the guards accompanying us on all trips. These socioeconomically poor rural areas lacked resources in many areas such as health care. Unemployment was high, especially among young men with very little opportunities for change. Family roles emphasized women assuming domestic responsibilities and being subservient to men.

Notable experiences: There were many cases of "jiggers" (*Tunga penetrans*) at the clinics. This sand flea burrows under the skin ("tungiasis"), causing inflammation and infection. Thousands of dollars were spent on prescription and nonprescription medications from donor funds. I wondered if this money should have been spent on sustainable initiatives. Our accommodations were basic; we were eight nurses sleeping in bunk beds in one room with no air-conditioning. We were in an isolated, rural area with limited electricity and used outside toilets and showers with our flashlights acting as guides. Boys from the local villages visited the compound and asked for money to complete their high school education, which is not government funded. It was clear men had few employment opportunities. We were told the girls were too busy working at home to seek similar financial support; the educational needs of the girls were not being addressed.

This has been an area marked by terrorist activity with bombings occurring in Mombasa.

Seeing elephants in Tsavo National Park and learning about their problems with poachers and the number of elephants killed each year was disturbing. Being attacked by a group of monkeys while we were in a transport truck was a unique and frightening experience.

Challenges: Ethical questions arose during this project. Would the money that was spent on prescription medications have helped more people if we had bought mosquito nets to prevent malaria in a high malaria area, or if we had bought large amounts of potassium permanganate solutions to treat the great number of sand flea infection cases? Could we have used the money to set up a sustainable educational program to treat sand flea infections among schoolchildren? The licensing status of those delivering care was unclear. Should we have been allowed to operate the mobile clinic? Children were given prescription medication to treat their condition when all efforts to reach parents failed. Should this have been done? There was a lack of clarity as to who was in charge of the daily functioning of the project and the NGO partner did not have a health care overseer, which led to a lack of cohesiveness and inefficiencies. There was no senior person to address the ethical concerns.

Treating Kenyans with tungiasis with a potassium-based soak was a major part of the project; it was and is a needed service as there is no known drug treatment. School principals asked to continue the treatment program for tungiasis but there was minimal opportunity to transfer skills and there was no plan for leaving supplies for long-term use.

Successes: Kenyans who came to the mobile clinic had access to nurse practitioners from a high-resource country, a local nurse, and a local medical doctor. They could be tested and treated for malaria. Some nurses financially sponsored male students so that they could complete their high school studies. Additionally, school principals saw the value of treating children who had the sand flea infections as they realized improved health would benefit their students scholastically and they wanted to do more for their students at their own cost.

Lessons Learned

Leaving Home

The first lesson is about the transition from home to a new country, leaving familiarity behind. There are several parts to familiarity: relationships, routines, values and ethics, communication style, and physical environment. The global nurse leaves behind a home with modern amenities and a work environment that is well equipped and spacious. She also leaves behind an established support network, which connects her to her environment.

In her new environment, there is a change of work routines, weekend routines, vacation routines, and family routines. Personal values and ethics affect work and home life; an example of value or ethics influencing work is a nurse's sense of justice when caring for a patient. She may see herself as a patient advocate in a system that embraces patient empowerment. The health care system she knows promotes and prioritizes best patient outcomes and best evidence-based clinical practice; this may not be prioritized in the same way in her new environment.

A nurse's communication style tends to become habituated to a new setting over time and through continual exposure to context, but is normally representative of his or her habits and past frame of reference. Similarly, nonverbal communication through body movements and facial expression is unique to her geographic location. When talking, she is used to a certain distance between herself and a colleague; that space etiquette may change in a different culture. She may feel uncomfortable with a person standing closer to her when she talks while others may not show facial expression in conversation. This lack of feedback may cause her to question how much of what she is saying is understood. In some settings, voices may sound loud and the tone harsh.

When a global nurse travels to a new country, her excitement about the approaching adventures is tempered by what she leaves behind. The global nurse is challenged to move beyond losses and embrace the future. Her new world has unfamiliar people, a changed support system, different routines, altered values and ethics, and a changed physical environment. Being aware of these factors can facilitate adaptive change.

New Arrival

The major theme on arrival is managing change. Addressing travel-related insomnia should be a priority; until sleep is normalized, daytime functioning remains suboptimal. Changed routines include: work start and finish times, transport to and from work, and work content and processes. What were once straightforward tasks at home become complex due to a lack of human and physical resources. For example, delivering a power point presentation can be delayed because there is no functioning projector or an extension cord is not available. In the clinical setting, drug availability may be minimal or standard equipment is broken, which prevents basic nursing assessment and care.

Home routines change and can be a source of frustration; electricity or Internet bills may shift to a pay-as-you-go system. The global nurse may need a new SIM card for phone and Internet services. Foods are different with questions about food safety, and privacy may be lost if she lives in a communal setting.

Each global nurse has a short time to develop relationships. Connectivity is important to preserve good physical and emotional health and Internet activity allows communication with those at home. Relationships facilitate her social life and can help her deal with death and dying in the workplace. Spending time with friends on the weekend gives the global nurse a chance to share her experiences, which may be common to others.

Values and ethics change when a nurse works in a different country. In a LMIC, a child may die of gastroenteritis because there are no available intravenous fluids or antibiotics. Women in the host country may not have the same rights, freedoms, or protections; and same-sex relationships may not be accepted. Health care in LMICs may be skewed toward a paternalistic and top-down hierarchy. Where does the global nurse's advocacy role begin and end? How does the nurse manage within a system that does not share the same values and ethics? What happens if the nurse's values clash with those of the employer? Each nurse needs to find his or her own answers and can gain insights from experienced colleagues. Resolving guilt at having more financial resources than local colleagues is an issue for some.

Verbal communication styles differ from country to country; the tone, language, and word context changes. Misunderstandings are common when starting a new position. English may be the second language in the host country and the global nurse may not be fluent in the local language. The global nurse's opinions and concerns may be less valued despite his or her training and knowledge, and the nurse's evidence-based views may be interpreted by local staff as, "You do not understand the culture." Host country participants may not share their opinions easily and may not be receptive to change.

Nonverbal communication is also different; facial expression may be wider or restricted depending on the culture. Consistently meeting a flattened affect can be distressing for global nurses. What does it mean? Does a local colleague's stoic expression after a patient death represent a lack of caring? Or, is it a protective shield to deal with frequent deaths? Nonverbal communication in the global nurse's personal life may change. A female nurse may be required to dress differently because of religious or country customs. Strangers, children, and adults may stare at her or touch a female Caucasian nurse out of curiosity.

At the nurse's new home, electricity, water, and Internet services may not be the same and the access to food and clothing changes. Isolation can be problematic in a rural setting while living in an urban center can have its challenges with limited personal space. Learning to live with less cleanliness, rodents, and insects is trying. Being in a work environment where there may be limited supplies or a lack of aseptic technique can create stress for the global nurse and she may be exposed to "needless deaths" comprising situations where patients die who would have been successfully treated in her resource-rich country. The contrast of care and outcomes can create disabling emotional turmoil.

Partnerships in Global Nursing

The global nurse is a key ingredient to international health partnerships. This next section emphasizes the partnerships that surround her and how they influence her daily activities.

Working With Partners

The global nurse works within partnerships and systems in her adopted country and may work for an employer who answers to governing bodies and legal entities. These partners assess a project's value, progress, and results and managing partners may be more concerned about big picture deliverables than field level events. The global nurse can feel forgotten or disempowered in this scenario.

A global nurse partners with governing agencies. The local nursing board reviews her licensing credentials and the Ministry of Health oversees scope of practice and patient contact. Immigration services control work permits, travel, and length of stays. Sponsoring partners, whether governmental, nongovernmental, or private, influence her work life. As financial aid diminishes globally, single-funder projects are reduced and multiple-funder projects become the new normal.

Challenges With Partners

When there are multiple partners, priorities differ, which can lead to a lack of direction and focus. The priorities may change as a project unfolds; thus, a nurse's job can change too. The change may not be to her liking and may not fit with her skill set. Communication about a project's content may be poor and as a result, the global nurse may not understand the fundamentals of her project. The theoretical plan and on-the-ground realities may differ making the nurse's role murky. If she asks questions, the answers may be, "Sorry that is as much as I can do . . . we do not have funding for that solution . . . somebody else will decide . . . " This situation can be distressing for a nurse trying to reach previously identified goals and she may question the value and sustainability of her project. This can lead to, "Why am I here" type thinking.

Partners may have different levels of commitment to a project. At a grassroots level, divergences of knowledge, skill, motivation, and financial compensation with local nurse partners can create discontent for both nurses and partners. A country's government officials may have imposed a project on local staff. When someone has had a program forced upon him or her, he or she may be less receptive to the global nurse's visit and an inadequately compensated local nurse partner is less motivated to participate in a project.

After a project starts, the managing partners may hand over a project to local managers; using training wheels to help someone ride a bike is an analogy that explains this concept. The local participants and host government are the ones riding the bike, the high-income funders and managers are the training wheels. When the training wheels come off, some projects manage and others do not. If the global nurse happens to be on the bike when it wobbles and falls, she is subjected to emotional cuts, scrapes, and burns. The global nurse needs to balance her well-being with her sense of duty to the project.

Global health projects are about helping countries meet their needs. The global nurse may be caught in an ethical dilemma when the overseeing partners' evaluation of needs differs from the countries' stated needs or her own assessment of needs.

The Value of the Global Nurse to Partners

Having looked at the experiences of the global nurse and the partnerships that surround him or her, this section expands on the value a global nurse brings to his or her partners. The global nurse is an integral and necessary part of rebuilding health care systems in LMICs. This reality behooves donors, fundraisers, private industry, governments, and nongovernmental partners to provide more roles for nurses in planning and executing projects.

A recently trained nurse brings fresh knowledge to her adopted country, which she can share with local partners while the experienced nurse brings wisdom with learned skills. A local nurse shares her concerns and needs and together the visiting nurse and the local nurse can apply solutions to educational, administrative, and clinical problems when given the power and freedom to do so. A global nurse has a chance to raise the profile of nursing, and in many cases women, in a LMIC. This raised profile may not result in immediate change but can provide the spark for future change. The global nurse can instill pride in her partners and encourage them to be leaders within health care and society.

The global nurse can help influence the delivery of health care. Many countries continue to work with a paternalistic, top-down, doctor-driven system that is not patient focused and tertiary care facilities remain the focus of attention. Nursing can show health systems how patient empowerment, patient education, and training local caregivers can be cost-effective and efficient. Nurses have a high level of public trust in high-income countries and can influence health care delivery; the global nurse has a chance to extend this level of influence abroad.

Final Thoughts

There are guiding principles a global citizen nurse can follow to reach his or her goals.

- **Helping:** A core feature of nursing is helping others. Wanting to "save and help" may be strong feelings but they may not be realistic; expectations should be tempered by pragmatism and environmental constraints.

- **Personal safety:** Be safe. Understand that no job is worth a nurse's health. It is the global nurse's choice to decide when she is working in an unacceptable situation and should carry out an evidence-based assessment of where she fits in the project and how much her skills are valued.

  The global nurse should be cautious about assuming that others have a satisfactory knowledge of the local medical system, facilities, and available care. Before leaving home, speak to someone who has knowledge of international travel. The health care system in a resource-poor country may not be able to support an easily managed condition in a high-income country.

  Police and laws vary in how they are enforced and applied; learn from your organization about the dos and don'ts. Some law enforcement groups look to expatriates to supplement their low incomes by asking for money; therefore do not assume law enforcement will act in your best interest. It is important to register with your embassy as they can help in an emergency. Learn to do a risk evaluation for personal safety such as assessing whether it is safe to go out at night. Can the antimalarial pill be stopped? How safe is it to have a relationship with a local partner? How safe is it to drink too much alcohol and be in a vulnerable state? Develop a social safety net for support; this can be done through relationships with employees of other organizations or joining expatriate groups.

- **The nurse as a guest:** Regardless of whether the global nurse agrees with the values, standards, and practices of the host country, he or she is a guest. The host country's rules apply regardless of their fairness. The global nurse is part of a revolving door of helpers in a LMIC. When he or she arrives, he or she does not know the context of his/her situation or his/her partners' past experiences. His or her local partner does not leave when he or she leaves. Therefore the issues that arise during his or her stay are left for his or her partner to manage after he or she is gone. Local peers or superiors may not share his or her enthusiasm for change; given this reality, a manager may limit his or her nurse partner's ability to make changes.

- **Having all the answers:** Do not assume the "way it is done at home" should be adopted in the host country. The host country's context, resources, and culture are different. The developed world's pushing of baby formula on LMICs is an example of how modern technology may not be best for everyone.

- **Making a difference:** Each global nurse wants to make a difference; sometimes making a difference means reevaluating original goals and resetting them. The global nurse can look beyond his or her job to improve the quality of life of those around him or her.

- **Expect the unexpected:** Working in a LMIC means there are daily inconveniences and problems that can derail the best-laid plans. Despite seeing an easy fix, local partners may not want to implement a suggested fix and the global nurse needs to respect the partner's voice even though it is not consistent with his or her own thinking.

- **Time flies:** The concept of time may differ in the host country. Start times and finish times for meetings and appointments may be relative and while planning may seem sensible and efficient, some countries are more spontaneous and work with short timelines. Long-term planning and systemizing may not work in a host country.

- **Flexibility:** The global nurse needs to be flexible about time, work environment, living conditions, values, ethics, communication styles, resource availability, local customs, and his or her interpretation of morbidity and mortality. Having said this, each nurse should know his or her limits and act quickly when the environment no longer supports him or her; a nurse's health is non-negotiable and should be the priority. There should be no shame in this philosophy; it is not a sign of weakness; it is good risk management.

CONCLUSION

A chain is only as strong as its weakest link; a strong nursing link supports healthy lives and a unified world. When true to one's profession, the global nurse brings a vital sense of caring, integrity, ethics, knowledge, and professionalism to his or her workplace. By engaging in global health projects, each nurse advances the UN SDGs.

As with Florence Nightingale's life, a nurse sometimes needs to challenge partners to improve health care. By doing this, patients and their families can have a better quality of life. Global nursing in LMICs can be difficult because partners may not value a nurse's opinion and be more rigid about making changes. Local nurses in LMICs still struggle for respect and decision making powers.

Global nursing gives each nurse a chance to learn about others and self. The global nurse faces situations that challenge him or her emotionally, intellectually, ethically, physically, personally, and professionally. As with all adventures, he or she does not know the outcome until the adventure is finished. Experiences can be eye-opening, life-changing, or a confirmation of held assertions.

We need global nurses to promote nursing and to improve health care systems. Our job, like Florence Nightingale, is to bring light to dark places.

REFLECTION AND DISCUSSION

- What is my global nursing story?

- How do I see my story as relevant to the UN 2030 Agenda? How can I more effectively integrate the SDGs into my story and my area of specialty?

- What are my judgments and reservations about using storytelling as a valid method of reflective practice?

- Global nurses share an ethical code that seeks to promote and protect human dignity, but each one of us does it differently. What aspects of the nurses' stories discussed earlier unite them as people and as professionals? How do they differ?

- In what ways am I, as a global nurse, integral to the sustainable advancement of People? Planet? Prosperity? Peace? Partnership?

REFERENCES

60 Million Girls. (n.d.). Empowering girls for a just and balanced world. Retrieved from http://60millionsdefilles.org/en

Alleyne, G., Binagwaho, A., Haines, A., Jahan, S., Nugent, R., Rojhani, A., & Stuckler, D. (2013). Embedding non-communicable diseases in the post-2015 development agenda. *The Lancet, 381*, 566–574.

Alsan, M., Westerhaus, M., Herce, M., Nakashima, K., & Farmer, P. (2011). Poverty, global health and infectious disease: Lessons from Haiti and Rwanda. *Infectious Disease Clinics North America, 25*(3), 611–622.

Alwan, A. (2011). *Global status report on noncommunicable diseases 2010*. Geneva, Switzerland: World Health Organization. Retrieved from http://www.who.int/nmh/publications/ncd_report_full_en.pdf

American Association of Colleges of Nursing. (2015). The impact of education on nursing practice. Retrieved from http://www.aacn.nche.edu/media-relations/fact-sheets/impact-of-education

American Nurses Association. (2016). Creating a culture of safety. Retrieved from http://www.nursingworld.org/CreatingSafetyofCulture

Bain, E. S. R., Gundry, W. S., Wright, J. A., Yang, H., Pedley, S., & Bartram, K. J. (2012). Accounting for water quality monitoring access to safe drinking-water as part of millennium development goals: Lessons from five countries. *Bulletin of the Organization, 90*, 228–235A.

Bajpai, P. (2016, July 18). The world's top 10 economies. Retrieved from http://www .investopedia.com/articles/investing/022415/worlds-top-10-economies.asp

Bartram, J., & Platt, J. (2010). How health professions can leverage health gains from improved water, sanitation and hygiene practices. *Perspectives in Public Health, 130*(5), 215–221.

Bausch, D. G., & Schwarz, L. (2014). Outbreak of Ebola virus disease in Guinea: Where ecology meets economy. *PLOS Neglected Tropical Diseases, 8*(7), e3056. doi:10.1371/journal.pntd .0003056

Benton, D. (2012). Advocating globally to shape policy and strengthen nursing's influence. *The Online Journal of Issues in Nursing, 17*(5), manuscript 5. doi:10.3912/OJIN.Vol17No01Man05

Bhengu, B. R. (2010). An investigation into the level of empowerment of rural women in Zululand District of KwaZulu-Natal. *Curationis, 33*(2), 4–12.

Bliss, E. K. (2009, September). Enhancing U.S. leadership on drinking water and sanitation: Opportunities within global health programs, a report on the CSIS global health policy center. Retrieved from http://www.csis.org

Brown, B. (2010). *The gifts of imperfections: Letting go of who we think we should be and embracing who we are.* Center City, MN: Hazelden.

Brown, B. (2012). *Daring greatly: How the courage to be vulnerable transforms the way we live, love, parent, and lead.* New York, NY: Gotham.

Brysiewicz, P., Hughes, T. L., & McCreary, L. L. (2015). Promoting innovation in global nursing practice. *Rwanda Journal Series F: Medicine and Health Sciences, 2*(2), 41–45.

Burkhardt, M. A., & Nagai-Jacobson, M. G. (2016). Spirituality and health. In B. M. Dossey & L. Keegan (Eds.), *Holistic nursing: A handbook for practice* (7th ed., pp. 135–163). Burlington, MA: Jones & Bartlett.

Burns, L. R. (Ed.). (2014). *India's healthcare industry: Innovation in delivery, financing, and manufacturing.* New York, NY: Cambridge University Press.

Campbell, M. R. O., Benova, L., Gon, G., Afsana, K., & Cumming, O. (2015). Getting the basic rights–the role of water, sanitation and hygiene in maternal and reproductive health: A conceptual framework. *Tropical Medicine and International Health, 20*(3), 252–267.

Clasen, T. F., Alexander, K. T., Sinclair, D., Boisson, S., Peletz, R., Chang, H. H., . . . Cairncross, S. (2015). Interventions to improve water quality f or preventing diarrhoea. *Cochrane Database of Systematic Reviews.* doi:10.1002/14651858.CD004794.pub3

Cumming, O., Elliot, M., Overbo, A., & Bartram, J. (2014). Does global progress on sanitation really lag behind water? An analysis of global progress on community- and household-level access to safe water and sanitation. *PLOS ONE, 9*(12). doi:10.1371/journal.pone.0114699

Das, J., Holla, A., Das, V., Mohanan, M., Tabak, D., & Chan, B. (2012). In urban and rural India, a standardized patient study showed low levels of provider training and huge quality gaps. *Health Affairs, 31*(12), 2774–2784.

DNA India. (2015). India clocks 7.5% growth in January–March, quarter, becomes world's fastest growing economy. Retrieved from http://www.dnaindia.com/money/report -india-clocks-75-growth-in-january-march-quarter-becomes-world-s-fastest-growing -economy-2090462

Doctors without Borders/Medecins Sans Frontieres. (n.d.). Charter. Retrieved from http:// www.doctorswithoutborders.org/about-us/history-principles/charter

Elliot, T. S. (1995). *The Four Quartets: "Little Gidding."* London, UK: Faber and Faber.

Extension Toxicology Network. (1993). Naled. Retrieved from http://pmep.cce.cornell.edu/ profiles/extoxnet/metiram-propoxur/naled-ext.html

Freshwater, D., Taylor, B., & Sherwood, G. (Eds.). (2008). The international textbook of reflective practice in nursing. London, UK: Blackwell/STTI.

Guarino, B. (2016, September 1). 'Like it's been nuked': Millions of bees dead after South Carolina sprays for Zika mosquitoes. *The Washington Post.* Retrieved from https:// www.washingtonpost.com/news/morning-mix/wp/2016/09/01/like-its-been-nuked -millions-of-bees-dead-after-south-carolina-sprays-for-zika-mosquitoes

Gupta, R. P. (2016). Health care reforms in India: Making up for the lost decades. New Delhi, India: Elsevier.

Heiman, H., & Artiga, S. (2015). Beyond healthcare: The role of social determinants in promoting health and health equity. Retrieved from http://kff.org/disparities-policy/issue-brief/beyond-health-care-the-role-of-social-determinants-in-promoting-health-and-health-equity

Helming, M. A. (2016). Relationships. In B. M. Dossey & L. Keegan (Eds.), *Holistic nursing: A handbook for practice* (7th ed., pp. 479–499). Burlington, MA: Jones & Bartlett.

Horton-Deutsch, S. (2016). Visionary and reflection centered: Remaining open to the possibilities of nursing praxis. In W. Rosa (Ed.), *Nurses as leaders: Evolutionary visions of leadership* (pp. 311–322). New York, NY: Springer Publishing.

Hutton, G., & Chase, C. (2016). The knowledge base for achieving the Sustainable Development Goal targets on water supply, sanitation and hygiene. *International Journal of Environmental Research and Public Health, 13*(6). doi:10.3390/ijerph13060536

Institute of Medicine. (2000). *To err is human: Building a safer health system.* Washington, DC: National Academies Press.

Institute of Medicine. (2001). *Crossing the quality chasm: A new health system for the 21st century.* Washington, DC: National Academies Press.

Institute of Medicine. (2011). *The future of nursing: Leading change, advancing health.* Washington, DC: National Academies Press.

Jha, D. N. (2015, September 12). 7-year-old dies of dengue, parents commit suicide. Retrieved from http://timesofindia.indiatimes.com/city/delhi/7-year-old-dies-of-dengue-parents-commit-suicide/articleshow/48934167.cms

Kinzer, S. (2008). *A thousand hills: Rwanda's rebirth and the man who dreamed it.* Hoboken, NJ: John Wiley.

Marmot, M. (2006). Harveian oration: Health in an unequal world. *The Lancet, 368,* 2081–2094.

Ministry of Health. (2013). Health management information system strategic plan. Retrieved from http://www.nationalplanningcycles.org/sites/default/files/country_docs/Lesotho/hmis_strategic_plan_2013-2017_final_-_01042013.pdf

Msiska, G., Smith, P., & Fawcett, T. (2014). The "lifeworld" of Malawian undergraduate student nurses: The challenge of learning in resource poor clinical settings. *International Journal of Africa Nursing Sciences, 1,* 35–42.

Mukamana, D., Dushimiyimana, V., Kayitesi, J., Mudasumbwa, G., Nibagwire, J., Ngendahayo, F., . . . Rosa, W. (2016). Nephrology nursing in Rwanda: Creating the future through education and organizational partnership. *Nephrology Nursing Journal, 43*(4), 311–315.

Mukamana, D., Karonkano, G. R., & Rosa, W. (2016). Advancing perioperative nursing in Rwanda through global partnerships and collaboration. *AORN Journal, 104*(6), 583–587.

Mukamana, D., Niyomugabo, A., & Rosa, W. (2016, June). Global partnership advances medical-surgical nursing in Rwanda. *Med-Surg Nursing Connection.* Retrieved from https://amsn.org/sites/default/files/documents/articles-events/amsn/msnc0616.pdf

Mulaudzi, F. M., & Chyun, D. A. (2015). Innovation in nursing and midwifery education and research. *Rwanda Journal Series F: Medicine and Health Sciences, 2*(2), 21–25.

National Cancer Institute. (2011). Agricultural health study. Retrieved from https://www.cancer.gov/about-cancer/causes-prevention/risk/ahs-fact-sheet

National Institute of Statistics of Rwanda. (2015). Rwanda demographic and health survey. Retrieved from http://www.statistics.gov.rw/publication/demographic-and-health-survey-dhs-20142015-key-findings

Nelson, M. L. (1988). Advocacy in nursing. *Nursing Outlook, 33*(3), 136–141.

Nyamidie, J. K. E. (1999). African proverb of the month September 1999. Retrieved from http://www.afriprov.org/african-proverb-of-the-month/25-1999proverbs/146-sep1999.html

Prüss-Ustün, A., Wolf, J., Corvalán, C., Bos, R., & Neira, M. (2016). *Preventing disease through health environments: A global assessment of the burden of disease from environmental risks.* Geneva, Switzerland: World Health Organization. Retrieved from http://apps.who.int/iris/bitstream/10665/204585/1/9789241565196_eng.pdf

Rao, M., Rao, K. D., Kumar, A. K. S., Chatterjee, M., & Sundararaman, T. (2011). Human resources for health in India. *The Lancet, 377*(9765), 587–598.

Roberts, E. M., English, P. B., Grether, J. K., Windham, G. C., Somberg, L., & Wolff, C. (2007). Maternal residence near agricultural pesticide applications and autism spectrum disorders among children in the California central valley. *Environmental Health Perspectives, 115*(10), 1482–1489.

Senior, K. (2010). Wanted 2.4 million nurses, and that's just in India. *Bulletin of the World Health Organization, 88*(5), 321–400. Retrieved from http://www.who.int/bulletin/volumes/88/5/10-020510/en

Shariff, N. (2014). Factors that act as facilitators and barriers to nurse leaders' participation in health policy development. *BMC Nursing, 13*(20). Retrieved from http://www.biomedcentral.com/1472-6955/13/20

Sherwood, G., & Horton-Deutsch, S. (Eds.). (2012). *Reflective practice: Transforming education and improving outcomes.* Indianapolis, IN: Sigma Theta Tau International.

Sherwood, G., & Horton-Deutsch, S. (Eds.). (2015). *Reflective organizations: On the frontlines of QSEN and reflective practice implementation.* Indianapolis, IN: Sigma Theta Tau International.

Shim, Y. K., Mlynarek, S. P., & van Wijngaarden, E. (2009). Parental exposure to pesticides and childhood brain cancer: U.S. Atlantic Coast Childhood Brain Cancer Study. *Environmental Health Perspectives, 117*(6), 1002–1006.

Sundar, D. K., Garg, S., & Garg, I. (Eds.). (2015). *Public health in India: Technology governance, and service delivery.* New Delhi, India: Routledge.

United Nations. (1948). *Universal declaration of human rights.* Retrieved from http://www.un.org/en/universal-declaration-human-rights

United Nations. (2015). Transforming our world: The 2030 Agenda for Sustainable Development. Retrieved from https://docs.google.com/gview?url=http://sustainabledevelopment.un.org/content/documents/21252030%20Agenda%20for%20Sustainable%20Development%20web.pdf&embedded=true

United Nations. (2016). Goal 14: Conserve and sustainably use the oceans, seas and marine resources: Facts and figures. Retrieved from http://www.un.org/sustainabledevelopment/oceans

United Nations Development Programme (2014). Socio-economic impact of the Ebola virus disease in Guinea, Liberia and Sierra Leone. Retrieved from http://www.africa.undp.org/content/dam/rba/docs/Reports/Ebola_policy_note_EN.pdf

Wagner, A. L. (2016). Engaged and expressed: Storytelling as a way to know and be known. In W. Rosa (Ed.), *Nurses as leaders: Evolutionary visions of leadership* (pp. 431–451). New York, NY: Springer Publishing.

World Health Organization. (1948). *Constitution of the World Health Organization.* Geneva, Switzerland: Author. Retrieved from http://www.who.int/governance/eb/who_constitution_en.pdf

World Health Organization. (2004). *Guidelines for drinking-water quality* (3rd ed., Vol. 1). Geneva, Switzerland: Author.

World Health Organization. (2016). *Global strategic directions for strengthening nursing and midwifery 2016–2020.* Geneva, Switzerland: Author. Retrieved from http://www.who.int/hrh/nursing_midwifery/global-strategic-midwifery2016-2020.pdf

Zimmerman, E., Woolf, S., & Haley, A. (2015). Understanding the relationship between education and health: A review of the evidence and an examination of community perspectives. Rockville, MD: Agency for Healthcare Research and Quality. Retrieved from http://www.ahrq.gov/professionals/education/curriculum-tools/population-health/zimmerman.html

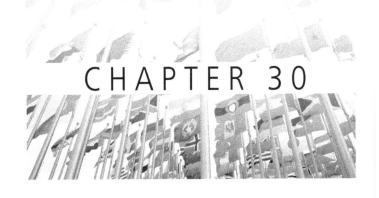

CHAPTER 30

The Role of Reflective Practice in Creating the World We Want

Sara Horton-Deutsch and William Rosa

Reflective practice is the vital and largely untapped resource for significant and sustained effectiveness. At its core, reflective practice is about tapping into things deeply human: the desire to learn, to grow, to be in community with others, to contribute, to serve, and to make sense of our time on earth. (York-Barr, Sommers, Ghere, & Montie, 2016, p. xxii)

On July 31, 2012, civil society and the United Nations (UN) joined forces to launch a web-based campaign entitled, "The World We Want" (Beyond 2015, 2015). It was an effort to give voice to people from every corner of the planet, to bring their lived experiences to the forefront and join like-minded others in creating a unified, collective vision beyond 2015. Through this platform, men, women, and children had the opportunity to participate in ongoing consultations regarding the keystones of what would later become the Sustainable Development Agenda; passionate discussions on everything from urbanization, food security, and environmental concerns to health, education, and governance emerged. The World We Want provided an opportunity for human beings to speak out and reflect on what was most important to them and the world they wanted to create by 2030. As global nurses continue to take on leadership and advocacy roles in achieving the 2030 Agenda, continued attention to personal–professional reflection will be necessary if we are to accomplish the Sustainable Development Goals (SDGs) and create an innovative, inspired, and informed vision for the post-2030 era.

REFLECTIVE PRACTICE: A GUIDE FOR THE BETTERMENT OF SELF AND SOCIETY

Reflective practice as a concept has been around since ancient times. The origins of reflection evolved many centuries ago from Eastern and Western philosophers, including Buddha, Plato, and Lao Tzu. They all emphasized human self-reflection as a willingness to learn more about one's fundamental nature, purpose, and essence. This form of inquiry leads to inquiry of the human condition and the philosophical consideration of consciousness and awareness.

The views of reflection and its use in more practical contexts originated from John Dewey, an influential 20th-century educational philosopher. He defined "reflection" as the active, persistent, and careful consideration of beliefs supported by knowledge. He emphasized not just rigor in practice, but the importance of incorporating scientific knowledge into reflection (Dewey, 1933). He equally valued external knowledge from research and internal knowledge that emerged when practitioners mindfully examine the impact of their practice. Building on these ideas, Donald Schön (1983, 1987), an expert in the field of organizational learning, identified learning as the foundation of individual and organizational improvement. His work authenticated both what was directly taught (explicit learning) and what was learned through experience (implicit learning), including observation and modeling. He emphasized that humans learn best when tapping into both internal and external resources to inform decisions. Concisely, these bodies of work characterize reflective practice as an active thought process intended to aid in understanding current truths of practice and at the same time seeing multiple possibilities for improvement. The fundamental importance is that reflective practice leads to informed action.

Christopher Johns, the leading nurse expert on reflective practice, has published widely on the topic for decades. Johns (2013) describes "reflective practice" as a mindful way of being within practice and a process to reflect on experience to appreciate and resolve contradiction with the intent of realizing one's own vision for practice as a lived reality. This definition grounds the practitioner in who he or she is as a learner and a practitioner. More broadly, Taylor (2000) describes "reflection" as a focused way of discerning practice and includes any type of attentive consideration such as thinking, contemplation, or meditation that helps clarify sense and leads to contextually appropriate changes. Freshwater (2008) extends this definition to not just discerning current practice but also questioning the underlying political, ethical, historical, and cultural traditions. More recently, reflection has been linked to the vital nursing skill and human attribute of self-awareness and authentic presence (Horton-Deutsch & Sherwood, 2008; Lombard & Horton-Deutsch, 2012).

Reflective practice contributes to working from our deeper sense of mission and purpose; where we consider what we know, believe, and value within the context of a particular situation in our work and/or life. It helps us to develop spiritual resources as we are encouraged to ponder meaning and our own way of being in the world. Being a reflective practitioner is an intentional strategy for professional development and expands our capacity for leadership. It supports and advances values clarification, an important reflective endeavor, and guides us to act and do the right thing, in our own leadership journey (Young, Pardue, & Horton-Deutsch, 2015).

WAYS OF REFLECTING

There is not one universal definition of "reflection" nor is there one universal way to reflect. No one person, group, or organization integrates reflective practice in precisely the same way. It is an active, iterative process that continually seeks to assess, understand, and adjust practices. Thus it is often framed as a cyclical or spiraling process—cycling forward and backward to challenge thinking and produce deeper practice knowledge (Gibbs, 1988; York-Barr et al., 2016). The Gibbs reflective cycle (1988) includes six stages and at each stage a question or cue is provided to aid in reflection. The model is wide-ranging and can be applied to numerous situations. The six stages are:

1. Describe what happened.
2. If it happened again what would you do?
3. What were you thinking/feeling?
4. What else could have been done?
5. What was good and bad about the experience?
6. What sense can you make of the situation?

The Reflective Practice Cycle (York-Barre et al., 2016) can be used in group settings and starts with being grounded in *purpose,* followed by being actively *present* to observe and learn, being open and partaking in the *inquiry,* acquiring *insights* from the learning and adding to the dialogue so others gain new insights, taking informed *action* based on the knowledge that is generated, and concludes with continually asking "Are we seeing the results we want to see?" If yes, the group asks "Now what?" And, if no, then the group asks "Now what?" This is a continual back and forth cycle to challenge thinking and harvest deeper knowledge and understanding. Contained between the purpose and the results are thought and regulatory cycles that circle back to previous steps to assess, challenge, and fine-tune the cycle. This iterative process helps to ensure that, however the process recycles, it remains rooted in the purpose.

A less prescriptive, more qualitative mode of reflection is offered by Christopher Johns (2006). The Model for Structured Reflection offers cues to assess the depth of reflection for learning through experience. The cues become internalized through time and can be continuously refined. The cues correspond to Carper's (1978) four fundamental ways of knowing: aesthetic, ethical, empirical, and personal. The map can be viewed in Johns (2006) and guides learners to frame learning through reflection. At the center of the map is the aesthetic response that encompasses four key processes:

1. Appreciating the pattern of the particular situation
2. Making judgments based on care needs
3. Responding in a particular way within the situation
4. Making judgments about the efficacy of response in meeting care needs

Next, asking the following three questions that are outlined in the periphery of the map respond to the other components of Carper's (1978) ways of knowing from ethical, empirical, and personal perspectives:

1. Did I act for the best?
2. What knowledge informed my practice? And, what knowledge should have informed my practice?
3. What personal factors were influencing me?

In addition to the ways of knowing proposed by Carper (1978) and addressed by Johns (2006) in his Model for Structured Reflection, other patterns of knowing have been proposed that may be incorporated into this model. For example, Munhall (1993) proposed a pattern of knowing titled "unknowing" while White (1995) added "sociopolitical knowing." More recently, Chinn and Kramer (2008) added "emancipatory knowing" to address issues of equity, justice, and transformation in all areas of practice. Inclusively, the seven patterns of knowing inform areas of nursing praxis including those that guide moral action. Additional reflective questions related to these ways of knowing include:

4. What else could it be?
5. What are the sociopolitical aspects of this situation?
6. Are there issues related to equity, justice, and transformation that I need to consider? If yes, what are they and how can they be addressed?

These three models for reflective practice are a representative sample; many others exist. However, they have particular value for both self-reflection and reflecting with others and represent contributions from nursing and educational scholars alike. The next three sections offer strategies for individual reflective practice, reflective practice with partners/groups, and reflective practice with organizations.

Individual Reflective Practice

Reflective practice is about tapping into the deepest part of ourselves: our compassion for ourselves, for others, and humanity. Put into action it is reflected in how we continuously learn, grow, contribute, serve, and "be" in community. As an individual practice, it is often triggered by a negative or uncomfortable experience projected into our conscious thought. As we become more self-aware, more of our experiences become available for reflection. Over time, individual reflection supports being a good listener, observing one's own and others' practices, viewing circumstances from multiple perspectives, thoughtfully interpreting events, and seeing possibilities for improvement. The value of individual reflection is that it (Johns, 2006; York-Barr et al., 2016):

- Supports access to and builds on experiential learning and other forms of knowledge;
- Expands awareness and insights that can lead to behavioral change;
- Resolves contradictions among actions and behaviors;
- Increases knowledge and skills that lead to personal and professional development;
- Restores balance and perspective by creating space for thoughtful consideration and learning;
- Renews clarity of personal and professional purpose by helping to align practice with intentions.

Likely the most important consideration for individual reflection is creating time and space in our lives to be fully present. Presencing is not easy but is essential for reflection to occur. Obstacles to creating space in our lives to be fully present include: our fear of vulnerability and going against social norms, our primitive stress reactions, and our challenge with not knowing how to nurture ourselves or honor vulnerability. By practicing compassion for ourselves and others we open ourselves to our own fear and vulnerability. This practice creates more space, which helps to develop greater presence with ourselves and others (Lombard & Horton-Deutsch, 2012).

To be a reflective practitioner, individually, we must choose to be reflective in our work and life. It is in the quiet and solitude that insights from life take on meaning and form. There are multiple ways to reflect alone including journaling, poetry, reading literature, exercising or walking in nature to clear our minds, meditation, contemplation, creating a piece of art, noticing and witnessing our own practice through video or webinars. Engaging in one of the many forms of reflection available is a commitment to our own growth and development. It is how we develop the expertise and insights that accumulate into wisdom. Becoming more reflective heightens awareness of the yearning to make sense of the world and to become the best one can be (York-Barr et al., 2016).

Reflective Practice With Partners and Groups

As we learn and grow as reflective practitioners, we increase our capacity to effectively engage, support, and facilitate others' personal–professional development. According to Johns (2006), working together demands a culture of mutual respect for each one's role and requires group learning. Group learning begins with dialogue and the capacity of individuals to suspend their assumptions and create space to think together. Through this process we recognize patterns of interaction in groups that may undermine learning. Reflection opens a space for individuals to express and nurture their voice so that it can be heard and respected. It also helps us to deliver our messages in a thoughtful and considerate manner. It is often said that what we say is not as important as how it is said. Through reflection we learn to carefully craft how we say something so that it is likely to be received in the intended manner. The value of reflecting with partners or groups (Johns, 2006; York-Barr et al., 2016):

- Enhances learning from varied experiences and expertise
- Increases professional and social support
- Supports the development of more effective interventions given shared purpose, responsibility, and expertise among partners and/or members
- Generates a sense of hope and encouragement for meaningful sustained improvements
- Increases collegiality and connections among partners/members through greater understanding of one's own and others' experiences, expertise, and perspectives

There are multiple ways to reflect with partners or in groups including traditional study groups and/or research projects, as well as less conventional ways to improve processes. Liberating Structures (LS) are a nonhierarchical collection of methods based on complexity science for thinking, relating, and working together (Lipmanowicz & McCandless, 2014). Reflection is an integral part of LS in a backward way. The idea is that we can act our way into thinking through LS to quickly make changes in our patterns of interaction, leading to reflection (Swenson & Sims, 2012). Changing the way we interact is about changing our culture, which is about changing our habits and behaviors. The goal of LS is to unleash the collective wisdom and creativity of everyone in the group. Through reflection we notice how much our relationships have changed through the use of LS. To learn more about LS and how ordinary people can use these methods based on complexity science, visit www.liberatingstructures.com

Reflective Practice With Organizations and Communities

Growing a reflective practice community means that at each level of a system, members listen and observe practice. Moving reflective practices to organizational and community levels can be challenging because of the complexity of working with entire systems and the complexity and particularity of different communities (Sherwood & Horton-Deutsch, 2015). However, when reflection becomes part of an overall way of doing and being, the value can result in (Johns, 2006; York-Barr et al., 2016):

- Greater coherence of the entire organization and/or community through a sense of common purpose and shared responsibility

- Alignment of resources for achieving system/community advances aimed at equitable outcomes for all

- Shared knowledge and planning so that issues are deeply understood and insights gained to guide next steps

- Coordination and collaboration across partners/groups within the organization or community to align work and development

- Increased support for the expanding network of relationships and sharing expertise with the larger organization or community

Similar to working with partners or groups, LS are methods that can be used with entire organizations. Again, based on complexity science, LS can unleash the power of everyone to think and act in new ways. Participants focus on letting go to foster cycles of self-organization versus control to foster a culture of dependence. When letting go is ascendant, the culture engages in interdependent work and shared accountability. Common behaviors in these reflective systems include listening, asking for help, removing barriers to innovation, taking more responsibility, seeking full participation, information sharing, and taking risks (Swenson & Sims, 2012). LS can be scaled up or down depending on the size of the organization/community and the nature of the work to be done. The key is they are open, inclusive, and thoughtful, and value all points of view.

MOVING GLOBAL NURSING FORWARD THROUGH REFLECTIVE PRACTICE

Reflective practice has ushered in renewed life energy for educational settings and organizations alike. As previously mentioned, it is a vital and available resource for significant and sustained effectiveness in communities as well. Experience by itself is not enough because it does not necessarily lead to informed knowledge, understanding, or wisdom. However, reflection as a means for examining our beliefs, assumptions, and practices can lead to insights. It can also help us to discover incongruities between beliefs and actions. The self-awareness gained through reflection can motivate us to initiate changes in our practice and in ways of being with others. Effective use of reflective practice requires continuous development of individual, organizational, and community learning capacities.

The SDGs create an opportunity for global collaboration such as the world has never witnessed. Their multifaceted call to improve the health and well-being for all people worldwide, end poverty and hunger, and eradicate barriers to equality and environmental sustainability may be a herculean task, but it is not impossible. The SDGs invoke a global commitment to the improvement of the quality of life for all human beings on the planet. And, as has been discussed throughout this text, global nurses are at the forefront of transforming this evolving transnational society toward a cross-cultural paradigm of progress, partnership, peace, and justice.

With an enhanced knowledge of SDG targets and a broadened global health perspective, it may be helpful to reflect on some key points:

- Which of the SDGs resonates most powerfully with my individual vision and passion?
- What are my strengths and unique skills that I can bring to these initiatives?
- In what areas can I continue to build my capacities for leadership and advocacy?
- Specifically, how will I take action based on my currently available resources and my ability/willingness to commit?
- What is the first step I can take toward realizing the SDG most important to me? With whom can I partner? When will I do this? How will I evaluate myself?

With strategic planning, and through the nurturing of our own self-awareness, we are capable of delivering the promise of equitable global health to the individuals and communities we serve: the belief that "everyone is entitled to the conditions that can maintain health" (R. L. Goldsteen, K. Goldsteen, & Dwelle, 2015, p. 36). These reflections on how to be purposeful in our influence, intentional in our behaviors, and active in our participation with others have been key characteristics and practices of nursing's greatest leaders (Forrester, 2016). Reflective practice is central to continued personal–professional development, aiding us to clarify purpose and providing us with the resilience to recommit to the demanding caliber of service that will be required for the Post-2015 Agenda.

The following is just one example of a reflective practice that can foster the values mentioned earlier and promote the awareness needed as the global community collaborates to achieve the 2030 Agenda.

The Sustainable Development Goals: A Reflective Inventory

Reflective inventory work has been employed in nursing to promote self-/community awareness and identify opportunities for self-/community growth. It is a method of reflection that allows the participant to use guided questions in relation to the topic at hand. For example, it has been offered as a reflective exercise for nurses in examining their self-care needs, evaluating the quality of care provided by systems at end of life, exploring the role of vulnerability in communication, and creating new meaning in professional roles and responsibilities (Rosa, 2014a, 2014b, 2017; Rosa & Santos, 2016; see Chapter 4). It can be used on an individual basis as a journaling or contemplation practice. It may also be used to facilitate group, organization, and/or community discussion.

Table 30.1 provides an SDG reflective inventory. Each of the SDGs is listed in abbreviated terms and accompanied by reflective questions for your own use. You are encouraged to move slowly through the questions, taking your time and challenging yourself to be as honest as possible. Pay particular attention to the question that repeats itself throughout and gets at the root of the role you will play in the global realizations of the SDGs: "Is it my responsibility. . . ?"

Table 30.1 Sustainable Development Goal Reflective Inventory

Sustainable Development Goals	Questions for Ongoing Reflection
1. No poverty	• How do I feel about the poor and economically disadvantaged? • What assumptions and judgments do I make about the poor that will prevent me from being an effective global nurse? • What are my fears related to poor people? • Which implications of poverty can I alleviate with a nursing sensibility? • Is it my responsibility to address and work for no poverty for all?
2. Zero hunger	• Do I know what it feels like to be hungry? To be without? • Am I willing to hear and see the impact of hunger on children and families, beyond statistics and research findings? • Are the experiences and feelings of the hungry included in my goals and plans? • In what ways do I contribute to hunger through wasting food or unconscious consumption/disposal? • Is it my responsibility to address and work toward zero hunger for all?
3. Good health and well-being	• What is my vision of a world where good health and well-being are experienced by all? • How do I define health and well-being? • Am I open to hearing definitions and perceptions of what health and well-being mean to others? • How can I change my approaches to advocacy so that colleagues and policy makers understand health and well-being as a human right? • Is it my responsibility to address and work toward good health and well-being for all?

(continued)

Table 30.1 Sustainable Development Goal Reflective Inventory (*continued*)

Sustainable Development Goals	Questions for Ongoing Reflection
5. Gender equality	• How has my own standing in the world been influenced by my gender? • What privileges and prejudices have I experienced based on my gender or gender identification? • What social misperceptions do I unconsciously ascribe to regarding gender and status? • How can I strive to heal the misunderstandings and social constructs around gender while remaining inclusive and respectful of cultural differences? • Is it my responsibility to address and work toward gender equality for all?
6. Clean water and sanitation	• How can I communicate the importance of clean water and sanitation to decision makers in a way that matters for them? • In what ways are clean water and sanitation human rights? • How can I educate about the value of clean water in settings where water access is limited? • How can I educate about the vital nature of sanitation in settings where sanitation is lacking or absent? • Is it my responsibility to address and work toward clean water and sanitation for all?
7. Affordable and clean energy	• How do I waste energy? • How do I promote the unconscious use of energy in my family and workplace? • In what ways can I raise awareness regarding energy consumption practice? • What are the strategies needed for a global commitment to clean energy use? • Is it my responsibility to address and work toward affordable and clean energy for all?
8. Decent work and economic growth	• What are the privileges that allow me to access and maintain decent and reliable work? • Do people in low- and middle-income countries share these opportunities? • How can I bridge the gaps between what people have, what they need, and what they deserve regarding economic disparities? • What is my global nursing contribution to responsible and safe economic growth for communities and countries? • Is it my responsibility to address and work toward decent work and economic growth for all?
9. Industry, innovation, and infrastructure	• In what ways do I take industry and innovation for granted? • What absences in infrastructure would impact the quality of my life? • How can I be proactive and preventative about the health needs of those communities without adequate infrastructure? • How do the concepts of innovation, cultural humility, and a client-centered approach to intervention relate? • Is it my responsibility to work toward industry, innovation, and infrastructure for all?

(continued)

Table 30.1 Sustainable Development Goal Reflective Inventory (*continued*)

Sustainable Development Goals	Questions for Ongoing Reflection
10. Reduced inequalities	• In what ways do I consider myself less than or greater than others? • How can I role-model equality in all I do and with all I have? • How bad do things need to get before I act on behalf of the oppressed? • Is equality foundational to health and health care delivery? • Is it my responsibility to address and work toward reduced inequalities for all?
11. Sustainable cities and communities	• In what ways does my community support/utilize sustainable practices? • What are the immediate areas for improvement on my street and in my town? • How do I advocate for the needs of those impacted by irresponsible urbanization? • Am I able to make the case between unsustainable practices and poor health outcomes? • Is it my responsibility to address and work toward sustainable cities and communities for all?
12. Responsible consumption and production	• How can I improve purchasing/spending practices in my work setting? • How can I translate environmentally conscious goals to administrators, leaders, and financial stakeholders? • Am I able to facilitate meaningful discussions regarding the role of environmentally friendly trends in health care among other global health workers? • Do I ignore the implications of irresponsible practices in the community or work settings? • Is it my responsibility to address and work toward responsible consumption and production for all?
13. Climate action	• How do I understand my individual role in climate change? • What personal lifestyle choices do I need to adapt to be more environmentally respectful? • Do I consider myself to be an environmental activist? • How do I close the gap between raising awareness and creating action? • Is it my responsibility to address and work toward climate action for all?
14. Life below water	• Do I believe biodiversity has an influence on my personal and community health? • How can I integrate biodiversity knowledge into community education? • In what ways do I misuse or waste water resources? • How can I promote awareness of marine preservation in my local/regional/national environments? • Is it my responsibility to address and work toward the preservation of life below water for all?

(continued)

Table 30.1 Sustainable Development Goal Reflective Inventory (*continued*)	
Sustainable Development Goals	**Questions for Ongoing Reflection**
15. Life on land	• In what ways are my goals as a global nurse tied to environmental justice? • What are my strategic plans to drive community-based change in policy regarding environmental preservation? • Are there efforts for land preservation that are relevant to my village, town, or city? • How can I help my family to better understand their relationship to all species and ecosystems? • Is it my responsibility to address and work toward the preservation of life on land for all?
16. Peace, justice, and strong institutions	• How have unjust laws and policies impacted my community? • In what ways does a lack of justice frustrate me? Anger me? Prevent me from taking action? • Am I conscious of peacemaking in my role as a global nurse? • Is peace a priority in my relationships? • Is it my responsibility to address and work toward peace and justice for all?
17. Partnerships for the goals	• Are my partnerships me-centered or other-centered? • Is it hard for me to remain authentically present to another's feelings and worldviews? • What are my barriers to surrendering my position and being flexible? • How do I show up in a spirit of true collaboration? • Is it my responsibility to address and work toward partnerships for the goals?

CONCLUSION

We are called to serve on a global scale so that all men, women, and children will feel seen, heard, and acknowledged as they strive for an improved quality of life. Throughout this process, it is important to remember that a nursing sensibility entails not only the science of knowledge and clinical applications, but also the art of caring and healing. An ongoing commitment to reflective practice supports us with the grounding and sense of self needed to enact real and meaningful progress. As we remain true to our nursing roots and intraprofessional identity, we will continue to identify opportunities to make our unique contributions toward the realization of the SDGs by 2030 and create the world we want.

REFLECTION AND DISCUSSION

- How can I promote an environment of reflection in professional settings?
- What fears, concerns, or hesitations do I have in reflecting upon my own practice?
- How can I provide a respectful, supportive environment for colleagues, clients, and communities to reflect in safety?

- What techniques are most comfortable for me to promote reflection? Journaling? Meditation? Quiet? Relaxation?

- How can I schedule reflection time into my daily or weekly schedule to promote integration of my personal–professional experiences?

REFERENCES

Beyond 2015. (2015). World we want 2015 web platform. Retrieved from http://www .beyond2015.org/world-we-want-2015-web-platform

Carper, B. (1978). Fundamental patterns of knowing in nursing. *Advances in Nursing Science, 1*(1), 13–23.

Chinn, P. L., & Kramer, M. K. (2008). *Integrated theory and knowledge development in nursing* (7th ed.). St. Louis: Mosby/Elsevier.

Dewey, J. (1933). *How we think: A restatement of the relation of reflective thinking to the educative process.* Boston, MA: D. C. Heath.

Forrester, D. A. (Ed.). (2016). *Nursing's greatest leaders: A history of activism.* New York, NY: Springer Publishing.

Freshwater, D. (2008). Reflective practice: The state of the art. In D. Freshwater, B. Taylor, & G. Sherwood (Eds.), *International textbook of reflective practice in nursing* (pp. 1–18). Oxford, UK: Blackwell.

Gibbs, G. (1988). Conditions under which assessment supports students' learning. Retrieved from http://www2.glos.ac.uk/offload/tli/lets/lathe/issue1/issue1.pdf#page=5

Goldsteen, R. L., Goldsteen, K., & Dwelle, T. L. (2015). Introduction and overview. In R. L. Goldsteen, K. Goldsteen, & T. L. Dwelle (Eds.), *Introduction to public health: Promises and practices* (2nd ed., pp. 1–41). New York, NY: Springer Publishing.

Horton-Deutsch, S., & Sherwood, G. (2008). Reflection: An educational strategy to develop emotionally competent nurse leaders. *Journal of Nursing Management, 16*(8), 946–954.

Johns, C. (2006). *Engaging reflection in practice: A narrative approach.* Oxford, UK: Blackwell Publishing.

Johns, C. (2013). *Becoming a reflective practitioner* (4th ed.). Hoboken, NJ: Wiley-Blackwell.

Lipmanowicz, H., & McCandless, K. (2014). *The surprising power of liberating structures.* Liberating Structures Press.

Lombard, K., & Horton-Deutsch, S. (2012). Creating space for reflection: The importance of presence in the teaching-learning process. In G. Sherwood & S. Horton-Deutsch (Eds.), *Reflective practice: Transforming education and improving outcomes* (pp. 43–61). Indianapolis, IN: Sigma Theta Tau International.

Munhall, P. (1993). Unknowing: Toward another pattern of knowing in nursing. *Nursing Outlook, 41*(3), 125–128.

Rosa, W. (2014a). Caring science and compassion fatigue: Reflective inventory for the individual processes of self-healing. *Beginnings, 34*(4), 18–20.

Rosa, W. (2014b). Conscious dying and cultural emergence: Reflective systems inventory for the collective processes of global healing. *Beginnings, 34*(5), 20–22.

Rosa, W. (2017). Change agent. In P. Dickerson (Ed.), *Nursing professional development core curriculum* (5th ed., pp. 211–222). Chicago, IL: Association for Nurses in Professional Development.

Rosa, W., & Santos, S. (2016). Introducing the engaged feedback reflective inventory in a preceptor training program. *Journal for Nurses in Professional Development, 32*(3), E1–E7.

Sherwood, G., & Horton-Deutsch, S. (2015). *Reflective organizations: On the frontlines of QSEN and reflective practice implementation.* Indianapolis, IN: Sigma Theta Tau International.

Schön, D. (1983). *The reflective practitioner.* New York, NY: Basic Books.

Schön, D. (1987). *Educating the reflective practitioner: Toward a new design for teaching and learning in the professions.* San Francisco, CA: Jossey-Bass.

Swenson, M., & Sims, S. (2012). Reflective ways of working together: Using liberating structures. In G. Sherwood & S. Horton-Deutsch (Eds.), *Reflective practice: Transforming education and improving outcomes* (pp. 229–244). Indianapolis, IN: Sigma Theta Tau International.

Taylor, B. (2000). *Reflective practice: A guide for nurses and midwives.* Buckingham, UK: Open University Press.

White, J. (1995). Patterns of knowing: Review, critique, and update. *Advances in Nursing Science, 17*(4), 73–86.

York-Barr, J., Sommers, W., Ghere, G., & Montie, J. (2016). *Reflective practice for renewing schools: An action guide for educators* (3rd ed.). Thousand Oaks, CA: Corwin.

Young, P., Pardue, K., & Horton-Deutsch, S. (2015). Practices of reflective leaders. In G. Sherwood & S. Horton-Deutsch (Eds.), *Reflective organizations: On the front lines of QSEN and reflective practice implementation* (pp. 49–67). Indianapolis, IN: Sigma Theta Tau International.

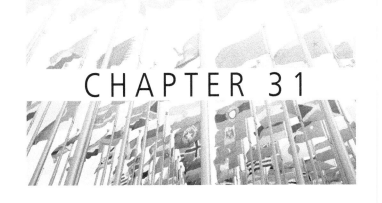

CHAPTER 31

A Call to Internationalization: The Global Advisory Panel on the Future of Nursing as Exemplar

Hester C. Klopper, Christine M. Darling, Cynthia Vlasich, Cathy Catrambone, and Martha Hill

International cooperation, multilateralism is indispensable. (Hans Blix)

Nurses make up 70% of the health care workforce, yet we often see that our voice is silent, or that we do not have a unified platform from which to speak. The perception exists by some organizations (mainly outside of nursing) that dividing and diluting the voice of nurses will bring about continued silence. However, what we have seen as a result of this divide is that many different voices are, in fact, heard, but then without a coherent message to move nursing forward.

Playing a prominent role in the global agendas of our time is critically important and essentially non-negotiable, more and more so since the acceptance of the Sustainable Development Goals (SDGs) on September 25, 2015, by all member states of the United Nations (UN), indeed creating a new era in global health. As a member of the Economic and Social Council (ECOSOC) of the UN, Sigma Theta Tau International (STTI) was frequently updated on the progress of the SDGs in the preceding 2 to 3 years of the development. Membership in ECOSOC also provided the opportunity to participate in policy documents during the process to influence the global agenda (see Chapter 3 for further information on ECOSON and how organizations obtain membership).

It was during this time we became aware that "health" would not be as prominent on the agenda as was the case with the Millennium Development Goals (MDGs). This resulted in several nursing organizations joining forces to advocate for health on the global agenda. The 17 SDGs and 169 targets integrate the three dimensions of sustainable development— economic, social, and environmental— giving rise to an integrated approach. It is anticipated that the SDGs and associated targets will encourage actions in areas of critical importance for humanity and the planet, and are to be achieved by 2030. Although only one goal gives pertinent focus to health (SDG 3), it is evident that the SDGs are paving the way to a new global era where the realization of the 169 outcomes is intertwined, multifaceted, and will require collaboration between various professions and sectors to ensure its transnational achievement.

It was against the backdrop of a fragmented voice and unfolding of a new global health agenda that STTI took the challenge to establish the Global Advisory Panel on the Future of Nursing (GAPFON) in November 2013. However, to arrive at a point where such an initiative can be established does not happen overnight, rather it demands time, resource investment (both human and financial), and the internationalization of STTI as a whole over a sustained period of time.

INTERNATIONALIZATION OF NURSING ORGANIZATIONS

Since the 1980s we have seen several nursing organizations' intent to expand internationally. It was during a time of increased awareness of a world that was opening up and becoming rapidly globalized, but characterized by uncertainty of how to embrace the international agenda. In the second chapter of this book, Rosa discusses the issues surrounding global health and global nursing and the shift toward planetary transformation. It is certain that this has now gained much momentum and, like a tsunami, will not be stopped; it is, therefore, important to consider how nursing organizations need to respond to internationalization and the broader global agenda in order to be leading health vanguards for the future.

Daly (1999) made an interesting differentiation between globalization and internationalization. He referred to *internationalization* as "the increasing importance of international trade, international relations, treaties, alliances, etc. International, of course, means between or among nations. The basic unit remains the nation, even as relations among nations become increasingly necessary and important" (p. 31). Within the nursing and health care context, this would imply building relationships between organizations, between regions, and between nations to contribute to the broader global health agenda. Moving toward a workable definition of "internationalization" of nonprofit organizations, Klopper (in press) states that it "is the process of integrating a global, and/or international dimension into the purpose of the organization, goals, activities, functions and the delivery system of services, products, membership benefits, capacity building initiatives, outreach opportunities, philanthropy efforts, and programme offerings." This implies a concerted internationalization effort in everything the organization does.

Why Internationalization?

Internationalization of nursing organizations is not a new trend, but is increasingly challenging, complex, and, most probably, confusing. We have seen over the past three decades an increase in initiatives with an aim to encourage collaboration among organizations and promote a mutual understanding of how to influence the global health agenda and elevate nursing from its marginalized status in many parts of the world. The accelerated rate of internationalization and globalization has focused attention on the use of technology to enhance interconnectedness and build networks; and the organization that has a high level of global awareness is seen as progressive, future-focused, and innovative. In embracing internationalization, there are guidelines that can be used by organizations. These include the following.

Integrated Approach

Internationalization should evolve as an integrated approach that affects the goal, activities, functions, and delivery system of services, products, membership benefits, capacity-building initiatives, outreach opportunities, philanthropy efforts, and program offerings to ensure lasting results, as noted earlier. It is anticipated that each institution will use processes unique to their operations to engage all stakeholders and role players, developing a coherent approach to achieve effectiveness and efficiency.

Global Citizenship

Several authors in this book emphasize the role of global citizenship and global nurse citizenship (see Chapters 4 and 8). Global citizenship nurtures personal respect and respect for others, wherever they live, and encourages individuals to think deeply and critically about what is equitable and just, and what will minimize harm to our planet (www.ideas-forum.org.uk/about-us/global-citizenship). Embedded in internationalization efforts should be the ideal to develop global citizenship. Oxfam (n.d.) suggests a *global citizen* is someone who is aware of the wider world and has a sense of his or her own role as a world citizen, respects and values diversity, has an understanding of how the world works, is outraged by social injustice, participates in the community at a range of levels from the local to the global, is willing to act to make the world a more equitable and sustainable place, and takes responsibility for his or her actions. The challenge for organizations is to determine how the development of global citizenship will be a main theme throughout the offering of programs and services and that the elements of learning, thinking, and acting are embedded.

Openness and Willingness to Experiment

There is no blueprint for internationalization, yet almost all nursing organizations set internationalization among their priorities for expansion. Due to the rapidly changing global environment, it is a challenge to generate strategies grounded in evidence in pursuit of a moving target. It is inevitable that organizations should have an appetite to experiment and the courage to use a trial and error approach, not ignoring the possible risks that may occur. The building of effective strategies should shift from unplanned to planned, reactive to proactive, opportunistic to systematic, and instinctive to rational.

Alignment

It is evident with internationalization that one size does not fit all. In terms of alignment, this also is the case. The institution should have an internationalization plan, but each of the departments or divisions will ideally use their individual strategies for internationalization aligned with the overarching plan.

Support System

Support for internationalization efforts is important on multiple levels. On an organizational level, central support in terms of finances, administrative services, and infrastructure needs to be established. Within departments or divisions, the focus is usually on providing information and advice, and sharing in the efforts to contribute to the overarching institutional strategy and planning and alignment with priority directions. Support systems are crucial to ensure on a short term that projects and initiatives are sustainable and that on a longer term systemic sustainability is achieved. One way to achieve a return on investment in a short turnaround time is to identify "low hanging fruits" and focus on those initiatives first. This would imply activation of activities in numerous smaller parts, aggregating them into more efficient programs.

Focus

It is important for institutions to decide how they want to focus. The focus could be within regions, countries, or specialty areas, or a mix of these. For example, an organization could decide to build priority relationships with certain countries and or regions, and invest energy in these. This approach would allow for concentrating efforts and mobilization of resources in a planned and phased manner, at the same time providing a basis to develop projects that allow for depth and breadth.

SIGMA THETA TAU INTERNATIONAL AS AN INTERNATIONAL ORGANIZATION

As this chapter is addressing GAPFON as an exemplar of how to embrace the global agenda, allow us to share the organizational growth experienced by STTI over the past four decades, as STTI has been instrumental in the establishment of this initiative. STTI in particular added the "I" for "international" to the name in 1980. This created opportunities to grow the organization outside of the boundaries of North America and facilitated membership across the globe. Although this was a slower than anticipated process, the organization persisted with the drive and has subsequently grown and now has 520+ chapters in 90+ countries, with more than 135, 000 active members (Sigma Theta Tau International, 2015). STTI, which holds special consultative status with the UN ECOSOC, has assumed an increasingly global role in advancing world health and promoting the nursing profession. STTI's contribution to the global health agenda has been through advocacy, policy influence, strengthening of health systems, scholarship development, and building leadership capacity. A part of the strategic positioning of STTI (2014–2020) is to be intentionally global in all aspects, thus applying an integrated approach.

Some pertinent decisions and actions in terms of serving this strategy include the following:

- Establishing a regional office for Africa in 2012, based in Pretoria, South Africa, to provide a one-stop service to members of the region and to build membership throughout the continent;
- Offering regional leadership conferences (since 2013 these have been conducted in Sweden, Sydney, and Amsterdam);

- Expanding the Maternal and Child Nursing Leadership Academy in partnership with Johnson and Johnson to include an Africa cohort, running since 2011;

- Holding associate membership status with International Council of Nurses (ICN), providing STTI the opportunity to participate in the World Health Assembly of the World Health Organization (WHO);

- Launching in November 2013 a Global Health Leadership Academy, offered for the first time in August of 2016 for emerging leaders who want to engage in global health initiatives.

This list gives some indication of actions taken to move forward on the global agenda, and the internationalization of the organization.

ESTABLISHMENT OF THE GLOBAL ADVISORY PANEL ON THE FUTURE OF NURSING AND MIDWIFERY

As discussed earlier, STTI has intentionally grown their international footprint over the past decade. On November 20, 2013, as part of the presidential call to action (2013–2015), *Serve Locally, Transform Regionally, Lead Globally*, STTI announced the creation of the GAPFON to establish a voice and vision for the future of nursing and midwifery to advance global health and the global health agenda. The creation of GAPFON represents a major advance in establishing strategic directions for improving global health. GAPFON seeks to align economic, social, and environmental pathways for the advancement of global health, and to identify how nursing and midwifery can take a lead in such endeavors (GAPFON, 2016). In conjunction with the SDGs, the advancement of world health through universal access to basic health care, and driven by the motive to create a unified voice for nursing, GAPFON intends to provide a communications conduit facilitating debates and conversations about the most important issues facing global health, nursing, and midwifery. This will be possible if we can demonstrate how nursing and midwifery contribute to strengthening health systems and attaining global health goals. These goals are congruent with the recent report released by Lord Nigel Crisp, chairperson of the All Party Parliamentary Group on Global Health. The report makes a very simple point that universal health coverage will not be achieved without strengthening nursing globally. And then the question arises: How will nursing be strengthened? By increasing the number of nurses, but also—crucially—by making sure their contributions are properly understood and enabling them to work to their full scope of practice and potential (Crisp et al., 2016).

GAPFON's main aim is to demonstrate how nursing and midwifery can contribute to strengthening health systems and attaining global health goals through the exchange of ideas and experiences across the different regions of the world. GAPFON's design was intended as a catalyst to promote and stimulate partnerships and collaborations to advance global health outcomes, and is a vehicle for thought leaders to share information, develop, and influence policy, and advance interprofessional efforts toward those goals (Klopper & Hill, 2015).

Having taken the initiative to host the inaugural meeting and additional regional meetings, STTI laid the foundation for GAPFON to continue in the future as a sustainable advisory entity.

Inaugural Meeting

The initial GAPFON meeting—an intense 3-day high-level gathering that facilitated discussion to identify and discuss strategies to positively influence global health—took place in Basel, Switzerland, March 27 to 29, 2014. The location was chosen to reflect the political neutrality of the organization. An inaugural panel of 17 members from nine countries and from all regions of the world was appointed in March 2014, selected to bring diverse perspectives of global nursing leaders to address the GAPFON purpose (Wilson et al., 2016). In addition, the composition of the panel was purposeful in nature to ensure that GAPFON would capitalize on the vast individual expertise and experience from diverse backgrounds. The members for 2013 to 2015 were:

- Dr. Martha Hill, PhD, RN, FAAN (chair), Dean Emerita and Professor, Nursing, Medicine, and Public Health, Johns Hopkins School of Nursing, Baltimore, Maryland

- Dr. Rowaida Al-Maaitah, PhD, Advisor for Her Royal Highness Princess Muna El Hussein for Health and Social Development; Former Senator and Minister of Higher Education; Member, Jordanian Nursing Council; Professor, Jordan University of Science and Technology, Amman, Jordan

- Dr. Cathy Catrambone, PhD, RN, FAAN, President, Sigma Theta Tau International, 2015–2017; Associate Professor, Rush University College of Nursing, Chicago, Illinois

- Dr. Eric Lu Shek Chan, DMgt, RN, FACN, Principal Nursing Officer, Hospital Authority, Kowloon, Hong Kong

- Dr. John Daly, PhD, RN, FACN, FAAN, Dean and Professor, Faculty of Health, University of Technology Sydney, Lindfield, New South Wales, Australia

- Dr. Hester C. Klopper, PhD, MBA, RN, RM, FANSA, FAAN, ASSAF, President, Sigma Theta Tau International, 2013–2015; Deputy Vice Chancellor: Strategic Initiatives and Internationalisation, Stellenbosch University, South Africa; Extra-ordinary Professor, INSINQ Research Unit, North-West University (Potchefstroom), South Africa

- Dr. Leslie Mancuso, PhD, RN, FAAN, President and CEO, Jhpiego, Baltimore, Maryland

- Dr. Isabel Amelia Costa Mendes, PhD, RN, Full Professor, University of Sao Paulo Ribeirao Preto College of Nursing, Ribeirao Preto, Brazil

- Dr. Mary E. Norton, EdD, APN-C, Associate Dean and Professor, Global Academic Initiatives, Felician College, The Franciscan College of New Jersey, Lodi, New Jersey

- Dr. Anne Marie Rafferty, CBE, DPhil (Oxon) RN, FRCN, FAAN, Professor of Nursing Policy, King's College London, United Kingdom

- Dr. Judith Shamian, PhD, RN, LLD, DSc (Hon), LLD (Hon), President, International Council of Nurses, Canada

- Dr. Wichit Srisuphan, DrPH, RN, Professor Emerita, Faculty of Nursing, Chiang Mai University, Chiang Mai, Thailand

- Dr. Patricia E. Thompson, EdD, RN, FAAN, Chief Executive Officer, Sigma Theta Tau International, Indianapolis, Indiana

- Dr. Roger Watson, PhD, RN, FRCN, FAAN, Professor of Nursing, Faculty of Health and Social Care, University of Hull, Hull, United Kingdom

- Dr. Lynda Wilson, PhD, RN, FAAN, Assistant Dean and Professor, International Affairs, Deputy Director, PAHO/WHO Collaborating Center on International Nursing University of Alabama Birmingham School of Nursing, Birmingham, Alabama (since the establishment of GAPFON, Dr. Wilson has retired)

- Ms. Cynthia Vlasich, MBA, BSN, RN, Director, Education and Leadership, Sigma Theta Tau International, Indianapolis, Indiana

- Administrative support and coordination was provided by Christine "Tina" Darling from Sigma Theta Tau International, Indianapolis, Indiana

In preparation for the inaugural meeting, a survey was developed with some key questions. The purpose of the survey was to solicit the key issues that the panel thought were most vital to unpack and discuss. These issues provided a point of departure and framework for further exploration. A consensus building methodology was used from the inaugural meeting and with all the regional meetings. Burgess and Spangler (2003) define "consensus building" as a collaborative problem-solving process that is used mainly to settle complex, multiparty interactions. It is particularly useful whenever multiple parties are involved in addressing complex issues and are seeking to find an agreement through active participation and taking ownership of decisions. Consensus is usually reached when participants agree they can live with what is proposed after every effort has been made to meet the interests of all stakeholding parties (Burgess & Spangler, 2003).

Key issues identified at this inaugural meeting included the need for reform, advocacy, and innovations in leadership, policy, practice, education, and work environments. While the specific context through which these efforts will be addressed is nursing and midwifery, recognition of the interprofessional and collaborative nature of the world's health care needs and systems was kept at the forefront of all discussions.

Regional Meetings

After the inaugural meeting, STTI addressed the core mission of GAPFON by convening a series of meetings in seven global regions:

- Pacific Rim and Asia/Oceania (Seoul, South Korea, June 15–16, 2015)

- The Caribbean (San Juan, Puerto Rico, July 17–18, 2015)

- Central-Latin America (San Juan, Puerto Rico, July 20–21, 2015)

- North America and Mexico (Washington, DC, February 22–23, 2016 and February 25–26, 2016)

- Middle East (Abu Dhabi, United Arab Emirates, March 23–24, 2016)

- Europe (Amsterdam, Netherlands, June 1–2, 2016)

- Africa (Cape Town, South Africa, July 16–17, 2016)

At each of the meetings thought and action leaders convened from a variety of disciplines, including representatives of the ministers of health and key nursing and midwifery associations, educational institutions, regulatory bodies, and leaders who are influential in global health. Limited space was made available for observers to register and attend the regional meetings as well. This inclusive approach reflects and recognizes a growing interdependence in all health matters, and the expansion of global health as a field of inquiry (ICN, 2014).

In preparation for each of the meetings, the same methodology was followed as for the inaugural group. The participants were sent a questionnaire to solicit the key issues of the region. The results were used to facilitate the discussion in terms of prioritization of issues and to add region-specific challenges. At each of the meetings, the identified issues were linked to the relevant MDGs (until the end of 2015) and in 2016 to the SDGs, ensuring that the work of GAPFON translates back to the global agenda. An overview of the regional meetings will follow, indicating the ranking of the issues as perceived by the region, as well as the identification of additional challenges in the region. In each case the four main themes are indicated in the order of importance ranking by the region. Table 31.1 provides a summary of the ranking of the themes by region. Press releases distributed publicly after each of the meetings were used to provide the details, and may be found online (www.gapfon.org). Testimonials of participants are also available on the same website and will provide valuable insight into the contribution GAPFON is making.

The *Asia/Pacific Rim* meeting took place in Seoul, South Korea, on June 15 and 16, 2015. The venue and time were deliberately scheduled to coincide with the ICN conference so that members would be able to attend both. The Korean Nursing Association cohosted the meeting and was represented by Dr. Oksoo Kim. Of note was that the meeting took place during the outbreak of Middle East respiratory syndrome (MERS) and that this had an impact as some countries in the region declared a moratorium on travel.

Table 31.1 Identified Priorities by Region and Ranking Order of Priority

Region	Policy	Leadership	Education/Curriculum	Workforce/Practice
Asia/Pacific	1	2	3	4
Caribbean	2	1	3	4
Latin/Central America	2	1	3	4
North America	2	1	3	4
Middle East	2	1	3	4
Africa	2	1	3	4
Europe	2	1	3	4

The Asia/Pacific nurse leaders confirmed that priority issues and action strategies must focus on (a) policy; (b) leadership; (c) education/curriculum; and (d) workforce/practice. In many settings, nurses and midwives are restricted from practicing to the full scope of their preparation and licensures. Removing these restrictions would allow nurses and midwives to care more comprehensively for patients, thus improving health care outcomes and reducing cost. In addition to the identified priority issues, the Asia/Pacific nurse leaders identified public and global health challenges, including maternal and child health; noncommunicable diseases (NCDs)/chronic diseases; disaster preparedness and emergency responses; and elderly care and mental health (GAPFON, 2016). As noted by the participants, all of these issues are opportunities for nurses and midwives to join other health professions in achieving universal health coverage, the Post-2015 UN SDGs and the Global Strategy for Health and Human Resources, and the future WHO Strategic Directions for Nursing and Midwifery.

The *Caribbean meeting* convened in San Juan, Puerto Rico, on July 17 and 18, 2015. It was evident that the nursing leaders from the Caribbean region were committed to continuing to contribute to global health and to strengthening human resources for health by ensuring active participation in the UN Post-2015 Agenda. The Caribbean nurse leaders confirmed that priority issues and action strategies must focus on: (a) leadership; (b) policy; (c) education/curriculum; and (d) workforce/practice. The Caribbean nurse leaders concurred that increased awareness around cultural diversity and its impact on health care and health systems should remain as an overarching theme for the four priority issues. In addition to the priority issues, the Caribbean nurse leaders spoke to the importance of strengthening the image of nursing, notably through evidence, and the immense value of multidisciplinary and intersectoral collaboration (GAPFON, 2016). They identified specific regional public health and global health challenges including NCDs; maternal–child health, including the need for increased education in midwifery and women's health care; improved treatment of substance abuse and mental health; preparedness for disasters and outbreaks of communicable diseases; and resources to promote and support healthy aging and healthy lifestyles. As noted by the participants, all of these issues are opportunities for nurses and midwives to join other health professions in achieving the WHO goal of universal health coverage, and are in alignment with the UN Post-2015 Agenda, the *Global Strategy on Human Resources for Health*, and the proposed WHO (2016a, 2016b) *Strategic Directions for Strengthening Nursing and Midwifery (2016–2020)*.

The *Latin/Central America meeting* was scheduled in San Juan, Puerto Rico for July 20 and 21, 2015. At this meeting, Dr. Silvia Cassiani, Advisor, Nursing and Allied Health Personnel Development, Unit of Human Resources for Health, Department of Health Systems and Services at the Pan American Health Organization (PAHO), noted that:

> GAPFON as a new initiative created by STTI brings together voices from the region to discuss issues related to nursing and health that will contribute to the goal of universal access to health and universal health coverage. It will create and strengthen partnerships and synergy to improve the health and quality of life in the American Region.

The Latin American nurse leaders confirmed that priority issues and action strategies must focus on the identified four priority issues. They also spoke strongly about the fact that these priority issues are interrelated and each is integral to the achievement of regional goals. They prioritized the issues as follows: (a) leadership; (b) policy; (c) education/curriculum; and (d) workforce/practice. The outcomes of this meeting reflected strong regional support for PAHO/WHO's nursing priority areas including education, research, policies and strategies, communication, and interprofessional collaboration (GAPFON, 2016).

In addition, the Latin American nurse leaders verbalized the importance of universal health care, and the value of leveraging technology and communication in all areas to assist in reaching this goal. They reiterated that ensuring access to health care—including community-based care—is an area where nurses can play a pivotal leadership role. Given the increase in aging populations and NCDs throughout the region, they agreed that health promotion is vital.

The Latin American nurse leaders identified the need to improve the workforce environment for nurses throughout the region, and suggested the establishment of regional standards of care and a broad nursing scope of practice that is tied to elevated levels of nursing preparation. They emphasized the importance of collaborating with colleagues from various professions, at all levels, regarding health care priorities. They noted that this collaboration is especially important to address the consequences from violence of various types across the region.

Due to the vast geographical area of North America, as well as the large number of stakeholders, two *North American meetings* were scheduled. These took place in Washington, DC, on February 22 and 23, 2016 and February 25 and 26, 2016. The strategic nurse leaders who participated in the meetings confirmed that priority issues and action strategies must focus on (a) leadership; (b) policy; (c) education/curriculum; and (d) workforce/practice. Participants spoke strongly about the fact that these priorities are interrelated and each is integral to the achievement of regional goals. They identified meaningful inclusion and evidence-based outcomes as essential components to be integrated within all strategies and recommendations. The stakeholders verbalized the importance of universal health care and the value of leveraging the return on investment that nursing contributes to the attainment of health. They reiterated that ensuring access to health care— including community-based care—is an area where nurses can play a pivotal leadership role. Given the role that healthy behaviors play in optimal health, they agreed that health promotion focused on disease prevention is vital (GAPFON, 2016).

During the discussions, stakeholders identified specific strategies to enhance health promotion, including promoting and engaging in advocacy in environmental and social justice issues that impact public health. These strategies are congruent with the UN SDGs. In addition, stakeholders were unanimous about the need for coalition building and interprofessional collaboration at all levels to improve health promotion. They noted that this collaboration is especially important to address the consequences of frequently overlooked or minimized mental health concerns, including those stemming from violence, poverty, and natural disasters.

The *Middle East meeting* was conducted in Abu Dhabi, United Arab Emirates, on March 23 and 24, 2016. More than 30 key nursing and midwifery leaders from 13 countries in the Middle East region participated under the patronage of Her Royal Highness Princess Muna Al-Hussein of Jordan. She said that this global partnership led by GAPFON was

> important . . . to identify and develop recommendations to address the most important issues facing health at the global level. Nurses and midwives will play an integral role in leading change to improve the quality of life of people globally by capitalizing on their best assets and collective potentials.

Nursing and midwifery leaders participated in the meeting and identified and prioritized professional issues and heath challenges of the Middle East Region. They confirmed that priority issues and action strategies to achieve global health must focus on (a) leadership; (b) policy/regulation; (c) education; and (d) workforce. Participants felt strongly that these priorities are interrelated and each is integral to the achievement of regional goals. Additionally, they noted that recommendations for action in any of these areas must be evidence-based and linked to achievement of outcomes. These stakeholders verbalized the importance of developing nursing and midwifery leaders and positioning them in roles where they can be most effective. They noted the importance of leveraging the return on investment that nurses and midwives contribute to the attainment of health. The stakeholders reiterated that promoting quality nursing/midwifery practice and education, including the development and promotion of community initiatives, social justice, and human rights, are areas where nurses and midwives have a pivotal leadership role. They agreed that health promotion focused on disease prevention is vital, along with the importance of adequate preparedness and response to natural and man-made disasters. They also agreed that education, awareness, and timely treatment of mental health issues are a priority in this region. During their discussions, stakeholders identified specific strategies to enhance health, including utilizing data and evidence to inform health policy and to increase national commitment and funding. They also stressed the importance of employing an accountability framework, including state-of-the-art technology, to monitor and evaluate performance against targets. In addition, the participants recognized the need for coalition building and interprofessional collaboration at all levels to improve health, along with the development of an adequate, competent nursing/midwifery workforce. These identified strategies are especially important to address the consequences of frequently overlooked or minimized mental health concerns, including those stemming from violence, poverty, and natural disasters. The strategies identified by the Middle East stakeholders are congruent with the UN SDGs (GAPFON, 2016).

The *Europe meeting* was scheduled in Amsterdam, the Netherlands, June 1 and 2, 2016. More than 25 key nursing and midwifery leaders from the European Union, Switzerland, and Albania met to identify the top regional health issues in Europe and determine strategies to allow nursing and midwifery professionals to impact those issues. During the meeting, participants confirmed that priority issues and action strategies to achieve global health must focus on (a) leadership; (b) policy; (c) education/curriculum; and (d) workforce/practice. Participants were passionate about the fact that these priorities are interrelated and each is integral to the achievement of regional goals. They identified quality of care as an essential overarching theme to be integrated within all strategies and recommendations (GAPFON, 2016). The stakeholders discussed the importance of universal health care and the value of leveraging the return on investment that nursing contributes to the attainment of health. They agreed that nurses and midwives can play a pivotal leadership role in ensuring access to health care—especially community-based care. Given the role that healthy behaviors play in optimal health, they agreed that health promotion focused on disease prevention is vital.

During their discussions, stakeholders identified specific strategies to cultivate and position nursing and midwifery leaders, whereby the evidence and value of the profession(s) can positively impact regional and global health policy. In addition, they identified supporting and promoting clinical academic careers as essential to quality nursing and midwifery practice, as well as the importance of patient/population and public involvement. These strategies are congruent with the UN SDGs. The health issues identified as primary concerns to the European region are NCDs, mental health, aging, and maternal–child health. In addition to the key health issues identified, the stakeholders also discussed a variety of other concerns, specifically noting challenges related to migrant/refugee health.

The *Africa meeting* took place in Cape Town, South Africa, on July 18 and 19, 2016. More than 20 key nursing and midwifery leaders met to identify Africa's top regional health issues and determine strategies to allow nursing and midwifery professionals to impact those issues. The participants identified maternal–child health, communicable diseases, and NCDs, including mental health, as primary issues of concern for the African region. To address these health concerns, the stakeholders felt strongly that nurses and midwives must engage communities in culturally relevant interventions to improve health outcomes. Participants were passionate about the fact that priority issues and action strategies must focus on health care: (a) leadership; (b) policy; (c) education/curriculum; and (d) workforce/practice, noting that these priorities are integral to the achievement of regional goals. The participants further emphasized that promotion of professionalism and capacity building for nursing and midwifery are essential overarching themes to be integrated within all strategies and recommendations (GAPFON, 2016). The stakeholders identified primary strategies congruent with the UN SDGs. They advocated for reform of educational programs to ensure innovative, interprofessional, and systems approaches to achieve global health care goals, along with reform of regulation and accreditation for nursing, midwifery, and health systems in Africa. They agreed that such steps will strengthen the nursing/midwifery workforce, while simultaneously improving quality of practice and building capacity for the professions in health policy and leadership.

The stakeholders discussed additional key strategies such as the need to use socially accountable approaches to train nurses and midwives to implement evidence-based interventions across all settings. Participants also stressed the importance of health policies and health care management that optimize the scope of evidence-based practice with a focus on patient outcomes, and identified that cultivation and positioning of nursing/midwifery leaders at all levels is vital to influence health policy and the global health agenda. The GAPFON Africa regional meeting outcomes also reflected strong regional support for the priority areas of the WHO, including education, research, policies and strategies, communication, and interprofessional collaboration.

Next Steps

The next step, which will lead to evidence-based recommendations, is to analyze both qualitative and quantitative data gathered from the regional meetings. This report will be available in early 2017. An implementation plan with measurable outcomes that can be customized by country will be developed for each recommendation. The full action plan, which will reflect the roles of both nursing and midwifery in influencing global health, will have specific implications for global and regional health policy. As these regional meetings have convened, new friends and partnerships have been made. STTI is proud to have launched and led this effort, and we look forward to exciting opportunities that await us in the project's next phases. Please monitor the GAPFON website (www.gapfon.org) for progress updates.

CONCLUSION

This chapter started off by making the case for a unified voice for nursing. The rationale for such a voice is to advocate for and demonstrate the indispensable value and impact of nursing to achieve universal access to health care for all. In order to achieve this, we have made arguments that internationalization of nursing organizations is both essential and inevitable. In addition, throughout this chapter we have demonstrated how one initiative, GAPFON as exemplar, can make a difference and bring about the achievement of several outcomes. These outcomes, among others, are building a unified voice that can guide nursing as a global force—without this force universal access to health care will not be possible. Another outcome is the contribution toward ensuring sustainable health and well-being beyond 2030, thus contributing to the greater goals of planetary health in the future. On reflection over the past 2 years since the inception of GAPFON and the journey across borders and regions, a quote from Walt Disney comes to mind . . . "if you can dream it, you can do it."

Let us all work toward the dream of building nursing into the global force that will strengthen health systems and provide health care for all on the planet.

REFLECTION AND DISCUSSION

- The SDGs provide an integrated approach to achieving global health, well-being, peace, and justice. How does nursing embody an integrated approach in research, education, practice, and policy?

- In what ways does the internationalization of nursing associations strengthen the profession? What obstacles face us in furthering unity among nurses and midwives worldwide?

- What does it mean, in my own words, to: *Serve Locally, Transform Regionally, Lead Globally*, as proclaimed in the STTI presidential call to action (2013–2015)?

- How do the efforts of GAPFON influence the outcomes of the SDGs? In what ways will outcomes related to the SDGs guide and inform the mission and vision of GAPFON?

- How does the local nursing experience inform regional nursing outcomes? In what ways do regional nursing priorities influence global nursing policies? How do global nursing goals usher in planetary health and well-being?

REFERENCES

Burgess, H., & Spangler, B. (2003). Consensus building. Retrieved from http://www.beyondintractability.org/essay/consensus-building

Crisp, N., Caulfield, M., Cox, C., Poulter, D., Ribeiro, B., Watkins, M., & Willis, P. (2016). All-Party Parliamentary Group on Global Health: Triple impact—How developing nursing will improve health, promote gender equality and support economic growth. Retrieved from http://www.appg-globalhealth.org.uk

Daly, H. E. (1999). Globalization versus internationalization. Retrieved from https://www.globalpolicy.org/component/content/article/162/27995.html

Global Advisory Panel on the Future of Nursing. (2016). Regional meetings press releases [Caribbean]. Retrieved from http://www.gapfon.org

International Council of Nurses. (2014). *Nurses: A force for change—A vital resource for health.* Geneva, Switzerland: Author.

Klopper, H. C. (2016, March). *Global Trends influencing nursing in the next decade.* Parry Distinguished Lecture. Texas Women's University, Houston, TX.

Klopper, H. C., & Hill, M. (2015). Global Advisory Panel on the Future of Nursing (GAPFON) and global health. *Journal of Nursing Scholarship, 47*, 3–4.

Oxfam. (n.d.). Global citizenship. Retrieved from http://www.oxfam.org.uk/education/global-citizenship

Sigma Theta Tau International. (2015). Biennial report 2013–2015. Retrieved from http://www.nursingsociety.org

Wilson, L., Mendes, I., Klopper, H. C., Catrambone, C., Al-Maaitah, R., Norton, M.E., & Hill, M. (2016). "Global health" and "global nursing": Proposed definitions from the Global Advisory Panel on the Future of Nursing. *Journal of Advanced Nursing, 72*(7), 1529–1540. doi:10.1111/jan.12973

World Health Organization. (2016a). *Global strategy on human resources for health: Workforce 2030.* Geneva, Switzerland: Author. Retrieved from http://apps.who.int/iris/bitstream/10665/250368/1/9789241511131-eng.pdf

World Health Organization. (2016b). *Global strategic directions for strengthening nursing and midwifery, 2016–2020.* Geneva, Switzerland: Author. Retrieved from http://www.who.int/hrh/nursing_midwifery/global-strategic-midwifery2016-2020.pdf?ua=1

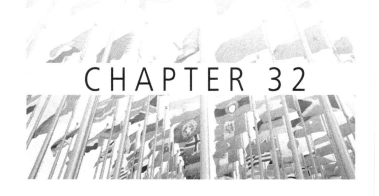

CHAPTER 32

Raising Consciousness Through Global Nursing Collaboration

Michele J. Upvall and Jeanne M. Leffers

> *If we have any role at all, I think it's the role of optimism . . . the kind which is meaningful, one that is rather close to that notion of the world which is not perfect, but which can be improved. (Chinua Achebe, cited in Wachtel, 1996, p. 115)*

Collaboration is a central component of true partnerships, as Rosa notes in Chapter 28. To achieve the Sustainable Development Goals (SDGs), in particular the broad implications of SDG 17, "Revitalize the global partnership for sustainable development," clear articulation of global health nursing partnerships is essential. While this goal addresses issues beyond health concerns, to effectively address sustainable development, partnerships for health must improve the health of populations worldwide. Looking ahead toward a post-2030 agenda requires that current understandings of partnerships be advanced not only to inform the work of nurses and other health professionals globally, but also to strengthen knowledge and practice of interprofessional collaboration. In this chapter, we are concerned with transforming health at the system or population level through the process of global collaboration (see Chapter 28 for additional tools and considerations in building individual partnerships across cultures and contexts).

Underpinning the 17 SDGs is the overall goal to end inequality and provide necessary resources for all in order to achieve sustainable development; in particular, SDG 1, "To end poverty in all forms everywhere"; SDG 3, "To ensure healthy lives and promote well-being for all at all ages"; SDG 5, "To achieve gender equality"; SDG 10, "To reduce inequality among countries"; and SDG 16, "To promote peaceful and inclusive societies for sustainable development" target equity for all people (United Nations [UN], 2015). Farmer, Kim, Kleinman, and Basilico (2013) argue that global health must address social and health inequalities and use a biosocial approach that considers cultural, social, political, and economic factors to ensure health equity. Therefore, partnerships and collaboration are both rooted in this human rights approach to equity.

THE MEANING OF GLOBAL COLLABORATION

Historical conceptualizations of collaboration focused on providing resources, including financial and human resources, for capacity building. There was an "us" and "them," with the "us" role consisting of imparting knowledge or skills to "them" who needed "development." Racine and Perron (2012) use the term, "cultural voyeurism" (p. 192) to describe a perspective of separateness or "distancing" by seeing groups of individuals as different or even "exotic." This perspective, pervasive in short-term health care projects including those with students in international service-learning experiences, implies a power-based relationship with the donor in full command of services provided. This imperialistic approach, sometimes called "duffel-bag" medicine, is the antithesis of the partnership process, a process that can begin with coordinating activities and culminating in the experience of close collaboration.

Partnership is a process existing along a spectrum from polite coordination, where partners have a common purpose and share information, to cooperation, where efforts are aligned to achieve the purpose. Close collaboration occurs when all partners are working together as an integrated team, achieving a shared goal. This experience of close collaboration is considered the most powerful form of partnership, but it is not always what is observed in global partnerships (Rosenberg, Hayes, McIntyre, & Neill, 2010). Figure 32.1 illustrates the continuum of partnership.

Recent conceptualizations of partnership (Everett, 2016) demonstrate its complexity and dynamic nature. Leadership is important in a partnership, but so too is being a follower. Roles may change throughout a partnership depending on the context of work to be done in achieving shared goals, but regardless of role, leader, or follower, both require commitment to the partnership goal. Shared knowledge

Figure 32.1 The continuum of partnership.

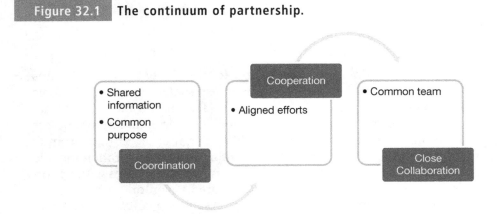

Source: Adapted from Rosenberg et al. (2010). Reprinted with permission, University of California Press.

and mutual respect are also critical to the partnership process and influence the sustainability or potential failure of a partnership. Lack of shared goals, knowledge, and mutual respect may signify issues of power that go unrecognized in a partnership. In this case, partners may say "yes," but their actions indicate "no."

Coordination and cooperation may constitute the beginning of a partnership, but transformation of individuals and systems can occur only through taking the next step: close collaboration. The World Health Organization (WHO) also recognizes that coordinating efforts does not necessarily imply a close collaborative partnership. WHO defines "collaboration" as,

> . . . not only about agreement and communication, but about creation and synergy. Collaboration occurs when two or more individuals from different backgrounds with complementary skills interact to create a shared understanding . . . something is there that was not there before. (WHO, 2010, p. 36)

This definition aligns with Lehman's perspective of collaboration (as quoted in Rosenberg et al., 2010, p. 7):

> Collaboration on the surface, is about bringing together resources, both financial and intellectual, to work toward a common purpose . . . The inner life of collaboration is about states of mind and spirit that are open—open to self-examination, open to growth, open to trust, and open to mutual action.

Both definitions of collaboration are rooted in shared mutuality and the potential for transformation among all partners. This worldview is consistent with Eisler's partnership model (Eisler & Potter, 2014) and perspectives of power, which Eisler terms "hierarchies of actualization" (p. 55). The essence of power within the context of collaboration signifies a sharing of power, with no partner dominating the relationship. All partners are considered equal within the relationship and have the potential to be transformed through the relationship. However, transformation is not a guarantee but, rather, depends upon the hearts and minds of those working in close collaboration.

BUILDING COLLABORATIVE PARTNERSHIPS

Movement from coordination and cooperation to close collaboration requires more than formal agreements between institutions, especially if the ultimate goals include transformation of individuals and systems. The significance of personal or informal relationships is continually highlighted as the foundation for success among partners (Barnes, Brown, & Harman, 2016; Beran et al., 2016; Corbin & Mittelmark, 2008; Downes, 2014). Other factors influencing collaboration include cultivating trust and respect in both formal and informal relationships with opportunities for frequent engagement, maintaining a shared vision or "unity through purpose," the ability to communicate through understanding cultural norms and variances in communication patterns, and making a commitment to meet the expected and unexpected challenges of the relationship (American Association of Colleges of Nursing, 2012; Downes, 2014).

MODELS OF PARTNERSHIP

The Partnership Pathway (Rosenberg et al., 2010) is one of the most detailed frameworks of partnership in global health and it is based on the continuum of partnership of coordination, cooperation, and close collaboration. Steps of the Partnership Pathway are conceived as a journey beginning with interested individuals or groups initiating a partnership to address a particular need. "The First Mile" of the journey, as outlined in the Partnership Pathway, culminates in agreement among foundational issues: choosing the right membership for achieving project goals; developing a shared goal among all partners; selecting the best structure to meet the goal(s); shaping a "big-picture" strategy that includes where, what, and how; and finally, agreeing on organizational roles. After developing a foundation in The First Mile, the group proceeds on the journey with the challenge of managing the project with flexibility, yet a sense of discipline for planning, and developing complementary leadership roles distinct from organizational leadership roles. "The Last Mile" includes adapting approaches to sustain momentum in meeting the goals, transferring control, communicating lessons learned, and dissolving the partnership when the goal is met. Ending the partnership may seem incongruent with a model of sustainability, but resources may be wasted and ongoing role confusion may occur if partners do not recognize when a goal has achieved sustainability (Rosenberg et al., 2010).

Partnership models applicable to global health issues are rare in nursing. The most comprehensive model in the literature is the Conceptual Model for Partnership and Sustainability in Global Health (Leffers & Mitchell, 2011). This model takes into account antecedents, which must be in place before the partnership process begins. These antecedents include consideration of both host and guest nurse partners and resources (human, financial, and material resources). The actual process of partnership begins with engagement and the core elements of cultural bridging, collaboration, capacity building, and mutual goal setting. Sustainability occurs when the hosts ultimately assume project ownership. However, ownership relies on a detailed community assessment with consideration of the political and social climate in the community, having enough resources for ongoing implementation of the project, and having a leadership champion to continue motivating those individuals responsible for project outcomes.

EXEMPLARS OF GLOBAL NURSING PARTNERSHIPS

As global nursing collaboration moves forward from the earlier perspectives of cultural arrogance, colonialism, and paternalism discussed earlier in this book, to a form of close collaboration and partnership, there are examples from large and small organizations that inform our future. Some of these are foundation funded or government sponsored such as the Regis College Haiti Partnership, the Human Resources for Health (HRH) Program, and Seed Global Health, while others are voluntary such as Health Volunteers Overseas (HVO) in the United States and Voluntary Services Overseas (VSO) from the United Kingdom. The use of exemplars facilitates a look at how strong working partnerships in 2017 can inform the post-2030 nursing and health agendas. While there are examples from other countries beyond the United States, each of the following partnerships brings nurses from the United States to collaborate with nurses in settings such as Haiti,

Guatemala, Rwanda, Uganda, Malawi, Liberia, Swaziland, and Tanzania. The three organizations are the Seed Global Health Service Partnership (GHSP), HRH, and Partners in Development, Inc. (PID), which represent: (a) academic and clinical medical and nursing education; (b) academic medical, nursing, public health, and medical management education; and (c) broader health and social service capacity building through direct service and education, respectively.

Exemplar 1: Seed Global Health Service Partnership

The first exemplar, the Seed GHSP, is an exciting partnership between governmental, private, academic, and global partners to increase clinical care capacity in low-resource settings. Founded in 2012 through the collaboration of Seed Global Health, the Peace Corps, and the U.S. President's Emergency Plan for AIDS Relief (PEPFAR), the program partners nurses and physicians with those in partner countries of Uganda, Tanzania, Malawi, Liberia, and Swaziland. Other sponsoring partners include the CDC, Medtronic, Bank of America, GE Foundation, Abbott Fund, Draper Richards Kaplan Foundation, ExxonMobil, FedEx, George Washington University, Gradian Health Systems, and Pfizer (Seed Global Health, 2016). U.S. volunteers spend 1 year working alongside their counterparts in the host settings. Through the collaboration with the Peace Corps, the volunteers are provided with a stipend to help with training, travel, and living expenses. While the U.S. GHSP professionals offer support clinically to the host country professionals, the collaboration seeks to: strengthen clinical education; expand continuing educational opportunities; share guidelines, protocols, and strategies; and invest in critical educational resource needs (Seed Global Health, 2016). Results from their first 2 years of the partnership show that the collaboration extended the training of 3,187 medical, assistant medical, and clinical officers; 3,060 nursing students; 287 medical and nursing postgraduates; 567 hospital staff and university faculty; and 118 other individuals (Seed Global Health, 2016).

Not to be confused with Partners in Health, which is a well-known organization that develops and supports partnerships in low-resource settings, PID is a U.S.-based program that supports programs in Haiti, Guatemala, and Glendora, Mississippi, to address the comprehensive economic, educational, housing, and health needs of the host partners. In Haiti and Guatemala, PID supports locally managed health clinics, social service programs, child sponsorship, and home construction services led by host-setting partners.

Exemplar 2: Human Resources for Health

The second exemplar, HRH, is one that also originated in 2012 as a collaboration between the Rwandan Ministry of Health; the Clinton Health Access Initiative; the Global Fund to Fight AIDS, Tuberculosis and Malaria; and the Centers for Disease Control and Prevention (CDC). The program sends approximately 100 faculty members annually from participating medical, nursing, public health, dentistry, and health management programs to partner (twin) with faculty in the Rwandan schools and hospitals to strengthen the capacity of health professionals. The 7-year initiative (currently in year 5 as of this writing) plans to almost double the 2012 number of physicians in Rwanda, advance the skill level and numbers of nurses and nursing faculty, offer support to strengthen capacity for public health, and increase the number of health managers who provide service in hospitals and district health centers from 7 to 157 (Binagwaho et al., 2013; Sliney & Uwimana, 2014; Uwiyeze et al., in press). During the first 2 years of the program, 313 U.S. faculty and 210 Rwandan faculty participated in the program.

Exemplar 3: Partners in Development

The final exemplar is a small nongovernmental organization (NGO) called Partners in Development, Inc. (PID). Nurses and other health professionals who come to Haiti or Guatemala partner in the medical clinics through collaborative education, by using the Haitian–American developed protocols for clinical care, or assisting with ongoing programs for prenatal care, family planning, diabetes, hypertension, and well-child screenings. Through the work of visiting teams of health providers, the Haitian nurses, physicians, and clinic providers are able to serve greater numbers of community members (PID, 2016). The medical clinic in Blanchard, Port au Prince, Haiti, works collaboratively with local Haitian public health, acute care, and social services. Presently, they are seeking to become a *Ministère de la Santé Publique et de la Population* (MSPP)-approved health facility. To date, PID funding supported eight of the Haitian clinic staff for advanced education and training in nursing, pharmacy, and laboratory areas. In addition, the clinic served 19,000 to 20,000 patient visits. This has been accomplished through the support of 10 to 12 medical service trips of volunteer health teams in addition to the permanent Haitian clinic staff. PID is funded primarily through donations (75%) and grants (25%) to accomplish the joint goals of these three program partnerships.

How the Exemplars Inform Global Health Nursing Partnerships

These exemplars are highlighted because hundreds of U.S. nurses and other medical volunteers participate in these programs. In looking at the models of partnership, they offer examples of what Leffers and Mitchell (2011) note as key components, partnering processes, and sustainability of interventions, and Sliney (2015) notes as elements of effective partnerships.

The importance of shared vision and goals is evident in the mission of each exemplar, the selection of volunteers, and the ongoing work of the organization (PID, Inc. and Seed Global Health) to align host country needs, the goals of the health professionals in the host country, joint planning and training, and efforts to ensure sustainability. PID relies upon donations and grants to support their programs and clinics in the three locations where they work while Seed Global Health has a broader range of sponsoring partners to meet their financial needs. PID hosts U.S. teams of volunteers, some to support construction and other programs, and the remaining medical volunteers to support the health programs.

Serving a broader mission to support families' economic, educational, housing, and health needs requires material resources of construction materials and laboratory and medical supplies. Whenever possible these are purchased in country or shipped from the United States to the locations in Guatemala and Haiti. In both Guatemala and Haiti, PID sponsors one U.S. field director to coordinate the resources (material, financial, and human volunteers) with the host country construction, social service, and medical directors. For example, in Haiti, the on-site U.S. field director works with the team of social service workers (to support the child sponsorship and Medical Mamba nutrition support program), the construction director, the business office staff, the medical director, staff physician, nurses, laboratory workers, pharmacy team, interpreters, and support staff totaling more than 30 Haitian workers 52 weeks a year. The field director also works with the visiting volunteer teams that offer human resources to extend the work that PID can provide year-round.

In-country leadership (Sliney, 2015) and host country ownership (Leffers & Mitchell, 2011) contribute to effective partnerships. Seed GHSP, HRH, and PID have leaders in their host settings who not only collaborate with the U.S. partners but direct the collaboration based upon the needs in the host country. Both HRH and GHSP have in-country training of U.S. volunteers (who typically serve for a minimum of 1 year) and PID has both an on-site field director and rotating clinic nurses from the United States to assist the host country health professionals with on-site orientation and supervision of nurse and medical volunteers.

Mutual respect is essential to the partnerships and each program ensures that the U.S. volunteers hold appropriate licensures and certifications and are licensed or registered in the host country settings. Further, efforts are made to promote cultural sensitivity through involvement of local medical staff and interpreters.

Outcome evaluation is essential to demonstrate the impact upon health to meet the SDGs and provide vision for post-2030 agendas. Each of the three exemplars has long-term goals to improve health outcomes in host settings. HRH and GHSP address the intermediate goal of capacity building for health professionals while PID works to improve health outcomes through broad approaches to address poverty for families and for the health care providers in their host setting. In a process evaluation of their program, HRH reports that in their first 2 years, they measured outcomes from U.S. faculty and Rwandan faculty partners for goal setting, effective skill transfer, and satisfaction with the twinning model. Ongoing evaluation helps to identify key areas for improvement (Ndenga et al., 2016).

Earlier in the chapter the elements of effective partnerships were offered. These include host and guest nurse partners' needs and resources; the process of engagement and the core elements of mutual respect, trust, cultural bridging, collaboration, capacity building, and shared vision and goals; joint planning, equity, accountability, ongoing assessment; and shared evaluation and sustainability as a goal to achieve in-country leadership and project ownership (Sliney, 2015; Leffers & Mitchell, 2011). Using exemplars illustrates how successful partnerships are built upon close collaboration, build host country capacity and ownership, and ensure sustainability for health and development.

A VISION FOR GLOBAL HEALTH COLLABORATION

Nursing is in a unique position to provide creative and transformative leadership in global health. Historically, there are a number of nursing leaders who understood close collaboration within the context of the individual and the community. Our role models of yesterday go beyond Florence Nightingale and include Mary Seacole, who braved the battlefields of the Crimea, Lillian Wald, Margaret Sanger, Mary Breckinridge, and Sister Elizabeth Kenney. These nursing leaders had a vision, committing their lives to achieving equity in health care while demonstrating principles of partnership and collaboration (Eisler & Potter, 2014). Moving forward toward the 2030 SDG target date, we anticipate that models of partnership will be better articulated and integrated into nursing and other health professional

| Box 32.1 | A Vision for Global Health Collaboration |

Concepts of collaboration, including interprofessional collaboration, informed by advanced models of partnership, will be integrated into all of nursing practice.

Nursing curricula at all levels will include concepts of global health, collaborative practice, and global health competencies.

Nurse volunteers for global health service, education, and research will demonstrate experience and skill in negotiating collaborative practice.

Preparticipation training programs will include global health competencies and evidence of participation from host countries.

All nurses who participate in global partnerships will adhere to ethical principles for global health nursing.

Nurses will participate across international boundaries through institutional-level partnerships at university, nongovernmental, or governmental level.

Nursing's relationship to sustainable development will be clearly defined and integrated into nursing practice.

practice. A vision for the future will be built upon advanced knowledge, evidence, and lessons learned from the next 15 years.

As technology shrinks our boundaries and we unite to achieve the SDGs, nurses must seek partnership opportunities for close collaboration in meeting the goals through practice, education, and research. Vision statements provide direction and those listed in Box 32.1, created by these authors, are only a beginning to addressing SDG 17: Revitalize the global partnership for sustainable development (UN, 2015). The vision statements in Box 32.1 are discussed in greater depth next.

Concepts of Collaboration, Including Interprofessional Collaboration, Informed by Advanced Models of Partnership, Will Be Integrated Into All of Nursing Practice

During the next decade, research and framework development will likely yield new and advanced models for partnership and collaboration. Further, efforts to address the SDGs will impact perspectives about partnership and collaboration to guide efforts of health professionals globally to advance health and well-being. In a post-2030 agenda, nurses and other health professionals must integrate knowledge and skills for partnership and collaboration into all levels and types of practice. Advances in health care, technology, and the ever-increasing demands on the profession of nursing require an ability to work within the context of a team. The team may be other health care professionals or the nurse with the patient and family in acute care, or nurses working in a team with community members to address a local concern. Regardless of the setting, collaboration with others will not just be a requirement, but a necessity.

The significance of collaboration was demonstrated on a global scale in research by the WHO (Mickan, Hoffman, & Nasmith, 2010), which used a case study approach to better understand collaborative practice. Ten countries from six WHO regions participated in the study and while this was only a small size, the commonalities in *how* collaboration was practiced was similar across settings. All participants agreed that collaboration with the entire health care team was crucial in complex cases and that regular team meetings were the appropriate venues for open dialogue and negotiation of interventions. Benefits to a collaborative approach included timely and appropriate patient care while the interprofessional team experienced stronger communication between members and an increase in confidence in managing complex care. There was a sense that being a member of a collaborative team enhanced one's ability to use professional skills.

What collaborative skills are needed?

The Canadian Interprofessional Competency Framework (Canadian Interprofessional Health Collaborative [CIHC], 2010) offers a unique approach to competency development by requiring an integration of ". . . knowledge, skills, attitude and values in arriving at judgments" (p. 8). Six competency domains are outlined in the framework (CIHC, 2010, p. 11):

- Interprofessional communication: includes communication with team members in a way that is collaborative, responsive, and responsible
- Patient/client/family/community-centered care: team members must actively seek, value, and engage with the patient, family, and/or community
- Role clarification: team members must have an understanding of each other's role
- Team functioning: the principles of team dynamics and group process must be understood
- Collaborative leadership: all members should work as a team with the patient/family/community to formulate, implement, and evaluate services and outcomes
- Interprofessional conflict resolution: team members must engage with all including the patient/family/community to effectively deal with interprofessional conflict

In any collaborative partnership, relationship building is the foundation of success. Trust and mutual respect develop over time and through our actions. The social–emotional learning skills of self-awareness, self-management (regulating and managing impulses), social awareness, relationship skills, and responsible decision making (Guerin, 2014, p. 39) support an individual's ongoing development within the context of the Canadian Interprofessional Competency Framework. These collaborative skills and interprofessional competencies require an attitude of lifelong learning as new ways of thinking about partnership continue to emerge through implementing the SDGs (Jones, 2016).

Nursing Curricula at all Levels Will Include Concepts of Global Health, Collaborative Practice, and Global Health Competencies

The SDGs require a nursing workforce ready to meet systems level targets both locally and globally. This will require nurses to have an understanding of global health and collaborative practice as they enter the profession. Nursing education can respond to this need in creative ways such as integrating simulated practice along with real-world clinical practice experiences into the curriculum. Simulation in particular offers a way for students to become collaborative practice-ready if simulation scenarios and case studies incorporate effective interprofessional experiences (WHO, 2010).

Incorporating global health concepts and competencies into the nursing curriculum may be one of the most effective ways to ensure graduates of all nursing programs are knowledgeable global citizens and collaborative practice-ready as a novice nurse. The Consortium of Universities for Global Health (CUGH) recognized the need to develop global health competencies for new curricula and training programs as interest in global health experiences increased since CUGH's inception in 2008.

The work of the subcommittee began in 2013 with a review of standards and existing competencies across disciplines including medicine, nursing, public health, physician's assistants, dentistry/oral health, nutrition, anthropology, pharmacy, mental health, engineering, and health economics. During the third of the four-phase subcommittee task, members identified the need to divide the competencies into four separate levels of training: global citizen, exploratory, basic operational, and advanced levels. Eventually, the subcommittee decided to focus only on competencies for the global citizen and basic operation levels. The global citizen level is considered to be a high school graduate who may not necessarily be working in global health in the future while the basic operation level assumes an individual has some interest in global health, but may not have a career in global health (Wilson et al., 2014). The subcommittee then divided 8 domains and 11 global health competencies into the two distinct levels using Bloom's taxonomy of knowledge, attitude, and skills for categorizing outcomes (see Table 32.1). CUGH encourages institutions to integrate the competencies into educational programs ensuring that all students have the opportunity to have a basic understanding of global health (Jogerst et al., 2015).

Incorporating competencies into curricula is challenging, especially within the context of interprofessional collaboration (Brown, 2014; Eichbaum, 2015). A few of the challenges include the possibility of changing scope of practices according to practice context and issues of power and hierarchy inherent to any collaborative relationship. The global health competencies developed by CUGH utilized the competencies already established in various professions and may, therefore, be at an advantage for curriculum integration. However, a greater challenge may be integrating interprofessional education for global health into preexisting educational programs. Resources and commitment may vary across programs within institutions and moving forward in interprofessional education, there must be a shared commitment to obtain resources and share risk as well (Pfeifle & Earnest, 2014).

Johnson, Riel, Ogbolu, Moen, Brenner, and Iwu (2014) shared their experience of developing an organizational capacity for global health learning at the University of Maryland School of Nursing (UMSON) with important lessons emerging. First, deep meaningful partnerships took time and, in fact, a number of years to develop; these partnerships were based on trust and respect. Second, power differentials exist among collaborators and must be addressed on an ongoing basis. Finally, there was a commitment among UMSON students, faculty, and administration, as well as leadership commitment from the university and other institutes within the university system.

Table 32.1 List of Competencies Categorized Into 8 Domains for Global Citizen and 11 Domains for Basic Operational Program-Oriented Levels

Domains and Competencies	Knowledge (K), Attitude (A), Skill (S)	Global Citizen Level	Basic Operational Program-Oriented Level
Domain 1. Global Burden of Disease Encompasses basic understandings of major causes of morbidity and mortality and their variations between high-, middle- and low-income regions, and with major public health efforts to reduce health disparities globally.			
1a. Describe the major causes of morbidity and mortality around the world, and how the risk for disease varies with regions.	K	X	X
1b. Describe major public health efforts to reduce disparities in global health (e.g., Millennium Development Goals and Global Fund to Fight AIDS, Tuberculosis and Malaria).	K	X	X
1c. Validate the health status of populations using available data (e.g., public health surveillance data, vital statistics, registries, surveys, electronic health records, and health plan claims data).	K, S		X
Domain 2. Globalization of Health and Health Care Focuses on understanding how globalization affects health, health systems, and the delivery of health care.			
2a. Describe different national models or health systems for provision of health care and their respective effects on health and health care expenditure.	K		X
2b. Describe how global trends in health care practice, commerce and culture, multinational agreements, and multinational organizations contribute to the quality and availability of health and health care locally and internationally.	K		X
2c. Describe how travel and trade contribute to the spread of communicable and chronic diseases.	K	X	X
2d. Describe general trends and influences in the global availability and movement of health care workers.	K		X
Domain 3. Social and Environmental Determinants of Health Focuses on an understanding that social, economic, and environmental factors are important determinants of health, and that health is more than the absence of disease.			
3a. Describe how cultural context influences perceptions of health and disease.	K	X	X

(continued)

Table 32.1 List of Competencies Categorized Into 8 Domains for Global Citizen and 11 Domains for Basic Operational Program-Oriented Levels (*continued*)

Domains and Competencies	Knowledge (K), Attitude (A), Skill (S)	Global Citizen Level	Basic Operational Program-Oriented Level
3b. List major social and economic determinants of health and their effects on the access to and quality of health services and on differences in morbidity and mortality between and within countries.	K	X	X
3c. Describe the relationship between access to and quality of water, sanitation, food, and air on individual and population health.	K	X	X
Domain 4. Capacity Strengthening "Capacity strengthening is sharing knowledge, skills, and resources for enhancing global public health programs, infrastructure, and workforce to address current and future global public health needs." (Association of Schools & Programs of Public Health, 2011)			
4a. Collaborate with a host or partner organization to assess the organization's operational capacity.	S		X
4b. Cocreate strategies with the community to strengthen community capabilities, and contribute to reduction in health disparities and improvement of community health.	K, S		X
4c. Integrate community assets and resources to improve the health of individuals and populations.	K, S		X
4d. Identify methods for ensuring program sustainability (proposed by members of the CUGH Global Health Competency Subcommittee).	K, S		X
Domain 5. Collaboration, Partnering, and Communication "Collaborating and partnering is the ability to select, recruit, and work with a diverse range of global health stakeholders to advance research, policy, and practice goals, and to foster open dialogue and effective communication" with partners and within a team. (Association of Schools & Programs of Public Health, 2011)			
5a. Include representatives of diverse constituencies in community partnerships and foster interactive learning with these partners.	S		X
5b. Demonstrate diplomacy and build trust with community partners.	A		X
5c. Communicate joint lessons learned to community partners and global constituencies.	S		X

Table 32.1 List of Competencies Categorized Into 8 Domains for Global Citizen and 11 Domains for Basic Operational Program-Oriented Levels (*continued*)

Domains and Competencies	Knowledge (K), Attitude (A), Skill (S)	Global Citizen Level	Basic Operational Program-Oriented Level
5d. Exhibit interprofessional values and communication skills that demonstrate respect for, and awareness of, the unique cultures, values, roles/responsibilities, and expertise represented by other professionals and groups that work in global health.	S	X	X
5e. Acknowledge one's limitations in skills, knowledge, and abilities.	S, A	X	X
5f. Apply leadership practices that support collaborative practice and team effectiveness.	S, A		X
Domain 6. Ethics Encompasses the application of basic principles of ethics to global health issues and settings.			
6a. Demonstrate an understanding of and an ability to resolve common ethical issues and challenges that arise when working within diverse economic, political, and cultural contexts as well as when working with vulnerable populations and in low-resource settings to address global health issues.	K, S, A	X	X
6b. Demonstrate an awareness of local and national codes of ethics relevant to one's working environment.	K		X
6c. Apply the fundamental principles of international standards for the protection of human subjects in diverse cultural settings.	K, S		X
Domain 7. Professional Practice Refers to activities related to the specific profession or discipline of the global health practitioner (domain definition proposed by members of the CUGH Global Health Competency Subcommittee).			
7a. Demonstrate integrity, regard, and respect for others in all aspects of professional practice.	S, A		X
7b. Articulate barriers to health and health care in low-resource settings locally and internationally.	K, S	X	X
7c. Demonstrate the ability to adapt clinical or discipline-specific skills and practice in a resource-constrained setting.	S, A		X
Domain 8. Health Equity and Social Justice "Health equity and social justice is the framework for analyzing strategies to address health disparities across socially, demographically, or geographically defined populations." (Association of Schools & Programs of Public Health, 2011)			

(*continued*)

Table 32.1 List of Competencies Categorized Into 8 Domains for Global Citizen and 11 Domains for Basic Operational Program-Oriented Levels (*continued*)

Domains and Competencies	Knowledge (K), Attitude (A), Skill (S)	Global Citizen Level	Basic Operational Program-Oriented Level
8a. Apply social justice and human rights principles in addressing global health problems.	K, S		X
8b. Implement strategies to engage marginalized and vulnerable populations in making decisions that affect their health and well-being.	K, S		X
8c. Demonstrate a basic understanding of the relationships between health, human rights, and global inequities.	K	X	X
8d. Describe role of WHO in linking health and human rights, the Universal Declaration of Human Rights, International Ethical Guidelines for Biomedical Research Involving Human Subjects.	K		X
8e. Demonstrate a commitment to social responsibility.	A	X	X
8f. Develop understanding and awareness of the health care workforce crisis in the developing world, the factors that contribute to this, and strategies to address this problem.	K		X
Domain 9. Program Management "Program management is ability to design, implement, and evaluate global health programs to maximize contributions to effective policy, enhanced practice, and improved and sustainable health outcomes." (Association of School & Programs of Public Health, 2011)			
9a. Plan, implement, and evaluate an evidence-based program.	K, S		X
9b. Apply project management techniques throughout program planning, implementation, and evaluation.	K, S		X
Domain 10. Sociocultural and Political Awareness "Sociocultural and political awareness is the conceptual basis with which to work effectively within diverse cultural settings and across local, regional, national, and international political landscapes." (Association of School & Programs of Public Health, 2011)			
10a. Describe the roles and relationships of the major entities influencing global health and development.	K	X	X
Domain 11. Strategic Analysis "Strategic analysis is the ability to use systems thinking to analyze a diverse range of complex and interrelated factors shaping health trends to formulate programs at the local, national, and international levels." (Association of School & Programs of Public Health, 2011)			

(*continued*)

Table 32.1 List of Competencies Categorized Into 8 Domains for Global Citizen and 11 Domains for Basic Operational Program-Oriented Levels (*continued*)

Domains and Competencies	Knowledge (K), Attitude (A), Skill (S)	Global Citizen Level	Basic Operational Program-Oriented Level
11a. Identify how demographic and other major factors can influence patterns of morbidity, mortality, and disability in a defined population.	K		X
11b. Conduct a community health needs assessment.	S		X
11c. Conduct a situation analysis across a range of cultural, economic, and health contexts.	S		X
11d. Design context-specific health interventions based on situation analysis.	S		X

CUGH, Consortium of Universities for Global Health; WHO, World Health Organization.
Source: Jogerst et al. (2015). Reprinted with permission, *Annals of Global Health.*

Nurse Volunteers for Global Health Service, Education, and Research Will Demonstrate Experience and Skill in Negotiating Collaborative Practice

Meeting the challenges of global health in any profession can feel overwhelming. Nursing is confronted with having the largest number of health care providers across the globe, but capacity remains far below need and demand. Regional differences exist, but the reality is that worldwide, over a billion people have no access to a health care provider (Crisp & Chen, 2014). Nursing is also experiencing a global faculty shortage further compromising the ability to educate more nurses. Solutions exist, but one overarching recommendation cited by Nardi and Gyurko (2013) is for nursing organizations to join together and take collective action to provide leadership needed at the global level. New models of education are needed and the apprenticeship style of nursing education may not be possible given the current context of health.

Leadership in organizations and institutions, academic or service providers, requires experience and skill in negotiating relationships and cocreating a vision with nurses globally for health care responsive to the needs of individuals, families, and communities. Even the most experienced faculty and researcher can be confronted with challenges in something as seemingly simple as working with an Institutional Review Board in another country. Eckhardt (2016) speaks frankly of her collaborative research experience in Japan. Challenges to the research planning and implementation processes included cultural differences in ethics, planning the budget, differences in medical records, errors in communication, and the importance of face-to-face presence. Eckhardt (2016) was able to negotiate through these challenges and she continues her partnership in Japan.

Preparticipation Training Programs Will Include Global Health Competencies and Evidence of Participation From Host Countries

Intentions to help others globally through volunteer and/or academic service experiences may come from the heart, but may result in harmful outcomes if adequate preparation is not provided. Numbers of volunteers through nongovernmental and faith-based organizations are unknown, but more and more "voluntourist" opportunities are being advertised. Websites such as Volunteer Forever (2017) rate these experiences and provide recommendations. More information is known about study abroad experiences and these experiences are increasing in popularity among all university students, not just nursing and other health profession students. The majority of students (32%) select the United Kingdom, Italy, and Spain, for their study abroad experience and they typically stay for under 8 weeks or they may go as part of a summer course (Institute of International Education, 2016).

In her study of short-term global health volunteer experiences, Lasker (2016) emphasizes the variety of preparation that volunteers may (or may not) receive. Most volunteers do receive some type of preparation, but it may occur only when the volunteer reaches the country or, if provided earlier, the amount of preparation may depend upon the motivation of volunteers to read the orientation packets before leaving. Lasker's study also asked hosts with what type of preparation they would like to see volunteers arrive for the experience. Most of the hosts spoke of the need for volunteers to have in-depth preparation in culture and language. In addition, hosts asked that volunteers have more knowledge of the specific needs within the country including health needs of the population.

Volunteers and global health care providers require extensive preparation and orientation to be effective and minimize the possibility of doing harm. Leffers and Plotnick (2011) provide detailed lists of requirements for becoming an effective volunteer at the end of each chapter in their textbook. The process of volunteering begins with making a personal commitment and then matching the volunteer's interest with a particular program. However, for maximum benefit, all organizations must require a thorough orientation that includes some level of mastery of global health competencies. For example, the GHSP program runs collaboratively through the Peace Corps, requires volunteers to complete 10 days of preservice training that includes work in a simulation laboratory there. During this training, their language and technical skills are evaluated prior to departure for their host country. They also begin to learn about the history, culture, and health care of the host setting. Once in the country, they complete approximately 1-month training for language and technical skills, continue their cross-cultural training to learn about history, politics, and culture and complete training to ensure their personal health, safety, and security (Peace Corps, 2016)

All Nurses who Participate in Global Partnerships Will Adhere to Ethical Principles for Global Health Nursing

At the present time, there are no formal guidelines or ethical principles for global health nursing. However, efforts are currently under way to develop guidelines for nursing and other health professions to address ethical concerns that emerge from current global exchanges.

At the beginning of the chapter, the broad ethical concerns for global health equity that underpins all humanitarian concerns were raised as foundational to all global health collaboration and partnerships. Breakey and Evans (2015) apply the traditional ethical principles of autonomy, beneficence, nonmaleficence, and justice to global health (see Chapter 6). Further, nurses are guided by the *Code of Ethics* of the International Council of Nurses (ICN) that is built upon the four principal elements that outline practice standards (nurses and people, nurses and practice, nurses and the profession, and nurses and coworkers; ICN, 2012). This document addresses ethical nursing practice but does not speak directly to collaborative practice that crosses international boundaries. In the United States, the American Nurses Association (ANA) published three versions of the *Code of Ethics for Nurses and Interpretive Statements* (ANA, 2015) since 2001. The nine provisions address nursing practice and scholarly inquiry, including provisions that address the right to dignity, the primacy of patient interests, protection of privacy and confidentiality, and the protection of human rights to promote health diplomacy and reduce health disparities as the most directly applicable to global health. One key element of the provision for primacy of patient interests is collaboration that includes mutual trust, respect, shared decision making, recognition, transparency, and open communication. While each of these guiding documents suggests ethical principles, the nursing professional lacks specific guidance for global health partnerships.

Critics of many volunteer nurse service experiences note that the principle of nonmaleficence or "first do no harm" is often compromised by the lack of defined partnerships because they often fail to meet the needs of those served (Crump & Sugarman, 2008), fail to address the roots of health inequalities, fail to address cultural norms (Crigger & Holcomb, 2007), and can increase dependency upon foreign donors and volunteers (Levi, 2009). While these comments most often address short-term or student learning experiences, the concerns can be applied to other international program experiences. Leffers and Plotnick (2011) note that, in addition to the ANA ethical provisions, the key factors for ethical practice experiences include transparency of all program aims and decisions, the need for nurse volunteers to be learners as well as providers, that services provided are controlled by the host country partners, and that all nurse volunteers have the proper credentials for their practice.

To address the limitations of specific guidelines for global health ethical principles, health professionals are developing guidance for their respective professions. For example, the Working Group on Ethics Guidelines for Global Health Training (WEIGHT) provides recommendations for sending and host institutions, students/trainees, and funding agencies. Important recommendations include (Crump & Sugarman, 2010) the following:

- Develop well-structured programs to derive mutual benefit.
- Clarify goals and expectations; be explicit in agreements.
- Develop, implement, and regularly update formal training for all trainees and mentors.
- Resolve ethical conflicts in real time.

Nurses are moving forward to address the ethical concerns raised regarding short-term mission trips and student experiential learning by developing more specific and detailed guidelines. Currently McDermott-Levy and Leffers (2017) are completing a Delphi study of more than 100 nurses from around the globe to address issues as broad as those related to human rights and partnerships to those as specific as related to privacy and Internet technology, appropriate donations, nursing practice and appropriate skill/credential level, and cross-cultural concerns with dress, communication, and privacy. By 2030, it is anticipated that the nursing profession (as well as other health care professions) will have articulated both principles and guidelines for global health nursing and that nursing education, practice, and scholarly inquiry will incorporate the guidance into practice.

Nurses Will Participate Across International Boundaries Through Institutional-Level Partnerships at University, Nongovernmental, or Governmental Level

Fragmented efforts of small organizations or individual contributions, while commendable, will not be enough to achieve the SDGs targeted toward system level changes. Organizations that are firmly established and demonstrate existing strong partnerships such as those discussed in the previous exemplars may offer the most benefit to achieving the SDGs (Dalmida et al., 2016). The University of Pennsylvania's global health program in the School of Nursing is an exemplar of university collaboration and interprofessional education. Students from nursing, medicine, public health, and dentistry participate in the same didactic global health course and may also participate in the same field experience (Lasker, 2016).

Nursing's Relationship to Sustainable Development Will Be Clearly Defined and Integrated Into Nursing Practice

Sustainability lacks clarity in nursing literature. One definition focuses on the environment (Anaker & Elf, 2014), while another, through an evolutionary concept analysis approach, discusses sustainability as a process, an outcome, and as social consciousness, which includes the goals of empowerment, capacity building, community mobilization, and health equity (McMillan, 2014). Within the context of global health nursing, sustainability requires a deeper understanding and commitment to social consciousness.

"Sustainability" is the core of "sustainable development" defined as meeting, ". . . the needs of the present without compromising the ability of future generations to meet their own needs" (UN, n.d.). Three integrated core elements encompassing sustainable development include: economic growth, social inclusion, and environmental protection. However, the UN further emphasizes that sustainable development cannot occur unless poverty is eradicated. Engebretsen, Heggen, Das, Farmer, and Ottersen (2016) caution that emerging conceptualizations of sustainability emphasize a focus on a nation's ability to self-manage resources and, therefore, may become a prerequisite for development aid. They write:

> Using sustainability as a selection criterion risks privileging recipients who have the capacity to gain control over health and living conditions and exclude others as unworthy needy. It would be a paradox if emphasis on sustainability ended up in preventing global equity and justice instead of promoting it. (p. e226)

Capitalizing on women's unique value to health care is one way to begin the journey. The Lancet Commission on Women and Health (Langer et al., 2015) described women's contribution to health as both unpaid and paid health care providers, and details the synergistic effect of women's influence on health and economics. Clearly, women are key to meeting the first SDG, ending poverty in all of its forms.

CONCLUSION

The nursing profession must look broadly at the SDGs in order to address the social determinants of health that either promote or adversely affect health and well-being. This requires focus upon the social determinants of health and a health in all policies approach (Benton & Ferguson, 2016; WHO, 2015). Benton and Ferguson (2016) summarize the SDGs through themes of justice, planet, partnership, dignity, prosperity, and people. This chapter began with a focus upon equity, partnership, and sustainability as central elements for nursing's response to the challenge of sustainable development. In particular, the key to successful partnerships to meet the SDGs requires a thorough understanding and consciousness of close collaboration.

Currently collaborative partnerships have moved from the earlier models of colonialism and paternalism to those of coordination and cooperation with an emphasis upon close collaboration (Rosenberg et al., 2010). While partnerships such as the HRH, Seed GHSP, PID, HVO, and the Regis College Haiti Partnership demonstrate stronger models to guide the future, the post-2030 agenda will require models that build upon advanced knowledge of ethical guidelines for global collaboration, key indicators of success for sustainable development, and essential components of strong collaborative partnerships. Nursing can help to achieve the 17 SDGs by raising consciousness of effective collaboration for strong, morally grounded, equitable partnerships that address the social determinants of health to end poverty (SDG 1), promote health and well-being for all, and strengthen transnational commitments toward sustainable development.

REFLECTION AND DISCUSSION

- How does my institution/organization incorporate partnership principles into collaborative efforts?
- What do I think I would need to change about myself in order to contribute fully to a collaborative relationship?
- How will integration of global health concepts and competencies into nursing education impact partnerships for sustainable development?
- What contributions could I make in realizing the vision statements for global collaboration?
- How will well-articulated ethical principles for global nursing practice change collaboration and partnerships?

REFERENCES

American Association of Colleges of Nursing. (2012). AACN-AONE Task Force on academic-practice partnerships. Retrieved from http://www.aacn.nche.edu/leading-initiatives/academic-practice-partnerships/GuidingPrinciples.pdf

American Nurses Association. (2015). *Code of ethics for nurses with interpretive statements.* Silver Spring, MD: Author.

Anaker, A., & Elf, M. (2014). Sustainability in nursing: A concept analysis. *Scandinavian Journal of Caring Sciences, 28,* 381–389. doi:10.1111/scs.12121

Association of Schools & Programs of Public Health. (2011). Global health competency model. Retrieved from http://www.aspph.org/educate/models/masters-global-health

Barnes, A., Brown, G. W., & Harman, S. (2016). Understanding global health and development partnerships: Perspectives from African and global health system professionals. *Social Science & Medicine, 159,* 22–29. doi:10.1016/j.socscimed.2016.04.033

Benton, D. C., & Ferguson, S. L. (2016). Windows to the future: Can the United Nations Sustainable Development Goals provide opportunities for nursing? *Nursing Economic$, 34*(2), 101–103.

Beran, D., Perone, S. A., Alcoba, G., Bischoff, A., Bussien, C.-L., Eperon, G., . . . Chappius, F. (2016). Partnerships in global health and collaborative governance: Lessons learnt from the Division of Tropical and Humanitarian Medicine at the Geneva University Hospitals. *Globalization and Health, 12*(1). doi:10.1186/s12992-016-0156-x

Binagwaho, A., Kyamanywa, P., Farmer, P. E., Nuthulaganti, T., Umubyeyi, B., Nyemazi, J. P., . . . Goosby, E. (2013). The Human Resources for Health Program in Rwanda: A new partnership. *New England Journal of Medicine, 369*(21), 2054–2059.

Breakey, S., & Evans, L. A. (2015). Global health ethics. In S. Breakey, I. Corless, N. L. Meedzan, & P. Nicholas, (Eds.), *Global health nursing in the 21st century* (pp. 49–71). New York: Springer Publishing.

Brown, L. D. (2014). Towards defining interprofessional competencies for global health education: Drawing on educational frameworks and the experience of the UW-Madison Global Health Institute. *Journal of Law, Medicine & Ethics, 42*(s2), 32–37.

Canadian Interprofessional Health Collaborative. (2010). *A national interprofessional competency framework.* Vancouver, Canada: University of British Columbia.

Corbin, J. H., & Mittelmark, M. B. (2008). Partnership lessons from the Global Programme for Health Promotion Effectiveness: A case study. *Heath Promotion International, 23*(4), 365–371. doi:10.1093/heapro/dan029

Crigger, N., & Holcomb, L. (2007). Practical strategies for providing culturally sensitive, ethical care in developing nations. *Journal of Transcultural Nursing, 18*(1), 70–76.

Crisp, N., & Chen, L. (2014). Global supply of health professionals. *New England Journal of Medicine, 4*(370), 950–957. doi:10.1056/NEJMra1111610

Crump, J. A., & Sugarman, J. (2008). Ethical considerations for short term trainees in global health. *The Journal of the American Medical Association, 300*(12), 1456–1458.

Crump, J. A., & Sugarman, J. (2010). Ethics and best practice guidelines for training experiences in global health. *American Journal of Tropical Medicine and Hygiene, 83*(6), 1178–1182.

Dalmida, S. G., Amerson, R., Foster, J., McWhinney-Dehaney, L., Magowe, M., Nicholas, P. K., . . . Leffers, J. (2016). Volunteer service and service learning: Opportunities, partnerships, and the United Nations Millennium Development Goals. *Journal of Nursing Scholarship, 48*(5), 1–10. doi:10.1111/jnu.12226

Downes, E. (2014). Selecting and negotiating partnerships for collaboration. In M. Upvall & J. Leffers (Eds.), *Global health nursing: Building and sustaining partnerships* (pp. 19–27). New York, NY: Springer Publishing.

Eckhardt, A. L. (2016). Transcultural collaborative research: Challenges and opportunities. *Western Journal of Nursing Research, 38*(6), 663–667. doi:10.1177/0193945915607362

Eichbaum, Q. (2015). The problem with competencies in global health education. *Academic Medicine, 90,* 414–417. doi:10.1097/ACM.0000000000000665

Eisler, R., & Potter, T. M. (2014). *Transforming interprofessional partnerships.* Indianapolis, IN: Sigma Theta Tau International.

Engebretsen, E., Heggen, K., Das, S., Farmer, P., & Ottersen, O. P. (2016). Paradoxes of sustainability with consequences for health. *The Lancet Global Health, 4*, e225–e226. Retrieved from http://www.thelancet.com/journals/langlo/article/PIIS2214-109X(16)00038-3/fulltext

Everett, L. Q. (2016). Academic-practice partnerships: The interdependence between leadership and followership. *Nursing Science Quarterly, 29*(2), 168–172. doi:10.1177/0894318416630106

Farmer, P., Kim, J. Y., Kleinman, A., & Basilico, M. (2013). *Reimaging global health: An introduction.* Berkeley: University of California Press.

Guerin, T. T. (2014). Relationships matter: The role for social-emotional learning in an interprofessional global health education. *Journal of Law, Medicine & Ethics, 42*(Suppl. 2), 38–44.

Institute of International Education. (2016). Opendoors® fast facts 2015. Retrieved from http://www.iie.org/Research-and-Publications/Open-Doors

International Council of Nurses. (2012). *The ICN code of ethics for nurses* (Revised 2012). Geneva, Switzerland: Author. Retrieved from http://www.icn.ch/images/stories/documents/about/icncode_english.pdf

Jogerst, K., Callender, M. D., Adams, V., Evert, J., Fields, E., Hall, T., . . . Wilson, L. L. (2015). Identifying interprofessional global health competencies for 21st-century health professionals. *Annals of Global Health, 81*(2), 239–247. doi:10.1016/j.aogh.2015.03.006

Johnson, J. V., Riel, R. F., Ogbolu, Y., Moen, M., Brenner, A., & Iwu, E. (2014). Organizational learning and the development of global health educational capabilities: Critical reflections on a decade of practice. *Journal of Law, Medicine & Ethics, 42*(s2), 50–59.

Jones, A. (2016). Envisioning a global health partnership movement. *Globalization and Health, 12*(1). Retrieved from https://globalizationandhealth.biomedcentral.com/articles/10.1186/s12992-015-0138-4

Langer, A., Meleis, A., Knaul, F. M., Atun, R., Aran, M., Arreola-Ornelas, H., . . . Frenk, J. (2015). Women and health: The key for sustainable development. *The Lancet, 386*, 1165–1220. doi:10.1016/S0140-6736(15)60497-4

Lasker, J. N. (2016). *Hoping to help: The promises and pitfalls of global health volunteering.* Ithaca, NY: Cornell University Press.

Leffers, J., & Mitchell, E. (2011). Conceptual model for partnership and sustainability in global health. *Public Health Nursing, 28*(1), 91–102. doi:10.1111/j.1525-1446.2010.00892.x

Leffers, J., & Plotnick, J. (2011). *Volunteering at home and abroad: The essential guide for nurses.* Indianapolis, IN: Sigma Theta Tau International.

Levi, A. (2009). The ethics of nursing student international clinical experiences. *Journal of Obstetric, Gynecologic & Neonatal Nursing, 38*(1), 94–99.

McDermott-Levy, R., & Leffers, J. (2017). *Ethical principles of global health nursing practice.* Presentation at Association of Community Health Nursing Educators (ACHNE) Annual Institute, Baltimore, MD. Retrieved from https://www.achne.org/i4a/pages/index.cfm?pageid=3533

McMillan, M. (2014). Sustainability: An evolutionary concept analysis. Exploring nursing's role within the sustainability movement. *Journal of Advanced Nursing, 70*(4), 756–767. doi:10.1111/jan.12250

Mickan, S., Hoffman, S. J., & Nasmith, L. (2010). Collaborative practice in a global health context: Common themes from developed and developing countries. *Journal of Interprofessional Care, 24*(5), 492–502.

Nardi, D. A., & Gyurko, C. C. (2013). The global nursing faculty shortage: Status and solutions for change. *Journal of Nursing Scholarship, 45*(3), 317–326. doi:10.1111/jnu.12030

Ndenga, E., Uwizeye, G., Thomson, D., Uwitonse, D. R., Mubiligi, J., Hedt-Gauthier, B. L., . . . Binagwaho, A. (2016). Assessing the twinning model in the Rwandan Human Resources for Health Program: Goal setting, satisfaction and perceived skill transfer. *Globalization and Health, 12*(4), 1–14. doi:10.1186/s12992-016-0141-4

Partners in Development. (2016). The history of PID. *Partners in Development*. Retrieved from http://www.pidonline.org/about/our-history

Peace Corps. (2016). Preparation & training. *Peace Corps*. Retrieved from https://www.peacecorps.gov/volunteer/preparation-and-training

Pfeifle, A., & Earnest, M. (2014). The creation of an institutional commons: Institutional and individual benefits and risks in global health interprofessional education [Special issue]. *Journal of Law, Medicine & Ethics, 42*, 45–49.

Racine, L., & Perron, A. (2012). Unmasking the predicament of cultural voyeurism: A postcolonial analysis of international nursing placements. *Nursing Inquiry, 19*(3), 190–201. doi:10.1111/j.1440-1800.2011.00555.x

Rosenberg, M. L., Hayes, E. S., McIntyre, M. H., & Neill, N. (2010). *Real collaboration: What it takes for global health to succeed*. Los Angeles: University of California Press.

Seed Global Health. (2016). Global health service partnership. Retrieved from http://seedglobalhealth.org/ghsp-volunteers-teach-300-courses-7000-individuals/#.V6-hJ67lfV0

Sliney, A. (2015). Global health partnerships. In S. Breakey, I. Corless, N. L. Meedzan, & P. Nicholas (Eds.), *Global health nursing in the 21st century* (pp. 103–111). New York, NY: Springer Publishing.

Sliney, A., & Uwimana, C. (2014). Rwanda human resources for health program. In M. Upvall & J. Leffers (Eds.), *Global health nursing: Building and sustaining partnerships* (pp. 208–218). New York, NY: Springer Publishing.

United Nations. (n.d.). Sustainable development goals: 17 goals to transform our world. Retrieved from http://www.un.org/sustainabledevelopment

United Nations. (2015). Transforming our world: The 2030 agenda for sustainable development. Retrieved from https://docs.google.com/gview?url=http://sustainabledevelopment.un.org/content/documents/21252030%20Agenda%20for%20Sustainable%20Development%20web.pdf&embedded=true

Uwizeye, G., Mukamana, D., Relf, M., Rosa, W., Kim, M. J., Munyiginya, P., . . . Moreland, P. (in press). Building nursing and midwifery capacity through the Human Resources for Health Program in Rwanda. *Journal of Transcultural Nursing*.

Volunteer Forever. (2017). 2017 best volunteer abroad programs, organizations, & projects. Retrieved from https://www.volunteerforever.com/article_post/2016-best-volunteer-abroad-programs-organizations-projects

Wachtel, E. (1996). *More writers & company*. Toronto, ON, Canada: Alfred A. Knopf.

Wilson, L., Callender, B., Hall, T. L., & Jogerst, K., Torres, H., & Velji, A. (2014). Identifying global health competencies to prepare 21st century global health professionals: Report from the Global Health Competency Subcommittee of the Consortium of Universities for Global Health [Special issue]. *Journal of Law, Medicine & Ethics, 42*, 26–31.

World Health Organization. (2010). *Framework for action on interprofessional education and collaborative practice*. Geneva, Switzerland: Author. Retrieved from http://www.who.int/hrh/resources/framework_action/en

World Health Organization. (2015). *Health in all policies: Training manual*. Geneva, Switzerland: Author. Retrieved from http://apps.who.int/iris/bitstream/10665/151788/1/9789241507981_eng.pdf?ua=1

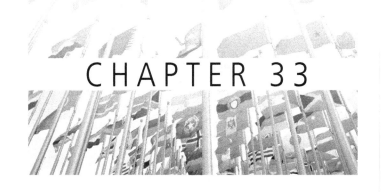

CHAPTER 33

A Post-2030 Agenda: The World Beyond the Sustainable Development Goals[1]

Ann E. Kurth

[Our] tremendous socio-economic progress is taking a heavy toll on the Earth's natural systems. Our patterns of highly inequitable, inefficient, and unsustainable resource consumption, together with population growth . . . are . . . undermining our well-being. There is growing evidence that the planet's capacity to sustain [humanity] is declining. . . . It is time for a new approach. (The Rockefeller Foundation, 2016. Reprinted with permission.)

Human health and economic development have improved but at the expense of undermining the very life-sustaining systems upon which all life on the planet relies for survival. In the 21st century the world has seen population level rises in life span and declines in child mortality and poverty. Yet this has been accompanied by increased carbon emissions and air pollutants; ocean acidification; unsustainable fossil-fuel, fertilizer, and water use; climate change; and losses in biodiversity, tropical forests, and arable land; in essence, mortgaging the ecosystems that sustain life. Gains for the current generation of humans are resulting in decimated ecosystems for future generations. As nurses, midwives, and other health professionals, we must be aware not only of these alarming trends but also incorporate advocacy and mitigation efforts into the work that we do in prevention and care of individuals and populations.

---

[1] This chapter is based in part on presentations by Kurth and grant proposal work collaboratively with Elizabeth Bradley and Anthony Leiserowitz of Yale University, with Kurth.

BACKGROUND AND CONTEXT: GLOBAL HEALTH FRAMEWORK EVOLUTION

Historically, what we now think of as "global health" work focused on single diseases—smallpox eradication, malaria campaigns, and so on. These efforts remained siloed by disciplines and sectors, generally health. A rise in funding to address the global HIV pandemic over the past decade has sparked a renaissance in global health, both as an academic discipline (over 150 global health programs at U.S. universities alone) and a practice. Improvements in population and economic health parameters in low- and middle-income countries, along similar trajectories to what high-income countries experienced earlier, have been pointed out as a "grand convergence" (Jamison et al., 2015). The organizing framework of the Millennium Development Goals (MDGs) has now transitioned to the Sustainable Development Goals (SDGs), setting out targets for 2030 in economic, educational, policy, infrastructure, environmental, and health indices for all nations, regardless of resource status. This emphasis on the engagement of all countries (as opposed to "donor" and "recipient" country relationships) in the enterprise of improving the human condition is new. Along with that has come increasing recognition of the interconnectedness of human and animal health, with a movement to merge the priorities of the health and environmental disciplines, known as "One Health." The latest iteration of global health thinking has most recently been summarized in a report from the Rockefeller Foundation–Lancet Commission (Whitmee et al., 2015) and explores *planetary health*, which stresses that advances in health cannot be sustained by damaging the planetary ecosystems on which all species depend for existence.

Planetary boundaries that support all life have been identified by colleague Dr. Johan Rockström and others (Demaio & Rockstrom, 2015) and include biosphere integrity, land-system and freshwater use, biogeochemical flows, ocean acidification, atmospheric aerosol loading, ozone depletion, climate change, and novel entities. Based on analysis of available data, three of these nine key boundaries are already at the breaking point (Steffen et al., 2015). This accelerated stress on the Earth's resource-carrying capacity in our *Anthropocene* era is not sustainable. Reputable scientists believe that we have the next 10 to 30 years (UK Foreign Office, 2016) in which to achieve substantial change, at the risk of species crash in the coming centuries—our own, this time. In the interim, numerous health impacts can be expected, as outlined in Figure 33.1 from the Lancet Planetary Health Commission report (reproduced from the Millennium Ecosystem Assessment [2005], by permission of World Health Organization [WHO], 2005). Already, 10% of global deaths are caused by poor air quality (Environmental Performance Index, 2016), and the term "climate refugees" has resonance not just in Micronesia but in high-income countries like the United States (Davenport & Robertson, 2016).

To have any hope of achieving the necessary scale of movement for planetary health, recognition of the scope of the problem needs to be rapidly expanded to the public, to industry (given the importance of businesses in contributing to relevant sustainability practices), and to policy makers, in order to support effective policy action. As of now there is no single governmental, academic, or nongovernmental organizational entity focused on both tracking planetary health data indices (to define the problem dynamically) or undertaking evidence-based approaches to communicating the need for action.

| Figure 33.1 | **Health effects of human ecosystem pressure.** |

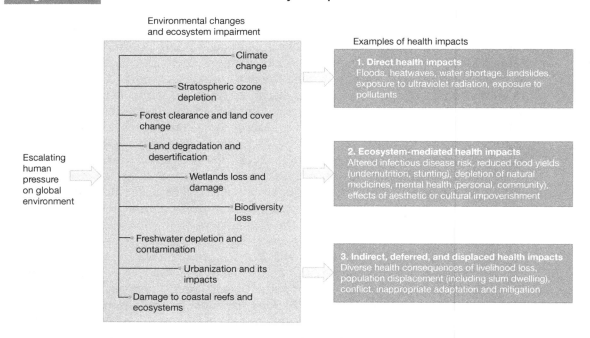

Source: Reproduced by permission of the WHO from Millennium Ecosystem Assessment (2005).

NURSING'S ROLE

Global health as a specialty area, encompassing local and international health inequities, and involving not only health but other disciplines and fields, is becoming an increasingly defined area of work, for nurses and others. Global health competencies have been defined by several groups, including Wilson and colleagues (Wilson et al., 2014) who outline 12 domains: Global Burden of Disease; Globalization of Health and Health Care; Social and Environmental Determinants of Health; Capacity Strengthening; Teamwork/Collaboration and Communication; Ethical Reasoning; Professional Practice; Health Equity and Social Justice; Program Management; Social, Cultural, and Political Awareness; Strategic Analysis; and Communication. It is important to point out that advocacy—for affected populations and for policy action to mitigate ecosystem damage—is an inherent skill needed and one for which nursing as a profession is uniquely prepared. As outlined by the American Nurses Association (ANA), the very definition of nursing includes "advocacy in the care of individuals, families, groups, communities, and populations" as an integral part of our professional identity and obligation (ANA, 2015). The enormity of the ecosystem crisis facing humanity—what has been noted by colleagues as a "superwickedly" complex problem (Levin, Cashore, Bernstein, & Auld, 2012, p. 124)—necessitates enhancing public awareness, and ensuring realistic policy action. These actions may be facilitated by emphasizing these planetary risks as ones that are actually "present, local, and personal" and that engage experiential and affective approaches to affect social group norms, while framing positive policy gains accrued from taking immediate action (van der Linden, Maibach, & Leiserowitz, 2015, p. 758). Nurses and midwives, as the single largest cadre of health providers worldwide, can be instrumental not only in addressing climate change and other ecosystem stress impacts on health but in advocating for action to reduce the damage to human and animal populations and the systems that support them.

The shift from MDGs to SDGs and beyond must therefore strive to ensure not only improved health outcomes for humans but also the planetary "must haves" (Griggs et al., 2013) of clean air, balanced nitrogen and phosphorus flow, climate stability, and so on. The SDGs are targets in a world affected by known challenges that include rising noncommunicable diseases, global urbanization, aging populations, income inequality, resource constraints, and social strife leading to forced population migration. Combined with the ecosystem stresses discussed earlier, there has never been a more urgent imperative for strong health systems that can be resilient and adaptive to coming needs (Whitmee et al., 2015). The projected shortage of 12.9 million health professionals by 2035 (WHO, 2014) is therefore doubly concerning, and highlights the need to support effective and scaled-up approaches to production, support, and retention of health workers over the coming few decades.

YOUR PERSONAL AND PROFESSIONAL ACTION PLAN

Nurses, midwives, and other health workers have the opportunity to take both personal and professional action for improving planetary health. Consider the following reflective questions as a starting point toward considering how you might engage in action to reduce ecosystem impact and build resilient health systems.

Ask yourself how we might help mitigate impact on ecosystem degradation in our own daily lives. Should we live in sustainable cities/use public transport rather than a car? Should we eat more plants and less or no meat? Should we choose smaller family size/increase contraceptive access?

Ask how we, as nurses, can influence policy and action to advocate for better governance and planning, and get engaged in elections, legislative agendas, and civil society movements.

Ask yourself how we can each be a part of realizing not only the Sustainable Development Agenda for 2030, but also the planetary, whole person/whole people, health and well-being that will ensure a truly safe, inclusive, and unified world for generations to come.

CONCLUSION

There has been progress made in health worldwide, but it has not always been equitable and a price has been paid. An evolution of approaches has occurred in "global health" work from (often) a single-disease or intervention focus (e.g., HIV, or agricultural subsidies) to appreciation of the interplay between living species and ecosystems. It is now more fully appreciated that we cannot mortgage progress in human health at the expense of planetary-level systems that sustain life. However, it is increasingly clear that beyond the development focus of the SDGs, we need action now that includes strengthening health systems as well as advocating for changes to address ecosystem support. Finally, nurses and midwives have a key role to play in this critical challenge facing us all, on the one place that we have to call home—planet Earth.

REFLECTION AND DISCUSSION

- How do I see planetary health relating to my own individual health? To the health of those I serve?
- What are some of the ways human beings can de-escalate their pressure on the global environment?
- Which of the environmental changes and ecosystem impairments shown in Figure 33.1 am I currently witnessing in my own home and country?
- What needs to be improved in the educational preparation of global nurses to advance from a single-disease focus to readily consider the interplay of species and factors described by the notion of planetary health?
- How can I use the resources listed in the reference section to develop an action plan for planetary health beyond 2030?

REFERENCES

American Nurses Association. (2015). *Nursing: Scope and standards of practice* (3rd ed.). Silver Springs, MD: Author.

Davenport, C., & Robertson, C. (2016, May 3). Resettling the first American "climate refugees." *The New York Times*. Retrieved from http://www.nytimes.com/2016/05/03/us/resettling-the-first-american-climate-refugees.html?_r=1

Demaio, A. R., & Rockstrom, J. (2015). Human and planetary health: Towards a common language. *The Lancet, 386*(10007), e36–e37. doi:10.1016/S0140-6736(15)61044-3

Environmental Performance Index. (2016). Global metrics for the environment. Retrieved from http://epi.yale.edu

Griggs, D., Stafford-Smith, M., Gaffney, O., Rockstrom, J., Ohman, M. C., Shyamsundar, P., . . . Noble, I. (2013). Policy: Sustainable development goals for people and planet. *Nature, 495*(7441), 305–307. doi:10.1038/495305a

Jamison, D. T., Summers, L. H., Alleyne, G., Arrow, K. J., Berkley, S., Binagwaho, A., . . . Yamey, G. (2015). Global health 2035: A world converging within a generation. *Salud Publica Mex, 57*(5), 444–467.

Levin, K., Cashore, B., Bernstein, S., & Auld, G. (2012). Overcoming the tragedy of super wicked problems: Constraining our future selves to ameliorate global climate change. *Policy Sciences, 45*(2), 123–152.

Millennium Ecosystem Assessment. (2005). *Ecosystems and human well-being: Synthesis.* Washington, DC: Island Press.

The Rockefeller Foundation. (2016). Planetary health. Retrieved from https://www.rockefellerfoundation.org/our-work/initiatives/planetary-health

Steffen, W., Richardson, K., Rockstrom, J., Cornell, S. E., Fetzer, I., Bennett, E. M., . . . Sorlin, S. (2015). Planetary boundaries: Guiding human development on a changing planet. *Science, 347*(6223), 1259855. doi:10.1126/science.1259855

UK Foreign Office. (2016). *Human Rights and Democracy: The 2015 foreign and commonwealth office report.* Retrieved from https://www.gov.uk/government/publications/human-rights-and-democracy-report-2015

van der Linden, S., Maibach, E., & Leiserowitz, A. (2015). Improving public engagement with climate change: Five "best practice" insights from psychological science. *Perspectives on Psychological Science, 10*(6), 758–763. doi:10.1177/1745691615598516

Whitmee, S., Haines, A., Beyrer, C., Boltz, F., Capon, A. G., de Souza Dias, B. F., . . . Yach, D. (2015). Safeguarding human health in the Anthropocene epoch: Report of the Rockefeller Foundation-Lancet Commission on planetary health. *The Lancet, 386*(10007), 1973–2028. doi:10.1016/S0140-6736(15)60901-1

Wilson, L., Callender, B., Hall, T. L., Jogerst, K., Torres, H., & Velji, A. (2014). Identifying global health competencies to prepare 21st century global health professionals: Report from the global health competency subcommittee of the Consortium of Universities for Global Health [Special issue]. *The Journal of Law, Medicine & Ethics, 42*, 26–31. doi:10.1111/jlme.12184

World Health Organization. (2005). *Ecosystems and human well-being: Health synthesis.* A Report of the Millenium Ecosystem Assessment. Geneva, Switzerland: Author. Retrieved from http://www.millenniumassessment.org/documents/document.357.aspx.pdf

World Health Organization. (2014). *A universal truth: No health without a workforce.* Geneva, Switzerland: Author. Retrieved from http://www.who.int/workforcealliance/knowledge/resources/GHWA-a_universal_truth_report.pdf

Resources

- Lancet Commission on Planetary Health (www.thelancet.com/commissions/planetary-health)
- Stockholm Resilience Centre (www.stockholmresilience.org/research/research-news/2013-03-27-redefining-sustainable-development.html)
- Consortium of Universities for Global Health (www.cugh.org)
- Planetary Health Alliance (planetaryhealthalliance.org)
- Sustainable Development Knowledge Platform (sustainabledevelopment.un.org/post2015/transformingourworld)

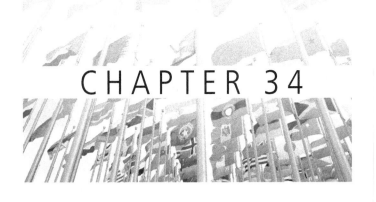

CHAPTER 34

One Mind, One Health, One Planet—A Pledge to Planetary Citizenship

William Rosa

Thank you for this day . . .
My blessings, my pain, my joy.
Bless all my family,
Bless all my friends.
Bless all the people I know,
Bless all the people I don't know.
Bless all the people I will know,
Bless all the people I will never know.
Bless all life on this earth and those who have gone.
Be in my thoughts, my actions, my words,
My deeds, my intentions, my livelihood,
My mindfulness, my concentration.
Help me be the change for peace, love, compassion, and light,
And may all beings be filled with loving kindness.
Namaste.

—*Elizabeth Anne Jones*

Dr. Larry Dossey (2013) has discussed in great detail, with impressively thorough references to the literature, countless case studies, and through his own experiences with the transcendent, the concept of the *One Mind*: a unitary and collective superior intelligence of which all beings are a part. He writes,

> [We have all] broken our responsibilities to our earth and environment, therefore to ourselves and to one another, a thousand times. Yet it is

> within our power to redeem [ourselves] by reclaiming . . . the One Mind
> that unites us with all else. . . ; the One Mind whose calling card is love,
> caring, affection. (L. Dossey, 2013, p. 259)

The One Mind suggests we are interconnected in ways not immediately visible to us, but that beneath the surface differences that plague and disillusion our ego minds, we are inextricably connected to a universal consciousness, linking us to each other, nature, animal species, and the Earth (L. Dossey, 2013). These views have been shared by nurse theorists and visionaries for many years, emphasizing a shared human experience that exists in our very being and belonging as a person on the planet (B. M. Dossey, 2016; Watson, 2008, 2012). It moves us from a reference to people and global health outcomes in terms of statistical data toward a deeper wisdom related to interconnectedness, the intention and purpose for our work as global nurses, and the ethical considerations that drive and guide us, both personally and professionally.

Unity and a unified consciousness has been a major theme throughout *A New Era in Global Health*: personal to planetary transformation (Sharma as cited by Rosa [Chapter 2]); global nurse citizenship (Rosa & Shaw [Chapter 4]); ethical considerations in global health (Breakey & Evans [Chapter 6]); the rationale for an integral worldview and the role of global human caring in building a safe and inclusive world (Dossey, Beck, Oerther, Manjrekar [Chapter 7]; Watson [Chapter 11]); reflective practice for global nursing (Rosa & Horton-Deutsch [Chapter 30]); raising consciousness through global nursing collaboration (Upvall & Leffers [Chapter 32]); and a Post-2030 Agenda for planetary health (Kurth [Chapter 33]); all through the lens of the greatest global agenda of human unity and betterment the world has ever seen: The United Nations (UN) 2030 Agenda for Sustainable Development. The previous contributions have provided ample resources and guideposts to aid us in being effective in the transnational arenas of global health and global nursing with the resources and opportunities available to us right now, today, as we are.

Discussions on global nurse citizenship as a means to accomplish the 2030 Agenda have also been prevalent throughout this text: global citizenship as a means to improved relations, increased environmental awareness, and developing a world based on respect and social justice. This can be achieved through concrete changes to policy, multisector equities for the global population, and the eradication of poverty. Teaching global citizenship may move us forward; role-modeling global citizenship may gain us some of the results we currently seek; but I believe that moving beyond global citizenship toward a One Mind–One Health–One Planet consciousness will create new possibilities in the realms of sustainable peace and optimal planetary well-being.

Planetary citizenship is now proposed herein as a way to invite healing to the fractured aspects of the human–animal–Earth experience, and to identify global nurses as planetary leaders, planetary advocates, and planetary change agents in this new era. "Healing" in this context may be defined as:

> a lifelong journey into understanding the wholeness of [planetary] existence. Healing occurs when we help [the planet] embrace what is feared most. . . . Healing is learning how to open what has been closed so that we can expand [new planetary] potentials. . . . It is accessing what we have forgotten about connections, unity, and interdependence. (B. M. Dossey, 2016, p. 23)

Planetary citizenship moves beyond man-made borders and limitations to the universal principles of a shared and reciprocal humanity and all-life relationship. It moves us from the notions of one woman, one man, one child, one country, or one continent, toward One Mind–One Health–One Planet.

In closing, I propose a pledge to planetary citizenship (Box 34.1) as just one way of recommitting our personal–professional lives to the work of achieving the UN 2030 Agenda for Sustainable Development, and to the values and ideals of global nursing practice: healing, health, human dignity, and peace for all beings everywhere and for the Earth itself.

Box 34.1 **A Pledge to Planetary Citizenship**

I pledge to be a Planetary Citizen,

> To strive continuously toward a universal experience of dignity,
>
> To embrace cultural differences and confront human inequalities and disparities in an effort to know and promote peace,
>
> And to lovingly, but directly, address all threats to Planetary well-being, be they human or environmental.

I pledge to be a Planetary Citizen,

> To be a global nurse in the highest sense of the word,
>
> Embracing nursing as the finest of arts and the most rooted of sciences,
>
> To wield safety, inclusiveness, and social justice as tools to elevate consciousness and role-model compassion,
>
> To be an advocate for healing and global activism,
>
> A conduit for transformation and unity,
>
> And a leader in the journey toward One Mind–One Health–One Planet.

I pledge to role-model kindness and respect as integral aspects of my Planetary Citizenship,

> To carry the intention of unity in my words and actions,
>
> To remain present to the global consequences of my choices,
>
> To commit to creating healing environments at all levels, in all spaces, for all beings everywhere,
>
> And to build relationships based on trust and awareness of a shared humanity.

I pledge to nurture a safe and inclusive world as a Planetary Citizen,

> To release prejudices, divisive judgments, and aggression,
>
> To forgive where it is needed and return myself to wholeness,

(continued)

| Box 34.1 | A Pledge to Planetary Citizenship (*continued*) |

To "Be the Change," live the virtues, and practice the values inherent to ethical engagement,

To accept people as they are and the world as it is in order to more fully embrace myself as I am.

I pledge to devote my energies to self-care, self-knowledge, and self-love as a Planetary Citizen,

Caring for myself as a sacred vessel,

Caring for my family as myself,

Caring for Others as my family,

And for the Planet as I do all Others,

And in this way, caring for the Planet as myself, and the sacred mystery that It is.

I pledge partnership with all beings in an effort to realize Planetary Citizenship and a Planetary World,

To remain open, available, and flexible,

To teach what I know and learn what I don't know,

To honor the light in all of life,

And to leave the Planet better than I found it.

This is my solemn pledge and commitment.

REFERENCES

Dossey, B. M. (2016). Nursing: Integral, integrative, and holistic—Local to global. In B. M. Dossey & L. Keegan (Eds.), *Holistic nursing: A handbook for practice* (7th ed., pp. 3–49). Burlington, MA: Jones & Bartlett.

Dossey, L. (2013). *One mind: How our individual mind is part of a greater consciousness and why it matters.* Carlsbad, CA: Hay House.

Watson, J. (2008). *Nursing: The philosophy and science of caring* (Rev. ed.). Boulder: University Press of Colorado.

Watson, J. (2012). *Human caring science: A theory of nursing* (2nd ed.). Sudbury, MA: Jones & Bartlett.

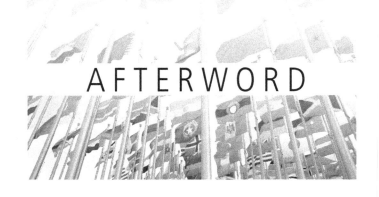

AFTERWORD

Nurses and Nursing Knowledge—Forces for Achieving the Sustainable Development Goals

Afaf Ibrahim Meleis

Throughout *A New Era in Global Health*, we have seen, again and again, that the stars are aligned for nurses to make substantive contributions to global health policies and to wield even greater impact than they have in the past. Evidence of this star alignment is manifested in advanced educational levels attained by nurses, cutting-edge research findings, and the policy-making positions they are holding with increased visibility. Nurses are well educated; national and international reports acknowledge their vital roles in health care and provide agreed-upon recommendations for political actions that guarantee nurses' scope of practice; and nursing research programs are yielding evidence used to provide quality care for diverse populations. Moreover, nurses are increasingly seeking and achieving appointments in leadership and decision-making positions in many corners of the globe.

Together, these are indicators that provide the platform for nurses' voices to be heard and to make a difference for more equitable and just quality care, for more sustainable environments, for supporting peace initiatives, and for pushing against acts that violate people's lives and freedoms.

What makes the stars so well aligned are also the many organized groups that provide mechanisms for partnerships and collaboration to ensure the articulation of shared health care goals. These lead to developing shared voices that ensure changes and implementation of policies based on human rights, environmental preservation, and equal access to resources. All of this provides a positive and powerful context for a much needed engagement and participation in the global progress toward meeting the United Nations (UN) Sustainable Development Goals (SDGs).

The profession at large must support and create more expanded roles for nurses in global health through direct participation in the UN Sustainable Development Agenda. While health may explicitly appear only in SDG 3, "Ensure healthy lives and promote well-being for all ages," it is easy to see health as a driver, an intervening variable, and/or a component in all of the other goals. Health and well-being are related to or a consequence of ending hunger and poverty; achieving quality education and gender equality; attaining access to clean water, energy and proper sanitation; promoting peace and environmental sustainability; and enhancing resilience and partnerships. There is much evidence that each of these profoundly influences, or are influenced by, the health and well-being of populations. Taking these health-related goals into consideration, nurses, as the largest global health care workforce, are essential and necessary components of achieving them by 2030. These goals are timely, ambitious, and essential for populations' health and quality of life, and without them, we cannot achieve sustainable health and well-being. To be achieved by 2030, they require deliberate and systematic efforts by all constituents, including leaders, professionals, as well as lay individuals. Among these constituents are nurses, individually and collectively.

In the final thoughts on this book, I hope to further provide a context and rationale for the engagement of nurses and the discipline of nursing in supporting progress toward the SDGs, and to provide some recommendations, and a few examples, for ways by which members of the discipline of nursing can contribute to and influence the achievement of the SDGs.

GLOBAL NURSING: AN ETHICAL OBLIGATION

Nurses have a moral and ethical obligation to ensure that the SDGs are met by 2030. Besides the obvious reason, which is that nurses are by far the largest global health care workforce (20.7 million globally), there are other equally compelling rationales why nurses must assume, if not leadership, then prominent roles in ensuring progress toward meeting many of the SDG targets across the spectrum.

Nursing is established on a social contract with society. That contract is to keep people healthy, to enhance their well-being, and to protect them from harm due to disease, environmental degradation, or violence. The well-accepted mission of the nursing profession is to enhance peoples' abilities to care for themselves, to decrease suffering, to contribute to populations' quality of life, to ensure effective transitions back to health and well-being, to facilitate populations' abilities to function and be productive up to their full capacities, and to provide compassionate care wherever it is needed regardless of race, culture, sexual orientation, socioeconomic class, or educational levels. Over many generations, and in many corners of the globe, nurses have provided care to the most vulnerable and needy, as well as to the least vulnerable and wealthy. Nurses practice from a framework driven by principles of human rights for equity, justice, inclusiveness, and access to fundamental resources that protect them from harm, the very principles that fortify and inform the SDGs. Nurses are concerned with what Ruger (2010) calls "health capability of individuals," which is people's ability to be healthy and function at their full capacities, to be able to use their own self-agency, and to lead lives they consider of value. This congruency between nursing ethics, principles, values, and mission, and those upon which the SDGs are established, provide one more strong impetus for nurses and the discipline of nursing to engage in ensuring systematic progress toward achieving these goals.

The discipline of nursing, as far back as Florence Nightingale in 1854, claims environment and its health as the cornerstones for ensuring and enhancing health care of populations and for bringing sick, invalid, or injured people back to wellness. Nightingale and her disciples strongly advocated for ensuring their immediate environment (e.g., air and lights) was attended to and maintained. Others followed suit and expanded the meaning of "environment" to be even more inclusive of energy, cultures, and family, social, economic, and political environments. Epistemologically, the discipline of nursing is based on the logical principles of holism and the connection of individuals with families, communities, and societies. The domain of nursing includes the inseparability of relationships between environment and individuals and the importance of community-based assessment for understanding human behavior and responses to health (Meleis & Glickman, 2014; Willis, Perry, LaCoursiere-Zucchero, & Grace, 2014). These relationships and connections are deemed essential conditions for the health and well-being of populations.

More recently, members of the nursing discipline went even further and investigated the effects of natural and man-made disasters, lead poisoning, pollution, and global warming, and their effects on lifestyle changes, and ultimately, their effects on cognition, inhalation, sleep, energy levels, and safety (Cusack, de Crespigny, & Athanasos, 2011; Liu et al., 2015; Noviana, Miyazaki, & Ishimaru, 2016). Once again, this provides rationale and credence to how vital it is to enhance and sustain an environment's health, which in turn profoundly influences populations' health and well-being.

The SDGs acknowledge these diverse aspects and components of environments and their impact on health and well-being while providing ambitious and transformative guidelines concerning their equitable development and sustainability. The 2030 Agenda calls for clean water and sanitation, clean energy, sustainable cities and communities, and actions for maintaining balanced climate ecosystems. This connection between the health and well-being of populations envisioned and promoted by the SDGs is totally and unequivocally congruent with nursing's mission and goals, and provides a platform for nursing's engagement in sustainable, healthy environments as conditions for achieving health and well-being of populations. Nursing's powerful voice, emanating from knowledge and research-based evidence and from expert practice, is needed to ensure progress for all the SDGs.

MAXIMIZING NURSING'S CONTRIBUTIONS AND INFLUENCE

I would like the readers to consider the ways by which nurses, and the discipline of nursing, may support and ensure that these progressive and futuristic Global Goals are achieved.

I propose that engaging, supporting, and influencing the achievement of these ambitious SDGs could happen if nurses, individually and collectively, *value and connect* their own goals and ongoing work with the SDGs, *focus* their efforts on specific goals and *advocate* for needed change, *monitor and evaluate* progress toward achieving them, and *disseminate findings globally*. I will briefly discuss each of these recommendations below and will provide specific guidelines and examples for each one. This discussion is not comprehensive and inclusive. It is provided to stimulate thoughts and challenge actions about ways by which the discipline of nursing may effectively engage and promote the achievement of the SDGs, taking the concepts contained in this text and translating them into deliberate leadership actions.

Value and Connect

It is essential that the nursing profession and nursing organizations recognize the significance of their role in achieving the SDGs (White, 2016). Therefore, students, faculty, clinicians, researchers, and administrators should recognize, study, and understand each of the 17 goals and 169 targets. While all goals should be reviewed in their totality, it may be prudent to identify different goals that are more specific for different organizations' focus and/or practice fields. For example, a course in global health may utilize all SDGs as a framework, while a course in a school of nursing about infant and children's health care may focus on hunger (SDG 2), a course in women's health may focus on equality (SDGs 5 and 10) and economic growth (SDG 8), and a course in community health may focus on making cities more inclusive, safe, resilient, and sustainable (SDG 11), and on the impact of climate change and how to affect changes to decrease global warming (SDG 13).

Theoretical and clinical assignments and classroom discussions may be geared toward how each of the SDGs may be achieved for individual patients, for families, for populations, or for communities. Similarly, nursing organizations, coalitions, or communities may also utilize similar approaches by integrating their strategic goals with the SDGs and critically addressing ways by which achieving organizational goals coincides with, or promotes progress in, SDG attainment. Another example may be that an organization, such as the American Academy of Nursing, may review edge runner nominees and their designation as edge runners by revising the criteria to include some of the goals and the targets outlined by the SDGs. The focus of edge runners then becomes the extent they contribute to progress in one or more of the Global Goals.

I challenge each and every institution or organization that is for or related to nursing to demonstrate how they have fostered a dialogue about the SDGs and how they will continue to integrate the targets into their own strategic goals.

Focus and Advocate

To make a substantive difference, organizations may choose to select one or two of the SDGs and systematically develop a plan to demonstrate how members may proceed to meet some (or all) of the relevant targets. An example may be members of a hospital selecting SDG 13, "Taking urgent action to combat climate change." One of the targets is 13.3, "Improve education, awareness-raising and human and institutional capacity on climate change mitigation, adaptation, impact reduction and early warning" (see the Appendix). By selecting this target, members of the organization could develop strategies to implement its relevant goals. Upon meeting target 13.3, the strategies could be used in other institutions developing the human capacity for planning, management, implementation, and evaluation of these strategies. Promoting these mechanisms, one institution at a time, the target of 13.3—enhancing institutions' human capacity—could be raised at the policy level, mandating human resources for all aspects of climate and environmental changes, first institutionally and organizationally, then citywide, statewide, nationally, and so on.

In addition to this selectivity of goals, it is vital that nurses and the nursing profession continue to honor commitment and resources to increasing access to health care, decreasing disparities, and attending to the needs of the most vulnerable and needy populations.

Monitor and Evaluate

The SDGs provide ample opportunities for both established and novice nurse investigators to develop mechanisms to monitor progress toward their achievement, as well as the metrics to measure the attainment of targets. By assuming leadership in the development of methodologies and metrics, nurses can evaluate progress in achieving the SDGs while demonstrating that nursing research and investigation are relevant to each of them. By focusing and making the necessary connective statements to the SDGs, a reservoir for findings is provided beyond singular research projects. By assuming ownership of some of the SDGs and integrating findings, these reviews may be used to determine progress toward SDG achievement. Nursing research findings, which inform health care policies in the United States, have not been as prominent in informing global health care polices. Developing measures and methodologies and programs of research for monitoring progress now and through to the completion of the year 2030 for achieving the SDGs provides a platform for nurse scientists to make a global impact on global health policies. It is strongly suggested that the SDGs could be a framework that informs the development of research themes and goals by members of institutions where nursing knowledge development is fostered. Among these are the universities that have PhD and postdoctoral programs in nursing, as well as organizations that support nursing science and scientists.

Similarly, a robust dialogue should be fostered by collaborative organizations such as the World Health Organization Collaborating Centres (WHOCCs) for Nursing and Midwifery that represent 42 centers in 25 countries. I may even go further by suggesting that a regular agenda item for each WHOCC, as well as for each meeting of the secretariat, may foster an exploratory dialogue about which SDGs may be selected for monitoring and evaluating.

Disseminate Findings Globally

Work in progress or completed by nurses, faculty, students, clinicians, or researchers, as well as work done related to the discipline of nursing mission and strategic goals that reflect the SDGs, should be disseminated widely through journals, books, and presentations. Several goals should drive the dissemination. One obvious goal is the sharing of knowledge that is expected in an established discipline. Another goal is to ensure that nursing knowledge is readily accessible through searches for those individuals who will be charged to evaluate progress in achieving the SDGs. Recognition of nursing knowledge and of clinicians' and researchers' roles in achieving the SDGs validates the discipline of nursing's mission and contributions. Often such acknowledgment and validation are lacking, particularly because nursing contributions are not included in the analyses and reports that integrate final indicators of the status of progress related to global initiatives.

In addition to developing programs of research that address questions and measures related to the SDGs, nursing organizations may periodically provide integrative analysis and interpretation of findings that address progress on SDG target achievement. This integrative analysis can become a precursor to final reviews, which will be conducted to determine whether and in what ways goals were attained by 2030. Different organizations may select different goals for such analysis and for producing reviews that integrate findings for a designated period. A framework for these reviews may utilize the format used for final reviews of the 2000–2015 Millennium Development Goals, which address such questions as: Where do we stand? What is working? How can we continue to "partner for success?" (UN, 2015).

MOVING FORWARD

Nurses, as global educators, researchers, and clinicians, are well positioned to use their strong moral commitment to the well-being of populations and their voice to advocate for, and participate in, achieving all of the SDGs. They could be the means, individually and collectively, to take full advantage of the multiple opportunities afforded to them through practice, community-based programs, and through mentoring and educating novices to influence progress toward meeting the SDGs. In addition, and as Benton and Ferguson (2016) articulated, nurses have an open window of opportunity to influence the outcomes of the SDGs because they have developed many tools to help governments achieve these goals. To be transformative agents, nurses must be fully aware of and value the SDG targets, and connect them to their own work, daily practices, and scientific investigations. But, they also must systematically and deliberately plan their work, actions, practice, and research toward supporting and/or advocating for the SDGs. By disseminating their findings, they can ensure that nurses' strategies and voices make a global difference in the SDGs and that they are included in the final analysis of progress toward SDG attainment.

Our many esteemed colleagues throughout this book serve as guideposts toward an emerging paradigm of global nursing leadership and advocacy. They remind us that we must create opportunities for ourselves to advance the profession in alignment with the UN Sustainable Development Agenda.

It is, after all, *A New Era in Global Health*.

REFERENCES

Benton, D. C., & Ferguson, S. L. (2016). Windows to the future: Can the United Nations Sustainable Development Goals provide opportunities for nursing? *Nursing Economics*, *34*(2), 101.

Cusack, L., de Crespigny, C., & Athanasos, P. (2011). Heatwaves and their impact on people with alcohol, drug and mental health conditions: A discussion paper on clinical practice considerations. *Journal of Advanced Nursing*, *67*(4), 915–922.

Liu, J., Liu, X., Pak, V., Wang, Y., Yan, C., Pinto-Martin, J., & Dinges, D. (2015). Early blood lead levels and sleep disturbance in preadolescence. *Sleep*, *38*(12), 1869–1874.

Meleis, A. I., & Glickman, C. (2014). A passion in nursing for justice: Toward global health equity. In P. N. Kagan, M. C. Smith, & P. L. Chinn (Eds.), *Philosophies and Practices of Emancipatory Nursing: Social Justice as Praxis* (pp. 309–322). New York, NY: Routledge.

Noviana, U., Miyazaki, M., & Ishimaru, M. (2016). Meaning in life: A conceptual model for disaster nursing practice. *International Journal of Nursing Practice*, *22*(Suppl. 1), 65–75.

Ruger, J. P. (2010). *Health and social justice*. Oxford, UK: Oxford University Press.

United Nations. (2015). *Millennium Development Goals Report 2015*. Retrieved from http://www
.un.org/millenniumgoals/2015_MDG_Report/pdf/MDG%202015%20rev%20(July%20
1).pdf

White, J. (2016). World Health Organization Global Strategy on Human Resources for Health in
the Era of the Post 2015 Sustainable Development Goals: Nursing's essential contribution:
ICN policy brief. Retrieved from http://www.who.int/workforcealliance/knowledge/
resources/ICN_PolicyBriefforNNAsNursingHRandSDGs.pdf

Willis, D., Perry, D., LaCoursiere-Zucchero, T., & Grace, P. (2014). Facilitating humanization:
Liberating the profession of nursing from institutional confinement on behalf of social
justice. In P. N. Kagan, M. C. Smith, & P. L. Chinn (Eds.), *Philosophies and practices of
emancipatory nursing: Social justice as praxis* (pp. 251–265). New York, NY: Routledge.

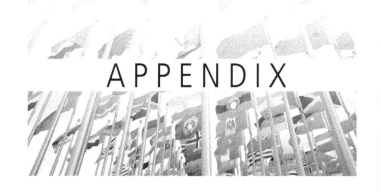

A P P E N D I X

Transforming Our World: The 2030 Agenda for Sustainable Development[1]

PREAMBLE

This Agenda is a plan of action for people, planet, and prosperity. It also seeks to strengthen universal peace in larger freedom. We recognize that eradicating poverty in all its forms and dimensions, including extreme poverty, is the greatest global challenge and an indispensable requirement for sustainable development.

All countries and all stakeholders, acting in collaborative partnership, will implement this plan. We are resolved to free the human race from the tyranny of poverty and want to heal and secure our planet. We are determined to take the bold and transformative steps which are urgently needed to shift the world on to a sustainable and resilient path. As we embark on this collective journey, we pledge that no one will be left behind.

The 17 Sustainable Development Goals and 169 targets which we are announcing today demonstrate the scale and ambition of this new universal Agenda. They seek to build on the Millennium Development Goals and complete what they did not achieve. They seek to realize the human rights of all and to achieve gender equality and the empowerment of all women and girls. They are integrated and indivisible and balance the three dimensions of sustainable development: the economic, social, and environmental.

The Goals and targets will stimulate action over the next 15 years in areas of critical importance for humanity and the planet.

People

We are determined to end poverty and hunger, in all their forms and dimensions, and to ensure that all human beings can fulfill their potential in dignity and equality and in a healthy environment.

---

[1] Copyright © 2015 United Nations. Reprinted with permission.

Planet

We are determined to protect the planet from degradation, including through sustainable consumption and production, sustainably managing its natural resources and taking urgent action on climate change, so that it can support the needs of the present and future generations.

Prosperity

We are determined to ensure that all human beings can enjoy prosperous and fulfilling lives and that economic, social, and technological progress occurs in harmony with nature.

Peace

We are determined to foster peaceful, just, and inclusive societies that are free from fear and violence. There can be no sustainable development without peace and no peace without sustainable development.

Partnership

We are determined to mobilize the means required to implement this Agenda through a revitalized Global Partnership for Sustainable Development, based on a spirit of strengthened global solidarity, focused in particular on the needs of the poorest and most vulnerable and with the participation of all countries, all stakeholders, and all people.

The interlinkages and integrated nature of the Sustainable Development Goals are of crucial importance in ensuring that the purpose of the new Agenda is realized. If we realize our ambitions across the full extent of the Agenda, the lives of all will be profoundly improved and our world will be transformed for the better.

DECLARATION

Introduction

1. We, the Heads of State and Government and High Representatives, meeting at United Nations Headquarters in New York from September 25 to 27, 2015, as the Organization celebrates its 70th anniversary, have decided today on new global Sustainable Development Goals.

2. On behalf of the peoples we serve, we have adopted a historic decision on a comprehensive, far-reaching, and people-centered set of universal and transformative Goals and targets. We commit ourselves to working tirelessly for the full implementation of this Agenda by 2030. We recognize that eradicating poverty in all its forms and dimensions, including extreme poverty, is the greatest global challenge and an indispensable requirement for sustainable development. We are committed to achieving sustainable development in its three dimensions—economic, social, and environmental—in a balanced and integrated manner. We will also build upon the achievements of the Millennium Development Goals and seek to address their unfinished business.

3. We resolve, between now and 2030, to end poverty and hunger everywhere; to combat inequalities within and among countries; to

build peaceful, just, and inclusive societies; to protect human rights and promote gender equality and the empowerment of women and girls; and to ensure the lasting protection of the planet and its natural resources. We resolve also to create conditions for sustainable, inclusive and sustained economic growth, shared prosperity, and decent work for all, taking into account different levels of national development and capacities.

4. As we embark on this great collective journey, we pledge that no one will be left behind. Recognizing that the dignity of the human person is fundamental, we wish to see the Goals and targets met for all nations and peoples and for all segments of society. And we will endeavor to reach the furthest behind first.

5. This is an Agenda of unprecedented scope and significance. It is accepted by all countries and is applicable to all, taking into account different national realities, capacities, and levels of development and respecting national policies and priorities. These are universal goals and targets which involve the entire world, developed and developing countries alike. They are integrated and indivisible and balance the three dimensions of sustainable development.

6. The Goals and targets are the result of over 2 years of intensive public consultation and engagement with civil society and other stakeholders around the world, which paid particular attention to the voices of the poorest and most vulnerable. This consultation included valuable work done by the Open Working Group of the General Assembly on Sustainable Development Goals and by the United Nations, whose Secretary-General provided a synthesis report in December 2014.

Our Vision

7. In these Goals and targets, we are setting out a supremely ambitious and transformational vision. We envisage a world free of poverty, hunger, disease, and want, where all life can thrive. We envisage a world free of fear and violence. A world with universal literacy. A world with equitable and universal access to quality education at all levels, to health care and social protection, where physical, mental, and social well-being are assured. A world where we reaffirm our commitments regarding the human right to safe drinking water and sanitation and where there is improved hygiene; and where food is sufficient, safe, affordable, and nutritious. A world where human habitats are safe, resilient, and sustainable and where there is universal access to affordable, reliable, and sustainable energy.

8. We envisage a world of universal respect for human rights and human dignity, the rule of law, justice, equality, and nondiscrimination; of respect for race, ethnicity, and cultural diversity; and of equal opportunity permitting the full realization of human potential and contributing to shared prosperity. A world which invests in its children and in which every child grows up free from violence and exploitation. A world in which every woman and girl enjoys full gender equality and all legal, social, and economic barriers to their empowerment have been removed.

A just, equitable, tolerant, open, and socially inclusive world in which the needs of the most vulnerable are met.

9. We envisage a world in which every country enjoys sustained, inclusive, and sustainable economic growth and decent work for all. A world in which consumption and production patterns and use of all natural resources—from air to land, from rivers, lakes, and aquifers to oceans and seas—are sustainable. One in which democracy, good governance, and the rule of law, as well as an enabling environment at the national and international levels, are essential for sustainable development, including sustained and inclusive economic growth, social development, environmental protection, and the eradication of poverty and hunger. One in which development and the application of technology are climate-sensitive, respect biodiversity, and are resilient. One in which humanity lives in harmony with nature and in which wildlife and other living species are protected.

Our Shared Principles and Commitments

10. The new Agenda is guided by the purposes and principles of the Charter of the United Nations, including full respect for international law. It is grounded in the Universal Declaration of Human Rights, international human rights treaties, the Millennium Declaration and the 2005 World Summit Outcome. It is informed by other instruments such as the Declaration on the Right to Development.

11. We reaffirm the outcomes of all major United Nations conferences and summits which have laid a solid foundation for sustainable development and have helped to shape the new Agenda. These include the Rio Declaration on Environment and Development, the World Summit on Sustainable Development, the World Summit for Social Development, the Programme of Action of the International Conference on Population and Development, the Beijing Platform for Action, and the United Nations Conference on Sustainable Development. We also reaffirm the follow-up to these conferences, including the outcomes of the Fourth United Nations Conference on the Least Developed Countries, the Third International Conference on Small Island Developing States, the Second United Nations Conference on Landlocked Developing Countries, and the Third United Nations World Conference on Disaster Risk Reduction.

12. We reaffirm all the principles of the Rio Declaration on Environment and Development, including, inter alia, the principle of common but differentiated responsibilities, as set out in principle 7 thereof.

13. The challenges and commitments identified at these major conferences and summits are interrelated and call for integrated solutions. To address them effectively, a new approach is needed. Sustainable development recognizes that eradicating poverty in all its forms and dimensions, combating inequality within and among countries, preserving the planet, creating sustained, inclusive, and sustainable economic growth and fostering social inclusion are linked to each other and are interdependent.

Our World Today

14. We are meeting at a time of immense challenges to sustainable development. Billions of our citizens continue to live in poverty and are denied a life of dignity. There are rising inequalities within and among countries. There are enormous disparities of opportunity, wealth, and power. Gender inequality remains a key challenge. Unemployment, particularly youth unemployment, is a major concern. Global health threats, more frequent and intense natural disasters, spiraling conflict, violent extremism, terrorism and related humanitarian crises, and forced displacement of people threaten to reverse much of the development progress made in recent decades. Natural resource depletion and adverse impacts of environmental degradation, including desertification, drought, land degradation, freshwater scarcity, and loss of biodiversity, add to and exacerbate the list of challenges which humanity faces. Climate change is one of the greatest challenges of our time and its adverse impacts undermine the ability of all countries to achieve sustainable development. Increases in global temperature, sea level rise, ocean acidification, and other climate change impacts are seriously affecting coastal areas and low-lying coastal countries, including many least developed countries and small island developing States. The survival of many societies, and of the biological support systems of the planet, is at risk.

15. It is also, however, a time of immense opportunity. Significant progress has been made in meeting many development challenges. Within the past generation, hundreds of millions of people have emerged from extreme poverty. Access to education has greatly increased for both boys and girls. The spread of information and communications technology and global interconnectedness has great potential to accelerate human progress, to bridge the digital divide and to develop knowledge societies, as does scientific and technological innovation across areas as diverse as medicine and energy.

16. Almost 15 years ago, the Millennium Development Goals were agreed. These provided an important framework for development, and significant progress has been made in a number of areas. But the progress has been uneven, particularly in Africa, least developed countries, landlocked developing countries, and small island developing States, and some of the Millennium Development Goals remain off-track, in particular those related to maternal, newborn, and child health and to reproductive health. We recommit ourselves to the full realization of all the Millennium Development Goals, including the off-track Millennium Development Goals, in particular by providing focused and scaled-up assistance to least developed countries and other countries in special situations, in line with relevant support programs. The new Agenda builds on the Millennium Development Goals and seeks to complete what they did not achieve, particularly in reaching the most vulnerable.

17. In its scope, however, the framework we are announcing today goes far beyond the Millennium Development Goals. Alongside continuing

development priorities such as poverty eradication, health, education, and food security and nutrition, it sets out a wide range of economic, social, and environmental objectives. It also promises more peaceful and inclusive societies. It also, crucially, defines means of implementation. Reflecting the integrated approach that we have decided on, there are deep interconnections and many cross-cutting elements across the new Goals and targets.

The New Agenda

18. We are announcing today 17 Sustainable Development Goals with 169 associated targets, which are integrated and indivisible. Never before have world leaders pledged common action and endeavor across such a broad and universal policy agenda. We are setting out together on the path toward sustainable development, devoting ourselves collectively to the pursuit of global development and of "win–win" cooperation, which can bring huge gains to all countries and all parts of the world. We reaffirm that every State has, and shall freely exercise, full permanent sovereignty over all its wealth, natural resources, and economic activity. We will implement the Agenda for the full benefit of all, for today's generation and for future generations. In doing so, we reaffirm our commitment to international law and emphasize that the Agenda is to be implemented in a manner that is consistent with the rights and obligations of States under international law.

19. We reaffirm the importance of the Universal Declaration of Human Rights, as well as other international instruments relating to human rights and international law. We emphasize the responsibilities of all States, in conformity with the Charter of the United Nations, to respect, protect, and promote human rights and fundamental freedoms for all, without distinction of any kind as to race, color, sex, language, religion, political or other opinion, national or social origin, property, birth, disability, or other status.

20. Realizing gender equality and the empowerment of women and girls will make a crucial contribution to progress across all the Goals and targets. The achievement of full human potential and of sustainable development is not possible if one half of humanity continues to be denied its full human rights and opportunities. Women and girls must enjoy equal access to quality education, economic resources, and political participation as well as equal opportunities with men and boys for employment, leadership, and decision making at all levels. We will work for a significant increase in investments to close the gender gap and strengthen support for institutions in relation to gender equality and the empowerment of women at the global, regional, and national levels. All forms of discrimination and violence against women and girls will be eliminated, including through the engagement of men and boys. The systematic mainstreaming of a gender perspective in the implementation of the Agenda is crucial.

21. The new Goals and targets will come into effect on January 1, 2016, and will guide the decisions we take over the next 15 years. All of us will work to implement the Agenda within our own countries and at the regional and global levels, taking into account different national realities,

capacities, and levels of development and respecting national policies and priorities. We will respect national policy space for sustained, inclusive, and sustainable economic growth, in particular for developing States, while remaining consistent with relevant international rules and commitments. We acknowledge also the importance of the regional and subregional dimensions, regional economic integration, and interconnectivity in sustainable development. Regional and subregional frameworks can facilitate the effective translation of sustainable development policies into concrete action at the national level.

22. Each country faces specific challenges in its pursuit of sustainable development. The most vulnerable countries and, in particular, African countries, least developed countries, landlocked developing countries, and small island developing States, deserve special attention, as do countries in situations of conflict and postconflict countries. There are also serious challenges within many middle-income countries.

23. People who are vulnerable must be empowered. Those whose needs are reflected in the Agenda include all children, youth, persons with disabilities (of whom more than 80% live in poverty), people living with HIV/AIDS, older persons, indigenous peoples, refugees, and internally displaced persons and migrants. We resolve to take further effective measures and actions, in conformity with international law, to remove obstacles and constraints, strengthen support, and meet the special needs of people living in areas affected by complex humanitarian emergencies and in areas affected by terrorism.

24. We are committed to ending poverty in all its forms and dimensions, including by eradicating extreme poverty by 2030. All people must enjoy a basic standard of living, including through social protection systems. We are also determined to end hunger and to achieve food security as a matter of priority and to end all forms of malnutrition. In this regard, we reaffirm the important role and inclusive nature of the Committee on World Food Security and welcome the Rome Declaration on Nutrition and the Framework for Action. We will devote resources to developing rural areas and sustainable agriculture and fisheries, supporting smallholder farmers, especially women farmers, herders, and fishers in developing countries, particularly least developed countries.

25. We commit to providing inclusive and equitable quality education at all levels—early childhood, primary, secondary, tertiary, technical, and vocational training. All people, irrespective of sex, age, race, or ethnicity, and persons with disabilities, migrants, indigenous peoples, children, and youth, especially those in vulnerable situations, should have access to lifelong learning opportunities that help them to acquire the knowledge and skills needed to exploit opportunities and to participate fully in society. We will strive to provide children and youth with a nurturing environment for the full realization of their rights and capabilities, helping our countries to reap the demographic dividend, including through safe schools and cohesive communities and families.

26. To promote physical and mental health and well-being, and to extend life expectancy for all, we must achieve universal health coverage and access to quality health care. No one must be left behind. We commit to accelerating the progress made to date in reducing newborn, child, and maternal mortality by ending all such preventable deaths before 2030. We are committed to ensuring universal access to sexual and reproductive health care services, including for family planning, information, and education. We will equally accelerate the pace of progress made in fighting malaria, HIV/AIDS, tuberculosis, hepatitis, Ebola, and other communicable diseases and epidemics, including by addressing growing antimicrobial resistance and the problem of unattended diseases affecting developing countries. We are committed to the prevention and treatment of noncommunicable diseases, including behavioral, developmental, and neurological disorders, which constitute a major challenge for sustainable development.

27. We will seek to build strong economic foundations for all our countries. Sustained, inclusive, and sustainable economic growth is essential for prosperity. This will only be possible if wealth is shared and income inequality is addressed. We will work to build dynamic, sustainable, innovative, and people-centered economies, promoting youth employment and women's economic empowerment, in particular, and decent work for all. We will eradicate forced labor and human trafficking and end child labor in all its forms. All countries stand to benefit from having a healthy and well-educated workforce with the knowledge and skills needed for productive and fulfilling work and full participation in society. We will strengthen the productive capacities of least developed countries in all sectors, including through structural transformation. We will adopt policies which increase productive capacities, productivity, and productive employment; financial inclusion; sustainable agriculture, pastoralist and fisheries development; sustainable industrial development; universal access to affordable, reliable, sustainable, and modern energy services; sustainable transport systems; and quality and resilient infrastructure.

28. We commit to making fundamental changes in the way that our societies produce and consume goods and services. Governments, international organizations, the business sector, and other non-State actors and individuals must contribute to changing unsustainable consumption and production patterns, including through the mobilization, from all sources, of financial and technical assistance to strengthen developing countries' scientific, technological, and innovative capacities to move toward more sustainable patterns of consumption and production. We encourage the implementation of the 10-Year Framework of Programmes on Sustainable Consumption and Production Patterns. All countries take action, with developed countries taking the lead, taking into account the development and capabilities of developing countries.

29. We recognize the positive contribution of migrants for inclusive growth and sustainable development. We also recognize that international

migration is a multidimensional reality of major relevance for the development of countries of origin, transit, and destination, which requires coherent and comprehensive responses. We will cooperate internationally to ensure safe, orderly, and regular migration involving full respect for human rights and the humane treatment of migrants regardless of migration status, of refugees, and of displaced persons. Such cooperation should also strengthen the resilience of communities hosting refugees, particularly in developing countries. We underline the right of migrants to return to their country of citizenship, and recall that States must ensure that their returning nationals are duly received.

30. States are strongly urged to refrain from promulgating and applying any unilateral economic, financial, or trade measures not in accordance with international law and the Charter of the United Nations that impede the full achievement of economic and social development, particularly in developing countries.

31. We acknowledge that the United Nations Framework Convention on Climate Change is the primary international, intergovernmental forum for negotiating the global response to climate change. We are determined to address decisively the threat posed by climate change and environmental degradation. The global nature of climate change calls for the widest possible international cooperation aimed at accelerating the reduction of global greenhouse gas emissions and addressing adaptation to the adverse impacts of climate change. We note with grave concern the significant gap between the aggregate effect of parties' mitigation pledges in terms of global annual emissions of greenhouse gases by 2020 and aggregate emission pathways consistent with having a likely chance of holding the increase in global average temperature below 2°C or 1.5°C above preindustrial levels.

32. Looking ahead to the 21st session of the Conference of the Parties in Paris, we underscore the commitment of all States to work for an ambitious and universal climate agreement. We reaffirm that the protocol, another legal instrument or agreed outcome with legal force under the Convention applicable to all parties, shall address in a balanced manner, inter alia, mitigation, adaptation, finance, technology development and transfer, and capacity building; and transparency of action and support.

33. We recognize that social and economic development depends on the sustainable management of our planet's natural resources. We are therefore determined to conserve and sustainably use oceans and seas, freshwater resources, as well as forests, mountains, and drylands and to protect biodiversity, ecosystems, and wildlife. We are also determined to promote sustainable tourism, to tackle water scarcity and water pollution, to strengthen cooperation on desertification, dust storms, land degradation, and drought and to promote resilience and disaster risk reduction. In this regard, we look forward to the 13th meeting of the Conference of the Parties to the Convention on Biological Diversity to be held in Mexico.

34. We recognize that sustainable urban development and management are crucial to the quality of life of our people. We will work with local authorities and communities to renew and plan our cities and human settlements so as to foster community cohesion and personal security and to stimulate innovation and employment. We will reduce the negative impacts of urban activities and of chemicals which are hazardous for human health and the environment, including through the environmentally sound management and safe use of chemicals, the reduction and recycling of waste, and the more efficient use of water and energy. And we will work to minimize the impact of cities on the global climate system. We will also take account of population trends and projections in our national rural and urban development strategies and policies. We look forward to the upcoming United Nations Conference on Housing and Sustainable Urban Development to be held in Quito.

35. Sustainable development cannot be realized without peace and security; and peace and security will be at risk without sustainable development. The new Agenda recognizes the need to build peaceful, just, and inclusive societies that provide equal access to justice and that are based on respect for human rights (including the right to development), on effective rule of law and good governance at all levels, and on transparent, effective, and accountable institutions. Factors which give rise to violence, insecurity, and injustice, such as inequality, corruption, poor governance, and illicit financial and arms flows, are addressed in the Agenda. We must redouble our efforts to resolve or prevent conflict and to support postconflict countries, including through ensuring that women have a role in peacebuilding and State building. We call for further effective measures and actions to be taken, in conformity with international law, to remove the obstacles to the full realization of the right of self-determination of peoples living under colonial and foreign occupation, which continue to adversely affect their economic and social development as well as their environment.

36. We pledge to foster intercultural understanding, tolerance, mutual respect, and an ethic of global citizenship and shared responsibility. We acknowledge the natural and cultural diversity of the world and recognize that all cultures and civilizations can contribute to, and are crucial enablers of, sustainable development.

37. Sport is also an important enabler of sustainable development. We recognize the growing contribution of sport to the realization of development and peace in its promotion of tolerance and respect and the contributions it makes to the empowerment of women and of young people, individuals, and communities as well as to health, education, and social inclusion objectives.

38. We reaffirm, in accordance with the Charter of the United Nations, the need to respect the territorial integrity and political independence of States.

Means of Implementation

39. The scale and ambition of the new Agenda requires a revitalized Global Partnership to ensure its implementation. We fully commit to this. This Partnership will work in a spirit of global solidarity, in particular solidarity with the poorest and with people in vulnerable situations. It will facilitate an intensive global engagement in support of implementation of all the Goals and targets, bringing together Governments, the private sector, civil society, the United Nations system, and other actors and mobilizing all available resources.

40. The means of implementation targets under Goal 17 and under each Sustainable Development Goal are key to realizing our Agenda and are of equal importance with the other Goals and targets. The Agenda, including the Sustainable Development Goals, can be met within the framework of a revitalized Global Partnership for Sustainable Development, supported by the concrete policies and actions as outlined in the outcome document of the third International Conference on Financing for Development, held in Addis Ababa from July 13 to 16, 2015. We welcome the endorsement by the General Assembly of the Addis Ababa Action Agenda, which is an integral part of the 2030 Agenda for Sustainable Development. We recognize that the full implementation of the Addis Ababa Action Agenda is critical for the realization of the Sustainable Development Goals and targets.

41. We recognize that each country has primary responsibility for its own economic and social development. The new Agenda deals with the means required for implementation of the Goals and targets. We recognize that these will include the mobilization of financial resources as well as capacity building and the transfer of environmentally sound technologies to developing countries on favorable terms, including on concessional and preferential terms, as mutually agreed. Public finance, both domestic and international, will play a vital role in providing essential services and public goods and in catalyzing other sources of finance. We acknowledge the role of the diverse private sector, ranging from microenterprises to cooperatives to multinationals, and that of civil society organizations and philanthropic organizations in the implementation of the new Agenda.

42. We support the implementation of relevant strategies and programs of action, including the Istanbul Declaration and Programme of Action, the SIDS Accelerated Modalities of Action (SAMOA) Pathway and the Vienna Programme of Action for Landlocked Developing Countries for the Decade 2014–2024, and reaffirm the importance of supporting the African Union's Agenda 2063 and the program of the New Partnership for Africa's Development, all of which are integral to the new Agenda. We recognize the major challenge to the achievement of durable peace and sustainable development in countries in conflict and postconflict situations.

43. We emphasize that international public finance plays an important role in complementing the efforts of countries to mobilize public resources

domestically, especially in the poorest and most vulnerable countries with limited domestic resources. An important use of international public finance, including official development assistance (ODA), is to catalyze additional resource mobilization from other sources, public and private. ODA providers reaffirm their respective commitments, including the commitment by many developed countries to achieve the target of 0.7% of gross national income for official development assistance (ODA/ GNI) to developing countries and 0.15% to 0.2% of ODA/GNI to least developed countries.

44. We acknowledge the importance for international financial institutions to support, in line with their mandates, the policy space of each country, in particular developing countries. We recommit to broadening and strengthening the voice and participation of developing countries— including African countries, least developed countries, landlocked developing countries, small island developing States, and middle-income countries—in international economic decision making, norm setting, and global economic governance.

45. We acknowledge also the essential role of national parliaments through their enactment of legislation and adoption of budgets and their role in ensuring accountability for the effective implementation of our commitments. Governments and public institutions will also work closely on implementation with regional and local authorities, subregional institutions, international institutions, academia, philanthropic organizations, volunteer groups, and others.

46. We underline the important role and comparative advantage of an adequately resourced, relevant, coherent, efficient, and effective United Nations system in supporting the achievement of the Sustainable Development Goals and sustainable development. While stressing the importance of strengthened national ownership and leadership at the country level, we express our support for the ongoing dialogue in the Economic and Social Council on the longer term positioning of the United Nations development system in the context of this Agenda.

Follow-Up and Review

47. Our Governments have the primary responsibility for follow-up and review, at the national, regional, and global levels, in relation to the progress made in implementing the Goals and targets over the coming 15 years. To support accountability to our citizens, we will provide for systematic follow-up and review at the various levels, as set out in this Agenda and the Addis Ababa Action Agenda. The high-level political forum under the auspices of the General Assembly and the Economic and Social Council will have the central role in overseeing follow-up and review at the global level.

48. Indicators are being developed to assist this work. Quality, accessible, timely, and reliable disaggregated data will be needed to help with the measurement of progress and to ensure that no one is left behind.

Such data is key to decision making. Data and information from existing reporting mechanisms should be used where possible. We agree to intensify our efforts to strengthen statistical capacities in developing countries, particularly African countries, least developed countries, landlocked developing countries, small island developing States, and middle-income countries. We are committed to developing broader measures of progress to complement gross domestic product.

A Call for Action to Change Our World

49. Seventy years ago, an earlier generation of world leaders came together to create the United Nations. From the ashes of war and division they fashioned this Organization and the values of peace, dialogue, and international cooperation which underpin it. The supreme embodiment of those values is the Charter of the United Nations.

50. Today we are also taking a decision of great historic significance. We resolve to build a better future for all people, including the millions who have been denied the chance to lead decent, dignified, and rewarding lives and to achieve their full human potential. We can be the first generation to succeed in ending poverty; just as we may be the last to have a chance of saving the planet. The world will be a better place in 2030 if we succeed in our objectives.

51. What we are announcing today—an Agenda for global action for the next 15 years—is a charter for people and planet in the 21st century. Children and young women and men are critical agents of change and will find in the new Goals a platform to channel their infinite capacities for activism into the creation of a better world.

52. "We the peoples" are the celebrated opening words of the Charter of the United Nations. It is "we the peoples" who are embarking today on the road to 2030. Our journey will involve Governments as well as parliaments, the United Nations system and other international institutions, local authorities, indigenous peoples, civil society, business and the private sector, the scientific and academic community—and all people. Millions have already engaged with, and will own, this Agenda. It is an Agenda of the people, by the people, and for the people—and this, we believe, will ensure its success.

53. The future of humanity and of our planet lies in our hands. It lies also in the hands of today's younger generation who will pass the torch to future generations. We have mapped the road to sustainable development; it will be for all of us to ensure that the journey is successful and its gains irreversible.

SUSTAINABLE DEVELOPMENT GOALS AND TARGETS

54. Following an inclusive process of intergovernmental negotiations, and based on the proposal of the Open Working Group on Sustainable

Development Goals,[2] which includes a chapeau contextualizing the latter, set out below are the Goals and targets which we have agreed.

55. The Sustainable Development Goals and targets are integrated and indivisible, global in nature, and universally applicable, taking into account different national realities, capacities, and levels of development and respecting national policies and priorities. Targets are defined as aspirational and global, with each Government setting its own national targets guided by the global level of ambition but taking into account national circumstances. Each Government will also decide how these aspirational and global targets should be incorporated into national planning processes, policies, and strategies. It is important to recognize the link between sustainable development and other relevant ongoing processes in the economic, social, and environmental fields.

56. In deciding upon these Goals and targets, we recognize that each country faces specific challenges to achieve sustainable development, and we underscore the special challenges facing the most vulnerable countries and, in particular, African countries, least developed countries, landlocked developing countries, and small island developing States, as well as the specific challenges facing the middle-income countries. Countries in situations of conflict also need special attention.

57. We recognize that baseline data for several of the targets remains unavailable, and we call for increased support for strengthening data collection and capacity building in Member States, to develop national and global baselines where they do not yet exist. We commit to addressing this gap in data collection so as to better inform the measurement of progress, in particular for those targets below which do not have clear numerical targets.

58. We encourage ongoing efforts by States in other forums to address key issues which pose potential challenges to the implementation of our Agenda, and we respect the independent mandates of those processes. We intend that the Agenda and its implementation would support, and be without prejudice to, those other processes and the decisions taken therein.

59. We recognize that there are different approaches, visions, models, and tools available to each country, in accordance with its national circumstances and priorities, to achieve sustainable development; and we reaffirm that planet Earth and its ecosystems are our common home and that "Mother Earth" is a common expression in a number of countries and regions.

---

[2]Contained in the report of the Open Working Group of the General Assembly on Sustainable Development Goals (A/68/970 and Corr.1; see also A/68/970/Add.1 and 2).

Sustainable Development Goals

Goal 1. End poverty in all its forms everywhere.

Goal 2. End hunger, achieve food security and improved nutrition, and promote sustainable agriculture.

Goal 3. Ensure healthy lives and promote well-being for all at all ages.

Goal 4. Ensure inclusive and equitable quality education and promote lifelong learning opportunities for all.

Goal 5. Achieve gender equality and empower all women and girls.

Goal 6. Ensure availability and sustainable management of water and sanitation for all.

Goal 7. Ensure access to affordable, reliable, sustainable, and modern energy for all.

Goal 8. Promote sustained, inclusive, and sustainable economic growth, full and productive employment, and decent work for all.

Goal 9. Build resilient infrastructure, promote inclusive and sustainable industrialization, and foster innovation.

Goal 10. Reduce inequality within and among countries.

Goal 11. Make cities and human settlements inclusive, safe, resilient, and sustainable.

Goal 12. Ensure sustainable consumption and production patterns.

Goal 13. Take urgent action to combat climate change and its impacts.*

Goal 14. Conserve and sustainably use the oceans, seas, and marine resources for sustainable development.

Goal 15. Protect, restore, and promote sustainable use of terrestrial ecosystems, sustainably manage forests, combat desertification, and halt and reverse land degradation and halt biodiversity loss.

Goal 16. Promote peaceful and inclusive societies for sustainable development, provide access to justice for all and build effective, accountable, and inclusive institutions at all levels.

Goal 17. Strengthen the means of implementation and revitalize the Global Partnership for Sustainable Development.

*Acknowledging that the United Nations Framework Convention on Climate Change is the primary international, intergovernmental forum for negotiating the global response to climate change.

Goal 1. End Poverty in All Its Forms Everywhere

1.1 By 2030, eradicate extreme poverty for all people everywhere, currently measured as people living on less than $1.25 a day.

1.2 By 2030, reduce at least by half the proportion of men, women, and children of all ages living in poverty in all its dimensions according to national definitions.

1.3 Implement nationally appropriate social protection systems and measures for all, including floors, and by 2030 achieve substantial coverage of the poor and the vulnerable.

1.4 By 2030, ensure that all men and women, in particular the poor and the vulnerable, have equal rights to economic resources, as well as access to basic services, ownership, and control over land and other forms of property, inheritance, natural resources, appropriate new technology, and financial services, including microfinance.

1.5 By 2030, build the resilience of the poor and those in vulnerable situations and reduce their exposure and vulnerability to climate-related extreme events and other economic, social, and environmental shocks and disasters.

1.a Ensure significant mobilization of resources from a variety of sources, including through enhanced development cooperation, in order to provide adequate and predictable means for developing countries, in particular least developed countries, to implement programs and policies to end poverty in all its dimensions.

1.b Create sound policy frameworks at the national, regional, and international levels, based on pro-poor and gender-sensitive development strategies, to support accelerated investment in poverty eradication actions.

Goal 2. End Hunger, Achieve Food Security and Improved Nutrition, and Promote Sustainable Agriculture

2.1 By 2030, end hunger and ensure access by all people, in particular the poor and people in vulnerable situations, including infants, to safe, nutritious, and sufficient food all year round.

2.2 By 2030, end all forms of malnutrition, including achieving, by 2025, the internationally agreed targets on stunting and wasting in children under 5 years of age, and address the nutritional needs of adolescent girls, pregnant and lactating women, and older persons.

2.3 By 2030, double the agricultural productivity and incomes of small-scale food producers, in particular women, indigenous peoples, family farmers, pastoralists, and fishers, including through secure and equal access to land, other productive resources and inputs, knowledge, financial services, markets, and opportunities for value addition and nonfarm employment.

2.4 By 2030, ensure sustainable food production systems and implement resilient agricultural practices that increase productivity and production, that help maintain ecosystems, that strengthen capacity for adaptation to climate change, extreme weather, drought, flooding, and other disasters, and that progressively improve land and soil quality.

2.5 By 2020, maintain the genetic diversity of seeds, cultivated plants, and farmed and domesticated animals and their related wild species, including through soundly managed and diversified seed and plant banks at the national, regional, and international levels, and promote access to and fair and equitable sharing of benefits arising from the utilization of genetic resources and associated traditional knowledge, as internationally agreed.

2.a Increase investment, including through enhanced international cooperation, in rural infrastructure, agricultural research and extension services, technology development, and plant and livestock gene banks in order to enhance agricultural productive capacity in developing countries, in particular least developed countries.

2.b Correct and prevent trade restrictions and distortions in world agricultural markets, including through the parallel elimination of all forms of agricultural export subsidies and all export measures with equivalent effect, in accordance with the mandate of the Doha Development Round.

2.c Adopt measures to ensure the proper functioning of food commodity markets and their derivatives and facilitate timely access to market information, including on food reserves, in order to help limit extreme food price volatility.

Goal 3. Ensure Healthy Lives and Promote Well-Being for All at All Ages

3.1 By 2030, reduce the global maternal mortality ratio to less than 70 per 100,000 live births.

3.2 By 2030, end preventable deaths of newborns and children under 5 years of age, with all countries aiming to reduce neonatal mortality to at least as low as 12 per 1,000 live births and under-5 mortality to at least as low as 25 per 1,000 live births.

3.3 By 2030, end the epidemics of AIDS, tuberculosis, malaria, and neglected tropical diseases and combat hepatitis, water-borne diseases, and other communicable diseases.

3.4 By 2030, reduce by one-third premature mortality from noncommunicable diseases through prevention and treatment, and promote mental health and well-being.

3.5 Strengthen the prevention and treatment of substance abuse, including narcotic drug abuse and harmful use of alcohol.

3.6 By 2020, halve the number of global deaths and injuries from road traffic accidents.

3.7 By 2030, ensure universal access to sexual and reproductive health care services, including for family planning, information and education, and the integration of reproductive health into national strategies and programs.

3.8 Achieve universal health coverage, including financial risk protection, access to quality essential health care services, and access to safe, effective, quality, and affordable essential medicines and vaccines for all.

3.9 By 2030, substantially reduce the number of deaths and illnesses from hazardous chemicals and air, water, and soil pollution and contamination.

3.a Strengthen the implementation of the World Health Organization Framework Convention on Tobacco Control in all countries, as appropriate.

3.b Support the research and development of vaccines and medicines for the communicable and noncommunicable diseases that primarily affect developing countries, provide access to affordable essential medicines and vaccines, in accordance with the Doha Declaration on the TRIPS Agreement and Public Health, which affirms the right of developing countries to use to the full the provisions in the Agreement on Trade-Related Aspects of Intellectual Property Rights regarding flexibilities to protect public health, and, in particular, provide access to medicines for all.

3.c Substantially increase health financing and the recruitment, development, training, and retention of the health workforce in developing countries, especially in least developed countries and small island developing States.

3.d Strengthen the capacity of all countries, in particular developing countries, for early warning, risk reduction, and management of national and global health risks.

Goal 4. Ensure Inclusive and Equitable Quality Education and Promote Lifelong Learning Opportunities for All

4.1 By 2030, ensure that all girls and boys complete free, equitable, and quality primary and secondary education leading to relevant and effective learning outcomes.

4.2 By 2030, ensure that all girls and boys have access to quality early childhood development, care, and preprimary education so that they are ready for primary education.

4.3 By 2030, ensure equal access for all women and men to affordable and quality technical, vocational, and tertiary education, including university.

4.4 By 2030, substantially increase the number of youth and adults who have relevant skills, including technical and vocational skills, for employment, decent jobs, and entrepreneurship.

4.5 By 2030, eliminate gender disparities in education and ensure equal access to all levels of education and vocational training for the vulnerable, including persons with disabilities, indigenous peoples, and children in vulnerable situations.

4.6 By 2030, ensure that all youth and a substantial proportion of adults, both men and women, achieve literacy and numeracy.

4.7 By 2030, ensure that all learners acquire the knowledge and skills needed to promote sustainable development, including, among others, through education for sustainable development and sustainable lifestyles, human rights, gender equality, promotion of a culture of peace and nonviolence, global citizenship, and appreciation of cultural diversity and of culture's contribution to sustainable development.

4.a Build and upgrade education facilities that are child, disability, and gender sensitive and provide safe, nonviolent, inclusive, and effective learning environments for all.

4.b By 2020, substantially expand globally the number of scholarships available to developing countries, in particular least developed countries, small island developing States, and African countries, for enrolment in higher education, including vocational training and information and communications technology, technical, engineering, and scientific programs, in developed countries and other developing countries.

4.c By 2030, substantially increase the supply of qualified teachers, including through international cooperation, for teacher training in developing countries, especially least developed countries and small island developing States.

Goal 5. Achieve Gender Equality and Empower All Women and Girls

5.1 End all forms of discrimination against all women and girls everywhere.

5.2 Eliminate all forms of violence against all women and girls in the public and private spheres, including trafficking and sexual and other types of exploitation.

5.3 Eliminate all harmful practices, such as child, early and forced marriage, and female genital mutilation.

5.4 Recognize and value unpaid care and domestic work through the provision of public services, infrastructure, and social protection policies and the promotion of shared responsibility within the household and the family as nationally appropriate.

5.5 Ensure women's full and effective participation and equal opportunities for leadership at all levels of decision making in political, economic, and public life.

5.6 Ensure universal access to sexual and reproductive health and reproductive rights as agreed in accordance with the Programme of Action of the International Conference on Population and Development and the Beijing Platform for Action and the outcome documents of their review conferences.

5.a Undertake reforms to give women equal rights to economic resources, as well as access to ownership and control over land and other forms of property, financial services, inheritance, and natural resources, in accordance with national laws.

5.b Enhance the use of enabling technology, in particular information and communications technology, to promote the empowerment of women.

5.c Adopt and strengthen sound policies and enforceable legislation for the promotion of gender equality and the empowerment of all women and girls at all levels.

Goal 6. Ensure Availability and Sustainable Management of Water and Sanitation for All

6.1 By 2030, achieve universal and equitable access to safe and affordable drinking water for all.

6.2 By 2030, achieve access to adequate and equitable sanitation and hygiene for all and end open defecation, paying special attention to the needs of women and girls and those in vulnerable situations.

6.3 By 2030, improve water quality by reducing pollution, eliminating dumping, and minimizing release of hazardous chemicals and materials, halving the proportion of untreated wastewater, and substantially increasing recycling and safe reuse globally.

6.4 By 2030, substantially increase water-use efficiency across all sectors and ensure sustainable withdrawals and supply of freshwater to address water scarcity and substantially reduce the number of people suffering from water scarcity.

6.5 By 2030, implement integrated water resources management at all levels, including through transboundary cooperation as appropriate.

6.6 By 2020, protect and restore water-related ecosystems, including mountains, forests, wetlands, rivers, aquifers, and lakes.

6.a By 2030, expand international cooperation and capacity-building support to developing countries in water- and sanitation-related activities and programs, including water harvesting, desalination, water efficiency, wastewater treatment, recycling, and reuse technologies.

6.b Support and strengthen the participation of local communities in improving water and sanitation management.

Goal 7. Ensure Access to Affordable, Reliable, Sustainable, and Modern Energy for All

7.1 By 2030, ensure universal access to affordable, reliable, and modern energy services.

7.2 By 2030, increase substantially the share of renewable energy in the global energy mix.

7.3 By 2030, double the global rate of improvement in energy efficiency.

7.a By 2030, enhance international cooperation to facilitate access to clean energy research and technology, including renewable energy, energy efficiency and advanced and cleaner fossil-fuel technology, and promote investment in energy infrastructure and clean energy technology.

7.b By 2030, expand infrastructure and upgrade technology for supplying modern and sustainable energy services for all in developing countries, in particular least developed countries, small island developing States, and landlocked developing countries, in accordance with their respective programs of support.

Goal 8. Promote Sustained, Inclusive, and Sustainable Economic Growth, Full and Productive Employment, and Decent Work for All

8.1 Sustain per capita economic growth in accordance with national circumstances and, in particular, at least 7% gross domestic product growth per annum in the least developed countries.

8.2 Achieve higher levels of economic productivity through diversification, technological upgrading, and innovation, including through a focus on high-value added and labor-intensive sectors.

8.3 Promote development-oriented policies that support productive activities, decent job creation, entrepreneurship, creativity and innovation, and encourage the formalization and growth of micro-, small- and medium-sized enterprises, including through access to financial services.

8.4 Improve progressively, through 2030, global resource efficiency in consumption and production and endeavor to decouple economic growth from environmental degradation, in accordance with the 10-Year Framework of Programmes on Sustainable Consumption and Production, with developed countries taking the lead.

8.5 By 2030, achieve full and productive employment and decent work for all women and men, including for young people and persons with disabilities, and equal pay for work of equal value.

8.6 By 2020, substantially reduce the proportion of youth not in employment, education, or training.

8.7 Take immediate and effective measures to eradicate forced labor, end modern slavery and human trafficking, and secure the prohibition and elimination of the worst forms of child labor, including recruitment and use of child soldiers, and by 2025 end child labor in all its forms.

8.8 Protect labor rights and promote safe and secure working environments for all workers, including migrant workers, in particular women migrants, and those in precarious employment.

8.9 By 2030, devise and implement policies to promote sustainable tourism that creates jobs and promotes local culture and products.

8.10 Strengthen the capacity of domestic financial institutions to encourage and expand access to banking, insurance, and financial services for all.

8.a Increase Aid for Trade support for developing countries, in particular least developed countries, including through the Enhanced Integrated Framework for Trade-Related Technical Assistance to Least Developed Countries.

8.b By 2020, develop and operationalize a global strategy for youth employment and implement the Global Jobs Pact of the International Labour Organization.

Goal 9. Build Resilient Infrastructure, Promote Inclusive and Sustainable Industrialization, and Foster Innovation

9.1 Develop quality, reliable, sustainable, and resilient infrastructure, including regional and transborder infrastructure, to support economic development and human well-being, with a focus on affordable and equitable access for all.

9.2 Promote inclusive and sustainable industrialization and, by 2030, significantly raise industry's share of employment and gross domestic product, in line with national circumstances, and double its share in least developed countries.

9.3 Increase the access of small-scale industrial and other enterprises, in particular in developing countries, to financial services, including affordable credit, and their integration into value chains and markets.

9.4 By 2030, upgrade infrastructure and retrofit industries to make them sustainable, with increased resource-use efficiency and greater adoption of clean and environmentally sound technologies and industrial processes, with all countries taking action in accordance with their respective capabilities.

9.5 Enhance scientific research, upgrade the technological capabilities of industrial sectors in all countries, in particular developing countries, including, by 2030, encouraging innovation and substantially increasing the number of research and development workers per one million people, and public and private research and development spending.

9.a Facilitate sustainable and resilient infrastructure development in developing countries through enhanced financial, technological, and technical support to African countries, least developed countries, landlocked developing countries, and small island developing States.

9.b Support domestic technology development, research, and innovation in developing countries, including by ensuring a conducive policy environment for, inter alia, industrial diversification and value addition to commodities.

9.c Significantly increase access to information and communications technology and strive to provide universal and affordable access to the Internet in least developed countries by 2020.

Goal 10. Reduce Inequality Within and Among Countries

10.1 By 2030, progressively achieve and sustain income growth of the bottom 40% of the population at a rate higher than the national average.

10.2 By 2030, empower and promote the social, economic, and political inclusion of all, irrespective of age, sex, disability, race, ethnicity, origin, religion, or economic or other status.

10.3 Ensure equal opportunity and reduce inequalities of outcome, including by eliminating discriminatory laws, policies, and practices and promoting appropriate legislation, policies, and action in this regard.

10.4 Adopt policies, especially fiscal, wage, and social protection policies, and progressively achieve greater equality.

10.5 Improve the regulation and monitoring of global financial markets and institutions and strengthen the implementation of such regulations.

10.6 Ensure enhanced representation and voice for developing countries in decision making in global international economic and financial institutions in order to deliver more effective, credible, accountable, and legitimate institutions.

10.7 Facilitate orderly, safe, regular, and responsible migration and mobility of people, including through the implementation of planned and well-managed migration policies.

10.a Implement the principle of special and differential treatment for developing countries, in particular least developed countries, in accordance with World Trade Organization agreements.

10.b Encourage ODA and financial flows, including foreign direct investment, to States where the need is greatest, in particular least developed countries, African countries, small island developing States, and landlocked developing countries, in accordance with their national plans and programs.

10.c By 2030, reduce to less than 3% the transaction costs of migrant remittances and eliminate remittance corridors with costs higher than 5%.

Goal 11. Make Cities and Human Settlements Inclusive, Safe, Resilient, and Sustainable

11.1 By 2030, ensure access for all to adequate, safe, and affordable housing and basic services, and upgrade slums.

11.2 By 2030, provide access to safe, affordable, accessible, and sustainable transport systems for all, improving road safety, notably by expanding public transport, with special attention to the needs of those in vulnerable situations, women, children, persons with disabilities, and older persons.

11.3 By 2030, enhance inclusive and sustainable urbanization and capacity for participatory, integrated, and sustainable human settlement planning and management in all countries.

11.4 Strengthen efforts to protect and safeguard the world's cultural and natural heritage.

11.5 By 2030, significantly reduce the number of deaths and the number of people affected and substantially decrease the direct economic losses relative to global gross domestic product caused by disasters, including water-related disasters, with a focus on protecting the poor and people in vulnerable situations.

11.6 By 2030, reduce the adverse per capita environmental impact of cities, including by paying special attention to air quality and municipal and other waste management.

11.7 By 2030, provide universal access to safe, inclusive and accessible, green, and public spaces, in particular for women and children, older persons, and persons with disabilities.

11.a Support positive economic, social, and environmental links between urban, peri-urban, and rural areas by strengthening national and regional development planning.

11.b By 2020, substantially increase the number of cities and human settlements adopting and implementing integrated policies and plans toward inclusion, resource efficiency, mitigation and adaptation to climate change, resilience to disasters, and develop and implement, in line with the Sendai Framework for Disaster Risk Reduction 2015–2030, holistic disaster risk management at all levels.

11.c Support least developed countries, including through financial and technical assistance, in building sustainable and resilient buildings utilizing local materials.

Goal 12. Ensure Sustainable Consumption and Production Patterns

12.1 Implement the 10-Year Framework of Programmes on Sustainable Consumption and Production Patterns, all countries taking action, with developed countries taking the lead, taking into account the development and capabilities of developing countries.

12.2 By 2030, achieve the sustainable management and efficient use of natural resources.

12.3 By 2030, halve per capita global food waste at the retail and consumer levels and reduce food losses along production and supply chains, including postharvest losses.

12.4 By 2020, achieve the environmentally sound management of chemicals and all wastes throughout their life cycle, in accordance with agreed international frameworks, and significantly reduce their release to air, water, and soil in order to minimize their adverse impacts on human health and the environment.

12.5 By 2030, substantially reduce waste generation through prevention, reduction, recycling, and reuse.

12.6 Encourage companies, especially large and transnational companies, to adopt sustainable practices and to integrate sustainability information into their reporting cycle.

12.7 Promote public procurement practices that are sustainable, in accordance with national policies and priorities.

12.8 By 2030, ensure that people everywhere have the relevant information and awareness for sustainable development and lifestyles in harmony with nature.

12.a Support developing countries to strengthen their scientific and technological capacity to move toward more sustainable patterns of consumption and production.

12.b Develop and implement tools to monitor sustainable development impacts for sustainable tourism that creates jobs and promotes local culture and products.

12.c Rationalize inefficient fossil-fuel subsidies that encourage wasteful consumption by removing market distortions, in accordance with national circumstances, including by restructuring taxation and phasing out those harmful subsidies, where they exist, to reflect their environmental impacts, taking fully into account the specific needs and conditions of developing countries and minimizing the possible adverse impacts on their development in a manner that protects the poor and the affected communities.

Goal 13. Take Urgent Action to Combat Climate Change and Its Impacts*

13.1 Strengthen resilience and adaptive capacity to climate-related hazards and natural disasters in all countries.

---

*Acknowledging that the United Nations Framework Convention on Climate Change is the primary international, intergovernmental forum for negotiating the global response to climate change.

13.2 Integrate climate change measures into national policies, strategies, and planning.

13.3 Improve education, awareness-raising, and human and institutional capacity on climate change mitigation, adaptation, impact reduction, and early warning.

13.a Implement the commitment undertaken by developed-country parties to the United Nations Framework Convention on Climate Change to a goal of mobilizing jointly $100 billion annually by 2020 from all sources to address the needs of developing countries in the context of meaningful mitigation actions and transparency on implementation and fully operationalize the Green Climate Fund through its capitalization as soon as possible.

13.b Promote mechanisms for raising capacity for effective climate change-related planning and management in least developed countries and small island developing States, including focusing on women, youth, and local and marginalized communities.

Goal 14. Conserve and Sustainably Use the Oceans, Seas, and Marine Resources for Sustainable Development

14.1 By 2025, prevent and significantly reduce marine pollution of all kinds, in particular from land-based activities, including marine debris and nutrient pollution.

14.2 By 2020, sustainably manage and protect marine and coastal ecosystems to avoid significant adverse impacts, including by strengthening their resilience, and take action for their restoration in order to achieve healthy and productive oceans.

14.3 Minimize and address the impacts of ocean acidification, including through enhanced scientific cooperation at all levels.

14.4 By 2020, effectively regulate harvesting and end overfishing, illegal, unreported, and unregulated fishing and destructive fishing practices, and implement science-based management plans, in order to restore fish stocks in the shortest time feasible, at least to levels that can produce maximum sustainable yield as determined by their biological characteristics.

14.5 By 2020, conserve at least 10% of coastal and marine areas, consistent with national and international law and based on the best available scientific information.

14.6 By 2020, prohibit certain forms of fisheries subsidies which contribute to overcapacity and overfishing, eliminate subsidies that contribute to illegal, unreported, and unregulated fishing and refrain from introducing new such subsidies, recognizing that appropriate and effective special and differential treatment for developing and least developed countries should be an integral part of the World Trade Organization fisheries subsidies negotiation.[3]

14.7 By 2030, increase the economic benefits to small island developing States and least developed countries from the sustainable use of marine resources, including through sustainable management of fisheries, aquaculture, and tourism.

14.a Increase scientific knowledge, develop research capacity, and transfer marine technology, taking into account the Intergovernmental Oceanographic Commission Criteria and Guidelines on the Transfer of Marine Technology, in order to improve ocean health and to enhance the contribution of marine biodiversity to the development of developing countries, in particular small island developing States and least developed countries.

14.b Provide access for small-scale artisanal fishers to marine resources and markets.

14.c Enhance the conservation and sustainable use of oceans and their resources by implementing international law as reflected in the United Nations Convention on the Law of the Sea, which provides the legal framework for the conservation and sustainable use of oceans and their resources, as recalled in paragraph 158 of "The future we want."

Goal 15. Protect, Restore, and Promote Sustainable Use of Terrestrial Ecosystems, Sustainably Manage Forests, Combat Desertification, and Halt and Reverse Land Degradation and Halt Biodiversity Loss

15.1 By 2020, ensure the conservation, restoration, and sustainable use of terrestrial and inland freshwater ecosystems and their services, in particular forests, wetlands, mountains, and drylands, in line with obligations under international agreements.

15.2 By 2020, promote the implementation of sustainable management of all types of forests, halt deforestation, restore degraded forests, and substantially increase afforestation and reforestation globally.

15.3 By 2030, combat desertification, restore degraded land and soil, including land affected by desertification, drought and floods, and strive to achieve a land degradation-neutral world.

15.4 By 2030, ensure the conservation of mountain ecosystems, including their biodiversity, in order to enhance their capacity to provide benefits that are essential for sustainable development.

15.5 Take urgent and significant action to reduce the degradation of natural habitats, halt the loss of biodiversity and, by 2020, protect and prevent the extinction of threatened species.

---

[3] Taking into account ongoing World Trade Organization negotiations, the Doha Development Agenda, and the Hong Kong ministerial mandate.

15.6 Promote fair and equitable sharing of the benefits arising from the utilization of genetic resources and promote appropriate access to such resources, as internationally agreed.

15.7 Take urgent action to end poaching and trafficking of protected species of flora and fauna and address both demand and supply of illegal wildlife products.

15.8 By 2020, introduce measures to prevent the introduction and significantly reduce the impact of invasive alien species on land and water ecosystems and control or eradicate the priority species.

15.9 By 2020, integrate ecosystem and biodiversity values into national and local planning, development processes, poverty reduction strategies, and accounts.

15.a Mobilize and significantly increase financial resources from all sources to conserve and sustainably use biodiversity and ecosystems.

15.b Mobilize significant resources from all sources and at all levels to finance sustainable forest management and provide adequate incentives to developing countries to advance such management, including for conservation and reforestation.

15.c Enhance global support for efforts to combat poaching and trafficking of protected species, including by increasing the capacity of local communities to pursue sustainable livelihood opportunities.

Goal 16. Promote Peaceful and Inclusive Societies for Sustainable Development, Provide Access to Justice for All and Build Effective, Accountable, and Inclusive Institutions at All Levels

16.1 Significantly reduce all forms of violence and related death rates everywhere.

16.2 End abuse, exploitation, trafficking, and all forms of violence against and torture of children.

16.3 Promote the rule of law at the national and international levels and ensure equal access to justice for all.

16.4 By 2030, significantly reduce illicit financial and arms flows, strengthen the recovery and return of stolen assets, and combat all forms of organized crime.

16.5 Substantially reduce corruption and bribery in all their forms.

16.6 Develop effective, accountable, and transparent institutions at all levels.

16.7 Ensure responsive, inclusive, participatory, and representative decision making at all levels.

16.8 Broaden and strengthen the participation of developing countries in the institutions of global governance.

16.9 By 2030, provide legal identity for all, including birth registration.

16.10 Ensure public access to information and protect fundamental freedoms, in accordance with national legislation and international agreements.

16.a Strengthen relevant national institutions, including through international cooperation, for building capacity at all levels, in particular in developing countries, to prevent violence and combat terrorism and crime.

16.b Promote and enforce nondiscriminatory laws and policies for sustainable development.

Goal 17. Strengthen the Means of Implementation and Revitalize the Global Partnership for Sustainable Development

Finance

17.1 Strengthen domestic resource mobilization, including through international support to developing countries, to improve domestic capacity for tax and other revenue collection.

17.2 Developed countries to implement fully their ODA commitments, including the commitment by many developed countries to achieve the target of 0.7% of ODA/GNI to developing countries and 0.15% to 0.20% of ODA/GNI to least developed countries; ODA providers are encouraged to consider setting a target to provide at least 0.20% of ODA/GNI to least developed countries.

17.3 Mobilize additional financial resources for developing countries from multiple sources.

17.4 Assist developing countries in attaining long-term debt sustainability through coordinated policies aimed at fostering debt financing, debt relief, and debt restructuring, as appropriate, and address the external debt of highly indebted poor countries to reduce debt distress.

17.5 Adopt and implement investment promotion regimes for least developed countries.

Technology

17.6 Enhance North–South, South–South, and triangular regional and international cooperation on and access to science, technology, and innovation and enhance knowledge sharing on mutually agreed terms, including through improved coordination among existing mechanisms, in particular at the United Nations level, and through a global technology facilitation mechanism.

17.7 Promote the development, transfer, dissemination, and diffusion of environmentally sound technologies to developing countries on favorable terms, including on concessional and preferential terms, as mutually agreed.

17.8 Fully operationalize the technology bank and science, technology, and innovation capacity-building mechanism for least developed countries by 2017 and enhance the use of enabling technology, in particular information and communications technology.

Capacity Building

17.9 Enhance international support for implementing effective and targeted capacity building in developing countries to support national plans to implement all the Sustainable Development Goals, including through North–South, South–South, and triangular cooperation.

Trade

17.10 Promote a universal, rules-based, open, nondiscriminatory, and equitable multilateral trading system under the World Trade Organization, including through the conclusion of negotiations under its Doha Development Agenda.

17.11 Significantly increase the exports of developing countries, in particular with a view to doubling the least developed countries' share of global exports by 2020.

17.12 Realize timely implementation of duty-free and quota-free market access on a lasting basis for all least developed countries, consistent with World Trade Organization decisions, including by ensuring that preferential rules of origin applicable to imports from least developed countries are transparent and simple, and contribute to facilitating market access.

Systemic Issues

Policy and Institutional Coherence

17.13 Enhance global macroeconomic stability, including through policy coordination and policy coherence.

17.14 Enhance policy coherence for sustainable development.

17.15 Respect each country's policy space and leadership to establish and implement policies for poverty eradication and sustainable development.

Multi-Stakeholder Partnerships

17.16 Enhance the Global Partnership for Sustainable Development, complemented by multi-stakeholder partnerships that mobilize and share knowledge, expertise, technology, and financial resources, to support the achievement of the Sustainable Development Goals in all countries, in particular developing countries.

17.17 Encourage and promote effective public, public–private, and civil society partnerships, building on the experience and resourcing strategies of partnerships.

Data, Monitoring and Accountability

17.18 By 2020, enhance capacity-building support to developing countries, including for least developed countries and small island developing States, to increase significantly the availability of high-quality, timely, and reliable data disaggregated by income, gender, age, race, ethnicity, migratory status, disability, geographic location, and other characteristics relevant in national contexts.

17.19 By 2030, build on existing initiatives to develop measurements of progress on sustainable development that complement gross domestic product, and support statistical capacity building in developing countries.

MEANS OF IMPLEMENTATION AND THE GLOBAL PARTNERSHIP

60. We reaffirm our strong commitment to the full implementation of this new Agenda. We recognize that we will not be able to achieve our ambitious Goals and targets without a revitalized and enhanced Global Partnership and comparably ambitious means of implementation. The revitalized Global Partnership will facilitate an intensive global engagement in support of implementation of all the Goals and targets, bringing together Governments, civil society, the private sector, the United Nations system, and other actors and mobilizing all available resources.

61. The Agenda's Goals and targets deal with the means required to realize our collective ambitions. The means of implementation targets under each Sustainable Development Goal and Goal 17, which are referred to earlier, are key to realizing our Agenda and are of equal importance with the other Goals and targets. We shall accord them equal priority in our implementation efforts and in the global indicator framework for monitoring our progress.

62. This Agenda, including the Sustainable Development Goals, can be met within the framework of a revitalized Global Partnership for Sustainable Development, supported by the concrete policies and actions outlined in the Addis Ababa Action Agenda,[4] which is an integral part of the 2030 Agenda for Sustainable Development. The Addis Ababa Action Agenda supports, complements, and helps to contextualize the 2030 Agenda's means of implementation targets. It relates to domestic public resources, domestic and international private business and finance, international development cooperation, international trade as an engine for development, debt and debt sustainability, addressing systemic issues and science, technology, innovation and capacity building, and data, monitoring and follow-up.

63. Cohesive nationally owned sustainable development strategies, supported by integrated national financing frameworks, will be at the heart of our efforts. We reiterate that each country has primary

[4] The Addis Ababa Action Agenda of the Third International Conference on Financing for Development (Addis Ababa Action Agenda), adopted by the General Assembly on July 27, 2015 (resolution 69/313).

responsibility for its own economic and social development and that the role of national policies and development strategies cannot be overemphasized. We will respect each country's policy space and leadership to implement policies for poverty eradication and sustainable development, while remaining consistent with relevant international rules and commitments. At the same time, national development efforts need to be supported by an enabling international economic environment, including coherent and mutually supporting world trade, monetary and financial systems, and strengthened and enhanced global economic governance. Processes to develop and facilitate the availability of appropriate knowledge and technologies globally, as well as capacity building, are also critical. We commit to pursuing policy coherence and an enabling environment for sustainable development at all levels and by all actors, and to reinvigorating the Global Partnership for Sustainable Development.

64. We support the implementation of relevant strategies and programs of action, including the Istanbul Declaration and Programme of Action, the SAMOA Pathway, and the Vienna Programme of Action for Landlocked Developing Countries for the Decade 2014–2024, and reaffirm the importance of supporting the African Union's Agenda 2063 and the program of the New Partnership for Africa's Development, all of which are integral to the new Agenda. We recognize the major challenge to the achievement of durable peace and sustainable development in countries in conflict and postconflict situations.

65. We recognize that middle-income countries still face significant challenges to achieve sustainable development. In order to ensure that achievements made to date are sustained, efforts to address ongoing challenges should be strengthened through the exchange of experiences, improved coordination, and better and focused support of the United Nations development system, the international financial institutions, regional organizations, and other stakeholders.

66. We underscore that, for all countries, public policies and the mobilization and effective use of domestic resources, underscored by the principle of national ownership, are central to our common pursuit of sustainable development, including achieving the Sustainable Development Goals. We recognize that domestic resources are first and foremost generated by economic growth, supported by an enabling environment at all levels.

67. Private business activity, investment, and innovation are major drivers of productivity, inclusive economic growth, and job creation. We acknowledge the diversity of the private sector, ranging from microenterprises to cooperatives to multinationals. We call upon all businesses to apply their creativity and innovation to solving sustainable development challenges. We will foster a dynamic and well-functioning business sector, while protecting labor rights and environmental and health standards in accordance with relevant international standards and agreements and other ongoing initiatives in this regard, such as the Guiding Principles on Business and Human Rights and the labor

standards of the International Labour Organization, the Convention on the Rights of the Child, and key multilateral environmental agreements, for parties to those agreements.

68. International trade is an engine for inclusive economic growth and poverty reduction, and contributes to the promotion of sustainable development. We will continue to promote a universal, rules-based, open, transparent, predictable, inclusive, nondiscriminatory, and equitable multilateral trading system under the World Trade Organization, as well as meaningful trade liberalization. We call upon all members of the World Trade Organization to redouble their efforts to promptly conclude the negotiations on the Doha Development Agenda. We attach great importance to providing trade-related capacity building for developing countries, including African countries, least developed countries, landlocked developing countries, small island developing States, and middle-income countries, including for the promotion of regional economic integration and interconnectivity.

69. We recognize the need to assist developing countries in attaining long-term debt sustainability through coordinated policies aimed at fostering debt financing, debt relief, debt restructuring, and sound debt management, as appropriate. Many countries remain vulnerable to debt crises and some are in the midst of crises, including a number of least developed countries, small island developing States, and some developed countries. We reiterate that debtors and creditors must work together to prevent and resolve unsustainable debt situations. Maintaining sustainable debt levels is the responsibility of the borrowing countries; however, we acknowledge that lenders also have a responsibility to lend in a way that does not undermine a country's debt sustainability. We will support the maintenance of debt sustainability of those countries that have received debt relief and achieved sustainable debt levels.

70. We hereby launch a Technology Facilitation Mechanism, which was established by the Addis Ababa Action Agenda in order to support the Sustainable Development Goals. The Technology Facilitation Mechanism will be based on a multi-stakeholder collaboration between Member States, civil society, the private sector, the scientific community, United Nations entities, and other stakeholders and will be composed of a United Nations interagency task team on science, technology, and innovation for the Sustainable Development Goals, a collaborative multi-stakeholder forum on science, technology, and innovation for the Sustainable Development Goals and an online platform.

  • The United Nations interagency task team on science, technology, and innovation for the Sustainable Development Goals will promote coordination, coherence, and cooperation within the United Nations system on science, technology, and innovation-related matters, enhancing synergy and efficiency, in particular to enhance capacity-building initiatives. The task team will draw on existing resources and will work with 10 representatives from civil society, the private sector, and the scientific community to prepare the meetings of the multi-stakeholder forum on science, technology, and innovation for the Sustainable Development Goals, as well as in the development and operationalization of the online platform, including preparing proposals for the modalities for the forum and the online platform. The 10 representatives will be appointed by the Secretary-General, for periods of 2 years. The task team will be open to the participation of all United Nations agencies, funds, and programs and the functional commissions of the Economic and Social Council and it will initially be composed of the entities that currently integrate the informal working group on technology facilitation, namely, the Department of Economic and Social Affairs of the Secretariat, the United Nations Environment Programme, the United Nations Industrial Development Organization, the United Nations Educational, Scientific and Cultural Organization, the United Nations Conference on Trade and Development, the International Telecommunication Union, the World Intellectual Property Organization, and the World Bank.

- The online platform will be used to establish a comprehensive mapping of, and serve as a gateway for, information on existing science, technology, and innovation initiatives, mechanisms, and programs, within and beyond the United Nations. The online platform will facilitate access to information, knowledge, and experience, as well as best practices and lessons learned, on science, technology, and innovation facilitation initiatives and policies. The online platform will also facilitate the dissemination of relevant open access scientific publications generated worldwide. The online platform will be developed on the basis of an independent technical assessment, which will take into account best practices and lessons learned from other initiatives, within and beyond the United Nations, in order to ensure that it will complement, facilitate access to, and provide adequate information on existing science, technology, and innovation platforms, avoiding duplications and enhancing synergies.

- The multi-stakeholder forum on science, technology, and innovation for the Sustainable Development Goals will be convened once a year, for a period of 2 days, to discuss science, technology, and innovation cooperation around thematic areas for the implementation of the Sustainable Development Goals, congregating all relevant stakeholders to actively contribute in their area of expertise. The forum will provide a venue for facilitating interaction, matchmaking, and the establishment of networks between relevant stakeholders and multi-stakeholder partnerships in order to identify and examine technology needs and gaps, including on scientific cooperation, innovation, and capacity building, and also in order to help to facilitate development, transfer, and dissemination of relevant technologies for the Sustainable Development Goals. The meetings of the forum will be convened by the President of the Economic and Social Council before the meeting of the high-level political forum under the auspices of the Council or, alternatively, in conjunction with other forums or conferences, as appropriate, taking into account the theme to be considered and on the basis of a collaboration with the organizers of the other forums or conferences. The meetings of the forum will be cochaired by two Member States and will result in a summary of discussions elaborated by the two co-Chairs, as an input to the meetings of the high-level political forum, in the context of the follow-up and review of the implementation of the post-2015 development agenda.

- The meetings of the high-level political forum will be informed by the summary of the multi-stakeholder forum. The themes for the subsequent multi-stakeholder forum on science, technology, and innovation for the Sustainable Development Goals will be considered by the high-level political forum on sustainable development, taking into account expert inputs from the task team.

71. We reiterate that this Agenda and the Sustainable Development Goals and targets, including the means of implementation, are universal, indivisible, and interlinked.

FOLLOW-UP AND REVIEW

72. We commit to engaging in systematic follow-up and review of the implementation of this Agenda over the next 15 years. A robust, voluntary, effective, participatory, transparent, and integrated follow-up and review framework will make a vital contribution to implementation and will help countries to maximize and track progress in implementing this Agenda in order to ensure that no one is left behind.

73. Operating at the national, regional, and global levels, it will promote accountability to our citizens, support effective international cooperation in achieving this Agenda, and foster exchanges of best practices and mutual learning. It will mobilize support to overcome shared challenges and identify new and emerging issues. As this is a universal Agenda, mutual trust and understanding among all nations will be important.

74. Follow-up and review processes at all levels will be guided by the following principles:

   a. They will be voluntary and country-led, will take into account different national realities, capacities, and levels of development and will respect policy space and priorities. As national ownership is key to achieving sustainable development, the outcome from national-level processes will be the foundation for reviews at the regional and global levels, given that the global review will be primarily based on national official data sources.

   b. They will track progress in implementing the universal Goals and targets, including the means of implementation, in all countries in a manner which respects their universal, integrated, and interrelated nature and the three dimensions of sustainable development.

c. They will maintain a longer term orientation, identify achievements, challenges, gaps, and critical success factors and support countries in making informed policy choices. They will help to mobilize the necessary means of implementation and partnerships, support the identification of solutions and best practices, and promote the coordination and effectiveness of the international development system.

d. They will be open, inclusive, participatory, and transparent for all people and will support reporting by all relevant stakeholders.

e. They will be people-centered, gender-sensitive, respect human rights, and have a particular focus on the poorest, most vulnerable, and those furthest behind.

f. They will build on existing platforms and processes, where these exist, avoid duplication, and respond to national circumstances, capacities, needs, and priorities. They will evolve over time, taking into account emerging issues and the development of new methodologies, and will minimize the reporting burden on national administrations.

g. They will be rigorous and based on evidence, informed by country-led evaluations and data which is high quality, accessible, timely, reliable, and disaggregated by income, sex, age, race, ethnicity, migration status, disability, and geographic location, and other characteristics relevant in national contexts.

h. They will require enhanced capacity-building support for developing countries, including the strengthening of national data systems and evaluation programs, particularly in African countries, least developed countries, small island developing States, landlocked developing countries, and middle-income countries.

i. They will benefit from the active support of the United Nations system and other multilateral institutions.

75. The Goals and targets will be followed up and reviewed using a set of global indicators. These will be complemented by indicators at the regional and national levels, which will be developed by Member States, in addition to the outcomes of work undertaken for the development of the baselines for those targets where national and global baseline data does not yet exist. The global indicator framework, to be developed by the Inter-Agency and Expert Group on Sustainable Development Goal Indicators, will be agreed by the Statistical Commission by March 2016 and adopted thereafter by the Economic and Social Council and the General Assembly, in line with existing mandates. This framework will be simple yet robust, address all Sustainable Development Goals and targets, including for means of implementation, and preserve the political balance, integration, and ambition contained therein.

76. We will support developing countries, particularly African countries, least developed countries, small island developing States, and landlocked developing countries, in strengthening the capacity of national statistical

offices and data systems to ensure access to high-quality, timely, reliable, and disaggregated data. We will promote transparent and accountable scaling up of appropriate public–private cooperation to exploit the contribution to be made by a wide range of data, including earth observation and geospatial information, while ensuring national ownership in supporting and tracking progress.

77. We commit to fully engage in conducting regular and inclusive reviews of progress at the subnational, national, regional, and global levels. We will draw as far as possible on the existing network of follow-up and review institutions and mechanisms. National reports will allow assessments of progress and identify challenges at the regional and global level. Along with regional dialogues and global reviews, they will inform recommendations for follow-up at various levels.

National Level

78. We encourage all Member States to develop as soon as practicable ambitious national responses to the overall implementation of this Agenda. These can support the transition to the Sustainable Development Goals and build on existing planning instruments, such as national development and sustainable development strategies, as appropriate.

79. We also encourage Member States to conduct regular and inclusive reviews of progress at the national and subnational levels, which are country-led and country-driven. Such reviews should draw on contributions from indigenous peoples, civil society, the private sector, and other stakeholders, in line with national circumstances, policies, and priorities. National parliaments as well as other institutions can also support these processes.

Regional Level

80. Follow-up and review at the regional and subregional levels can, as appropriate, provide useful opportunities for peer learning, including through voluntary reviews, sharing of best practices, and discussion on shared targets. We welcome in this respect the cooperation of regional and subregional commissions and organizations. Inclusive regional processes will draw on national-level reviews and contribute to follow-up and review at the global level, including at the high-level political forum on sustainable development.

81. Recognizing the importance of building on existing follow-up and review mechanisms at the regional level and allowing adequate policy space, we encourage all Member States to identify the most suitable regional forum in which to engage. United Nations regional commissions are encouraged to continue supporting Member States in this regard.

Global Level

82. The high-level political forum will have a central role in overseeing a network of follow-up and review processes at the global level, working

coherently with the General Assembly, the Economic and Social Council, and other relevant organs and forums, in accordance with existing mandates. It will facilitate sharing of experiences, including successes, challenges, and lessons learned, and provide political leadership, guidance, and recommendations for follow-up. It will promote system-wide coherence and coordination of sustainable development policies. It should ensure that the Agenda remains relevant and ambitious and should focus on the assessment of progress, achievements, and challenges faced by developed and developing countries as well as new and emerging issues. Effective linkages will be made with the follow-up and review arrangements of all relevant United Nations conferences and processes, including on least developed countries, small island developing States, and landlocked developing countries.

83. Follow-up and review at the high-level political forum will be informed by an annual progress report on the Sustainable Development Goals to be prepared by the Secretary-General in cooperation with the United Nations system, based on the global indicator framework and data produced by national statistical systems and information collected at the regional level. The high-level political forum will also be informed by the *Global Sustainable Development Report*, which shall strengthen the science–policy interface and could provide a strong evidence-based instrument to support policy makers in promoting poverty eradication and sustainable development. We invite the president of the Economic and Social Council to conduct a process of consultations on the scope, methodology, and frequency of the global report as well as its relation to the progress report, the outcome of which should be reflected in the ministerial declaration of the session of the high-level political forum in 2016.

84. The high-level political forum, under the auspices of the Economic and Social Council, shall carry out regular reviews, in line with General Assembly resolution 67/290 of July 9, 2013. Reviews will be voluntary, while encouraging reporting, and include developed and developing countries as well as relevant United Nations entities and other stakeholders, including civil society and the private sector. They shall be State-led, involving ministerial and other relevant high-level participants. They shall provide a platform for partnerships, including through the participation of major groups and other relevant stakeholders.

85. Thematic reviews of progress on the Sustainable Development Goals, including cross-cutting issues, will also take place at the high-level political forum. These will be supported by reviews by the functional commissions of the Economic and Social Council and other intergovernmental bodies and forums, which should reflect the integrated nature of the Goals as well as the interlinkages between them. They will engage all relevant stakeholders and, where possible, feed into, and be aligned with, the cycle of the high-level political forum.

86. We welcome, as outlined in the Addis Ababa Action Agenda, the dedicated follow-up and review for the financing for development

outcomes as well as all the means of implementation of the Sustainable Development Goals, which is integrated with the follow-up and review framework of this Agenda. The intergovernmentally agreed conclusions and recommendations of the annual Economic and Social Council forum on financing for development will be fed into the overall follow-up and review of the implementation of this Agenda in the high-level political forum.

87. Meeting every 4 years under the auspices of the General Assembly, the high-level political forum will provide high-level political guidance on the Agenda and its implementation, identify progress and emerging challenges, and mobilize further actions to accelerate implementation. The next high-level political forum under the auspices of the General Assembly will be held in 2019, with the cycle of meetings thus reset, in order to maximize coherence with the quadrennial comprehensive policy review process.

88. We also stress the importance of system-wide strategic planning, implementation, and reporting in order to ensure coherent and integrated support to the implementation of the new Agenda by the United Nations development system. The relevant governing bodies should take action to review such support to implementation and to report on progress and obstacles. We welcome the ongoing dialogue in the Economic and Social Council on the longer term positioning of the United Nations development system and look forward to taking action on these issues, as appropriate.

89. The high-level political forum will support participation in follow-up and review processes by the major groups and other relevant stakeholders in line with resolution 67/290. We call upon those actors to report on their contribution to the implementation of the Agenda.

90. We request the Secretary-General, in consultation with Member States, to prepare a report, for consideration at the 70th session of the General Assembly in preparation for the 2016 meeting of the high-level political forum, which outlines critical milestones toward coherent, efficient, and inclusive follow-up and review at the global level. The report should include a proposal on the organizational arrangements for State-led reviews at the high-level political forum under the auspices of the Economic and Social Council, including recommendations on voluntary common reporting guidelines. It should clarify institutional responsibilities and provide guidance on annual themes, on a sequence of thematic reviews, and on options for periodic reviews for the high-level political forum.

91. We reaffirm our unwavering commitment to achieving this Agenda and utilizing it to the full to transform our world for the better by 2030.

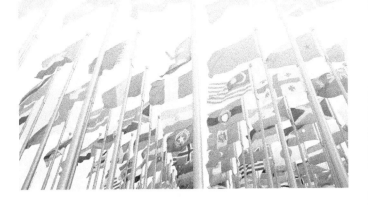

Contributor Biographies

Sarah Abboud, PhD, RN, is an assistant professor at the University of Illinois at Chicago, College of Nursing, Department of Women, Children, and Family Health Science. Her research interests are health promotion and disease prevention, with focus on (sexual) health disparities among immigrants and ethnic minorities in the United States. Dr. Abboud's research interests developed from her clinical and research work in Lebanon, Kuwait, and the United States, as well as her Lebanese background. Dr. Abboud uses feminist and health equity lenses to inform her research and to address the several components of sexual health at the intersectionality of different social determinants such as gender, ethnic identity, family, religion, education, immigration, among several other categories. Dr. Abboud completed her BS and MS (adult care) in nursing at the American University of Beirut School of Nursing, Lebanon, and her PhD and postdoctoral fellowship at the University of Pennsylvania, School of Nursing.

Julie K. Anathan, RN, MPH, is the associate chief nursing officer at Seed Global Health. In this role, she develops and evaluates Seed Global Health's nursing programs and supports volunteers in the field from a clinical and educational perspective. Previously, Ms. Anathan worked with Partners in Health and their sister organization Zamni Lasante in Haiti. She partnered with Haitian clinical nurse educators to support an in-service educational strategy to provide professional development opportunities for nurses aimed at improving patient outcomes and encourage nurse retention at l'Hôpital Saint Nicolas. She holds a bachelor of science degree in nursing from Boston College and a Master of Public Health degree with a concentration in international health from Boston University.

Olivia Bahemuka, DNP, MSN, RN-BC, is a postdoc alumnus with honorable mention from the Afya Bora Consortium (ABC) Global Health Leadership Fellowship. She received her doctor of nursing practice (DNP) at the University of Alabama at Birmingham (UAB). She is currently a University of Illinois at Chicago (UIC) visiting clinical instructor with the Human Resource for Health Program at the College of Medicine and Health Sciences in Kigali, Rwanda. Her previous background includes such roles as advanced nurse coordinator for Hematology-Oncology & Bone Marrow Transplant at UAB Hospital. She has led numerous interdisciplinary medical teams to work on a voluntary basis in Uganda for over 15 years, starting from her nursing school days. She has held positions on the North Carolina Nurses Association, Central Alabama Chapter Oncology Nurses Association (CACONS) and has served one term as board member on the Uganda North American Association (UNAA) national board.

Deva-Marie Beck, PhD, RN, is a nurse educator, multimedia journalist, keynote speaker, author, and Nightingale scholar, and serves in all these roles as international codirector of Nightingale Initiative for Global Health (NIGH) and as editor-in-chief of NIGH's "Global Online Portal." She mentors and collaborates with a volunteer team of nurses who serve as youth representatives at the United Nations in New York. In 2014, Dr. Beck was commissioned by the World Health Organization (WHO) to create a video, At the Heart of It All: Nurses & Midwives for Universal Health Coverage, which premiered at a WHO Global Forum for Chief Nursing & Midwifery Officers in Geneva, Switzerland. In 2008, she collaborated with WHO-affiliated nurses to produce the video Health Professions' Role in Primary Health Care, Featuring Nurses and Midwives—Now More Than Ever for a Healthy World, to celebrate WHO's 60th anniversary.

Busisiwe Rosemary Bhengu, PhD, RN, is an honorary associate professor at the University of KwaZulu-Natal (UKZN) and a critical care nurse who holds a PhD in nursing. She is the former head of the School of Nursing at UKZN, Durban. She is currently the chairperson of the South African Nursing Council and also served in the Council of the Critical Care Society of Southern Africa for 2 years. As the director of the World Health Organization Collaborating Centres (WHOCCs) at UKZN, she also represented the Afro Region of the WHOCCs in the Global Network of the WHOCCs. Dr. Bhengu is currently working for the Human Resources for Health Program developing specialist nurses at the graduate level (Critical Care Nursing track) at the University of Rwanda.

Suellen Breakey, PhD, RN, is assistant professor at the Massachusetts General Hospital (MGH) Institute of Health Professions, Boston, Massachusetts, where she teaches accelerated BSN students. She completed her BS in biology at Salem State University, Salem, Massachusetts, an MSN in critical care nursing at the MGH Institute of Health Professions, and a PhD in nursing at Boston College Connell School of Nursing. Dr. Breakey's global nursing efforts are focused on prevention and treatment of rheumatic heart disease in resource-limited settings. She is a leader in Team Heart, a nonprofit organization that works in Rwanda. Dr. Breakey led a team that developed the teaching modules, both written materials and videos, which were translated into Kinyarwanda language for their patients. Dr. Breakey was a member of a screening team to study the prevalence of rheumatic heart disease in school-aged children in Rwanda.

Kelly Burke, MPH, BSN, RN, is a public health professional and nurse who has worked in global health for the majority of her career. She has worked in various nursing capacities overseas as a clinical trials coordinator, clinical manager, trainer and clinical mentor in locations such as Malawi, Uganda, Ethiopia, China, and Rwanda. She has also worked on the Navajo Nation. She has a passion and dedication to improving the health of vulnerable populations through training, capacity building, and health system strengthening.

Cathy Catrambone, PhD, RN, FAAN, is an associate professor at Rush University College of Nursing, Chicago, Illinois. Following 10 years of distinguished service at the international level, Dr. Catrambone is currently president of Sigma Theta Tau International (STTI) for 2015–2017. She is a leader in the STTI Global Advisory Panel for the Future of Nursing (GAPFON) that will establish a voice and vision for the future of nursing and midwifery and advance global health. She was awarded the Herbert De Young Medal for her leadership in advancing the lung health mission in Chicago.

Maureen E. Connell, MPH, BSc (Hons), RN, was born in 1955 into a working class family in Northern England. From an early age, she was drawn to the spiritual life with two main desires: to become a nun and to serve the poor and marginalized. At the age of 18, she entered a convent and trained as a nurse. After 10 years, Ms. Connell left the convent, trained as a midwife, and went to work in Sudan for 2 years, during the great Ethiopian famine of 1985–86. She has worked for several public health organizations, namely Save the Children, Oxfam, and Children's Aid Direct. Ms. Connell has been deployed on short contracts to emergency situations in Nepal, South Sudan, Rwanda (1994), Democratic Republic of Congo, Azerbaijan, Haiti, Albania, Burundi, and Tajikistan. She currently works in a volunteer capacity as a nurse educator in Rwamagana, Rwanda.

Christine M. Darling, MPA, has served as senior operations administrator for the Honor Society of Nursing, Sigma Theta Tau International, headquartered in Indianapolis, Indiana. There, she manages a variety of special projects pertaining to the organization's presence on the global health care stage, including the Global Advisory Panel on the Future of Nursing (GAPFON). In addition to academic program management at the university, she directed interdisciplinary program development of statewide community outreach initiatives, lay and professional (medical) education, statewide and national conferences, and fund development. Her community commitment is reflected in her volunteer and board service for local nonprofit organizations that address domestic violence prevention and the empowerment of women and girls. She is also an active member of the Indiana Rural Health Association.

Barbara Montgomery Dossey, PhD, RN, AHN-BC, FAAN, HWNC-BC, is internationally recognized as a pioneer in the holistic nursing and nurse coaching movements. She is codirector of the International Nurse Coach Association (INCA) and a core faculty of the Integrative Nurse Coach Certificate Program (INCCP) in North Miami, Florida. She is the international codirector and a board member of the Nightingale Initiative for Global Health (NIGH), Washington, DC, and Neepawa, Manitoba, Canada, and the director of Holistic Nursing Consultants (HNC), Santa Fe, New Mexico. Dr. Dossey is a Florence Nightingale scholar and has authored or coauthored 26 books.

Carole Ann Drick, PhD, RN, AHN-BC, is presently the director of Conscious Awareness, Austintown, Ohio, and the codirector of Golden Room Advocates. She has authored or coauthored four books and numerous professional publications. As an author, consultant, educator, and metaphysician, her national and international presentations have been numerous. Dr. Drick's teaching experience has been broad and inclusive: University of Pittsburgh graduate maternity faculty, Pittsburgh, Pennsylvania, Department of Health, Education, and Welfare (DHEW) project grant coordinator to develop a BSN completion program at Youngstown State University, Youngstown, Ohio, University of Cincinnati maternal–child graduate faculty, Cincinnati, Ohio, and University of Akron School of Nursing graduate faculty, Akron, Ohio. The next 10 years Dr. Drick spent traveling internationally, speaking and working with natural healers, professional organizations, the Prison Reform Movement in England, and widely throughout Russia and Australia. Her seminal experience with the Apache Indians laid the groundwork for her seventh generation perspective on decision making and greatly assisted deepening her connection with nature and the mind–body–spirit connection.

Linda A. Evans, PhD, RN, has expertise in nursing practice, leadership, and education attained largely at Brigham and Women's Hospital, Boston, Massachusetts, a large, renowned academic medical center. She currently serves as the program director at the Center for Nursing Excellence at Brigham and Women's Hospital. Additionally she coordinates relationships and learning activities with approximately 30 schools of nursing and the 1,300 nursing students who are welcomed each year at Brigham and Women's Hospital. Dr. Evans holds a master's degree in nursing education from Salem State University, Salem, Massachusetts, and a PhD in nursing with a concentration in nursing research from the University of Massachusetts Worcester. Dr. Evans's area of research expertise is as one of the leading nurse scientists who has studied the experiences related to facial transplantation.

Helen Ewing, DHSc, MN, RN, is the senior manager for Nursing and Midwifery and the clinical training specialist with the Clinton Health Access Initiative. She is working in Liberia on the Health Workforce Program This position facilitates building the health education infrastructure, faculty, and health workforce necessary to create a high-quality, sustainable health care system in Liberia. Dr. Ewing holds a nursing diploma, and bachelor's and master's degrees in nursing specializing in management and quality improvement. She completed her doctorate degree in health science from Nova Southeastern University, Fort Lauderdale, Florida, specializing in the evaluation of health care in developing countries. She has experience working in resource-poor countries and in various leadership, academic, and clinical roles including curriculum development and delivery for bachelor's-, master's-, and doctorate-level nursing and health science programs as well as leading programs as a program chair. Dr. Ewing's research interests focus on studying issues impacting global health, quality of life of nurses, health care leadership, online education, and academic integrity.

Joyce J. Fitzpatrick, PhD, MBA, RN, FAAN, FNAP, is Elizabeth Brooks Ford Professor of Nursing, Frances Payne Bolton School of Nursing, Case Western Reserve University (CWRU), Cleveland, Ohio, where she was dean from 1982 to 1997. She is also adjunct professor, Department of Geriatrics, Icahn School of Medicine, New York, New York. She earned a BSN (Georgetown University, Washington, DC), MS in psychiatric–mental health nursing (The Ohio State University, Columbus, Ohio), PhD in nursing (New York University, New York, New York), and MBA (CWRU). In 1990, Dr. Fitzpatrick received an honorary Doctor of Humane Letters from Georgetown University. In 2011, she received an honorary Doctor of Humane Letters from

Frontier University of Nursing, Hyden, Kentucky. She received the *American Journal of Nursing* Book of the Year Award 20 times and the Sigma Theta Tau International (STTI) Elizabeth McWilliams Miller Founders Award for Excellence in Nursing Research. In 2016, she was named a Living Legend by the American Academy of Nursing (AAN). Dr. Fitzpatrick is widely published in nursing and health care literature with over 300 publications, including more than 75 authored/edited books. She edits the journals *Applied Nursing Research, Archives of Psychiatric Nursing,* and *Nursing Education Perspectives.* Dr. Fitzpatrick founded and led the Bolton School's World Health Organization Collaborating Centre for Nursing. From 1997 to 1999 she served as president of the AAN. During 1998–1999, while on sabbatical from CWRU, she directed a Nursing Care Quality Initiative, a multisystem, 10-hospital project focused on improving care for hospitalized elders and their families. She served as global nursing consultant to the Dreyfus Health Foundation, with nursing programs in 15 countries, and as senior advisor, Center for Nursing Research and Education, Mount Sinai Department of Nursing and School of Medicine.

Martha Hill, PhD, RN, served as dean for the Johns Hopkins University School of Nursing, Baltimore, Maryland, from 2001 until early 2014 and has been a member of the faculty since the school was established in 1983, most recently as professor of nursing, medicine, and public health. Dr. Hill is a member of the National Academy of Medicine of the National Academy of Sciences (formerly the Institute of Medicine [IOM]). Dr. Hill served as the co-vice chair of the institute's committee that produced the 2002 publication, *Unequal Treatment: Confronting Ethnic and Racial Disparities in Health Care.* She served on the IOM Council 2007–2013 and currently serves on the academy's board on Health Sciences Policy.

Elizabeth Holguin, MPH, MSN, FNP-BC, RN, is enrolled as a doctoral student at the University of New Mexico, Albuquerque, New Mexico, pursuing a PhD in nursing and health policy. She is a Robert Wood Johnson Foundation Nursing and Health Policy Collaborative Fellow and a Jonas Nurse Leader Scholar. She received her master's degree of public health from Tulane University, New Orleans, Louisiana, as a master's degree international student and served in the Peace Corps in Ethiopia. During her graduate studies, she also implemented an infection control program in a government hospital in Kenema, Sierra Leone, West Africa. While working as a nurse, she managed a research program dedicated to reducing transport to a level one trauma center and increasing access to specialty care with telemedicine with a focus on mild traumatic brain injuries for Indian Health Service hospitals. She then went on to receive a master of science degree in nursing from Duke University, Durham, North Carolina, and became certified as a family nurse practitioner. She is currently collaborating with the International Council of Nurses on various projects and fulfilling a health policy field placement with the Centers for Disease Control and Prevention focusing on health policy implementation. Current research interests include increasing access to care and resource sustainability through policy implementation at the national and global levels as well as feasibility and cost-effectiveness of health care coverage for undocumented immigrants within the United States.

Sara Horton-Deutsch, PhD, RN, PMHCNS, FAAN, ANEF, Caritas Coach, Heart-Math Trainer, graduated in 1986 with a BSN from the University of Evansville, Evansville, Indiana. She then moved to Chicago, Illinois, to take a position in inpatient adult and geropsychiatry at Rush Presbyterian St. Luke's Medical Center, where she simultaneously began work on her master's degree in psychiatric–mental health nursing at Rush University. After completing her doctorate and a 1-year postdoctorate in psychoneuroimmunology there, she spent 7 years on the faculty at Rush. In 2011, she was inducted as an Academy of Nursing Education Fellow (ANEF) by the National League for Nursing (NLN), and in 2014 as a Fellow of the American Academy of Nursing (FAAN). She is a graduate of the Watson Caring Science Institute Caritas Coach Education Program (CCEP).

Frances Hughes, RN, BA, MA, DNurs, Col (ret), JP, ONZM, was appointed as chief executive officer of the International Council of Nurses in February 2016. Immediately prior to this, she held the role of chief nursing and midwifery officer, Queensland, Australia, and also served as chief nurse for New Zealand. From 2005 to 2011, Dr. Hughes worked for the World Health Organization with 16 countries in the Pacific region, supporting them to develop policy and plans to improve mental health for consumers in the Pacific. Qualified as a general and psychiatric health nurse, Dr. Hughes has a Doctor of Nursing degree from the University of Technology, Sydney. She has held senior roles for many years across a range of organizations and served as the commandant colonel for the Royal New Zealand Nursing Corps.

Lynn Keegan, PhD, RN, AHN-BC, FAAN, is one of the founders of the holistic health focus in nursing and a leader in holistic nursing. She currently works as director of Holistic Nursing Consultants (HNC) in Port Angeles, Washington. Dr. Keegan was inducted in 1996 as a Fellow of the American Academy of Nursing (FAAN) and is board certified as an advanced holistic nurse by the American Holistic Nurses Association (AHNA). In 1991, she received the Distinguished Alumnus Award from Cornell University–New York Hospital School of Nursing and later was named Holistic Nurse of the Year by the AHNA. She is a six-time recipient of the *American Journal of Nursing* Book of the Year Award.

Hester C. Klopper, PhD, RN, MBA, FAAN, ASSAf, is the deputy vice chancellor of Strategic Initiatives and Internationalization at Stellenbosch University, Cape Town, South Africa. She is an international academic leader with extensive networks globally. She is also the immediate past president of Sigma Theta Tau International (2013–2015), the first non-North American to hold this position. She was the first South African to be inducted as Fellow of the American Academy of Nursing (FAAN), and is also a Fellow of the Academy of Science of South Africa (ASSAf) and a Fellow of the Academy of Nursing of South Africa (FANSA). Dr. Klopper is an inductee into the International Hall of Fame of Sigma Theta Tau International for Research Excellence. She received a Doctor of Nursing (honoris causa) degree from Oxford Brookes University, Oxford, England, on September 2, 2016 in recognition of her contribution to nursing education and research globally.

Ann E. Kurth, PhD, CNM, MPH, FAAN, is dean and Linda Koch Lorimer Professor (inaugural chair) of the Yale University School of Nursing, New Haven, Connecticut. She previously held the inaugural Paulette Goddard Chair in Global Health Nursing at New York University (NYU) College of Nursing and was associate dean for research at the NYU College of Global Public Health. Her work has been funded by the National Institutes of Health (NIH), the Bill & Melinda Gates Foundation, Joint United Nations Programme on HIV and AIDS (UNAIDS), Centers for Disease Control and Prevention (CDC), Health Resources and Services Administration (HRSA), and others, for studies conducted in the United States and internationally. Dr. Kurth has consulted for the NIH, Gates Foundation, World Health Organization (WHO), United States Agency for International Development (USAID), and CDC, among others. Dr. Kurth is vice chair of the Consortium of Universities for Global Health (the first nonphysician in this role), and a Fellow of the American Academy of Nursing and of the New York Academy of Medicine. She is a member of the 2014–2018 U.S. Preventive Services Task Force, which sets screening and primary care prevention guidelines for the United States.

Jeanne M. Leffers, PhD, RN, FAAN, is professor emeritus at the University of Massachusetts Dartmouth. An educator for more than 30 years, Dr. Leffers taught nursing, sociology, environmental health, and global health courses at the University of Rhode Island, Kingston, Rhode Island, the University of Massachusetts Dartmouth, and Villanova University, Villanova, Pennsylvania. Dr. Leffers worked with the American Public Health Association (APHA) Public Health Nursing Section and served on the executive board of Association of Community Health Nursing Educators (ACHNE) and as the former Health Volunteers Overseas (HVO) Nursing Education Program director for Uganda as well as on two Sigma Theta Tau International Task Force groups. She now serves on the Nursing Education Steering Committee at HVO and on the board of directors of the Global Nursing Caucus. Dr. Leffers has more than 20 years of experience in global health nursing in settings in the United States, Uganda, Honduras, and Guatemala, serving with HVO in Uganda and as a faculty leader of academic service-learning programs in the Dominican Republic and Haiti. She coauthored *Volunteering at Home and Abroad: Essential Guide for Nurses (2011)* and coedited *Global Health Nursing: Building and Sustaining Partnerships (2014).* In her environmental health work, she serves on the steering committee for the Alliance of Nurses for Healthy Environments (ANHE), as cochair of the ANHE Education Workgroup, as an author/editor of the ANHE Environmental E-Textbook, with the ANA-RI Environmental Health Task Force, the Education Advisory Committee of the Children's Environmental Health Network (CEHN), and on the Environmental Protection Agency (EPA) Children's Health Protection Advisory Committee (CHPAC).

Susan Luck, MA, RN, HNB-BC, CCN, HWNC-BC, is a holistic nurse educator and integrative nurse coach, medical anthropologist, clinical nutritionist, and a national speaker, writer, and consultant for organizations pioneering the emerging integrative health care paradigm. She is the clinical nutritionist for special immunology services at Mercy Hospital, Miami, Florida, and maintains a private practice in Miami as a wellness nurse coach and clinical nutritionist. She is codirector of International Nurse Coach Association (INCA) and core faculty for the Integrative Nurse Coach Certificate Program (INCCP). Ms. Luck is on the editorial board of the *Alternative Therapies in Health and Medicine* journal and is a founding member of and consultant to the *Integrative Practitioner* newsletter. She is the founder and program director of EarthRose Institute (ERI), a nonprofit organization dedicated to women's and children's environmental health education.

Phalakshi Manjrekar, MScN, RN, is the distinguished nursing director and board member at the P. D. Hinduja National Hospital & Medical Research Centre, Mumbai, India. She has served as a coresearcher on a team from the Missouri University of Science & Technology, Rolla, Missouri, the University of Cincinnati, Cincinnati, Ohio, and the Sardar Patel University in Gujarat, India. She has conferred with global and regional nursing leaders in Canada, Great Britain, and other Commonwealth nations, as well as in Switzerland and India, and has attended World Health Organization (WHO) briefings in Geneva and at the WHO South East Asian Regional Office (SEARO) in New Delhi. She has served as chairperson of Nurses' Welfare for the Maharashtra State Chapter of the national Trained Nurses Association of India (TNAI). Ms. Manjrekar presently serves on the executive committee of the Nightingale Initiative for Global Health (NIGH) world board of directors and oversees the development of the NIGH's worldwide presence in India.

Tamara H. McKinnon, DNP, APHN, RN, is an internationally recognized leader in global service learning for nursing. She started her career as an international volunteer at the age of 19 (in the Tijuana jail) and continues her international work to this day. Promoting sustainable service programs and encouraging the integration of interdisciplinary teams, Dr. McKinnon developed and leads credit-toward-major global clinical courses in a public university school of nursing. In 2000, she founded the Beach Flats Nurse Managed Center, Santa Cruz, California. This vibrant center is now an integral part of the community, serving Spanish-speaking, low-resource clients in their homes. Dr. McKinnon's students carry the lessons learned about collaborative, competent care "around the corner and across the globe" into their work as nurses in hospitals and communities across the country.

Afaf Ibrahim Meleis, PhD, FAAN, LL, is a professor of nursing and sociology at the University of Pennsylvania, where she was the Margaret Bond Simon Dean of Nursing and director of the school's WHO Collaborating Center for Nursing and Midwifery Leadership (2002–2014). This followed her 34-year tenure as a professor at the University of California, San Francisco and Los Angeles. She developed Transitions Theory, which is translated into policy, research, and evidence-based practice. Dr. Meleis is the author of more than 200 articles and her books continue to be used internationally. Her leadership in the International Council on Women's Health Issues played a central role in bringing together world leaders to form partnerships to improve the lives of women. She is a member of the National Academy of Medicine and cochaired its Global Forum on Innovation in Health Professional Education, as well as a board member of The Josiah Macy Jr. Foundation Faculty Scholars Program. She cochaired the *Lancet* Commission on Women and Health, the results of which were published in a full *Lancet* issue in 2015. She is also a member of a Center for Strategic and International Studies (CSIS) Global Health Policy Center Task Force on Women's and Family Health.

Patricia Moreland, PhD, CPNP, RN, is visiting faculty in the Master of Science in Nursing Program, Pediatric Track, School of Nursing and Midwifery, College of Medicine and Health Sciences, University of Rwanda in partnership with the University of Illinois at Chicago College of Nursing. Dr. Moreland graduated from Columbia University School of Nursing, New York, New York, with a PhD and completed her postdoctoral fellowship at the University of North Carolina,

Chapel Hill. Her area of expertise is pediatrics, and her research interests include young adults with congenital heart disease and health outcomes of HIV-exposed infants.

Karen H. Morin, PhD, RN, ANEF, FAAN, is professor emeritus, the University of Wisconsin–Milwaukee, and visiting professor, the University of West Georgia, Tanner System School of Nursing. Over the course of the past 35 years, Dr. Morin has held teaching positions at the University of Alabama at Birmingham, Thomas Jefferson University, Philadelphia, Pennsylvania, Widener University, Chester, Pennsylvania, the Pennsylvania State University, Centre County, Pennsylvania, and Western Michigan University, Kalamazoo, Michigan. Dr. Morin also is the director of the Center for Nursing Inquiry, Bronson Methodist Hospital, Kalamazoo, Michigan, where she assists staff nurses with the development and implementation of quality improvement projects and research projects. She also serves as associate editor for the *Journal of Nursing Education*. She has given numerous presentations addressing the need to develop leaders including succession planning, the need for practice based on evidence, faculty development, and caring for obese pregnant women. She is a founding faculty of the Sigma Theta Tau International (STTI) and J & J Maternal-Child Health Leadership Academy. She is a fellow in the Academy of Nursing Education (ANEF) and the American Academy of Nursing (FAAN).

Jasintha T. Mtengezo, MPH, BSN, RN, is a certified midwife who received her MPH from College of Medicine and her BSN/M from Kamuzu College of Nursing in Malawi. She is currently a nursing PhD student in the Population Health Track at the University of Massachusetts in Boston. Her experience includes over 20 years in nursing and midwifery training, education, and practice. Jasintha transitioned to nursing administration in 2003 and has held roles with progressive leadership responsibilities, including the director of Nursing Education Programs at Nurses and Midwives Council and dean of Nursing Faculty at Deayang College of Nursing in Malawi. She has been involved in program planning, management, and monitoring and evaluation of nursing activities at both national and international levels.

Sarah Oerther, MSN, MEd, RN, CSPI, is a Jonas Nurse Leader Scholar and currently enrolled as a PhD student at the School of Nursing, Saint Louis University, St. Louis, Missouri. Sarah earned her BSN from the University of Cincinnati, Cincinnati, Ohio (2004) and two master's degrees (nursing and education) from Xavier University, Cincinnati, Ohio (2008). She is certified in terrorism response, trained in drug abuse prevention, and is a certified specialist in poison information (CSPI). As a nurse educator, Sarah has partnered with nurses, engineers, and other professionals to address the United Nations Millennium Development Goals (MDGs) through her work in India, Kenya, Tanzania, Guatemala, and Brazil.

Melissa T. Ojemeni, MA, RN, PCCN, is a fourth-year PhD student at New York University (NYU) Rory Meyers College of Nursing, New York City, New York. Melissa was recently named an occupational and environmental health nursing trainee. This training grant will prepare her to conduct interdisciplinary occupational and environmental health focused research that will advance nursing science. Her dissertation will focus on comparative policy responses from the United States and United Kingdom and how they have managed international nurse migration from 2004 to 2014. Ms. Ojemeni holds a master's of arts in international peace and conflict resolution with a global health concentration from Arcadia University, Montogomery County, Pennsylvania, and a bachelor's of science in nursing from Gwynedd Mercy University, Gwynedd Valley, Pennsylvania. Melissa has acquired 2 years of international experience working in Rwanda, Tanzania, and Haiti. Her global health work has centered on human resources for health development, health systems, and educational capacity building focused on the nursing workforce.

Laura Ridge, ANP-BC, RN, obtained her bachelor of arts degree from Harvard University in Social Studies. She went on to complete a second bachelor's degree in nursing at Columbia University, New York, New York, where she also obtained her master's in adult primary care. She has practiced in addiction medicine and primary care settings and is a specialist in HIV, certified by the American Academy of HIV Medicine. Laura cofounded Nursing for All, a small nonprofit that supports nurse-led public health initiatives in Liberia in 2013. She is currently a PhD candidate at NYU Rory Meyers College of Nursing, New York, New York, and her dissertation work will focus on nursing human resources capacity building in Liberia.

William Rosa, MS, RN, LMT, AHN-BC, AGPCNP-BC, CCRN-CMC, is a nurse, author, and educator. He graduated with his bachelor of science in nursing, magna cum laude, from NYU, Rory Meyers College of Nursing, New York, New York, in 2009. After graduating as valedictorian of his master of nursing program at the Hunter–Bellevue School of Nursing at Hunter College, New York, New York in 2014, he moved into the role of nurse educator for critical care services at NYU Langone Medical Center. He is a graduate of the Caritas Coach Education Program (CCEP) offered by the Watson Caring Science Institute (WCSI), the Integrative Nurse Coach Certificate Program (INCCP) offered by the International Nurse Coach Association, and the Clinical Scene Investigator (CSI) Academy of the American Association of Critical-Care Nurses (AACN). Mr. Rosa is a fellow of the New York Academy of Medicine. He has been recognized with the Association for Nursing Professional Development's National 2015 Excellence in Professional Development Change Agent/Team Member Award and the 2015 national AACN Circle of Excellence Award, and he was the winner of the 2012 National League for Nursing (NLN) Student Excellence Paper Competition. As of this writing, Mr. Rosa is a Palliative Care Nurse Practitioner Fellow at Memorial Sloan Kettering Cancer Center in New York, New York. He is a fellow of the New York Academy of Medicine.

Judith Shamian, PhD, RN, LLD (Hons), DSci (Hons), FAAN, is the president of the International Council of Nurses (ICN). She also serves as president emeritus, immediate past president and chief executive officer of the Victorian Order of Nurses, and past president of the Canadian Nurses Association (CNA). Dr. Shamian serves on the United Nations Secretary-General's High-Level Commission on Health Employment and Economic Growth, which is cochaired by H.E. Mr. Francois Hollande, president of France, and H.E. Mr. Jacob Zuma, president of South Africa. Previously, she held the position of professor of nursing at the University of Toronto and established the Office of Nursing Policy at Health Canada. Dr. Shamian obtained her PhD from Case Western Reserve University, Cleveland, Ohio; her master's in public health from New York University, New York, New York, and a baccalaureate in community nursing from Concordia University in Montreal. She is the recipient of numerous awards including Canada's Most Powerful Women: Top 100 award; the Golden Jubilee Medal from the governor general of Canada; and the CNA's Centennial Award. Dr. Shamian is also an international fellow with the American Academy of Nursing.

Holly K. Shaw, PhD, RN, is a graduate of the Harvard Medical School master's certificate program in global mental health, trauma, and recovery. She earned her BS at Boston University and MS and PhD at Adelphi University, Garden City, New York, where she is an adjunct associate professor in the College of Nursing and Public Health. Her clinical and advocacy work is well known within the United Nations (UN) System where she was the first to represent Sigma Theta Tau International (STTI), the Honor Society of Nursing, and currently the Nightingale Initiative for Global Health (NIGH) in the UN nongovernmental organization (NGO) community. She is a director on the UN NGO Department of Public Information (DPI) Executive Committee and vice chair of the NGO Committee on Mental Health, Inc. where she is the coconvener of the Working Group on Refugee and Immigrant Mental Health. She developed with NIGH colleagues *The World Nurses Want,* an online, platform endeavor facilitating worldwide nurses' participation in the UN World We Want Campaign and Sustainable Development Goals. Her current research and clinical practice interests focus on the UN and NGO advocacy; the resilience and healing experiences of children and adolescents, refugees, and survivors of armed conflict and violence; global nursing workforce issues; and collaborative, reciprocal mentorship. Dr. Shaw has a clinical mental health practice in Sea Cliff, New York.

Allison P. Squires, PhD, RN, FAAN, is an associate professor and director of international education at the Rory Meyers College of Nursing at New York University, New York, New York. She is widely published with over 120 publications. Dr. Squires began her nursing career at the University of Pennsylvania's School of Nursing, Philadelphia, Pennsylvania, where she received her bachelor of science in Nursing with a minor in Latin American studies in 1995. At Duquesne University's School of Nursing, Pittsburgh, Pennsylvania, she focused her graduate work on nursing education and received her Master of Science in nursing. While at Duquesne, she worked with their International Nursing Center on projects in Nicaragua, the Dominican Republic, and Peru while also practicing as a medical-surgical staff nurse in the University of Pittsburgh Medical Center's health system, Pittsburgh, Pennsylvania. She moved on to PhD study at Yale University School of Nursing, New Haven, Connecticut, in 2002 where she focused her studies on global health policy. While at Yale, she was selected as an associate fellow for the Yale World Fellows Program. To date, she remains the only nurse selected for the program. Through this program, she had the opportunity to collaborate on projects with fellows from Iraq, Pakistan, and the country of Georgia. Finally, she completed a postdoctoral fellowship at the Center for Health Outcomes and Policy Research at the University of Pennsylvania.

Michele J. Upvall, PhD, RN, CRNP, is professor of nursing and coordinator of the MSN Nurse Educator programs at the University of Central Florida in Orlando, Florida. She has studied the collaborative practices of nursing with indigenous healers in southern Africa and with the Navajo Nation in southwestern United States. Other populations with which she has worked include Somali refugee women and their families; nurses and other health care providers in Bhutan, Cambodia, Vietnam, and Botswana; and rural populations in Ghana. Dr. Upvall developed and coordinated the first baccalaureate nursing (BSN) program for Navajo and Hopi students in Ganado, Arizona, while on faculty at Northern Arizona University. Dr. Upvall then traveled to the Aga Khan University School of Nursing in Karachi, Pakistan, where she served as director of the prelicensure BSN and RN-to-BSN programs. Dr. Upvall returned and facilitated growth of the nursing programs division at Carlow University, Pittsburgh, Pennsylvania, into a school of nursing as associate dean and director. She is active in the Commission on Collegiate Nursing Education serving as an evaluator and she is a member of Health Volunteers Overseas (HVO) Nursing Education Steering Committee, the American Nurses Association, and Florida Nurses Association. Dr. Upvall has many publications in the area of global health including coeditor of the book, *Global Health Nursing: Building and Sustaining Partnerships*. Most recently, Dr. Upvall completed a Fulbright scholarship in Thailand.

Cynthia Vlasich, MBA, RN, BSN, is the director of Global Initiatives at the Honor Society of Nursing, Sigma Theta Tau International (STTI). She was promoted to this role after directing education and leadership at STTI for 6 years, successfully leading it through one of its most extensive periods of growth and expansion. She provides direction for the global regional offices and relationships with global organizations such as the United Nations and the World Health Organization, oversees the Institute for Global Healthcare Leadership, and leads initiatives to enhance the global recognition and reputation of the organization. She has been both a member and chair of the United States Federal Nursing Chiefs Council, and has coordinated nursing involvement for domestic and international disaster relief missions.

Jean Watson, PhD, RN, AHN-BC, FAAN, is distinguished professor and dean emerita, University of Colorado Denver, College of Nursing Anschutz Medical Center campus, where for 16 years she held the Murchison-Scoville Chair in Caring Science, the nation's first endowed chair in caring science. She is founder of the original Center for Human Caring in Colorado and is a fellow of the American Academy of Nursing, past president of the National League for Nursing (NLN), and founding member of the International Association of Human Caring (IAHC) and International Caritas Consortium (ICC). Dr. Watson is founder and director of the nonprofit Watson Caring Science Institute (WCSI). Dr. Watson has earned undergraduate and graduate degrees in nursing and psychiatric–mental health nursing and holds a PhD in educational psychology and counseling. She is the recipient of many awards, including 11 honorary doctoral degrees. As author/ coauthor of more than 20 books on caring, she seeks to bridge paradigms as well as point toward transformative models for the 21st century. In October 2013, Dr. Watson was inducted as a Living Legend by the American Academy of Nursing

Deborah Wilson, BSN, RN, CRNI, has been working as a registered nurse internationally for the past 30 years. Her specialties are emergency medicine and neuroscience, with a focus on trauma. Over the past 6 years, Ms. Wilson has worked with Médecins Sans Frontières/Doctors Without Borders, establishing a malnutrition project during an emergency hunger gap in Chad, and setting up a medical clinic in Haiti during the cholera epidemic. In October 2014 she returned from Liberia, where she worked in a 120-bed Ebola treatment center. Since her return, Ms. Wilson has been speaking on the ethical and treatment issues involved when there is an epidemic and has been awarded the Clinical Excellence award for 2015 by Berkshire Health Systems and was the recipient of the 2016 Praxis award in professional ethics at Villanova University, Villanova, Pennsylvania, in March 2016. She is currently pursuing an MSN/MPH at Johns Hopkins University, Baltimore, Maryland.

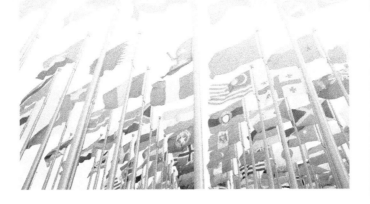

Index

Unite for Sight's Global Health University, 188
Universal Declaration of Human Rights (UDHR), 130–131
Universal Health Coverage (UHC), 75
universal health coverage approach, 6
U.S. President's Emergency Plan for AIDS Relief (PEPFAR), 405
utilitarian theories of justice, 138

Victorian Order of Nurses (VON), 70

Watson Caring Science Institute (WCSI)
  active programs, 231
  goals, 232
  Middle East Nurses and Partners on armed forces, 238

as caregivers, 236
challenges, 234–235
conferences, 233
as educators, 236
as leaders, 236
opportunities, 235
Palestinian and Israeli nurses, 233–234
safety and security, 236–237
violence reframing, 238–239
UN sustainability agenda, 232–233
well-functioning health systems, 143
Working Group on Ethics Guidelines for Global Health Training (WEIGHT), 505
World Food Programme (WFP), 257, 259
World Health Organization Collaborating Centres (WHOCCs), 525